White Coat Companion

White Coat Companion

Michael Lorinsky, MD
Hospital Medicine Unit, Massachusetts General Hospital
Instructor of Medicine, Harvard Medical School
Boston, Massachusetts

Jason Ryan, MD
Associate Professor of Medicine
University of Connecticut School of Medicine
Farmington, Connecticut

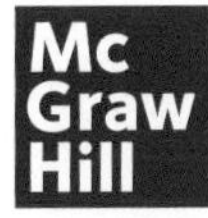

White Coat Companion 2024–2025

2 3 4 5 6 7 8 9 DSS 29 28 27 26 25 24

ISBN 978-1-265-45596-5
MHID 1-265-45596-1

This book was set in Kepler by KnowledgeWorks Global Ltd.
The editors were Bob Boehringer and Kim J. Davis.
The production supervisor was Jeffrey Herzich.
Project management was provided by Nitesh Sharma of KnowledgeWorks Global Ltd.

Contents

Acknowledgments and Contributors

Since the initial version of the White Coat Companion was published in 2019, the text has gone through major changes on a yearly basis in response to feedback that we have received from students. This edition marks one of the biggest transitions yet, as the 2024–2025 edition will be the first that is published by McGraw Hill. We would like to thank the team at Boards and Beyond for help with previous editions, including Anthea Strezze and Amy Snyder. We would also like to thank the publishing team at McGraw Hill for their great support in this new 2024–2025 edition of the White Coat Companion, including Rachel Norton, Jeffrey Herzich, Kim Davis, and Bob Boehringer.

We acknowledge all who provided content for this book. A special thanks to Dr. Sana Majid for her contributions in prior editions and for many of the images and radiographs in the book. Thanks to Dr. Richard Usatine for providing many outstanding clinical images.

We would also like to thank all the students that have submitted errata and content updates. This includes Liyan Mazahreh, Yasmine Choroomi, Vincent Okine, Sebastien Jette, Or Dayan, Aman Kalra, James Nguyen, and countless others. If you submit an update that is accepted for the next edition of the book, we will recognize it in future acknowledgments.

About the Authors

Dr. Michael Lorinsky is a hospitalist at Massachusetts General Hospital and an instructor of medicine at Harvard Medical School. He completed internal medicine residency at Beth Israel Deaconess Medical Center in Boston, MA, where he was a member of the Clinician-Educator Track. He received his undergraduate degree in biophysics from Brown University and his MD from the University of Connecticut School of Medicine, where he graduated with the Dean's Award for most outstanding academic achievement. He has also been extremely successful on the USMLE exams, scoring 275 on Step 1, 283 on Step 2 CK, and 274 on Step 3.

Dr. Jason Ryan is the creator of the website Boards and Beyond. Thousands of students from around the globe use his online videos and practice questions to prepare for the USMLE Step 1 exam. Dr. Ryan trained in internal medicine and cardiology at Harvard's Beth Israel Deaconess Medical Center, where he also served as a chief resident. In addition to his MD, he holds a Master of Public Health degree and a Bachelor of Science degree in Chemical Engineering. He has been a faculty member at the University of Connecticut School of Medicine in Farmington, Connecticut for over 10 years.

Introduction

While studying during my clinical years of medical school, I found there was a lack of succinct, well-structured, and current resources. I wanted a single book that I could use to consolidate all my knowledge from clinical rotations. Ultimately, that led to the creation of this review text. The information provided here is synthesized from a variety of textbooks, online videos, and formal teaching that I received as a medical student. It then was refined using primary resources to ensure that everything contained is as updated and evidence-based as possible. The book undergoes frequent reviews to ensure the content reflects the latest clinical guidelines. It is designed to be a singular comprehensive resource that can serve as your foundation while going through core clerkships, and later can be used as a review for Step 2CK and Step 3.

Each topic in this book is presented in the same basic format, focusing on general pathophysiology, risk factors, clinical presentation, diagnostics, and disease management. The content is stripped down to be as succinct as possible. As a result, this book is not going to explain any complex topics, but rather should be used as a resource that can organize and consolidate all that you learn during the clinical years of medical school. Once you have a deep understanding of a topic, the book can be used to efficiently review for shelf and board examinations.

One note of caution—clinical medicine changes rapidly. Although this book is updated frequently, it may not reflect recent changes in clinical guidelines. In addition, there are some areas of medicine in which multiple societies release differing guidance (e.g., asthma). This book does not contain the full breadth of all clinical knowledge, but focuses on what I believe to be the most high-yield information needed for examinations.

I hope you find this book fills the void for which it was created.

Michael Lorinsky, MD

Coronary Artery Disease

Asymptomatic Coronary Artery Disease

General: Gradual narrowing of arteries by atherosclerosis. Generally asymptomatic until > 75% stenosis.

Risk: Obesity, diabetes, hypertension, hyperlipidemia, CKD, smoking, ↑ age (> 45 y/o M/ 55 y/o F), family history of premature CAD (1° relative, < 55 y/o M/ 65 y/o F)

Management: Aspirin + statin. Lifestyle modifications.

Stable Angina (Stable CAD)

General: Fixed atherosclerotic lesions → Inadequate perfusion (O_2 demand > supply)

Clinical: Chest pain occurring with exertion, relieved with rest or nitroglycerin
- Typical features: Squeezing/pressure diffuse substernal pain. Brought on by exertion, stress, sex, cold.

Diagnosis: Clinical (classic symptoms + risk factors)
- ECG (perform on all with symptoms, but generally nonspecific or normal at rest)
- Stress testing (identifies flow-limiting stenosis), coronary CTA

Management:
- **Preventative Therapy**: Aspirin, statin, smoking cessation, hypertension/diabetes control
- **Angina**: Beta-blockers, calcium channel blockers, nitrates, ranolazine
- Revascularization (PCI or CABG) only indicated if:
  - (1) Functional impairment despite medical therapy
  - (2) High risk lesions (such as left-main, 3-vessel, proximal LAD)

PCI	Single-vessel disease (circumflex, RCA, some single-vessel LAD)
CABG	Multivessel disease, left-main, some single-vessel LAD

Diagnostic Testing for CAD

Type	Features
Coronary CTA	- **High sensitivity**, best used to rule out CAD in low-risk patients
Exercise Stress	- Must be able to achieve target HR/interpret ECG - ECG always used (look for ST changes) - Can add imaging modality (ECHO/MPI) to increase sensitivity

Pharm Stress	- Use if unable to exercise
	- Must have imaging (ECHO or MPI)
	- <u>Drug choice</u>:
	  - Adenosine/Dipyridamole/Regadenoson (contraindicated with reactive airway disease)
	  - Dobutamine (risk for ventricular arrhythmias)

Myocardial Perfusion Imaging (MPI): Tc-99/SPECT or Rb-82/PET
- Visualize myocardial perfusion before/after stress[A]
- Defects that occur with stress but improve with rest → Likely ischemia
- Stable defects (poor perfusion throughout study) → Likely old scar tissue

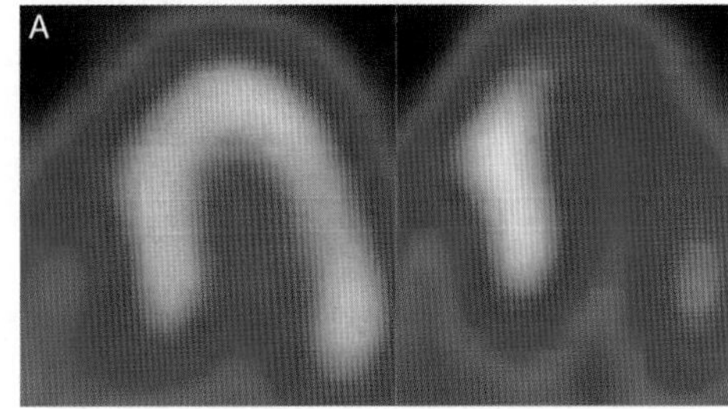

Acute Coronary Syndrome

Unstable Angina/NSTEMI

General:

- **Unstable Angina**: Ischemic symptoms without elevation in biomarkers
- **NSTEMI**: Ischemic symptoms with elevated cardiac biomarkers
    - **Type I NSTEMI**: Acute plaque rupture → Thrombus formation, subtotal occlusion
    - **Type II NSTEMI**: Imbalance of oxygen supply/demand

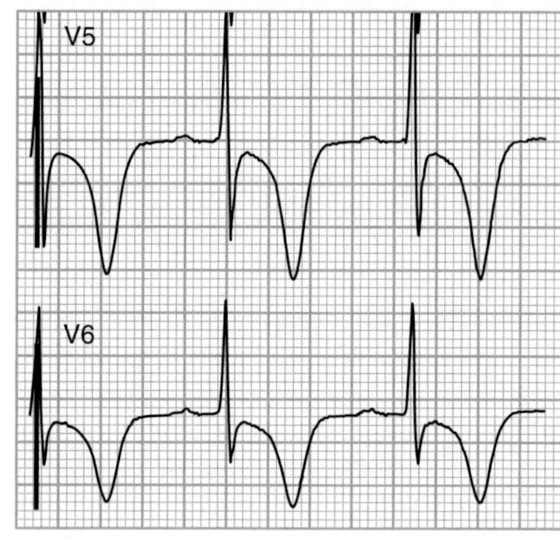

Clinical:

- Chest pain (at rest, new onset with physical limitation, or angina increasing in frequency or duration)
- Other symptoms: Dyspnea, nausea/vomiting (especially in elderly/women)

Diagnosis: Clinical features

- ECG: ST depressions, T-wave inversions
- + Biomarkers with NSTEMI (troponin I/T)

Management:

Initial (Acute)	- ASA 325 mg - Statin (as early as possible) - O_2 (to maintain O_2 saturation > 90%) - Nitroglycerin (persistent pain, HTN, or HF) - Beta-blocker (contraindicated with HF, bradycardia) - 2nd ("Dual") antiplatelet agent (ticagrelor or clopidogrel) - Anticoagulation (heparin or LMWH)
Reperfusion (Coronary Angiography)	- Immediate PCI: Indicated if shock, severe CHF, ventricular arrhythmias, structural complications - Reperfuse others within 24-48 hours depending on risk (i.e., TIMI risk score)

STEMI (ST-Elevation Myocardial Infarction)

General: Defined as chest pain + ECG Δ + cardiac enzyme ↑ (troponin). Most commonly due to acute plaque rupture.

Location	Artery	ECG
Anteroseptal	LAD	V1-V2
Anteroapical	LAD	V3-V4
Anterolateral	LCX	I, aVL, V5-V6
Inferior	RCA	II, III, aVF
Posterior	PDA	V1-V3 ST Dep.
Left Main		aVR ST elevation

Clinical:

- Persistent substernal chest pain > 20 min
- Radiation of pain (jaw, arm, or neck), diaphoresis, dyspnea

Diagnosis:

- Cardiac biomarkers (troponin appears within 2-3 hours)
- ECG: **ST elevation in ≥ 2 contiguous leads**, > 0.1 mV (> 0.2 mV in V2/V3)

Management: Initial management similar to UA/NSTEMI above

Reperfusion (PCI)	- Ideally door-to-balloon of 90 min or 120 min if transferred - Benefits all within 12 hours of symptom onset - 12-24 hours: Reperfuse if ongoing ischemia, HF, hypotension
Fibrinolysis (Tenecteplase, alteplase)	- Used if PCI not available in timely manner - Contraindications similar to those in stroke [See: Neuro]

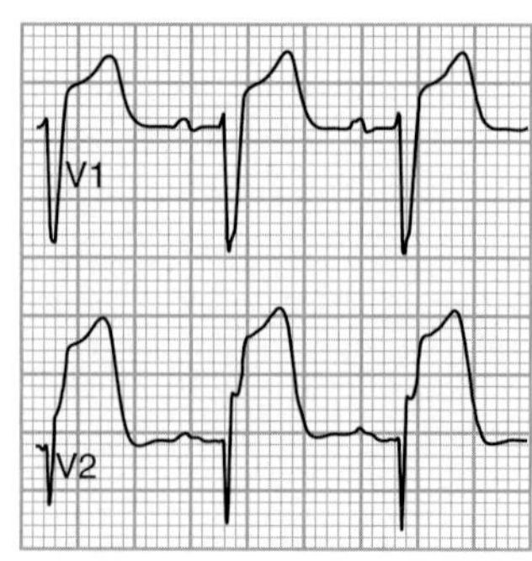

Stent management

- Drug eluting/bare metal stents require at least 6-12 months of DAPT
    - If DAPT missed, at risk for in-stent thrombosis (presents like STEMI)

Acute Coronary Syndrome

Myocardial Infarction Complications

Disorder [Timing]	Clinical Features
Arrhythmia [any time]	- Commonly **ventricular arrhythmias** - Most common cause of death within 24 hours - [See: Arrhythmia] for management of VTach/VFib
RV Failure [any time]	- Seen with RCA territory MI - Presents with hypotension, elevated JVP, peripheral edema - Tx: Avoid nitroglycerin (preload dependent), watch for AV block or bradycardia, gentle IV fluids for preload, inotropes if severe
LV Failure [any time]	- Can present with **cardiogenic shock** - Tx: Diuresis (furosemide), avoid beta-blockers. Inotropic or mechanical support if severe.
Fibrinous Pericarditis [< 1 week]	- Extension of myocardial inflammation after MI - Tx: ASA plus colchicine (rarely life-threatening)
Papillary Muscle Rupture [< 1 week]	- Presents with acute onset HF due to mitral regurgitation (holosystolic murmur) - Dx: TTE - Tx: Surgical repair
Interventricular Septal Rupture [< 1 week]	- Presents with VSD formation (holosystolic murmur at LLSB), biventricular CHF - Dx: TTE - Tx: Surgical repair
Ventricular Free Wall Rupture [1-2 weeks]	- Complete rupture presents with hemopericardium, cardiac tamponade, chest pain - Often results in PEA arrest - Dx: TTE, +/− pericardiocentesis - Tx: Surgical repair (but usually fatal)
Ventricular Pseudoaneurysm [1-2 weeks]	- Free wall rupture contained by scar/pericardium - Dx: TTE, angiography - Tx: Surgical repair (high risk of rupture)
True Ventricular Aneurysm [weeks to months]	- Dyskinetic, scarred LV wall that balloons during systole. Risk of thrombus. - Persistent ST elevations after MI - Tx: Medical (ACEi +/− anticoagulation)
Dressler Syndrome [weeks to months]	- Post MI autoimmune pericardial inflammation - Tx: NSAIDs or ASA + colchicine

Variant (Prinzmetal) Angina

General: Episodic vasoconstriction of coronary vessels

Risk: Associated with smoking

Clinical: Episodic chest pain at rest, often in early morning

Management: Calcium channel blockers, nitrates

Heart Failure

Heart Failure: Overview, Chronic Management

General: Clinical syndrome of dyspnea resulting from cardiomyopathy that impairs ventricular filling or ejection

Subtype	Definition	Causes
HFpEF (diastolic)	Ejection fraction > 50%	- Diastolic dysfunction (associated w/ obesity, HTN, DM, aging) - Hypertrophic and restrictive cardiomyopathy
HFrEF (systolic)	Ejection fraction < 40%	- Dilated cardiomyopathy (ischemic or nonischemic) - Myocarditis - Stress cardiomyopathy

Clinical:

- Right sided: Peripheral edema, jugular venous distension (JVD) elevation, hepatomegaly
- Left sided: Pulmonary edema, orthopnea, paroxysmal nocturnal dyspnea
- Exam: S3, displaced PMI, rales, JVD
- CXR: Interstitial edema, Kerley B lines, pleural effusion, alveolar edema[A]
- BNP: High sensitivity, high negative predictive value

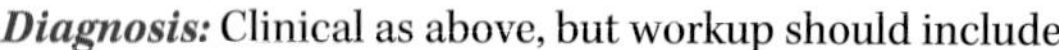

Diagnosis: Clinical as above, but workup should include:

- **TTE**: Evaluates systolic ejection fraction, diastolic function, and valves
- Coronary angiogram to assess for underlying CAD in new HF presentation
- **Right heart cath**: ↑ PCWP (left-sided HF) and ↑ RA pressure, RVEDP (right-sided HF)

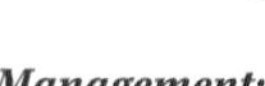

Management:

Reduced EF	Symptomatic interventions: - Salt restriction - Loop diuretic (furosemide, torsemide) - Digoxin (if symptomatic despite above measures) Guideline-directed medical therapy (GDMT): *Initial Therapy:* - ACEi, ARB, or angiotensin receptor-neprilysin inhibitor - Beta-blocker (carvedilol, metoprolol, bisoprolol) *Secondary Therapy:* - Aldosterone antagonists (spironolactone) - Hydralazine + nitrates - SGLT-2 inhibitor - Ivabradine Other interventions: - ICD (implantable defibrillator): Indicated if EF < 35% or aborted SCD - BiV-pacer: Indicated if EF < 35% + LBBB with QRS (> 120 ms) Advanced treatments: - Inotropes (dobutamine, milrinone), LVAD, heart transplant
Preserved EF	- Treat underlying disease - Diuretics (if volume overloaded) - SGLT-2 inhibitor, spironolactone in some

New York Heart Classification

Stage	Symptoms	Management
I	Asymptomatic	ACEi/ARB/ARNI + beta-blocker
II	Symptoms with moderate exertion	Spironolactone, hydralazine + nitrate, SGLT-2 ICD/BiV pacer if indicated
III	Symptoms with activities of daily living	
IV	Symptoms at rest	Advanced therapies

Heart Failure

Acute HF Exacerbation

General: Acute worsening of new or underlying heart failure

Risk: Precipitated by **dietary indiscretion, medication noncompliance**, infection, trauma, surgery, ischemia, arrhythmias, NSAIDs

Clinical: Dyspnea, peripheral edema, exercise intolerance, weight gain, rales, ↑ JVP
- CXR: Interstitial edema

Diagnosis: Clinical

Management:
- Respiratory support: Supplemental O_2, with NIPPV/intubation if required
- Diuretics: Furosemide (2.5 × home oral dose, generally as IV)
    - Monitor for hypokalemia, renal failure, hypotension
- Afterload reduction: Nitroglycerine, hydralazine in some cases
- Inotropic agents (dobutamine, milrinone) if refractory to above

High Output Heart Failure

General: Elevated cardiac output, usually secondary to chronically increased volume status OR decreased peripheral vascular resistance

Etiology: Severe anemia, hyperthyroidism, arteriovenous shunting (congenital [PDA], AV fistulas), beriberi, sepsis, pregnancy, erythroblastosis fetalis

Clinical: Heart failure (elevated JVP, pulmonary edema)

Management: Diuretics, treat underlying condition

Cor Pulmonale (Right-heart Failure)

General: Isolated right heart failure. Caused by **advanced pulmonary hypertension** (due to mechanism other than left heart failure).

Clinical:
- Exertional dyspnea, angina, and syncope
- Right heart failure (JVD, peripheral edema), prominent S2, RV heave, hepatomegaly
- ECG: RBBB, RVH, right axis
- TTE: Right ventricular dilatation[A], possible tricuspid regurgitation

Diagnosis: Right heart catheterization

Management: Diuretics. Treat underlying pulmonary hypertension.

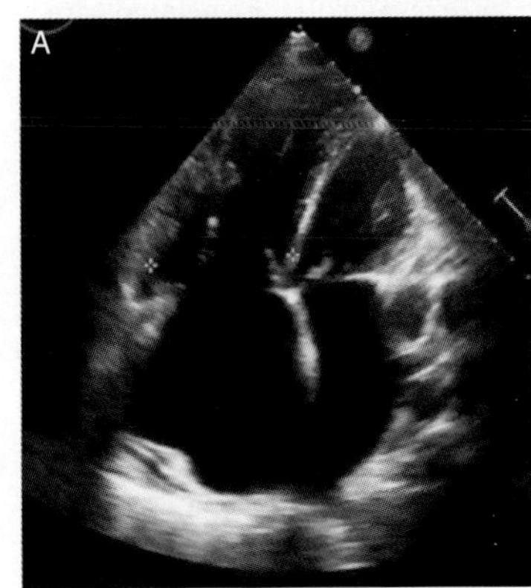

Cardiomyopathy

Type	Definition/Etiology	Clinical/Diagnosis/Management
Dilated	- Dilation and impaired contraction of one or both ventricles (EF < 40%) Etiology - **Ischemia** (focal areas of abnormal wall motion) - **Nonischemic** (global hypokinesis) - Infectious (viral, HIV, Chagas, Lyme) - Peripartum - Toxic (alcohol, cocaine) - Meds (anthracyclines, trastuzumab) - Familial/genetic - Tachycardia-mediated	- Presents with systolic HF - Diagnosis: TTE - Tx: HFrEF management
Restrictive	- Process infiltrates myocardium, resulting in impaired ventricular diastolic relaxation Causes - Amyloid, sarcoid, hemochromatosis, Fabry - Eosinophilic myocarditis - Endocardial fibroelastosis (children)	- Presents with diastolic HF - Prominent right heart symptoms - Diagnosis: TTE (diastolic dysfunction with restrictive filling pattern, biatrial enlargement[A]) - Tx: HFpEF management
Hypertrophic	- Disorder of sarcomere proteins resulting in disorganized/hypertrophied myocytes - Commonly AD b-myosin heavy chain or myosin binding protein C mutations	Presents with: - Heart failure (dyspnea), chest pain - Syncope or sudden cardiac death - Harsh systolic murmur (LLSB) - Diagnosis: TTE (asymmetric septal hypertrophy, LVH, systolic anterior motion of the mitral valve) Management - Beta/calcium channel blocker - Cautious diuretics (for edema) - ICD Note: Avoid preload or afterload reducers - Myectomy or alcohol ablation for persistent symptoms despite therapy
Takotsubo (Stress CM)	- Nonischemic temporary hypokinesis of myocardium - Occurs after severe emotional distress, high catecholamines	- Presents with chest pain and symptoms of acute HF - ↑ Troponin, possible EKG changes - TTE shows apical ballooning[B] (diagnostic), ↓ EF - Treatment is supportive, as cardiac function often returns
Right Ventricular Arrhythmogenic Cardiomyopathy	- Genetic nonischemic RV cardiomyopathy associated with ventricular arrhythmias	- Can present as cardiogenic syncope or sudden cardiac death in young adults - EKG with epsilon wave[C], diagnosis by cardiac MRI

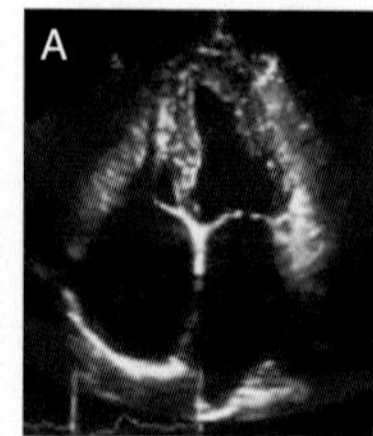

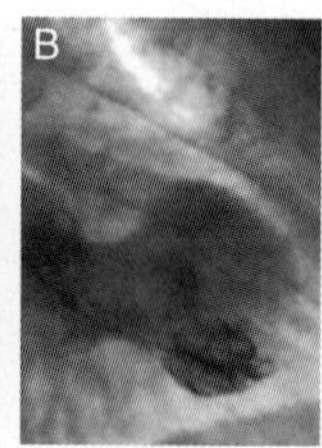

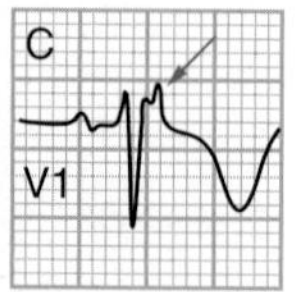

Cardiac/Vascular Malignancy

Cardiac/Vascular Malignancy	
Cardiac Malignancies	
Metastases	- 75% of cardiac neoplasm - Common primary sites include melanoma, liquid tumors (leukemia/lymphoma)
Atrial Myxoma	***General:*** Benign mesenchymal growth, often pedunculated and located in the left atrium. Most common primary cardiac tumor. ***Clinical:*** Cardiovascular symptoms (chest pain, dyspnea, palpitations), embolization (stroke, arterial occlusion), constitutional (fever, weight loss). Low-pitched diastolic murmur (diastolic plop). ***Diagnosis:*** TTE[A] ***Management:*** Surgery
Papillary Fibroelastoma	- Benign valvular growth - Often asymptomatic, but can embolize (stroke/TIA)
Rhabdomyomas	- Almost entirely in children - Associated with tuberous sclerosis
Vascular Malignancies	
Angiosarcoma	- Rare blood vessel malignancy typically occurring in the head, neck, and breast areas (sun-exposed areas). Usually in elderly. - Associated with radiation therapy, chronic postmastectomy lymphedema

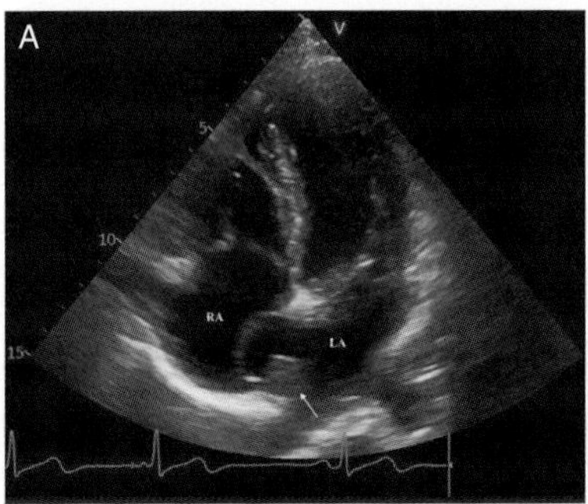

Pericardial Disease

Acute Pericarditis

General: Inflammation of the pericardial sac

Etiology:

- Viral (coxsackie, echovirus, adenovirus), bacterial (TB), fungal
- Uremia
- Acute MI, Dressler
- Autoimmune (collagen vascular diseases)
- Surgery/trauma/radiation

Clinical:

- **Severe, pleuritic chest pain** (improves leaning forward)
- Fever, leukocytosis, ↑ ESR/CRP
- Pericardial friction rub (specific)
- ECG (PR depressions, ST elevation)
- TTE (~50% have pericardial effusion)

Diagnosis: Clinical criteria (≥ 2/4 of the following)

(1) Classic positional chest pain; (2) friction rub; (3) typical ECG changes; (4) pericardial effusion

Management: Generally self-limited (1-3 weeks resolution)

- Idiopathic → NSAIDs (ibuprofen or indomethacin) + colchicine
- Post MI → ASA + colchicine
- Uremic → Dialysis

Note: Glucocorticoids reserved for those with contraindication for NSAIDs

Constrictive Pericarditis

General: Fibrous scarring of pericardium resulting in rigid and thick pericardium. Restricts diastolic filling of the heart. Increased ventricular interdependence.

Etiology: Bacterial (TB), connective tissue disease, surgery, radiation

Clinical:

- Presents with dyspnea, **prominent right heart failure**, congestive hepatopathy ("nutmeg liver")
- Elevated JVP, Kussmaul sign (JVP up with deep breath), pericardial knock

Diagnosis: CXR, cardiac MRI or CT (pericardial thickening +/− calcification)[A]

Management: Pericardiectomy

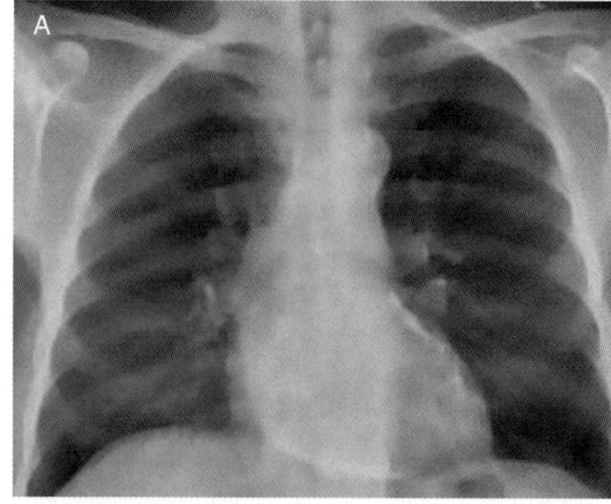

Pericardial Disease

Pericardial Effusion

General: Fluid between the visceral and parietal layers of the pericardial sac

Risk:

- Pericarditis (of any cause)
- Malignancy
- Hypervolemia (as seen with CHF, cirrhosis, nephrotic syndrome)

Clinical:

- Often asymptomatic, but can develop signs of impaired cardiac function
- Muffled heart sounds, soft PMI, dullness at left lung base (compressed by pericardial fluid), friction rub
- CXR (water bottle appearance)
- ECG (low voltage, electrical alternans)

Diagnosis: TTE[A] (best at establishing effusion and assess hemodynamic compromise)

- Pericardial fluid analysis (if etiology is unknown)

Management: Treat underlying disease. Can sample fluid if etiology unclear. Avoid diuretics. Follow with TTE.

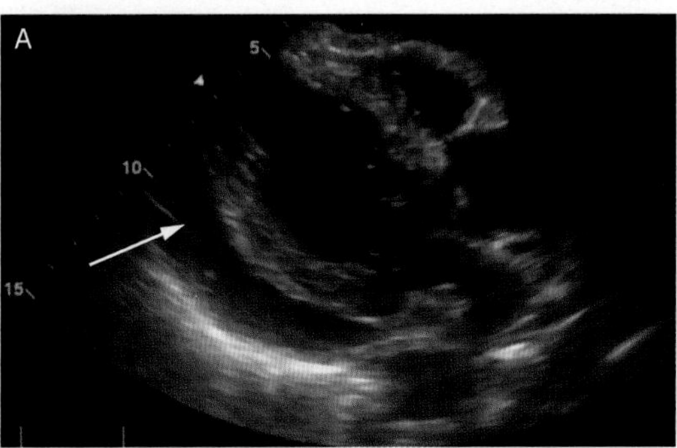

Cardiac Tamponade

General: Impaired diastolic function of heart due to pericardial effusion that is under pressure. Results from either a large effusion (> 2L) OR rapid accumulation of smaller effusion.

- Equalization of cardiac pressures and decreased cardiac output (ventricular interdependence)

Clinical:

- Presents with signs of hemodynamic compromise, chest pain, dyspnea
- Cardiogenic shock without pulmonary edema
- Pulsus paradoxus, narrowed pulse pressure, distant heart sounds
- **Beck's triad**: (1) Hypotension; (2) JVD; (3) muffled heart sounds
- ECG with decreased voltage, electrical alternans[B]

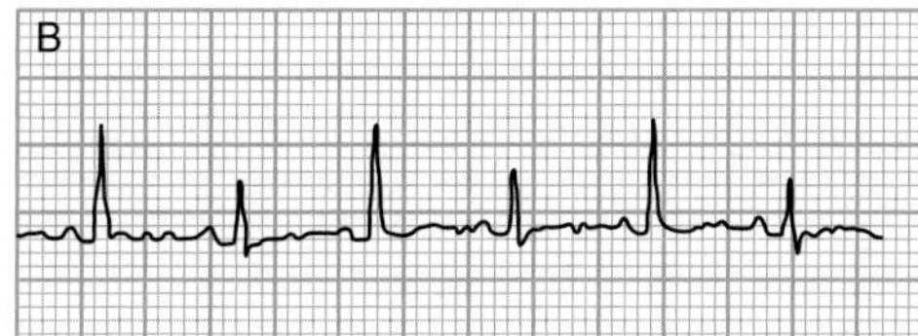

Diagnosis: TTE (confirms effusion) + elevated pulsus paradoxus

Management:

- IV fluids
- Nonhemorrhagic → Urgent pericardiocentesis or surgical drainage
- Hemorrhagic (traumatic) → Surgical drainage and repair

	Tamponade	Constriction	Restrictive
Pulsus	Yes	No	No
Kussmaul	No	Yes	Yes

Inflammatory Cardiac Disease

Myocarditis

General: Myocardial inflammation, that may be accompanied by cardiac dysfunction

Etiology:

- Idiopathic/viral (coxsackie B, adenovirus, influenza, CMV, EBV, parvovirus)
- Giant cell myocarditis
- Eosinophilic myocarditis

Clinical:

- Variable presentation. Ranges from subclinical to highly symptomatic (chest pain, heart failure, shock).
- Nonspecific ECG changes, TTE with diffuse wall motion abnormalities

Diagnosis:

Clinical criteria:
(1) Elevated cardiac biomarkers
(2) ECG changes (myocardial injury)
(3) Abnormal cardiac function (on TTE/MRI)
PLUS low suspicion for CAD (based on clean cardiac catheterization or age)

- Myocardial biopsy gold standard for diagnosis (not always obtained)

Management: Supportive if viral/idiopathic, immunosuppression for giant cell/eosinophilic

Rheumatic Fever

General: Sequella (~2-4 weeks) of group A *Streptococcus* pharyngitis, from M protein cross reactivity (molecular mimicry). Acute rheumatic fever presents as below, which can lead to chronic rheumatic valvular disease.

Clinical/Diagnostic Criteria: Either 2 major OR 1 major + 2 minor

Major (JONES)	Minor
1) **J**oints (migratory polyarthritis) 2) Pancarditis (endocarditis, pericarditis, myocarditis) 3) **N**odules (subcutaneous) 4) **E**rythema marginatum 5) **S**ydenham chorea	1) Fever 2) Elevated ESR 3) Polyarthralgias 4) Prolonged PR

*Evidence of previous *Streptococcus* infection (helpful, but not necessary) with either (+) throat *Streptococcus* test or ASO titer

Management:

- *Streptococcus* eradication: Penicillin G
- Joint pain: NSAIDs

Prophylaxis: Penicillin G (IM q4 weeks), Penicillin V (daily), or Azithromycin (daily)

Rheumatic fever w/ carditis + valve disease	Until 40 y/o OR 10 years
Rheumatic fever w/ carditis	Until 21 y/o OR 10 years
Rheumatic fever w/o carditis	Until 21 y/o OR 5 years

Nonbacterial Thrombotic Endocarditis

General: Noninfectious endocarditis characterized by thrombi deposition on valves. Associated with advanced malignancy ("Marantic") and SLE ("Libman-Sacks").

Clinical: Typically asymptomatic until embolization. Diagnosed with TTE.

Management: Anticoagulation (Heparin). Surgery.

Inflammatory Cardiac Disease

Infectious Endocarditis

General: Infection of the endocardial surface of the heart (generally of a valve)
- Location (in order of frequency): (1) Mitral; (2) Aortic; (3) Tricuspid (IVDU)
- Can be acute (rapidly progressive symptoms) or subacute

Risk: Prosthetic valve, cardiac devices, valvular disease, congenital heart disease, IVDU, poor dentition

Etiology:

Organism	Presentation
Staphylococcus aureus	- IV drug use, prosthetic valve, cardiac device
Streptococci viridans	- Gingival manipulation or poor dentition. Subacute presentation.
Enterococcus	- Genitourinary problems. Subacute presentation.
Streptococcus gallolyticus (bovis)	- Associated with colon cancer
Coagulase negative *Staph*	- Prosthetic devices, valves
HACEK: *Haemophilus aphrophilus, Actinobacillus actinomyc. Cardiobacterium hominis, Eikenella corrodens, Kingella kingae*	- *Eikenella*: Found in human mouths
Fungi (*Candida*)	- IV drug use, immunocompromised status
Brucella, Coxiella	- Animal exposures

Clinical:
- Constitutional: Fever, weight loss, night sweats. Dyspnea, cough, pleuritic chest pain.
- New murmur, petechiae, splinter hemorrhage (nails)
- **Janeway lesions** (nontender macules on extremities), **Osler nodes** (tender nodules fingers/toes), **Roth spots** (exudative lesions of retina). All highly specific but rare findings.

Diagnosis: Modified Duke Criteria

Definite IE: 2 Major OR 1 major + 3 minor OR 5 minor	**<u>Major criteria</u>** 1) Positive blood culture of typical organism 2) Echo evidence of endocardial lesion
Possible IE: 1 Major + 1 minor OR 3 minor	**<u>Minor criteria</u>** 1) Risk factor (IV drug, prosthetic valve) 2) Fever > 38°C 3) Vascular event (arterial emboli, septic infarcts, etc.) 4) Immunologic (glomerulonephritis, Osler, Roth, RF+) 5) Atypical blood cultures or serologic evidence of infection

Management:
- Workup → 3 × Blood cultures, prior to empiric therapy
- Antibiotics: Empiric (acutely ill patients) → Vancomycin
    - Transition to specific drug once blood cultures result. 4-6 weeks total therapy.
- Surgery: Indicated if severe valve dysfunction, abscess, or persistent infection

Complications:
- Heart failure, perivalvular abscess (suspect in patients developing conduction defects or persistent bacteremia), septic embolization (strokes, pulmonary infarcts), mycotic aneurysms, glomerulonephritis

Endocarditis Prophylaxis Guidelines:

Drug Choice (single dose preprocedure)	Indicated Conditions	Indicated Procedures
- Amoxicillin (alt: Cephalexin, clindamycin, azithromycin)	1) Prosthetic valves/cardiac material 2) History of endocarditis 3) Unrepaired cyanotic congenital heart disease	1) Dental (with gingival manipulation: extraction, implants, periodontal, cleaning with bleeding) 2) Respiratory biopsy 3) Procedure on infected GI/GU tract or skin 4) Heart surgery involving prosthetic valves or intracardiac materials

Valvular Heart Disease

Aortic Stenosis

General: Left ventricular outflow obstruction at the aortic valve

Risk: Idiopathic "wear & tear" (age > 65), bicuspid valve (~50 y/o), rheumatic valve (rare)

Clinical:

- Asymptomatic or nonspecific findings early in disease
- Severe disease → Classic triad of **heart failure, angina, syncope**
- Systolic ejection (crescendo-decrescendo) murmur at second right intercostal, radiates to carotids, soft S2
    - Carotid pulse ("parvus et tardus" or weak and delayed), sustained PMI

Diagnosis: TTE

S1 S2

Management: Aortic valve replacement if severe grade stenosis/highly symptomatic

- Transcatheter aortic valve replacement (TAVR) or surgical valve replacement (SAVR)

Aortic Insufficiency

General: Inadequate closure of aortic valve leaflets with regurgitation, increasing LV diastolic pressure/volume, resulting in dilatation and eccentric hypertrophy of the LV to maintain cardiac output, but eventually leading to heart failure

Risk:

- <u>Acute</u>: Endocarditis, aortic dissection
- <u>Chronic</u>: Valve issues (bicuspid valve, rheumatic disease), root issues (syphilis aortitis, Marfan)

Clinical:

- Presents with heart failure symptoms (more severe with acute AI)
- **Diastolic decrescendo murmur** at lower left sternal border, wide pulse pressure, water hammer pulse, head/uvula bobbing, Austin-Flint murmur

Diagnosis: TTE

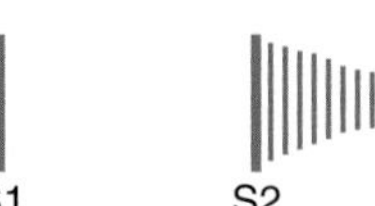

Management:

- <u>Acute</u>: Emergent aortic valve replacement/repair
- <u>Chronic</u>: Manage heart failure medically
    - Severe/highly symptomatic disease → Aortic valve replacement

Tricuspid Regurgitation

General: Reflux during systole from right ventricle to right atrium

Risk:

- Functional (from dilation of right atrium/ventricle)
- Valve damage (from endocarditis, rheumatic disease, carcinoid, injury from cardiac device)
- Ebstein's anomaly

Clinical:

- Right-sided CHF signs (JVD, RV heave, hepatomegaly, peripheral edema)
- Holosystolic murmur heard best at the left mid sternal border

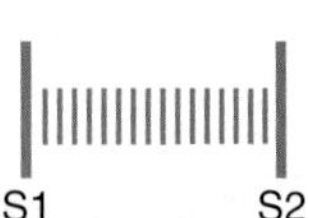

Diagnosis: TTE

Management: Functional regurgitation → Treat underlying disorder. Rarely repair/replace valve if severe.

Valvular Heart Disease

Mitral Regurgitation

General: Reflux during systole from left ventricle to left atrium

Risk:

- Primary: Degenerative valve disease (MVP, myxomatous), endocarditis, rheumatic valve disease
- Secondary: Ischemic (papillary muscle/chordae rupture), functional (HF), hypertrophic CM (SAM)

Clinical:

- Ranges from asymptomatic to left-sided heart failure (dyspnea, fatigue)
- **Holosystolic murmur** at apex, radiates to axilla

S1 S2

Diagnosis: TTE (regurgitation, LA dilatation)

Management:

- Acute: Emergent valve repair or replacement
- Chronic: Medical therapy (for heart failure), surgery if severe

Mitral Valve Prolapse

General: Myxomatous degeneration of mitral valve leaflets, with excessive or redundant tissue, leading to prolapse into LA. Can develop mitral regurgitation.

Risk: Primary MVP (idiopathic/familial) or secondary MVP (connective tissue disorders like Marfan, Ehlers-Danlos)

Clinical:

- MVP syndrome: Nonspecific symptoms (chest pain, palpitations, dyspnea)
- **Midsystolic click and murmur**
    - Standing/valsalva increases the murmur, makes click earlier; squatting decreases click/murmur

Diagnosis: TTE

Management: Reassurance

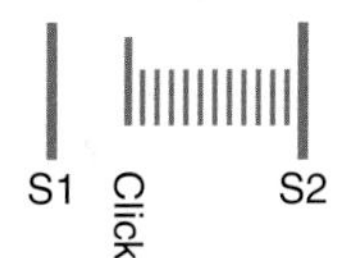

Mitral Stenosis

General: Obstruction of blood flow from left atrium to the ventricle, with resulting ↑ pressure in the left atrium and pulmonary circulation

Risk: Rheumatic heart disease

Clinical:

- Exertional dyspnea, decreased exercise tolerance, hemoptysis, AF
- **Opening snap followed by mid-diastolic rumble** (Loud S1, P2)
- ECG: Can show RVH, atrial enlargement

S1 S2 OS

Diagnosis: TTE (MV thickening/calcification, decreased valve mobility, LA enlargement)

Management:

- Surgery definitive therapy (balloon valvuloplasty)
- Medical treatment for AF/HF
    - Warfarin first-line anticoagulant for valvular AF

EP: Bradycardias

Sinus Bradycardia

General: Sinus rhythm with rate < 60 bpm

Etiology:

- **Benign** (sleep, well-conditioned athletes)
- **Drugs** (beta-blockers, CCBs)
- **Pathologic** (SA node disease, increased ICP, OSA, hypothyroidism)

Clinical: Generally asymptomatic until < 45 bpm, then possible fatigue, dizziness, or syncope

Diagnosis: ECG (sinus origin of P waves, HR < 60 bpm)

Management:
Hemodynamically stable: Workup for underlying cause

Hemodynamically unstable: Defined as bradycardia causing CHF, altered mentation, shock, hypotension, or chest pain. Follow ACLS bradycardia algorithm [on right].

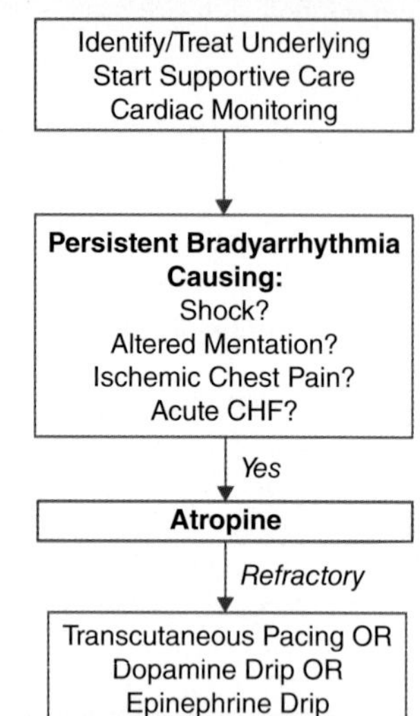

Atrioventricular Block

General: Abnormal conduction through the AV/His system

Etiology: Idiopathic, ischemia, drugs (beta-blocker, calcium channel blocker), congenital abnormalities, athletes, Lyme

Degree	ECG Findings	Management
1°[A] (AV delay)	PR > 0.2 sec (AV Nodal delay)	Reassurance
2° Mobitz I[B] (Wenckebach)	Progressive PR lengthening into dropped beat (usually at level of AV node)	Reassurance (generally benign)
2° Mobitz II[C]	Consistent PR interval with dropped beats (usually at level of HIS)	Pacemaker (risk to progress to complete block)
3°[D] (Complete)	Complete P/QRS disassociation	Pacemaker

Note: If reversible cause of heart block is identified (ischemia, drugs, vagal tone), pacemaker not indicated.

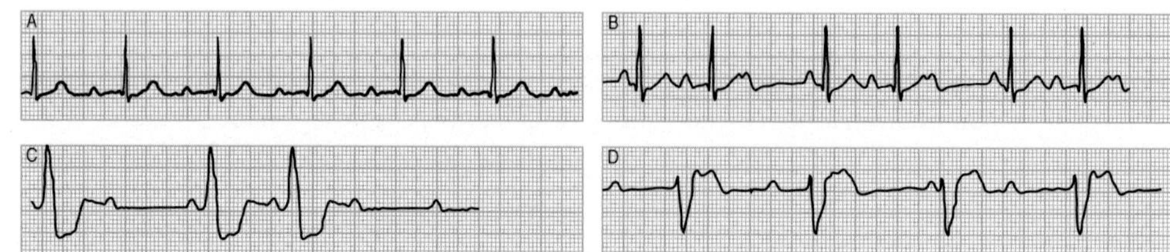

Sick Sinus Syndrome

General: SA nodal dysfunction, resulting in a wide range of abnormal heart rhythms (including sinus pauses and tachy-brady syndrome)

Clinical: Fatigue, presyncope, palpitations, dizziness, dyspnea, angina

Diagnosis: Telemetry (sinus bradycardia, sinus pauses[E]/conversion pause, alternating tachy/bradycardia)

Management: Permanent pacemaker (for symptomatic patients)

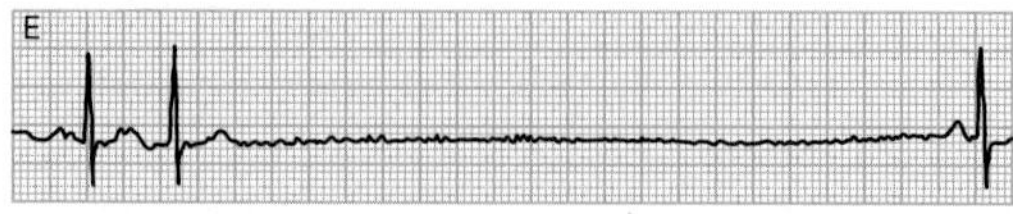

EP: Tachycardias

Atrial Fibrillation

General: Ectopic atrial rhythm, most commonly originating from abnormal foci near pulmonary veins. Atrial HR ~400, but AV nodal conduction is variable, so ventricular rate is ~75-125.

- Can be paroxysmal (comes and goes), persistent (lasts days to weeks), or permanent.

Risk: Age > 80, HTN, CAD, atrial abnormalities (HF, valvular disease), hyperthyroidism

- Can be triggered by EtOH, or increased catecholamines (infection, surgery, pain)

Clinical: Can be asymptomatic or symptomatic (palpitations, presyncope, dyspnea)

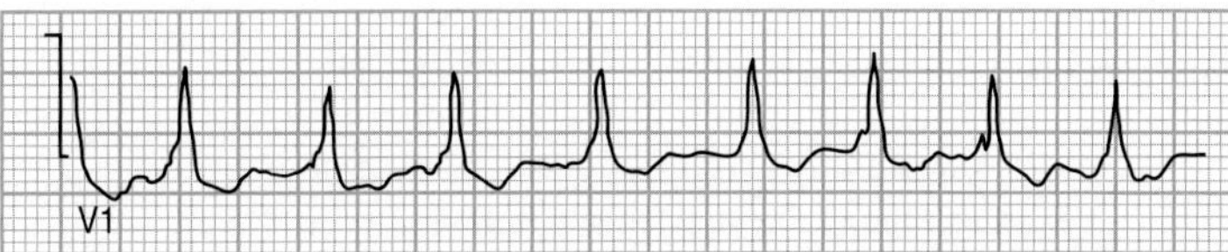

Diagnosis: ECG (irregularly irregular rhythm without distinct P waves)

Management:

<u>New onset</u>:

Step 1: Rate control (if necessary: Beta-blocker or calcium channel blocker)

Step 2: Cardioversion (if still in AF after trial of rate control)

- DC electrical cardioversion preferred to pharmacologic (flecainide, propafenone, or ibutilide)

Note: Patient must be anticoagulated for at least 3 weeks OR have developed AF within last 48 hours

Step 3: Chronic therapy (as below)

If in RVR (rapid ventricular response): IV beta-blocker, calcium channel blocker, digoxin or amiodarone

- Emergent cardioversion if unstable

<u>Chronic therapy</u>:

<u>Rate control</u> (Rate control = Rhythm control)

- Goal HR: < 85 (symptomatic) and < 110 (asymptomatic)
- Drug choice: Beta-blocker (e.g., Metoprolol) (alt: calcium channel blocker, digoxin)

<u>Rhythm control</u>

- Used for: < 65 y/o, symptomatic patients that need restoration of sinus rhythm
- Flecainide or propafenone. If CAD → Sotalol. If HF → Amiodarone.

<u>Anticoagulation</u>

Indications [CHA2DS2-VASc]	
CHF (1 point) HTN (1 point) Age ≥ 75 (2 points) DM (1 point) Stroke/TIA/Thromboembolism (2 points) Vascular disease (1 point) Age 64-75 (1 point) Sex female (1 point)	Score: ≥ 2 → Anticoagulate = 1 → Clinical judgment = 0 → No anticoagulation. Consider aspirin. **<u>Drug Choice</u>** 1) DOAC (dabigatran, rivaroxaban, apixaban) Note: Contraindicated in renal insufficiency 2) Warfarin (INR 2-3)

<u>Surgical</u>: Pulmonary vein isolation for severe cases

Complications:

- **Tachyarrhythmia-induced cardiomyopathy**: Dilated cardiomyopathy from prolonged tachycardia
- **Embolic events**: Stroke, mesenteric ischemia, limb ischemia

EP: Tachycardias

Atrial Flutter

General: Rapid, regular atrial depolarizations with an atrial rate ~300 bpm and ventricular rate of 150 bpm. Caused by re-entrant circuit that revolves around the tricuspid annulus or atrial scar tissue.

Clinical: Palpitations, dyspnea, fatigue, dizziness, presyncope. Risk for atrial thrombus.

Diagnosis: ECG (atrial rate 300 bpm [**saw-tooth-shaped waves**], with variable levels of conduction across the AV node [most commonly 2:1], resulting in a ventricular rate around 150 bpm)

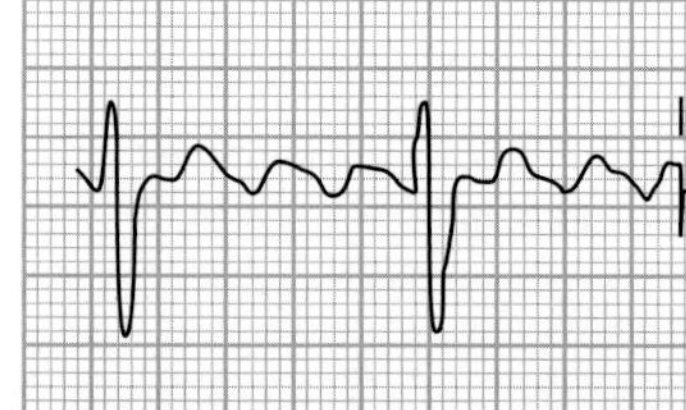

Management:

Medical:
- Rate control with beta-blocker or nondihydropyridine calcium channel blocker
- Anticoagulate as in atrial fibrillation

Interventions:
- DC cardioversion (if ablation is delayed/not planned)
- Radiofrequency catheter ablation (definitive therapy)

Multifocal Atrial Tachycardia

General: Arrhythmia with **HR > 100 bpm PLUS variable P-wave morphology**

Note: Variable P-wave morphology with normal rate is called wandering pacemaker

Risk: COPD (most common), heart failure

Clinical: Generally asymptomatic

Diagnosis: ECG (rate > 100 bpm with P waves of at least 3 different morphologies)

Management: Usually self-limited

AV Nodal Reentry Tachycardia

General: Most common paroxysmal SVT, caused by a reentry circuit in the AV node

Risk: Idiopathic, generally with onset in young adulthood

Clinical: Acute onset palpitations, dizziness, dyspnea

Diagnosis: ECG (regular narrow complex tachycardia without P waves, +/− retrograde P waves)

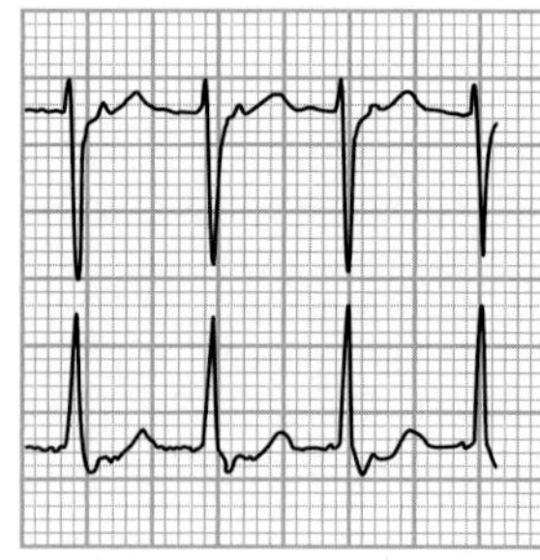

Management:
- Unstable: DC cardioversion
- Stable: Valsalva maneuvers, carotid massage, IV adenosine to terminate
    - Long-term treatment with beta-blockers or surgical ablation

EP: Tachycardias

Ventricular Tachycardia

General: Rapid firing of > 3 PVCs (originating below the bundle of His), with HR of 120-250 bpm. Subtypes:

- **Nonsustained** (< 30 sec, but > 3 beats, generally asymptomatic)
- **Sustained** (> 30 sec, generally symptomatic)
- Can also be classified as **monomorphic** or **polymorphic**

Risk: Ischemic heart disease, nonischemic cardiomyopathy, structural abnormalities

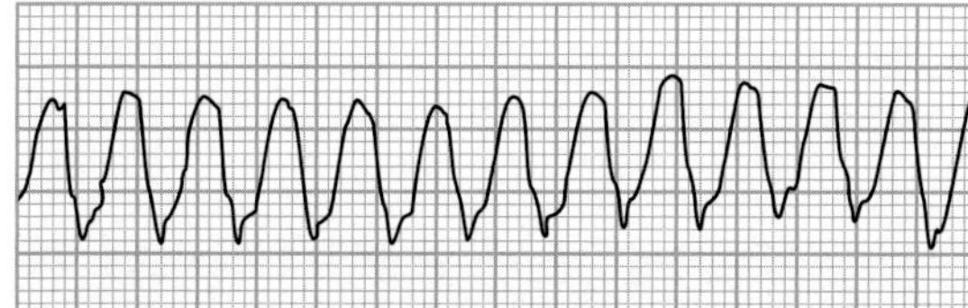

Management:

Nonsustained VT: Search for underlying etiology and treat

Sustained VT:

- No pulse → ACLS
- Pulse found: **Stable → IV amiodarone** (alt: Lidocaine, procainamide)
  Unstable → Synchronized cardioversion

Long-term

- ICD placement
- Meds: Beta-blocker or amiodarone may be indicated

Torsades de Pointes

General: Polymorphic VT with cyclic, sinusoidal changes in the QRS. Occurs with prolonged QT.

Risk:

- Congenital long QT
- Drugs: Macrolides/fluoroquinolones, antipsychotics/TCA, methadone, antiemetics, antiarrhythmics
- Electrolytes: Hypocalcemia, hypokalemia, hypomagnesemia

Management: Stable → IV magnesium.
Unstable → Electric defibrillation.

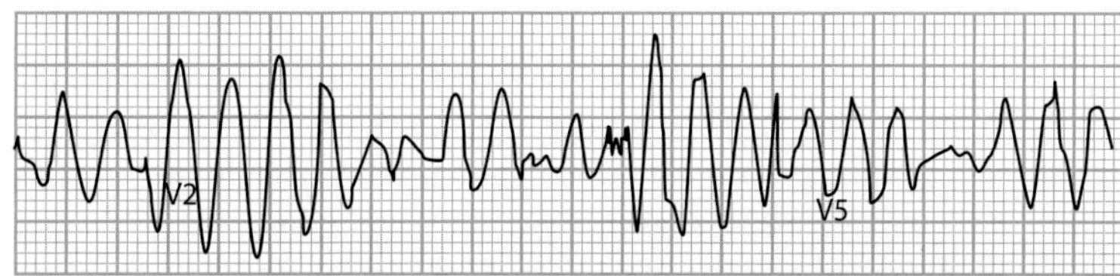

Ventricular Fibrillation/ACLS

General: Arrest of systolic cardiac function from disorganized electrical activity in the ventricles

Management: See ACLS algorithm below

- ICD indicated for patients that survive

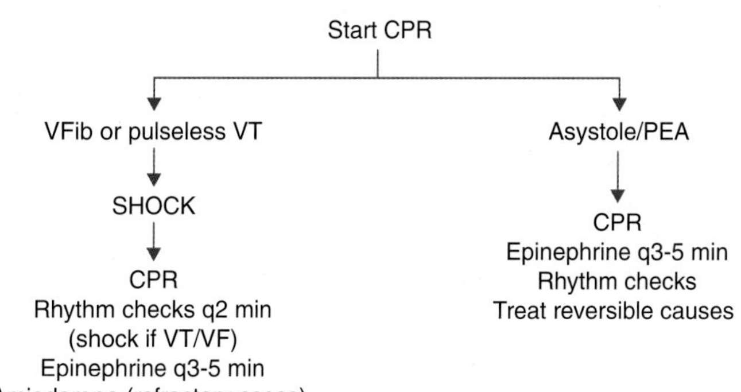

Reversible causes (5 Hs/Ts):
Hs: Hypovolemia, hyper/hypokalemia, hypoxemia hydrogen ion (acidosis), hypothermia
Ts: Thrombosis (pulmonary/coronary), tension pneumothorax, tamponade, toxins

Electrophysiology

Approach to Tachycardias

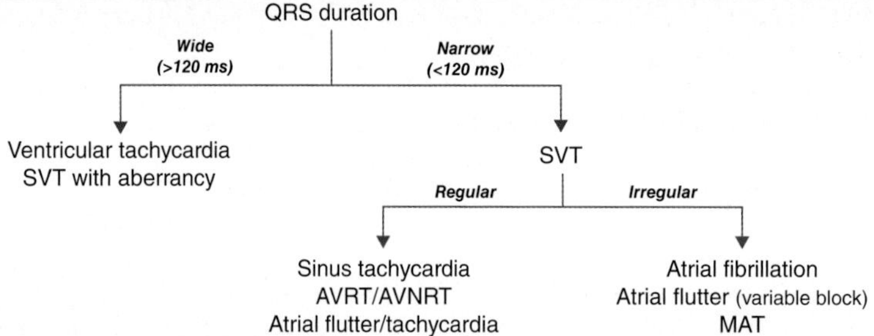

PAC/PVC

Premature Atrial Complex: Generally benign and asymptomatic ectopic (nonsinus) atrial beats. No treatment necessary. Beta-blocker if symptomatic.

Premature Ventricular Complex: Ectopic ventricular beats. Generally asymptomatic, but can experience palpitations. Workup patients with unexplained PVCs with 24-hour ambulatory monitoring/TTE/exercise stress test. Beta-blocker if symptomatic.

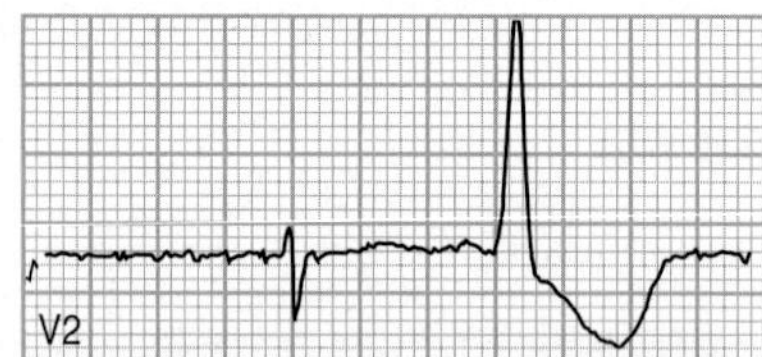

Pacemaker Basics

Types:

- **Single-chamber pacemaker** – 1 pacing lead is implanted in the RA or RV
- **Dual-chamber pacemaker** – 2 pacing leads are implanted (1 in RV, 1 in RA)
- **Biventricular pacing** (cardiac resynchronization therapy [CRT])
  - Single or dual-chamber leads, PLUS coronary sinus lead

Indications:

ICD

1) Anyone who suffers a cardiac arrest or sustained ventricular tachycardia (unless reversible cause was identified)
   - Includes structural causes, such as ischemic or hypertrophic cardiomyopathy
2) EF < 35% in NYHA Class II/III HF
3) EF < 30% and recent MI (> 40 days ago)
4) Channelopathies, including long QT and Brugada

Resynchronization therapy (CRT)

1) LVEF ≤ 35% + QRS > 0.12-0.15 sec, with HF symptoms on medical therapy

Permanent pacemaker

1) Symptomatic bradycardia (for any reason, including sinus node dysfunction)
2) Chronic heart rate < 40 while awake
3) Irreversible Mobitz type II heart block or complete heart block
4) Symptomatic chronotropic incompetence

Cardiac Event Monitors

Types:

1) Holter (1-2 days continuous ECG monitor)
2) Loop event monitor (weeks long, patient activated when symptomatic)
3) Implantable loop recorder (months of monitoring, subcutaneous recorder)
4) Mobile cardiac outpatient telemetry [MCOT] (up to 30 days continuous ECG monitor)

Indications:

1) Unexplained syncope, near syncope
2) Recurrent unexplained palpitations
3) Monitor for atrial fibrillation
4) Screen for ventricular arrhythmia in structural heart disease

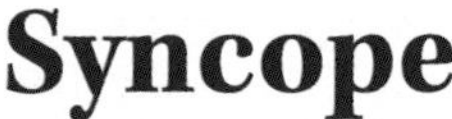

Syncope

General: Transient loss of consciousness due to inadequate cerebral blood flow

Etiology: See below
- Nonsyncopal mimics of syncope: Seizures, pseudoseizures, mechanical falls (subsequent LOC from head trauma)

Clinical:
- Transient loss of consciousness (usually for ~10 sec)
- Can result in fall (loss of postural tone) or accident if driving
- Prodromal features specific to syncopal etiology

Workup: History/physical is key. Labs, ECG/telemetry, orthostatics, TTE if concerned for structural abnormality.

Management: Risk stratification
- Low risk (clear vasovagal syncope, no red flags): Discharge home
- High risk (syncope during exercise, palpitations, abnormal ECG findings [VTach, sinus bradycardia, prolonged QT, heart block, bifascicular block])
  - Requires admission for further evaluation

	General/Clinical	Management
Neurocardiogenic		
Vasovagal	- Increased parasympathetic outflow (vagus nerve), resulting in transient bradycardia and hypotension - Triggers: Emotional stress, pain, fear, heat, prolonged standing - Clinical: Presents with prodrome of nausea, diaphoresis, pallor, and feeling faint, followed by syncope - Rapid return to consciousness	Dx: Usually clinical. Tilt-table testing reserved for special circumstances. Tx: Reassurance. If prodromal symptoms, try counterpressure maneuvers or laying down.
Situational	- Variant of vasovagal syncope - Syncope with one of the following situations: - Cough, sneeze, urination, swallowing, defecation - Carotid sinus syncope: Specific situational subtype from hypersensitive carotid sinus to stimulation. Significant drop in BP/HR with carotid massage.	Tx: Reassurance - Pacing rarely required for carotid sinus syncope
Orthostatic	- Exaggerated fall in blood pressure due to gravity - Cause: Hypovolemia, autonomic failure (diabetes, Parkinson), and medications (alpha, beta-blockers) - Clinical: Lightheadedness, dizziness upon standing, with syncopal episode upon standing or prolonged standing	Tx: - Fluids (if hypovolemic) - Fludrocortisone/midodrine (if neurogenic)
Cardiogenic (arrhythmias)	- Cause: Bradycardia (heart block, sick sinus syndrome) or ventricular arrhythmias - Clinical: Syncope often sudden (without prodrome) - Sometimes preceded by palpitations or chest pain	Dx: ECG, cardiac monitoring
Cardiogenic (structural)	- Causes: Aortic stenosis, hypertrophic cardiomyopathy - Clinical: Generally presents during exertion	Dx: TTE
Other	- Pulmonary embolism, subarachnoid hemorrhage	

Hyperlipidemia

General: Elevated levels of LDL are known to be atherogenic, while HDL is anti atherogenic. Triglycerides do not have clear association with atherosclerosis, but at very high levels (> 1000) are associated with pancreatitis.

Clinical: Generally asymptomatic. **Risk factor for coronary disease and stroke.** If very high, can develop deposition:
- Xanthoma (lipid deposit, commonly of tendon and eyelid ["xanthelasma"])
- Corneal arcus (lipid deposit in cornea)

Management:
- Lifestyle modification for all (healthy diet, exercise, quit smoking)
- Statin therapy (see USPSTF indications)
- If patient extremely high risk and LDL remains > 70-100 mg/dL, can consider ezetimibe or PCSK-9 inhibitor

Indication	Statin
Known ASCVD (CAD/CVA/PAD)	High intensity
LDL > 190	High intensity
40-75 y/o diabetics	Moderate to high intensity
ASCVD risk > 10%	Moderate to high intensity

Notes on statins:
- If patient develops myalgias or transaminitis on statins, stop drug, retry at lower dose
- Obtain baseline LFTs and CK, but no need to screen for LFTs/CK unless symptomatic

Drug	LDL	HDL	Trig	Mechanism	Adverse Reaction
Statin Atorva, rosuva simva, prava	↓↓	↑	↓	HMG-CoA inhibitor	Hepatotoxicity Myopathy, rhabdomyolysis
Bile Resin Cholestyramine, Colestipol	↓	↑	↔	Inhibit bile resorption	GI disturbance Drug malabsorption
Ezetimibe	↓	↔	↔	Inhibit cholesterol absorption (NPC1L1)	Diarrhea
Fibrate Gemfibrozil Fenofibrate	↔	↑	↓↓	Upregulate LPL Activate PPAR-a	Myositis (gemfibrozil) Cholesterol gallstone
Niacin	↓	↑	↓	Inhibit lipolysis	Flushing (use ASA) Hyperglycemia, uricemia
Omega-3	↔	↑	↓	Decrease hepatic fat secretion	
PCSK-9 Inhibitor Evolocumab Alirocumab	↓↓↓	↑	↓	Prevent LDL-R uptake/breakdown	Reaction at injection site

Genetic Dyslipidemia:

Class	Name	Mechanism	Clinical
I (AR)	Hyperchylomicronemia	LPL deficiency	↑ TG → Pancreatitis
IIa (AD)	Hypercholesterolemia	LDL-R deficiency	↑ LDL → Severe atherosclerosis
III (AR)	Dysbetalipoproteinemia	APO-E mutation	↑ Chol/TG → Premature CAD
IV (AD)	Hypertrigliceridemia	VLDL overproduction	↑ TG/VLDL → Premature CAD

Hypertension

Stage	SBP mmHg	DBP mmHg	Management
Normotensive	< 120	< 80	
Prehypertensive	120-129	< 80	- Lifestyle modification, routine follow-up
Stage 1	130-139 or	80-89	- Lifestyle (all) - Pharm (for high risk individuals[$])
Stage 2	> 140 or	> 90	- Lifestyle + pharm (for all)
Severe	> 180	> 110	- Management below
[$]High risk: CAD, HF, diabetes, CKD, age > 65, ASCVD 10 year risk > 10%			
Hypertensive Urgency	- Severe grade hypertension with possible mild headache, but no end organ damage		
Hypertensive Emergency	- Severe grade hypertension with evidence of **end organ damage**, including: - **CNS:** Encephalopathy, stroke, elevated ICP, retinal hemorrhage - **Renal:** AKI, hematuria, proteinuria - **Cardiovascular:** ACS, angina, worsening CHF, aortic dissection		
White Coat Hypertension	- Elevated blood pressure in doctor's office - Diagnose with either 24-hour ambulatory or home BP monitoring		
Secondary Hypertension	- Etiologies: CKD, renal arterial stenosis, hyperaldosteronism, pheochromocytoma, Cushing, aortic coarctation, meds (OCP), OSA - Workup for secondary hypertension indicated if: Young (age < 35), severely elevated or refractory BP, or sign/symptom specific to secondary disorder		

Risk: Family history, Black, high salt intake, alcohol use, obesity, physical inactivity

Diagnosis: Two separate clinic readings over 4 weeks
- Ambulatory or home blood pressure monitoring preferred to confirm

Management:

Essential	- Lifestyle change (in order of efficacy): Weight loss > DASH diet > Exercise > Salt restriction > ↓ Alcohol - Pharm indicated if > 140/90 in average risk adult, or > 130/80 in high risk adult - First-line meds: Include **ACEi/ARB, thiazides, or calcium channel blockers** - Med choice should be tailored based on patient's comorbid conditions
Severe	Overall goal for either is either 25% reduction from baseline or < 160/100 mmHg <u>Emergency</u> - Drop MAP by ~20% in first hour, with total of no more than 25% in 24 hours - Overly aggressive reduction can lead to ischemic end organ damage (unable to autoregulate in time) - Drug choice: IV hydralazine, esmolol, nitroprusside, labetalol, nicardipine <u>Urgency</u> (**Asymptomatic severe hypertension**) - Lower within 24 hours using oral meds

Congenital Defects (Acyanotic)

	General/Risk	Clinical/Management
Ventricular septal defect (VSD)	- Most common congenital defect, typically located in the membranous septum - Often idiopathic, associated with Down and fetal alcohol syndrome	- Small defects often asymptomatic, while larger defects can lead to tachypnea, failure to thrive within 1-2 months of birth - **Harsh holosystolic murmur** at left sternal border, which can be louder with smaller defects - Severe defects cause diastolic rumble (high mitral flow), sternal lift (RV enlargement) ***Management:*** - Surgically close if large/symptomatic
Atrial septal defect (ASD)	- Congenital defect of the atrial septum - **Secundum:** Arrested growth of the septum secundum or excessive septum primum absorption - **Primum:** Septum primum does not fuse with the endocardial cushions, associated with AV canal defects Note: Patent foramen ovale not considered an atrial septal defect - ***Risk:*** Down (primum)	- Asymptomatic until middle age, then can develop dyspnea, fatigue, exercise intolerance - Systolic ejection murmur at pulmonary area (due to increased pulmonary blood flow), fixed split S2, diastolic flow rumble murmur across tricuspid area ***Management:*** - Children: Monitor if small/asymptomatic, surgically close if large/symptomatic - Adults: Symptomatic / RV overload / embolic stroke: Surgical or percutaneous closure - Severe PAH → No surgical closure
Patent ductus arteriosus (PDA)	- Communicating vessel from aorta to pulmonary artery, which remains open in-utero due to low O_2 and elevated PGE2 levels, but closes shortly after birth. If it remains patent, a left-to-right shunt occurs. - ***Risk:*** Prematurity, rubella infection	- Ranges from asymptomatic to HF. Persistent large shunts can lead to shunt reversal and Eisenmenger. - **Continuous "machinery murmur,"** wide pulse pressure/bounding pulse, differential cyanosis ***Management:*** - Preterm infants: Indomethacin/ibuprofen - Term infants and older: Surgical closure
Coarctation of the aorta	- Narrowing of the descending aorta, typically just distal to the left subclavian artery origin - ***Risk:*** Generally an idiopathic, congenital structural abnormality. Associated with Turner syndrome or acquired with Takayasu arteritis.	- Upper-lower body blood pressure differential, brachial-femoral pulse delay, upper body hypertension (headaches, epistaxis) - Interscapular murmur (from collateral circulation) - CXR can show rib notching (arterial collaterals). ECG can show LVH. ***Management:*** - In patients with significant stenosis (causing elevated pressure gradient), correction via surgery or balloon angioplasty is indicated
Vascular rings	- Congenital anomaly of the aortic arch that results in compression of the trachea or esophagus - ***Risk:*** Idiopathic. Can be associated with Down or DiGeorge.	- Can present with respiratory distress, tachypnea, cyanosis (arching back and extending head relieves obstruction) ***Management:*** Surgical correction

Congenital Defects (Cyanotic)

	General/Risk	Clinical/Management
Truncus arteriosus	- Common truncal artery that gives rise to aorta and pulmonary arteries - Often have VSD - ***Risk:*** DiGeorge	- Presents within first weeks of life with cyanosis, heart failure, respiratory distress - Dx: TTE ***Management:*** - Surgical repair
D-transposition of the great vessels	- Aorta arises from RV, pulmonary artery from the LV - Utilizes some combination of VSD, ASD, PFO, PDA to survive - ***Risk:*** Preexisting maternal diabetes	- Presents within hours of birth with cyanosis and respiratory distress - Dx: TTE. CXR ("eggs on a string" narrowed mediastinum). ***Management:*** - Alprostadil (PGE1), which maintains patent ductus - Balloon atrial septostomy (allow for blood mixing) - Surgical correction (arterial switch)
Tricuspid atresia	- Absence of the tricuspid valve, with no direct connection between RA/RV - All have ASD, RV hypoplasia - Many also have PDA, VSD	- Presents within days of birth with cyanosis +/– murmur - Dx: TTE. CXR (minimal pulmonary markings). ECG (left axis). ***Management:*** - Alprostadil (PGE1), which maintains patent ductus - Surgical correction
Tetralogy of Fallot	- Syndrome of: **(1) RVH** **(2) VSD** **(3) Overriding aorta** **(4) Obstructed RV outflow**	- Clinical severity varies with degree of outflow obstruction - Can present immediately to within weeks of birth with cyanosis, distress - **"Tet Spell" or hypercyanotic spells** with periods of agitation. Squatting relieves symptoms. - Harsh systolic murmur from RV outflow - Dx: TTE. CXR (boot-shaped heart). ***Management:*** - Medical stabilization: Alprostadil - Tet spell: Knee-chest position, O_2, pain control - Surgical closure (3-6 months of life)
Total anomalous pulmonary venous return	- Four pulmonary veins fail to make connection to LA → drain to systemic system, mixing oxygenated blood with deoxygenated from venous return	- Can have acute or subacute presentation of cyanosis and heart failure - Dx: TTE. CXR ("snowman" sign from enlarged vein). ***Management:*** - Surgical repair

Congenital Defects

Hypoplastic Left Heart Syndrome

General: Hypoplasia of the LV and abnormal development of mitral/aortic valves. Requires RV to help deliver both pulmonary and systemic circulation.

Clinical: Presents with cyanosis, respiratory distress, decreased peripheral pulses

Diagnosis: TTE

Management: Alprostadil and transcatheter septoplasty to maintain shunting, followed by surgical repair

Ebstein's Anomaly

General: Malformed and displaced tricuspid valve displaced through the valve annulus and attached to the RV endocardium

Clinical: Severe disease presents with cyanosis and heart failure in infants

Diagnosis: TTE (tricuspid regurgitation and RV dilatation)

Management: Surgical repair

Supravalvular Aortic Stenosis

General: Rare cause of aortic stenosis, due to thickening of the ascending aorta

Risk: Characteristic of William's syndrome, but can be idiopathic

Clinical: Features are variable depending on the degree of obstruction, but causes a systolic ejection murmur

Management: Surgical repair for high grade stenosis

Approach to Pediatric Murmurs

Innocent murmurs

1) Vibratory Still's (most common innocent murmur)
    - Low-pitched vibratory crescendo-decrescendo systolic murmur at left lower sternal border

2) Cervical venous hum
    - Low-pitched crescendo-plateau-decrescendo, continuous, below clavicle
    - Begins in mid systole, crosses S2, and is loudest in diastole

3) Pulmonary or aortic flow
    - Systolic ejection murmurs

"Red flags" (that workup is indicated)

- If > 3/6 in intensity and harsh in quality
- Diastolic or continuous
- Holosystolic murmurs
- S3 or S4 gallop

Pediatric Arrhythmia

Wolff Parkinson White

General: Accessory electrical pathway ("Bundle of Kent") that can lead to premature ventricular excitement. Tachycardia can be caused by either AFib/Flutter OR reentry of normal conduction (atrioventricular reentrant tachycardia or AVRT).

Clinical: Asymptomatic unless arrhythmia develops

Diagnosis: ECG shows **shortening PR interval and presence of delta wave**

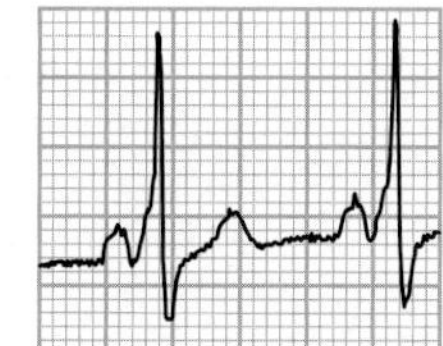

Management:

- Unstable arrhythmia → Cardioversion
- AVRT → Vagal maneuvers, adenosine
- Atrial fibrillation → Ibutilide or procainamide
- Definitive therapy → Catheter ablation of accessory pathway

Brugada Syndrome

General: AD genetic condition with increased risk of ventricular arrhythmias and sudden cardiac death

Diagnosis: ECG typically shows **pseudo-right bundle branch block with ST elevations in V1-V3**

Management: ICD placement

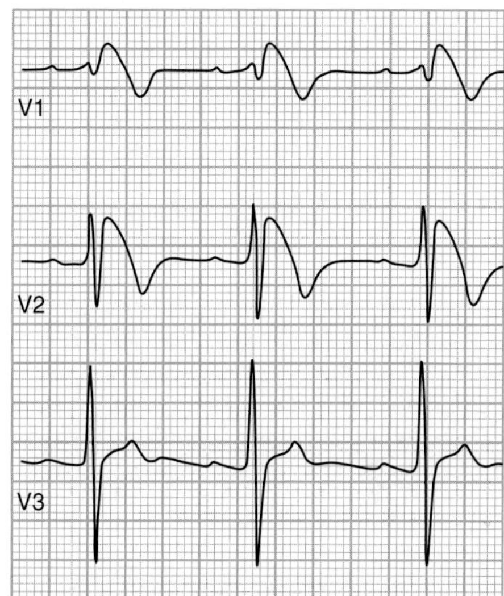

Congenital Long QT

General: Congenital defect in sodium or potassium channels resulting in delayed cardiac repolarization. High risk for ventricular tachycardia (Torsades).

Etiology: Many mutations in Na/K channels have been implicated

- **Romano-Ward:** AD LQTS without deafness
- **Jervell and Lange Nielsen:** AR LQTS with sensorineural deafness

Management: Exercise avoidance, beta-blocker, with ICD in certain situations

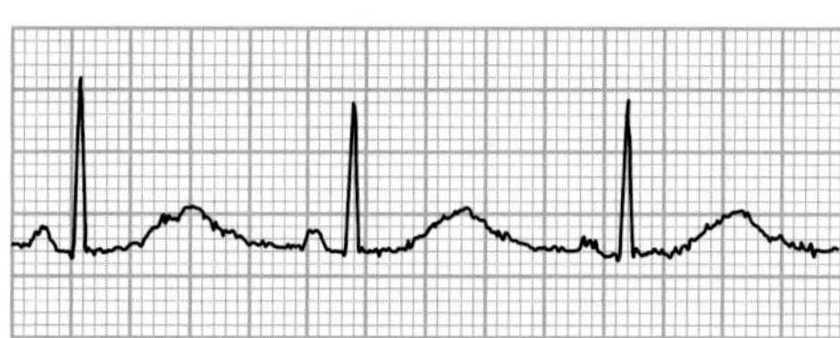

Peripheral Artery Disease

Peripheral Artery Disease

General: Atherosclerosis of peripheral vessels, usually in the lower extremities

Risk: Smoking, hypertension, hyperlipidemia, diabetes mellitus, CKD, history of CAD

Clinical:
- Initial symptom is **claudication, induced by walking, relieved with rest**
    - Quads, calves, and gluteal muscles most commonly involved
- Severe symptoms: Rest pain, purple/blue, hairless legs, ulcers, shiny skin, atrophy of muscles
- Buerger sign: Elevation turns foot pale, then dangling turns in bright red
- Rutherford symptom scale (see right)

Category	Symptoms
0	Asymptomatic
1	Mild claudication
2	Moderate claudication
3	Severe claudication
4	Rest pain
5	Minor tissue loss
6	Major tissue loss

Diagnosis:
- ABI (ankle-brachial index): ≤ 0.9 is abnormal
    - Can add exercise to test if equivocal
    - Elevated values can be seen with calcified vessels
- Imaging: US, CT/MRI angiography

Management:
- Medical therapy (prevention):
    - Antiplatelets (ASA/clopidogrel)
    - Smoking cessation
    - Statin
- Medical therapy (claudication):
    - **Exercise Therapy**
    - Cilostazol
- Revascularization (either surgical bypass or endovascular stenting)
    - Indications: Disabling symptoms refractory to medical therapy OR limb-threatening ischemia

Leriche syndrome

General: Obstruction of aortoiliac vessels

Clinical: Presents as bilateral thigh/quad claudication, erectile dysfunction, and absent/diminished femoral pulse

Acute Limb Ischemia

General: Sudden decrease in limb perfusion leading to tissue ischemia

Etiology:
- **Thrombosis** (at site of atherosclerosis, aneurysm)
- **Embolism**
- **Phlegmasia** (extensive venous backup, very rare)
- Trauma [See: Trauma]

Clinical: Six Ps (pain, pallor, pulselessness, poikilothermia, paresthesia, paralysis)
- Sensory symptoms occur early, while motor loss is severe

Diagnosis: CTA

Management: Fluids, heparin, place limb in dependent position

Class	Definition	Intervention
Viable (I)	Mild pain, but intact capillary refill, peripheral pulses	None
Marginally threatened (IIa)	Moderate pain, diminished pulses, possible sensory deficit	Urgent revascularization
Immediately threatened (IIb)	Severe pain, sensory/motor deficits, no pulses	Emergent revascularization
Irreversible ischemia (III)	Complete paralysis/no sensation. Signs of dead tissue.	Amputation

*Depending on type of obstruction, procedure could be open embolectomy, endovascular thrombectomy, medical thrombolysis.

Aortic Disease

Aortic Dissection

General: Separation of the layers of the aortic wall, due to an intimal tear. Stanford subtypes:
- **A (ascending/arch)**: Involves ascending aorta
- **B (arch/descending)**: Distal to the subclavian artery

Risk:
- Aortic damage (**hypertension**, thoracic aneurysm, atherosclerosis)
- Marfan/Ehlers-Danlos
- Bicuspid valve, Turner syndrome, syphilis aortitis

Clinical:
- **Severe chest pain, radiating to back, "tearing" quality**
- Asymmetric BP (> 20 mmHg)
- CXR: Widened mediastinum
- Type A: Risk for MI, stroke, aortic regurgitation, tamponade, Horner, vocal cord paralysis
- Type B: Risk for limb, renal, mesenteric ischemia

Diagnosis:
- CTA[A] (test of choice in hemodynamically stable patients)
- TEE (test of choice in hemodynamically unstable patients)

Management:

Both Subtypes	- Maintain HR < 60 and BP between 100 and 120 mmHg systolic
	  - IV beta-blockers: Esmolol or labetalol
	  - Add nitroprusside if BP still elevated
	- IV opioid analgesia

Type A	- Surgical emergency
Type B	- Medically managed, unless develops complication - Surgery indicated if evidence for ischemic complication or disease propagation/progression (Note: Intervention can be either endovascular or open surgery)

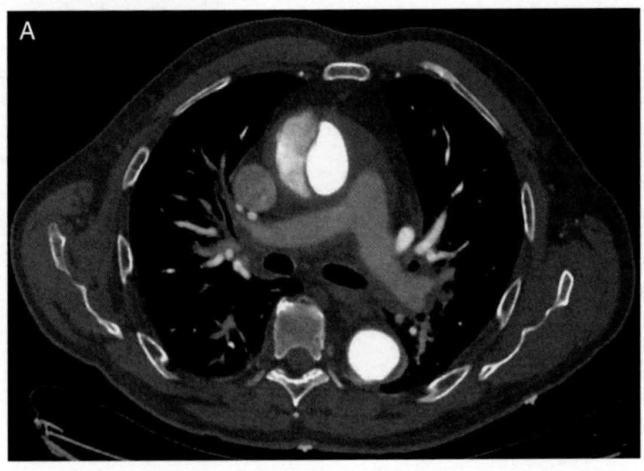

Aortic Disease

Abdominal Aortic Aneurysm

General: Focal aortic dilatation, generally > 3 cm in size

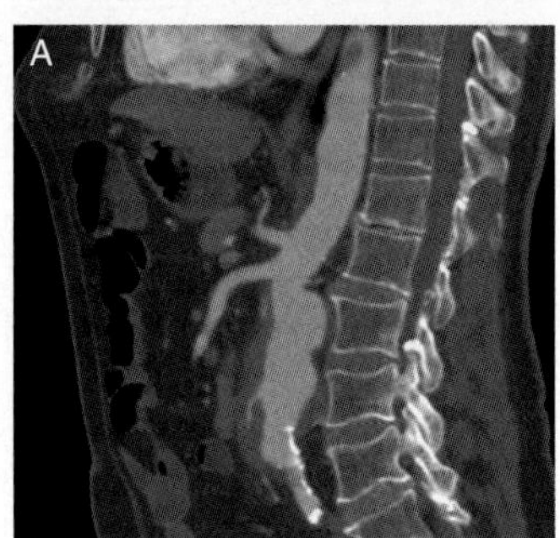

Risk: **Atherosclerotic disease**, smoking, ↑ age, males, HTN, HLD

Clinical:
- Usually asymptomatic if AAA is stable
- Symptomatic, but not ruptured: Can cause pressure/pain in back

Diagnosis: Abdominal US (initial modality of choice), CT[A]

Management:
- Symptomatic: Elective repair
- Asymptomatic:
    - Surgery (EVAR or TAVR): ≥ **5.5 cm or rapidly expanding (> 1 cm/yr)**
    - Observation: In anyone not meeting surgical criteria
        - q6-12 months screening ultrasounds
        - Treat modifiable risk factors (e.g., smoking cessation)

Ruptured Abdominal Aortic Aneurysm

Clinical: Classic triad: Abdominal pain, shock, pulsatile abdominal mass

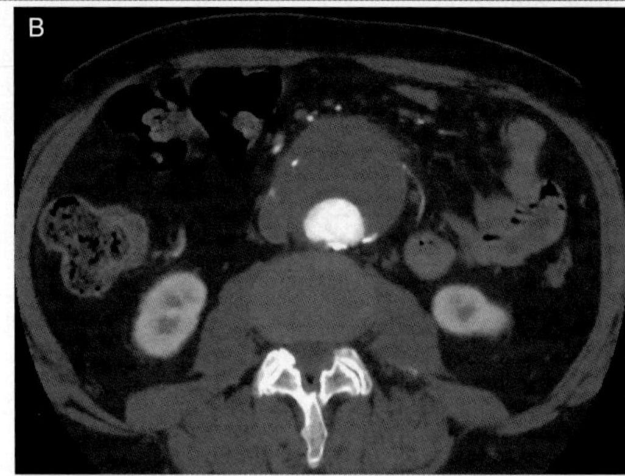

Diagnosis:
- Stable: Abdominal CT[B]
- Unstable: Bedside US

Management: Endovascular or open surgical repair

Complications: Aortoenteric fistula (causes large GI bleed)

Thoracic Aortic Aneurysm

General: Localized dilatation of thoracic aorta, > 50% larger in diameter than normal

Risk: Hypertension, hyperlipidemia, atherosclerosis, smoking
- Marfan, Ehlers-Danlos, Turner syndrome, bicuspid aortic valve, vasculitis, tertiary syphilis

Clinical: Most commonly asymptomatic
- **Rupture, or imminent rupture:** Chest/back pain, nerve compression, thromboembolism, aortic dissection
- XR: Can show widened mediastinum

Diagnosis: Echocardiography, CTA, or MRA

Management:
- Surgery (open or endovascular): **> 5.5 cm or rapid expansion (> 1 cm/yr)**
- Observation/serial monitoring if does not meet surgical criteria

Cardiovascular Pharm

	Mechanism	Indication	Side Effects/Management
Antiarrhythmics			
Class Ia Quinidine Procainamide Disopyramide	- Na^+ channel inhibitor - ↑ QRS, ↑ QT duration	- Ventricular arrhythmias - Atrial arrhythmias	- ↑ QT → Torsades, ventricular arrhythmias (all) - Quinidine: Cinchonism (tinnitus, confusion, psychosis) - Procainamide: Drug-induced SLE - Disopyramide: Myocardial depression, anticholinergic
Class Ib Lidocaine Mexiletine	- Na^+ channel inhibitor - ↑ QRS, ↑ QT duration	- Ventricular arrhythmias	- Ventricular arrhythmias - Lidocaine: CNS (tremor, agitation, etc)
Class Ic Flecainide Propafenone	- Na^+ channel inhibitor - ↑ QRS duration	- Atrial arrhythmias	- Ventricular arrhythmias *Not used if structural heart disease
Class II **Beta-blockers** Atenolol Bisoprolol Carvedilol Esmolol Labetalol Metoprolol Propranolol	- β-adrenergic antagonist β1-Selective: "A-M" Nonselective: "N-Z" Carvedilol/labetalol: α/β block	- Atrial fibrillation/flutter - AVNRT - Angina/ACS Hypertension - Heart failure - Migraine PPX (propranolol) - Thyrotoxicosis (propranolol) - Variceal PPX (nadolol) - Glaucoma (timolol)	- Fatigue, erectile dysfunction, depression, mild HLD - Bradyarrhythmias - Caution with acute exacerbation of HF, asthma, COPD <u>Beta-blocker overdose</u>: - Presents with bradycardia, AV block, shock - Tx: Fluids, atropine, glucagon
Class III Amiodarone Ibutilide Dofetilide Sotalol	- K^+ channel blocker	- Ventricular arrhythmias - Atrial arrhythmias	- ↑ QT → Torsades, ventricular arrhythmias (all) <u>Amiodarone</u>: - Pulmonary fibrosis, hepatotoxicity - Hypo or hyperthyroidism - Bradyarrhythmias - Corneal deposits, blue/gray skin, sun hypersensitivity
Class IV Diltiazem Verapamil	- Ca^{2+} channel blocker (nondihydropyridine)	- Atrial fibrillation/flutter - AVNRT - Angina - Hypertension	- Constipation - Edema - Bradyarrhythmias - Hyperprolactinemia (verapamil)

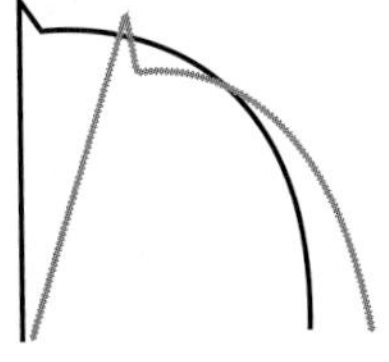
Class IA

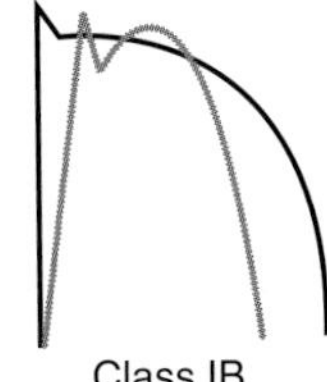
Class IB

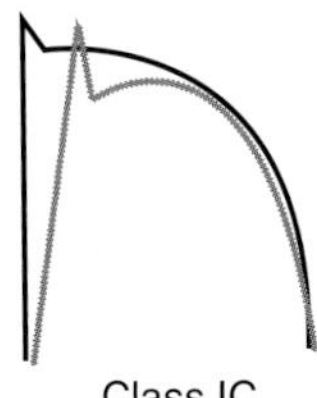
Class IC

- Class IA-IC antiarrhythmics exhibit "use dependency." They bind more regularly to on/off Na^+ channels, rather than resting channels.
- Class C > A > B in terms of strength of effect.

Cardiovascular Pharm

	Mechanism	Indication	Side Effects/Management
Ca^{2+} Channel Blocker Amlodipine Nicardipine Nifedipine Nimodipine	- Ca^{2+} channel blocker (Dihydropyridine)	- Hypertension - Angina - Raynaud	- Peripheral edema - Flushing, headache, hypotension
Hydralazine	- Arteriolar vasodilation	- Hypertension	- Reflex tachycardia - Headache, edema - Angina - Drug-induced SLE
Nitroprusside	- Arterial/venous dilator (NO release → ↑ cGMP)	- Hypertension (emergency)	- Cyanide toxicity - Methemoglobinemia
Nitrovasodilator Nitroglycerine Isosorbide mono/di-nitrate	- Vasodilatation (veins > arterial)	- Angina - HF	- Reflex tachycardia - Flushing, headache, hypotension - Contraindicated if on PDE inhibitor
Glycosides Digoxin	- Inhibitor of Na^+/K^+ ATPase - Results in increased cardiac calcium and contractility - Increased vagal tone	- HF - Atrial fibrillation	- GI (nausea, vomiting, abdominal pain) - Hyperkalemia - Neurologic (confusion and weakness) - Visual disturbances (scotomas, change in color vision) - Arrhythmias: Ventricular arrhythmias, heart block, bradycardia Toxicity: - ↑ Risk for toxicity with renal failure, hypokalemia - Reverse severe toxicity with digoxin Fab
Adenosine	- Transient induction of heart block by activating K^+ channels, increasing K^+ efflux, hyperpolarizing cells	- Supraventricular tachycardia	- Effects blunted by caffeine and theophylline - Flushing, chest pain, sense of impending doom - Bronchospasm
Atropine	- Muscarinic receptor antagonist	- Bradycardia	- Dry mouth, constipation, urinary retention, confusion
Sacubitril	- Neprilysin inhibitor, ↑ levels of ANP/BNP	- HFrEF	- Hypotension - Hyperkalemia, AKI - Angioedema
Ivabradine	- Inhibits funny channel, slowing heart rate	- HF requiring rate control	- Bradycardia - Visual changes (phosphenes)
Ranolazine	- Inhibits late Na current, reducing diastolic wall tension /O_2 consumption	- Angina	- QT prolongation

Physical Exam/PFTs

Pulmonary Physical Exam

	Sounds	Percussion	Fremitus	Trachea
Pleural Effusion	Decreased	Dull	Decreased	Midline (away from large effusions)
Consolidation	Increased (Rales)	Dull	Increased	Midline
Pneumothorax	Decreased	Hyperresonant	Decreased	Away from tension pneumothorax
Atelectasis	Decreased	Dull	Decreased	Toward large atelectasis
COPD (emphysema)	Decreased	Hyperresonant	Decreased	Midline

Clubbing

General: Associated with pulmonary or cardiovascular diseases, including lung cancer, interstitial pulmonary fibrosis, pulmonary tuberculosis, pulmonary lymphoma, HF, infective endocarditis, and cyanotic congenital heart disease. Unknown pathophysiology, thought to involve excess growth factor production in the lungs (PDGF).

Clinical: Increased convexity of the nail bed[A]. Can progress to hypertrophic osteoarthropathy, which presents with focal distal extremity bone and joint pain.

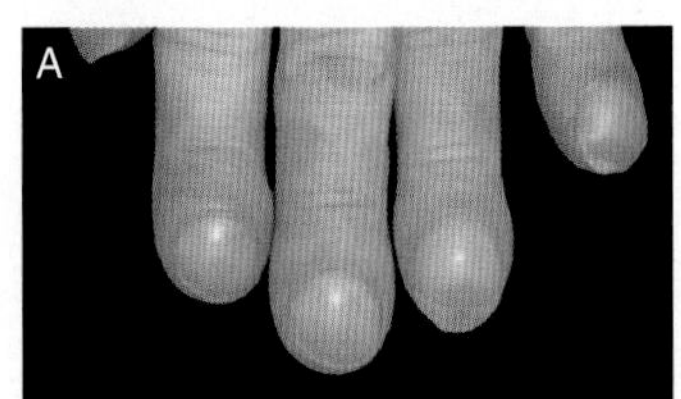

Pulmonary Function Tests

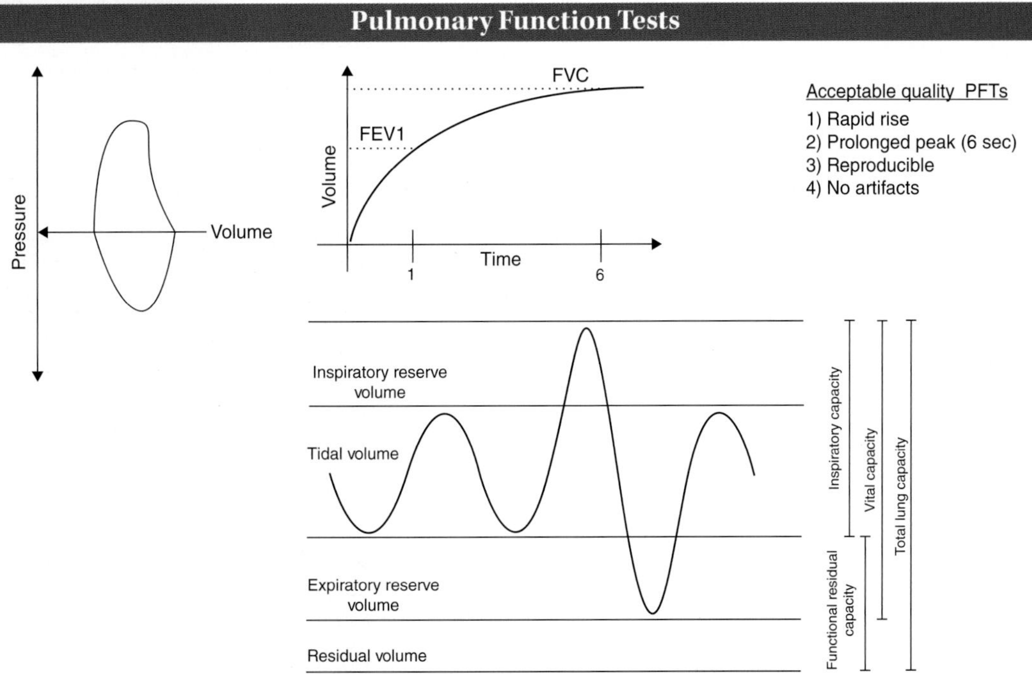

Acceptable quality PFTs
1) Rapid rise
2) Prolonged peak (6 sec)
3) Reproducible
4) No artifacts

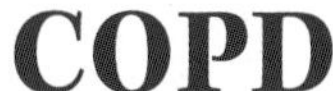

COPD

Overview of COPD

General: Chronic lung disease, with multiple subtypes:

Chronic Bronchitis	- Cough > 3 months for at least 2 years - Caused by excessive mucus production
Emphysema	- Enlarged air spaces with alveolar destruction, secondary to excess protease activity - Centrilobular (smokers) vs Panlobular (α1-antitrypsin)
Asthma-COPD Overlap	- Asthma with persistent airflow obstruction

Risk: Smoking, genetic (α1-antitrypsin), environmental (occupational exposure, air pollution, second-hand smoke), chronic poorly controlled asthma

Clinical: **Dyspnea, cough, sputum, wheezing, or chest tightness**

- Chronic bronchitis (prolonged expiration, rhonchi, wheeze)
- Emphysema (decreased breath sounds, hyperinflation, barrel chest, pursed lip breathing)
- X-ray[B]: **Hyperinflation**, increased lung translucency, flat diaphragm, subpleural blebs

Diagnosis: Pulmonary function testing (PFTs)
(Original GOLD Classification, see right)
- **FEV1/FVC ratio < 0.70**
- ↓ FEV1, FVC
- ↑ TLC, FRC, RV
- ↓ DLCO
- Obstructive flow-volume curve[A]

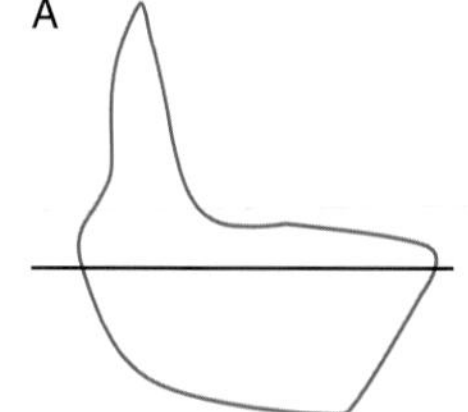

Class	Severity	FEV1
1	Mild	≥ 80%
2	Moderate	50-79%
3	Severe	30-49%
4	Very severe	< 30%

Management: Revised GOLD Classification (used to determine management)

	mMRC 0-1	mMRC ≥ 2	mMRC Dyspnea Scale 0: Dyspnea with strenuous exercise 1: Dyspnea with hills or brisk walk 2: Walks slower than others due to dyspnea 3: Takes break after 100 yard walk 4: Dyspneic with dressing, can't leave house due to symptoms
0 or 1 Exacerbation	Class A	Class B	
≥ 2 Exacerbation or > 1 Hospitalization	Class E		

Inhaled therapy:

- Class A: LAMA + as needed SABA
- Class B: LAMA-LABA + as needed SABA
- Class E: LAMA-LABA + as needed SABA +/– inhaled corticosteroid

SABA (short-acting β agonist): Albuterol
SAMA (short-acting muscarinic antagonist): Ipratropium
LABA (long-acting β agonist): Formoterol, salmeterol
LAMA (long-acting muscarinic antagonist): Aclidinium, tiotropium

Other measures:

- Smoking cessation (decreases mortality)
- Group B and above: Pulmonary rehab
- Roflumilast: PDE4 inhibitor (in severe chronic bronchitis)
- Supplemental oxygen, if O_2 saturation < 55 mmHg or 88%

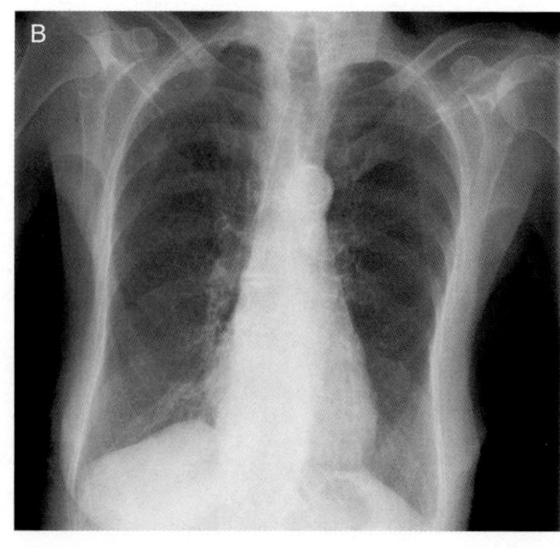

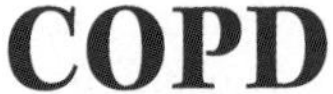

Acute Exacerbation of COPD

General: Worsening of respiratory symptoms, characterized by one or more of the following:

(1) Increased cough/cough severity
(2) Increased sputum production
(3) Increased dyspnea

Risk: High-severity COPD at higher risk. Trigger most commonly bacterial or viral infection.

Diagnosis: Clinical diagnosis (worsening respiratory status, exam, and vitals)

Management:

- **Short-acting β-agonists** (albuterol) +/– anticholinergic (ipratropium)
- **Systemic glucocorticoids**
- IV magnesium sulfate
- Oxygen goal of 88-92% (to avoid CO_2 retention from loss of hypoxemic respiratory drive, Haldane effect)
- If necessary, NIPPV preferred to invasive mechanical ventilation
- No evidence for mucoactive agents or mucus clearance techniques

<u>Antibiotics</u>

- Indicated if ≥ 2/3 cardinal symptoms
- **Uncomplicated COPD** (age < 65, FEV1 > 50%, < 2 exacerbations a year)
    - Azithromycin or 2nd/3rd gen cephalosporin (e.g., ceftriaxone or cefpodoxime)
- **Complicated COPD** (age > 65, FEV1 < 50%, > 2 exacerbations a year)
    - Cover *Pseudomonas* if patient has risk factors (levofloxacin, cefepime)

Alpha-1 Antitrypsin Deficiency

General: Deficiency in **antiprotease protein**, which results in ↑ elastase activity

- M allele (normal protein levels), Z allele (deficient alpha-1 antitrypsin)
- MM (normal), MZ (normal or mild increase in COPD risk), ZZ (high-risk)

Clinical:

(1) Early onset panacinar COPD (Age ~ 40s)
(2) Liver disease (on a spectrum from mild transaminitis to cirrhosis)
(3) Panniculitis (rare complication)

Diagnosis:

- **AAT Levels**
- Genotype (PCR)

Management:

- Avoid cigarette smoke and occupational exposures
- Normal COPD management
- IV human AAT

Asthma

Asthma Overview

General: Condition of bronchial hyperresponsiveness → inflammation causes episodes of reversible airflow obstruction

Risk:

- History of atopy (most commonly IgE against environmental allergens)
- Triggers include allergens, tobacco smoke, air pollution, respiratory infections, cold, and exercise

Clinical:

- Intermittent **dyspnea, wheezing**, chest tightness, and cough
- Wheezing may or may not be present

Diagnosis:

- Most often a clinical diagnosis (confirmed by improvement with albuterol)
- Spirometry: **Reversible airflow obstruction** (> 12%/200 cc improvement in FEV1 after bronchodilator)
    - If inconclusive: Methacholine or exercise challenge testing

Management: Note: For > 12 y/o

	Intermittent	**Mild Persistent**	**Moderate Persistent**	**Severe Persistent**
Symptoms	≤ 2 days/week	> 2 days/week	Daily	Constant
Short Acting Agent Use	≤ 2 days/week	> 2 days/week	Daily	Multiple times per day
Nighttime Awakenings	≤ 2 times/month	3-4 times/month	Multiple nights weekly	Most nights
Lung Function	FEV1 normal (outside of episodes)	FEV1 > 80%	FEV1 60-80%	FEV1 < 60%
Exacerbations	0-1 per year	≥ 2 per year	≥ 2 per year	≥ 2 per year
Management	Step 1	Step 2	Step 3	Step 4 or 5

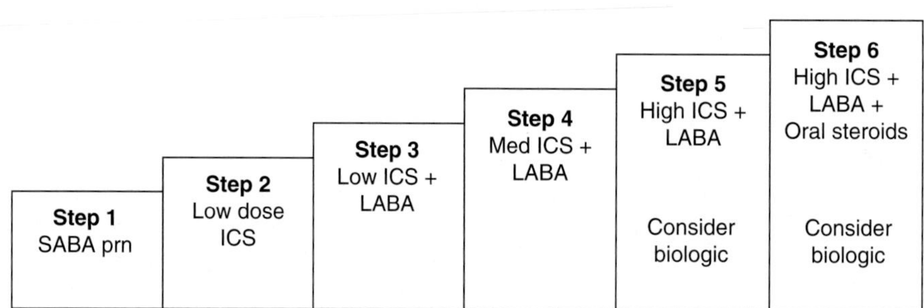

SABA: Albuterol
LABA: Formoterol, salmeterol

Alternative agents:

- LTRA (montelukast)
- Omalizumab (if known allergies/↑ IgE)
- Mepolizumab/dupilumab (if eosinophilia)

- If uncontrolled, step up
- If under good control, consider step down in therapy (if stable > 3 months)

*Steps based on 2020 NAEPP guidelines. 2022 GINA guidelines slightly different, utilize ICS-LABA in Steps 1/2.

Asthma

Acute Asthma Exacerbation

Clinical:

- Dyspnea, wheezing, coughing, chest tightness
- Decreased I:E ratio, accessory muscle use, tachypnea

Diagnosis: Primarily clinical

- Peak flow testing (> 10% worsening from baseline suggests exacerbation)

Management:

- **β Agonists +/– Ipratropium**
- Supplemental oxygen (goal O_2 > 92%). NIPPV/mechanical ventilation if this goal cannot be achieved.
- **Early steroids** (Oral prednisone or IV methylprednisolone for ICU)
- Severe exacerbations: **Intravenous Mg**

Note: Patients with normal/increasing CO_2 may have impending respiratory failure

Aspirin Exacerbated Respiratory Disease

General: Imbalance in which leukotrienes > prostaglandins, due to NSAIDs or ASA use, leading to respiratory symptoms and airway hyperreactivity

Clinical: **(1) Rhinosinusitis (2) Nasal polyposis (3) Asthma**

Management: NSAID/ASA avoidance, normal asthma management, plus addition of leukotriene antagonists (montelukast, zileuton)

Bronchiectasis

General: Permanent, abnormal dilation and destruction of bronchial walls with inflammation and airway collapse. Due to chronic inflammation with impaired mucous clearance.

Risk:

- Recurrent infections (airway obstruction, immunodeficiency, allergic bronchopulmonary aspergillosis)
- **Cystic fibrosis**, primary ciliary dyskinesia, or autoimmune (RA/SLE)

Clinical: Chronic cough (with lots of mucopurulent sputum), dyspnea, hemoptysis, halitosis

Diagnosis:

- High Res CT (Study of choice) → **Bronchial dilatation/wall thickening**
- PFTs (show obstructive disease)
- Workup for underlying etiology (CF test, sputum culture, Ig quantification)

Management:

<u>Acute exacerbations</u>

- Antibiotics (tailored to previous infectious agents; normally amoxicillin-clavulanate or fluoroquinolone, but *Pseudomonas*/MRSA coverage if history)
- If history of asthma → May require oral glucocorticoids/bronchodilators

<u>Chronic</u>

- Chest physiotherapy/mucus clearance techniques
- Azithromycin if ≥ 2 exacerbations per year

Restrictive Lung Disease

Overview (Pulmonary Processes)

General: Heterogenous group of processes that distort the pulmonary interstitium and alveolar walls, resulting in fibrosis, distortion of the lung structure, and impaired gas exchange

Etiologies:

- Environmental (pneumoconiosis)
- Granulomatous (sarcoid, vasculitis, histiocytosis X)
- Alveolar filling disease (goodpasture, alveolar proteinosis)
- Hypersensitivity (pneumonitis, eosinophilic pneumonia)
- Drug induced (amiodarone, nitrofurantoin, bleomycin, methotrexate)
- Autoimmune CT disorders (RA, SLE, scleroderma)
- Others (idiopathic pulmonary fibrosis, cryptogenic organizing pneumonia)

Clinical:

- Dyspnea, nonproductive cough, +/– symptoms of a specific above etiology
- Rales, clubbing

Workup:

- **High resolution CT**
- Pulmonary function testing
    - Decreased lung volumes (TLC)
    - **FEV1/FVC ≥ 85%, ↓ FEV1 and FVC**
- Bronchiolar lavage (if hemoptysis)
- Lung biopsy (if workup is inconclusive of etiology)

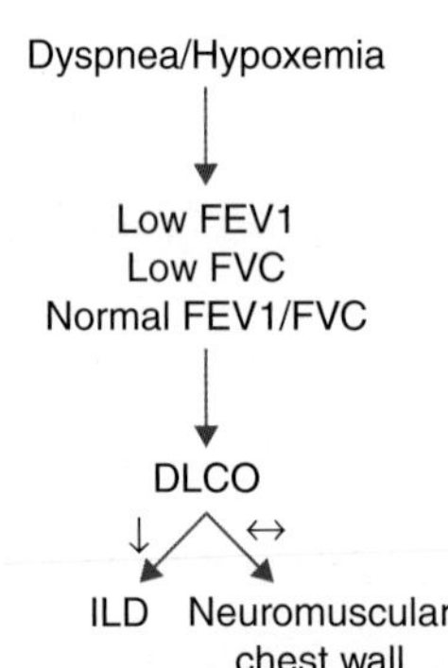

Classifying Interstitial Lung Disease

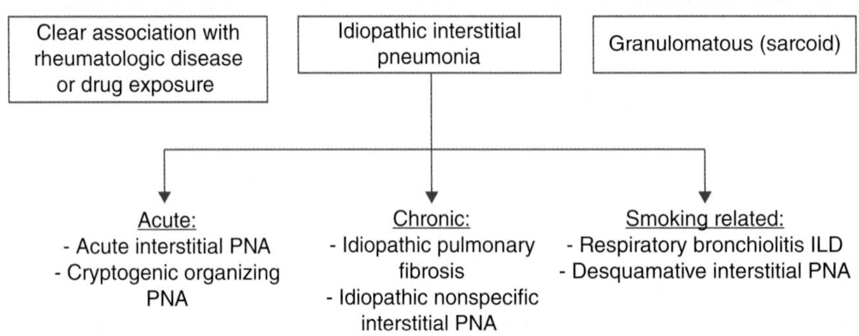

Overview (Extrinsic Processes)

General: Restrictive disease due to abnormalities in chest wall structure or respiratory musculature

Etiologies:

- **Neuromuscular** (myasthenia gravis, ALS, multiple sclerosis)
- **Chest-wall** (obesity hypoventilation, kyphoscoliosis)

Restrictive Lung Disease

	Definition/Risk	Clinical/Diagnosis/Management
Extrinsic Disease		
Obesity Hypoventilation Syndrome	- Alveolar hypoventilation due to obesity (BMI generally > 30)	- Dyspnea - Restrictive PFTs, normal Aa gradient/DLCO - ABG: **Hypercapnia + compensatory ↑ HCO_3** - Tx: Weight loss
Idiopathic Interstitial PNA		
Acute Interstitial Pneumonia	- Rare, fulminant form of diffuse lung injury without clear cause	- Presents with acute respiratory failure (very **similar to ARDS**), but without trigger - Dx: Clinical above, plus biopsy showing diffuse alveolar damage - Tx: High-dose corticosteroids
Cryptogenic Organizing Pneumonia	- Idiopathic, noninfectious inflammatory pneumonia of the distal bronchioles and alveolar walls	- Two month onset of cough, dyspnea, fever, malaise (often starts with flu-like illness) but does not respond to antibiotics - Dx: CT (patchy interstitial opacities, ground glass, nodular opacities). Biopsy for definitive diagnosis. - Tx: Corticosteroids

Idiopathic Pulmonary Fibrosis ("Usual Interstitial Pneumonia")	- Chronic fibrosing interstitial pneumonia
	- Can be idiopathic (6th/7th decade) or genetically based (earlier onset)
		- Gradual onset dyspnea, cough, rales, clubbing
		- Dx: CT (classic **honeycombing/reticular opacities**). Biopsy for definitive diagnosis.
		- Tx: Supportive (supplemental O_2, vaccines, pulmonary rehab)
		  - Pirfenidone or nintedanib
		  - Lung transplant

Granulomatous		
Sarcoid	- Idiopathic disorder characterized by noncaseating granuloma formation in multiple systems, especially lung	- [See: Rheum] for full discussion
Histiocytosis X	[See: Heme-Onc]	
Vasculitis	[See: Rheum]	
Alveolar Filling Disorders		
Goodpastures	- Circulating antibodies against alpha-3 chain of type IV collagen (expressed in GBM and alveoli)	- Rapidly progressive glomerulonephritis and alveolar hemorrhage - Dx: Kidney biopsy (linear IgG deposits), serology (for **anti-GBM**) - Tx: Plasmapheresis, prednisone + cyclophosphamide
Alveolar Proteinosis	- Intraalveolar accumulation of phospholipids and apoproteins. There is no disturbance of lung architecture.	- Progressive dyspnea, cough, sputum production, fatigue, weight loss. Exam with crackles, clubbing, cyanosis. - Dx: CT, bronchiolar lavage - Tx: Supportive care, whole lung lavage (if severe)
Pneumoconiosis		
Coal Miner's Lung	- Inhalation of coal dust, resulting in formation of nodular opacities, fibrosis, and areas of necrosis	- Simple disease: Most commonly asymptomatic - Can develop fibrosis, restrictive lung disease
Silicosis	- Inhalation of silica particles that results in pulmonary fibrosis - Sandblasting, mining, masonry - Increased risk for TB, lung malignancy	- Can present acutely (months to years after exposure) or chronically (> 10 years after exposure) with dyspnea/cough - Dx: CT (upper lobe opacities, "eggshell" calcifications of nodes)
Asbestosis	- Inhalation of asbestos fibers, resulting in progressive pulmonary fibrosis - Exposures include older, asbestos-containing buildings/shipbuilding	- Presents 20-30 years after exposure with dyspnea, dry cough - Elevated risk of bronchogenic carcinoma and mesothelioma - Dx: CT (subpleural linear opacities, fibrosis, pleural plaques)
Berylliosis	- Beryllium exposure → Noncaseating lung granulomas (looks like sarcoid) - Seen in aerospace, computers, automotive industries	- Presents with progressive dyspnea, cough

Restrictive Lung Disease

Hypersensitivity Pneumonitis

General: Alveolar inflammation due to type III/IV hypersensitivity against inhaled organic dusts

Etiologies:

- **Farmer's lung** (moldy hay, or thermophilic actinomycetes)
- Silo filler's
- Bird breeder's lung (avian droppings)
- Bagassosis (moldy sugar cane)
- Byssinosis (textiles)

Clinical: Can present acutely (within hours) or chronically with cough, dyspnea, fatigue, weight loss

Diagnosis:

- Inhalation challenge (reexposure)
- CT (ground glass/nodular opacities)
- BAL (marked lymphocytosis with decreased CD4/CD8 ratio)
- Biopsy (poorly formed granulomas)

Management:

- Avoid exposure
- If severely symptomatic → Steroids
- If severe, irreversible fibrosis develops → Transplant

Eosinophilic Pneumonia

General: Eosinophilic infiltration of the pulmonary parenchyma, thought to be hypersensitivity against inhaled antigen

Clinical:

- Acute (< 4 week) illness with cough, dyspnea, fever, and systemic symptoms
- Hypoxemic respiratory failure

Diagnosis: CT (diffuse pulmonary opacities), BAL with > 25% eosinophils

Management:

- Supportive care
- Glucocorticoids

Pulmonary Hypertension

Pulmonary Hypertension (Overview)

General: Mean pulmonary arterial pressure ≥ 25 mmHg

	Etiology	Description
Class 1	Pulmonary arterial hypertension	[See below]
Class 2	Left heart disease	- Elevated left ventricular EDP (PCWP)
Class 3	Chronic lung disease	- COPD, ILD, OSA, etc
Class 4	Chronic thromboembolism (CTEPH)	- Occurs after PE/multiple PEs - V/Q scan can aid in diagnosis
Class 5	Multifactorial/Unclear mechanism	- Variety of causes (sickle cell, systemic disorders, metabolic disorders)

Clinical:

- Progressive exertional dyspnea, presyncope/syncope, exertional angina
- Signs of **right heart failure** (peripheral edema, elevated JVP, loud P2)
    - Right-sided S3, RV heave, holosystolic tricuspid regurgitation murmur

Diagnosis: **Right heart catheterization**

- Note: TTE can be used for noninvasive evaluation of pressures

Management:

- Treat underlying (i.e., treat heart failure for Class 2, manage lung disease for Class 3)
- Class 4: Warfarin and surgical thromboendarterectomy

Pulmonary Arterial Hypertension (PAH)

General: Pulmonary hypertension from proliferation of smooth muscle in pulmonary arterioles

Etiology:

- Idiopathic
- Familial: BMPR-2 mutation (commonly young adult females)
- Drugs, toxins, connective tissue disease, HIV, schistosomiasis

Clinical/Diagnosis: Overview above

Management:

- CCB (diltiazem)
- Oral endothelin antagonists (bosentan)
- Oral phosphodiesterase inhibitors (sildenafil, tadalafil)
- Oral prostacyclin agonists (selexipag)
- For severe: IV prostacyclin agonists (epoprostenol or treprostinil)

Note: Transplantation is last line for severe refractory cases

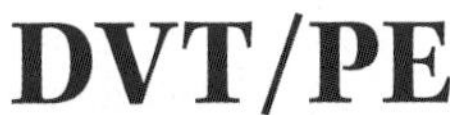

DVT/PE

DVT

General: Formation of blood clot within a deep vein of the legs. 90% are proximal (most commonly femoral, iliac), 10% distal (posterior tibial).

Risk: Virchow triad (endothelial injury, stasis, and hypercoagulability)

- Hypercoagulability risks: Cancer, surgery, obesity, smoking, oral contraceptives, pregnancy, genetic thrombophilia

Clinical:

- ~50% have **calf pain, tenderness, erythema**, and superficial vein dilatation
- Homan sign: Calf pain on ankle dorsiflexion

Diagnosis: Lower extremity US. Risk stratify utilizing modified Wells score below.

Simplified Wells Score (Pretest Probability of DVT)	
- Previous DVT - Active cancer diagnosis - Recent immobilization or bedridden - Localized tenderness along venous distribution - Leg swelling - Asymmetric calf swelling - Pitting edema - Collateral superficial nonvaricose veins *Alternative diagnosis more likely (-2 points)	< 1: Low probability (DVT unlikely) 1-2: Moderate probability 3-8: High probability (DVT likely) - **Low/Moderate Probability** → D-dimer: If elevated, then US. - **High Probability** → US

Old methods: CTV, MRV, contrast venography, impedance plethysmography rarely used

Management:

Proximal DVT	- Anticoagulate (**heparin, warfarin, LMWH, or DOAC**) - Contraindication to anticoagulation → IVC filter
Massive proximal DVT	- Defined by severe swelling, soft tissue ischemia - Thrombolytic or surgical thrombectomy
Distal DVT	- Anticoagulate (if contraindication, then observe closely with LE US)

- Follow-up:
  - Workup for underlying cause (age-appropriate cancer screening, if young then hereditary thrombophilia panel)
  - 3 months of anticoagulation required, continue indefinitely if cause is unknown or irreversible

Complications:

Phlegmasia cerulea dolens: Severe pain/edema/blue discoloration due to ischemia from extensive proximal DVT. Indication for thrombolytic/surgical thrombectomy.

Post-thrombotic syndrome: Chronic venous insufficiency that can occur after DVT. Presents as chronic extremity pain, edema, and venous changes. Manage with symptomatic therapy, such as limb elevation, compression therapy, exercise.

Inpatient DVT/PE Prophylaxis:

- Indications: Hospitalized patients with ≥ 1 following risk factor deserve prophylaxis
  - Risks: ICU, cancer, stroke, CHF, MI, age > 75, hx of VTE, renal failure, obesity, immobility
- Pharm: **LMWH, subQ unfractionated heparin** (contraindicated if bleeding risk/current active bleeding)
- Nonpharm: Mechanical (intermittent pneumatic compression or graduated compression stockings)

DVT/PE

Pulmonary Embolism

General: Embolization of a thrombus into the pulmonary vasculature. Subtypes:
- **Massive** (high-risk): Hemodynamically unstable
- **Submassive** (intermediate-risk): Hemodynamically stable with RV strain
- **Low Risk**: Hemodynamically stable, no RV dysfunction

Can also be characterized by anatomic location: Saddle, lobar, segmental, subsegmental

Clinical:
- Dyspnea, pleuritic chest pain, hemoptysis. Syncope possible.
- Tachypnea, tachycardia. Small pleural effusions possible.
- ECG: Sinus tachycardia, t-wave inversions, S1Q3T3

Wells Criteria [Pretest Probability of PE]	
Clinical symptoms of DVT	3 points
Other diagnoses less likely	3 points
HR > 100 bpm	1.5 points
Immobilization or recent surgery	1.5 points
Hx of DVT/PE	1.5 points
Hemoptysis	1 point
Malignancy	1 point
High probability: ≥ 6 points Medium probability: 2-6 points Low probability: < 2 points	

Low probability → PERC ruleout? —yes→ No workup indicated
PERC ruleout? —no→ D-dimer
Intermediate probability → D-dimer
D-dimer —Neg→ No workup indicated
D-dimer —Pos→ Imaging indicated
High probability → Imaging indicated

PERC (Ruleout criteria)	
Age < 50	No prior PE/DVT
BPM < 100	No leg swelling
O_2 Sat > 95%	No recent surgery/trauma
No hemoptysis	No estrogen use

Diagnosis:
- **Spiral CT angiography**[A] (first line)
- V/Q scan (for those who cannot tolerate contrast)
- If patient is unstable despite resuscitation → TTE [McConnells sign: Mid RV free wall hypokinesis]

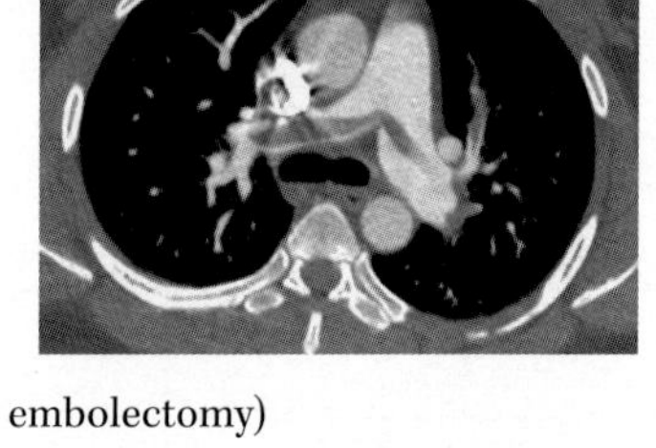

Management:
- Initial:
    - Suspected PE: Supplemental O_2, ventilation, hemodynamic support
    - If high probability for PE and low bleeding risk → empiric anticoagulation
- Unstable:
    - Thrombolytic therapy, followed by anticoagulation (Alternative: Catheter or surgical embolectomy)
- Stable: Anticoagulation
    - Initial: Heparin, LMWH, fondaparinux, apixaban/rivaroxaban
    - Long term: DOAC (Factor Xa or thrombin inhibitor), warfarin, LMWH
    - If anticoagulation contraindicated → IVC filter

Other Embolic Syndromes

Fat Emboli	- Often occurs after a long bone fracture - Presents with lung symptoms (dyspnea, ARDS), neurologic symptoms (confusion), and petechiae
Amniotic Fluid Emboli	- Amniotic fluid, fetal cells, fetal debris enter maternal circulation - Respiratory failure followed by DIC

Pleural Effusion

Pleural Effusion (Overview)

General: Excess fluid in pleural cavity, from either increased fluid production or impaired drainage

Etiology:

- **Transudative** (HF, hypoalbuminemia, cirrhosis)
- **Exudative** (parapneumonic, malignancy, TB, autoimmune [RA, SLE], trauma)
- Chylothorax (rupture of thoracic ducts)

Clinical:

- Often asymptomatic, but can cause dyspnea
- Decreased breath sounds, dullness to percussion, decreased fremitus

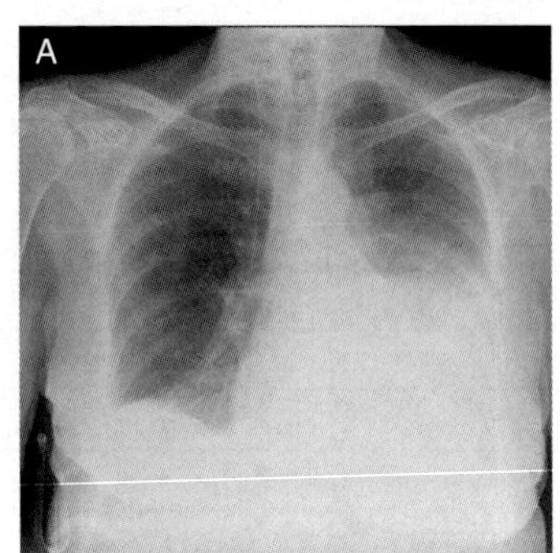

Diagnosis:

- CXR[A] (blunting of costophrenic angle)
- CT (can confirm/reveal small effusions)
- **Thoracentesis** (diagnostic/therapeutic, obtain on all large effusions unless clear HF)
- Lights criteria:
    - (1) Pleural protein/serum protein ratio > 0.5
    - (2) Pleural LDH/serum LDH > 0.6
    - (3) Pleural LDH > ⅔ upper limit of normal serum LDH
- Other pleural fluid findings:
    - Glucose low in infection, malignancy
    - pH (7.6 normal, 7.4-7.55 transudative, 7.3-7.45 exudative)
    - Cytology
    - Amylase (esophageal rupture)

Management:

Transudative	- Treat underlying condition - Therapeutic thoracentesis may be useful in large effusions
Exudative	- Depends on etiology, but in general thoracentesis, +/– chest tube - Surgical intervention for those that are loculated/difficult to drain

Parapneumonic Effusions

	Uncomplicated	Complicated	Empyema
General	Sterile exudate	Bacterial invasion	Frank pus
Pleural Fluid	WBC < 50k pH > 7.2	WBC > 50k pH < 7.2	Pus
Gram Stain/Culture	Negative	Positive ~50%	Positive
Management	Antibiotics	Antibiotics +/– Drainage	Antibiotic + Drainage

Pneumothorax/Hemoptysis

Pneumothorax (Overview)

General: Accumulation of air in the pleural space

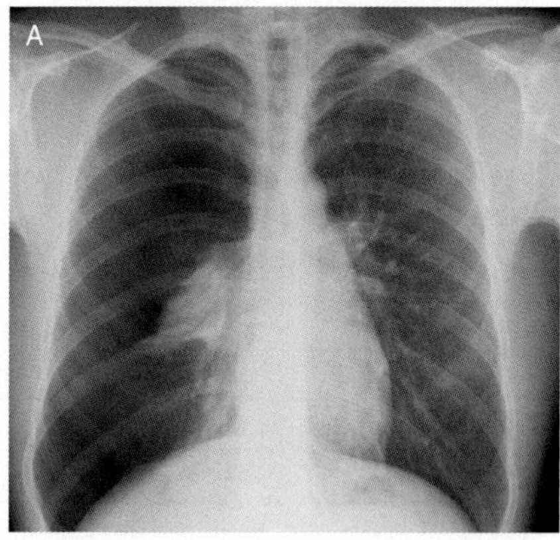

Etiology:

- **Spontaneous**
  - Primary (due to subpleural bleb rupture, young tall male)
  - Secondary (due to underlying lung disease, like COPD)
- **Traumatic**
- **Iatrogenic** (mechanical ventilation, thoracentesis, central lines, CPR)

Clinical:

- Acute onset ipsilateral chest pain, dyspnea, cough
- Decreased breath sounds, hyperresonance

Diagnosis: CXR[A] (**absent lung markings**, with pleural line)

Management:

- Small (< 2 cm): Observation and supplemental oxygen +/– drainage of air
- Large (> 2 cm or >15% lung volume) or Clinically Unstable: Chest tube placement

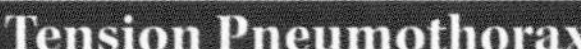

Tension Pneumothorax

General: Subtype of pneumothorax characterized by accumulation of subpleural air resulting in increased pressure and collapse of lung tissues. Elevated thoracic pressures result in hemodynamic compromise.

Etiology: Trauma or mechanical ventilation

Clinical:

- Hemodynamic collapse, hypotension (impaired venous return)
- Decreased breath sounds, hyperresonance, plus possible tracheal deviation, distended neck veins

Diagnosis: CXR will confirm, but treat if high clinical suspicion

Management: Emergent needle thoracostomy or chest tube placement

Hemoptysis

General: Expectoration of blood, most commonly from bronchial arteries. Classified based on amount of blood.

< 500 mL: Mild to moderate

> 500 mL or 100 mL/hr: Massive

Etiology:

- Airway disease (bronchitis, bronchiectasis, neoplasm, trauma, iatrogenic)
- Parenchymal disease (infection, autoimmune/genetic connective tissue disorders)
- Vascular (PE, AV malformation)

Management:

Mild/Moderate	- Workup/treat underlying cause - CT scan or flexible bronchoscopy reserved for cases of active bleeding
Massive	- Establish airway, maintain hemodynamics (ABCs) - Flexible bronchoscopy (electrical cautery or balloon tamponade) - Arteriographic embolization (if bronchoscopy fails to identify and reverse bleed)

Respiratory Failure

Acute Respiratory Failure

General: Inadequate ventilation leading to hypoxemia. Subtypes:
- Hypoxemic (V/Q mismatch, shunting, or decreased diffusion)
    - Associated with high A-a gradient
- Hypercapnic (decreased alveolar ventilation from decreased respiratory rate, minute ventilation, or ↑ dead space)

Clinical: Dyspnea, accessory muscle use, inability to complete sentences, hypoxemia

Diagnosis: ↓ O_2 saturation on pulse oximeter, ABG

Management:

	Method	Oxygen Delivery
Floors	Nasal cannula	- 2-6 L/min (FiO_2: 24-40%)
	Face mask	- 5-8 L/min (FiO_2: 30-50%)
	Venti mask	- 5-10 L/min (FiO_2: 30-60%)
	Nonrebreather	- 10-15 L/min (FiO_2: 60-80%)
ICU	High-flow nasal cannula	- 10-60 L/min (FiO_2: up to 100%)
	CPAP	- Provides positive end-expiratory pressure
	BIPAP	- Provides positive end-expiratory pressure AND additional pressure support with breaths
	Mechanical ventilation	- FiO_2: up to 100%

Mechanical Ventilation

Indications: Apnea, acute respiratory failure, impending respiratory failure, or need for airway protection

Note: Typically start in volume-control, with V(t) of 6-8 mL/kg, RR 12-16, FiO_2 100%, PEEP 5 cm H_2O

Mode	Description	Rate	Set
Assist control (volume control)	Set tidal volume delivered at set rate, fully machine supported. Pressure varies with compliance.	Set	Volume
Pressure control (PCV)	Set inspiratory positive pressure administered over a set time. Tidal volume varies with compliance.	Set	Pressure
Pressure support	No set tidal volume or rate, but set inspiratory pressure to reduce work of breathing.	Patient	Pressure

Sedation: Utilize medication pairings with analgesic and amnesic effects:
- Analgesia: Opiates (fentanyl or hydromorphone)
- Sedation: Propofol, midazolam, dexmedetomidine

Respiratory Failure

Mechanical Ventilation (Management Basics)

After intubation, check for proper placement (2-5 cm above carina) and ABG

Situation	Adjustment
$paCO_2$ is high + respiratory acidosis	Increase RR/ V(T) to increase ventilation
$paCO_2$ is low + respiratory alkalosis	Decrease RR/ V(T) to decrease ventilation
paO_2 is low	FiO_2 and PEEP in steps to achieve $PaO_2 > 60$ mmHg
paO_2 is high	Decrease FiO_2 in steps to 50% and then slowly reduce PEEP in 3-5 mmHg increments, maintaining $PaO_2 > 60$
Refractory hypoxemia	Pressure control mode, prone ventilation, or ECMO
↑ Peak pressure	Can be elevated with low lung compliance, but also ↑ airway resistance (mucus plugging, obstructed ET tube)
↑ Plateau pressure	Sign of low lung compliance

Weaning:

- Patient should have low settings ($FiO_2 < 50\%$ and PEEP < 5 cm H_2O) prior to considering extubation
- **Spontaneous Breathing Trial:** Most commonly trial of pressure support
    - RSBI (rapid shallow breathing index) < 105 (RR/Vt)

Complications:

- Barotrauma (can lead to pneumothorax)
- Oxygen toxicity:
    - Absorptive atelectasis
    - Parenchymal injury (worsening lung disease due to high O_2 sats)

Acute Respiratory Distress Syndrome (ARDS)

General: Hypoxemic respiratory failure secondary to alveolar injury, which results in accumulation of proteinaceous fluid in the alveoli, impairing gas exchange and decreasing compliance. Results in massive pulmonary shunt physiology.

Etiology: Sepsis, aspiration, pneumonia, trauma, transfusions (TRALI), pancreatitis

Clinical: Respiratory distress, dyspnea, hypoxemia, cyanosis, tachypnea, rales

Diagnosis:

Berlin definition

(1) **Acute** onset < 1 week
(2) **Bilateral infiltrates** on chest imaging[A]
(3) Pulmonary edema **not explained by fluid overload or CHF** (no CHF and PCWP is < 18 mmHg)
(4) Abnormal **PaO_2/FiO_2 ratio < 300** (Mild: 200-300, Moderate: 100-200, Severe: 100)

Management:

- Mechanical ventilation (high PEEP, low tidal volume ventilation)
    - Neuromuscular blockade (helps ventilator synchrony)
    - Conservative fluid strategy (to avoid worsened pulmonary edema)
- Treat underlying condition

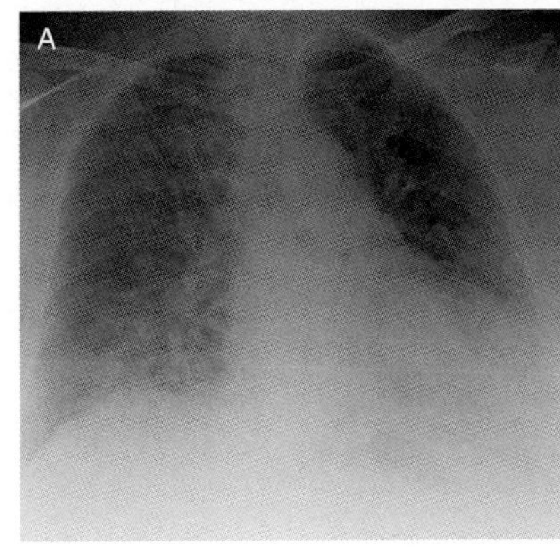

Shock

Shock Overview

General: Low tissue perfusion, resulting in cellular injury and tissue hypoxia

Subtypes	Cause	Clinical	PCWP	CO	SVR
Hypovolemic	Hemorrhage, dehydration, burns	Cold, clammy	↓	↓	↑
Cardiogenic	MI, HF, valvular, arrhythmia	Cold, clammy	↑	↓	↑
Distributive	Sepsis, anaphylaxis	Warm, dry	↓	↑	↓
Obstructive	Cardiac tamponade, PTX, PE	Cold, clammy	–/↓	↓	↑

Clinical: **Hypotension (MAP < 70 mmHg)**, clinical signs of hypoperfusion (cool skin, altered mental status, low urine output), ↑ lactate

Management:

- Hypovolemic: Fluids or blood
- Cardiogenic: Inotropes
- Distributive: Fluids, vasopressors
- Obstructive: Fix obstruction

Drug	Activity	Effect	Indications
Norepinephrine	α1 > α2 > β1	↑ SVR, CO	- Initial vasopressor of choice in septic, cardiogenic and hypovolemic shock
Phenylephrine	α1 > α2	↑ SVR	- Alternative or add on to norepinephrine - Indicated if norepi induces tachyarrhythmia
Vasopressin	V_1, V_2	↑ SVR	- Used primarily as adjunctive agent to others
Epinephrine	β > α	↑ SVR, HR, CO	- Agent of choice in anaphylaxis, cardiac arrest - High doses → α effects predominate - Low doses → Decreases peripheral tone
Dopamine	D1 > β1 > α1	↑ SVR, CO	- Second line agent. Used for bradycardia. - Low dose: Dilates renal veins (D1) - Medium dose: Increase heart contractility (β) - High dose: Vasoconstriction (α)
Midodrine (PO)	α1	↑ SVR	- Mild vasoconstrictor, only oral agent
Inotropic Agents			
Dobutamine	β1 > β2 > α	↑ CO	- Initial agent of choice in cardiogenic shock with low cardiac output and normal blood pressure - Inotropic > chronotropic. Also causes mild peripheral vasodilation (so can ↓ BP).
Milrinone	PDE3 inhibitor	↑ CO	- Cardiogenic shock

Sepsis

Sepsis

Definitions: (Note: SIRS and severe sepsis no longer used)

- **Infection:** Invasion of sterile tissue by organisms
- **Bacteremia:** Bacteria in bloodstream
- **Sepsis:** Organ dysfunction from infection (≥ 2 SOFA score from baseline)
- **Septic shock:** Sepsis plus hemodynamic compromise. Despite resuscitation, requires pressors to maintain MAP and have elevated lactate (> 2 mmol/L).

Diagnosis:

SIRS Criteria	qSOFA
≥ 2/4 of the following:	≥ 2 of the following:
(1) Temperature > 38°C or < 36°C (2) HR > 90 bpm (3) RR > 20 or $paCO_2$ < 32 mmHg (4) WBC > 12k, < 4k, or > 10% bands	(1) RR > 22 (2) Altered mentation (3) SBP < 100 mmHg Note: Applies to patients outside the ICU

SOFA Score (ICU mortality increases with increased score)

Variable	0	1	2	3	4
Respiratory - PaO_2/FiO_2	> 400	≤ 400	≤ 300	≤ 200	≤ 100
Coagulation - Platelets × 10^3	> 150	≤ 150	≤ 100	≤ 50	≤ 20
Liver - Bilirubin	< 1.2	1.2-1.9	2.0-5.9	6.0-11.9	> 12.0
CV - Hypotension	None	MAP < 70	Dop < 5 Dob (any)	Dop > 5 Epi ≤ 0.1 Norepi ≤ 0.1	Dop > 15 Epi > 0.1 Norepi > 0.1
CNS - Glasgow Coma	15	13-14	10-12	6-9	< 6
Renal - Creatinine/UO	< 1.2	1.2-1.9	2.0-3.4	Cr 3.5-4.9 UO < 500 mL/d	Cr > 5.0 UO < 200 mL/d

*Dop=Dopamine, Dob=Dobutamine, Epi=Epinephrine, Norepi=Norepinephrine. All rates in ug/kg/min

Management:

- **Early antibiotic therapy**
  - Broad spectrum with gram positive and negative coverage
- **Vascular access and IV fluids** (bolus 30 mL/kg of NS or LR)
  - Give fluids to maintain > 65 mmHg MAP and urine > 0.5 mL/kg/hr
  - RBC transfusion if Hgb < 7 g/dL
- **Vasopressors if MAP goal (> 65 mmHg) not achieved**

Lung Malignancy

Lung Cancer (Overview)		
Subtype	**Location**	**Characteristics**
Small cell carcinoma	Central	- Undifferentiated → very aggressive - Associated with paraneoplastic syndromes
Non-Small Cell Lung Cancer (NSCLC)		
Squamous cell carcinoma	Central	- Arises from bronchus - Associated with cavitation, hypercalcemia
Adenocarcinoma	Peripheral	- Most common lung cancer (and most common in non smokers) - Bronchioloalveolar (low-grade subtype with improved prognosis)
Large cell carcinoma	Peripheral	- Highly anaplastic, undifferentiated tumor
Bronchial carcinoid	Either	- Excellent prognosis with rare metastasis - Symptoms due to mass effect or carcinoid syndrome - Flushing, diarrhea, wheezing

Risk: Smoking (~90% of cases), second-hand smoke, radon (basements), asbestos

Clinical: Variable presentation. Can present as cough, hemoptysis, wheezing, dyspnea, recurrent pneumonia, weight loss, fever, or with complication/paraneoplastic syndrome.

Diagnosis:

- CT chest[A]
- **Confirm diagnosis with biopsy or cytology**
    - Bronchoscopy, CT-guided biopsy or VATS for tissue sample

Management:

- **SCLC**: Chemotherapy, +/− prophylactic cranial irradiation
- **NSCLC**: Surgery +/− Chemo and/or Radiation

Complications:

- Paraneoplastic:
    - SCLC: SIADH, lambert-eaton, ectopic ACTH production
    - Squamous: PTHrP → hypercalcemia
- Pleural effusions
- Horner syndrome (ptosis, miosis, anhidrosis from cervical chain invasion)
- Recurrent laryngeal nerve compression (hoarseness)
- Superior vena cava syndrome [See: Heme-Onc]

- Pancoast (superior sulcus) tumors:
    - Upper lobe tumors
    - Arm edema
    - Horner
    - Brachial plexus invasion (shoulder pain, weakness, paresthesias)

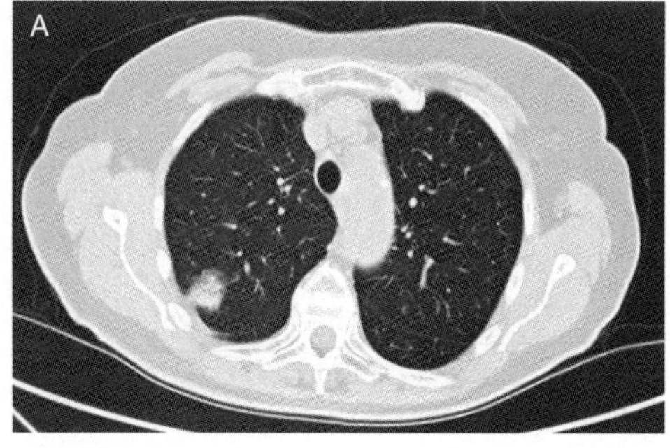

Lung Malignancy

Lung Nodules

Note: Any nodule found on CXR should be evaluated with CT

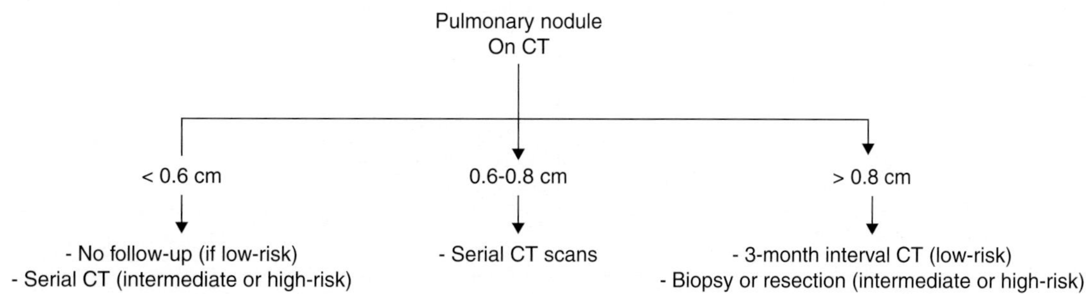

Risk	Age	Smoking	Size (cm)	Characteristics
Low	< 40	Never	< 0.8	Smooth, fat inside (hamartoma), or calcifications (granuloma)
Intermediate	40-60	Current or quit 5-15 yr	0.8-2.0	Scalloped
High	> 60	Current or quit < 5 yr	≥ 2.0	Spiculated

- Benign nodules most commonly hamartomas, granulomas, or focal pneumonia
- Any growing nodule should undergo biopsy or resection

Mediastinal Mass

Compartment	Major Structures	Masses
Anterior mediastinum	Thymus, internal mammary arteries, lymph nodes	Teratoma, thyroid mass, thymoma, lymphoma
Middle mediastinum	Pericardium, heart, aorta, trachea, esophagus	Bronchogenic cyst, lymph nodes, pericardial or enteric cyst
Posterior mediastinum	Spine, nerves, and spinal ganglia	Neurogenic tumors

Mesothelioma

General: Rare neoplasm arising from mesothelial surface of pleural cavity. Associated with **asbestos** exposure.

Clinical: Generally insidious, with symptoms including dyspnea, chest pain, cough

Diagnosis:

- CT (unilateral pleural thickening, calcification, pleural effusion)
- Cytology (thoracentesis, closed biopsy, or VATS)

Management: Surgery (pleurectomy or radical pneumonectomy) + Chemotherapy

Lower Respiratory Infections

Pneumonia

	Definition	Organisms
Community-Acquired	Within 72 hours of hospitalization	- *S. pneumoniae* - *H. influenzae* - *Moraxella* - *S. aureus* - Atypicals (see below)
Hospital-Acquired	> 72 hours after hospitalization	- MSSA/MRSA/*Strep* - *Pseudomonas* - *E. Coli, Klebsiella, Enterobacter*
Ventilator-Acquired	> 48 hours after ventilation	

Etiology:

Group	Organism	Group	Organism
< 4 weeks old	*E. Coli*, Group B *Strep*	***IV Drug Use***	MSSA/MRSA, *Pseudomonas*
4 weeks-18 y/o	*Mycoplasma, Chlamydia* Virus (RSV), Pneumococcus	***Alcohol Use***	*Klebsiella*, anaerobes
Postviral	MSSA/MRSA, Pneumococcus	***Cystic Fibrosis***	MSSA/MRSA, *Pseudomonas*

Clinical:
- Acute onset fever/chills, productive cough, dyspnea, pleuritic chest pain
- Hypoxemia, rales, dullness to percussion, increased tactile fremitus

Diagnosis:
- **Chest x-ray**[A] (GOLD standard, infiltrates are classic)
- Sputum culture, blood culture, pneumococcal/*Legionella* urine antigen test
    - Check if critically ill or in some selected floor-level patients

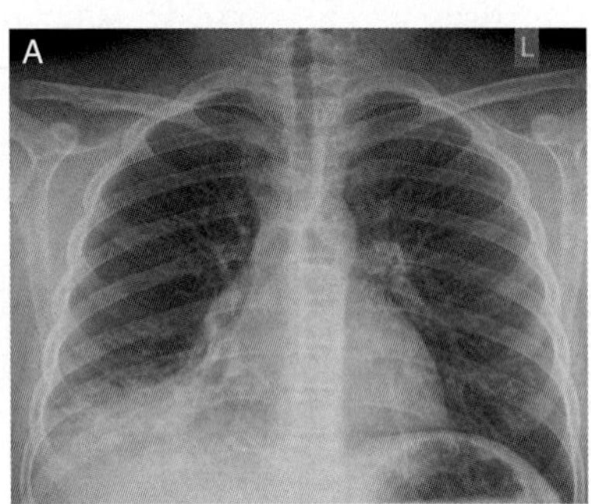

Curb-65 (aid for disposition)	
- Confusion - Urea (BUN) > 19 mg/dL - RR > 30 - BP < 90/60 mmHg - Age > 65	0-1 → Outpatient ≥ 2 → Inpatient

Atypical Pneumonia

Etiology:
- *Mycoplasma pneumoniae, Chlamydia pneumoniae, Chlamydia psittaci, Coxiella* (Q fever), *Legionella*
- Viruses: Influenza, adenoviruses, RSV

Clinical:
- Insidious onset (headache, sore throat, fatigue), dry cough, fever
- Diffuse wheezing, rhonchi, or rales
- CXR (**Diffuse reticulonodular infiltrates**)

Lower Respiratory Infections

Pneumonia Management

Subgroup	Intervention
Outpatient	- Empiric antibiotic: Macrolide or doxycycline. - If high rate of resistance to above, or antibiotic use within the last 3 months→β-lactam (e.g., amoxicillin) PLUS azithromycin or levofloxacin - 5-day course. Must be afebrile for > 48 hours upon termination of antibiotics.
Inpatient CAP	Empiric antibiotics: - **β-lactam (ceftriaxone, ampicillin-sulbactam) PLUS macrolide (azithromycin)** - OR respiratory fluoroquinolone (levo/moxifloxacin)
ICU CAP	- Empiric antibiotics: β-lactam (ceftriaxone, ampicillin-sulbactam) PLUS macrolide (azithromycin) or respiratory fluoroquinolone (levo/moxifloxacin) - **MRSA coverage (vancomycin or linezolid)** IF: Septic shock/mechanically ventilated, known MRSA colonization or risk for colonization - **Pseudomonas coverage (piperacillin-tazobactam, cefepime, meropenem)** IF: Structural lung disease (bronchiectasis), GNRs on gram stain, frequent COPD exacerbations
HAP or VAP	- MRSA coverage (vancomycin or linezolid) PLUS *Pseudomonas* coverage: Pip-tazo, cefepime

Follow-up:

- Narrow therapy based on culture results, change to oral meds when stable
- X-ray will not improve for 4-6 weeks after treatment
    - High risk individuals should receive follow up x-ray in ~ 7 weeks (i.e., male smokers, age > 50)

Recurrent PNA:

Same location	- Most likely anatomical abnormality (neoplasm, or bronchial abnormality like bronchiectasis) - If right lower or middle lobe: Consider recurrent aspiration
Different location	- Primary or secondary immunodeficiency

Lung Abscess

General: Local area of necrotic pulmonary parenchyma

Risk: Most commonly due to aspiration with anaerobes (*Bacteroides, Peptostreptococcus, Prevotella*), MRSA, *Klebsiella*

Clinical: Presents with subacute onset of fever and productive cough, with systemic symptoms such as night sweats/weight loss. Can also present as a secondary complication of pneumonia in hospitalized patients.

Diagnosis: CXR or CT: **Pulmonary infiltrate with cavitary area**

Management: Antibiotics (with anaerobic coverage: Ampicillin-sulbactam, piperacillin-tazobactam, or a carbapenem)

Aspiration Pneumonitis/Pneumonia

General: Pulmonary consequences resulting from the entry of exogenous fluid or particles into the lower airway. Syndromes attributed to aspiration include chemical pneumonitis, bacterial pneumonia, and simple mechanical obstruction.

Risk: Reduced consciousness, dysphagia, esophageal disorders, vomiting, seizure, alcohol use

	Pneumonitis	Pneumonia
Gen	- "Flash burn" from aspiration of gastric acid	- Aspiration of oropharyngeal or upper airway contents (anaerobes, common airway bacteria)
Clin	- Acute onset of dyspnea, often after witnessed aspiration - Hypoxemia, respiratory distress	- Insidious onset of classic pneumonia symptoms, in someone with risk factors
Dx	- Clinical diagnosis, based on the presentation above, presence of risk factors, and XR demonstrating infiltrates	
Tx	- Tracheal suctioning, supplemental O_2 - Antibiotics are controversial	- Antibiotics (amp-sulbactam, pip-tazo)

Lower Respiratory Infections

Tuberculosis

General: Infection due to *Mycobacterium tuberculosis*. Spread by respiratory droplets. Bacteria can be immediately cleared, or result in primary infection, latent infection, or reactivation disease.

Risk: Prisoners, healthcare workers, recent immigrants (within 5 years), close contact with someone with TB, IV drug use, immunodeficiency (HIV, glucocorticoid use, hematologic malignancy)

	Primary	Reactivation
Definition	- New TB infection in naive host	- Reactivation of previous TB infection - Occurs with immunocompromise (HIV, TNF-α inh.)
Clinical	- Often asymptomatic - Acute pneumonia possible (fever, cough, fatigue, hilar lymphadenopathy)	- Fever, night sweats, weight loss, dyspnea, cough
Diagnosis	- Positive PPD or IFN-γ assay	- Positive CXR (pulmonary infiltrate, most commonly upper lobe) PLUS sputum culture/AFB smear

Latent TB: Asymptomatic chronic infection (controlled by immune response). Picked up via screening.

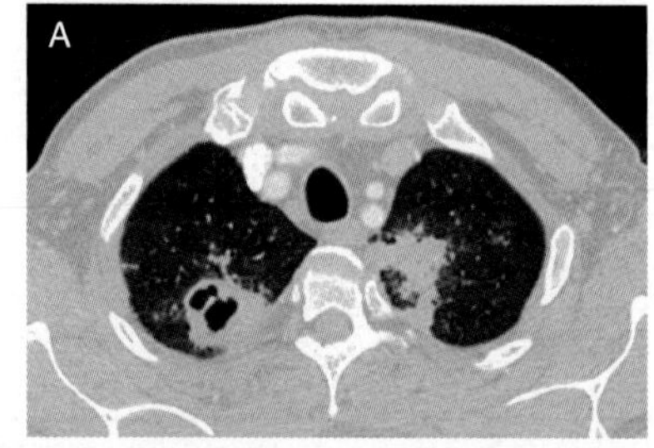

Diagnosis:

Screening:

- Positive PPD (or IFN-γ release assay), with normal x-ray → Latent TB
- Positive PPD with abnormal x-ray → active TB or reactivation

Suspicion for active disease:

- CXR (Looking for: Focal infiltrates most commonly in apex, +/− cavitation[A])
- Cultures (three sputum cultures, taken at various times)
    - Test with **AFB smear, mycobacterial culture, and NAA test**

Tuberculin Skin Testing (PPD) Interpretation	
Induration	Group
≥ 5 mm	- HIV, recent TB contact, immunosuppressed, evidence of prior TB infection
≥ 10 mm	- Recent (< 5 years) immigrant from endemic country, IV drug use, high-risk exposure (prison, healthcare, TB lab) - High risk for reactivation (DM, CKD, leukemia, glucocorticoid use)
≥ 15 mm	- Everyone else

Management:

Latent: Isoniazid + rifapentine (3 months) or rifampin (4 months) or isoniazid + pyridoxine (6-9 months)

Active: 2 months of RIPE (rifampin, isoniazid, pyrazinamide, ethambutol) + 4 months of isoniazid + rifampin

Complications and Disseminated Disease:

- Hemoptysis, bronchiectasis, pneumothorax
- Can involve: Bone ("Pott disease"), pleura, pericardium (constrictive pericarditis), peritoneum, CNS (meningitis)

Miliary TB

- Hematogenous dissemination of TB, resulting in multiorgan failure and septic shock
- Pulmonary disease with small "millet seed-like" lesions
- Can involve bones, adrenal, CNS, GU (sterile pyuria)
- Diagnosis: Acid-fast blood cultures, tissue biopsy (culture/NAA testing)
- Treat similarly to pulmonary tuberculosis

Vaccination:

- BCG vaccine is attenuated live strain of *Mycobacterium bovis*
- > 80% efficacy early on, but immunity wanes
- + PPD within first 10 years of vaccination, IFN-γ release assay can be used to differentiate
- Can cause disseminated infection if immunocompromised

Lower Respiratory Infections

Acute Bronchitis

General: Large airway inflammation resulting in syndrome defined by a cough > 5 days that can last up to 3 weeks

Risk: Typically follows viral URI, with < 10% of cases bacterial

Clinical:

- **Cough +/– sputum production**. URI symptoms can overlap early on.
- **Cough can be subacute (multiple weeks)**
- Physical exam typically unremarkable. Wheezing/rhonchi possible.

Diagnosis: Clinical diagnosis. CXR in those with suspicion for PNA (no infiltrates with bronchitis).

Management:

- Reassurance/Education (antibiotics not indicated)
- Nonpharm options preferred (tea, lozenges)
- Dextromethorphan or guaifenesin for refractory cough, albuterol if wheezing component

Upper Respiratory Infection (Common Cold)

General: Common, self-limited syndrome from upper respiratory virus infection. Term URI includes viral rhinosinusitis, pharyngitis.

Etiology: Rhinovirus, coronavirus, influenza, parainfluenza, RSV

Clinical:

- **Rhinitis, nasal congestion, sore throat, cough, malaise**
- Can be complicated by bacterial sinusitis/otitis, bronchitis

Diagnosis: Clinical

Management:

- Self-limited (1-1.5 weeks)
- Symptomatic care: NSAIDs for pain, antihistamine/decongestant combination for congestion
    - If severe cough: Dextromethorphan

Influenza

General: Acute respiratory illness due to influenza A or B virus. Transmitted via respiratory droplets/aerosols.

Clinical:

- Sudden onset of **malaise, fever, headache, myalgia**
- URI symptoms possible (cough/sore throat/rhinitis)
- Pneumonia (can be primary viral or secondary bacterial) [Pneumococcus, *S. aureus*]

Diagnosis:

- Molecular Tests: **RT-PCR** (Alt: Rapid molecular assay)
    - Both are sensitive, can reveal subtype of flu
- Antigen tests (rapid antigen assay) less sensitive (possible false negative)

Management:

- Antiviral therapy (**oseltamivir**, zanamivir, peramivir [IM]). Indicated if:
    - < 48 hours of symptoms
    - > 48 hours of symptoms, if high risk for complications
- Consider prophylactic antivirals if close contact AND high risk for influenza complication or if member of long-term care facility

Upper Respiratory Infections

Rhinosinusitis

General: Inflammation in the nasal cavity and paranasal sinuses. Sinusitis most commonly viral/associated with common cold, but can be bacterial (most common organisms Pneumococcus, *H. influenzae,* and *Moraxella*).

Risk: Often associated with polyps, deviated septum, foreign body

Clinical:

Acute (< 4 weeks):

- Facial pain/pressure
- Nasal congestion with purulent nasal discharge
- Maxillary tooth discomfort
- Other symptoms (fever, malaise, headache, ear pain/pressure)

Key bacterial features:

(1) **> 10 days without improvement**
(2) **"Double Worsening"** (gets worse after seems to improve)
(3) Severe symptoms for ≥ 3 days (**T > 102°F, heavy purulent drainage**)

Chronic (> 12 weeks):

- Purulent drainage, nasal obstruction, facial pain, decreased olfaction

Diagnosis: Clinical (see key bacterial features above to differentiate from viral)

- Imaging (head CT) only indicated if concerned about complication
- Chronic disease: Require clinical symptoms plus imaging or endoscopic evidence of inflammation

Management:

Viral	- Self-limited - Symptomatic (analgesia, saline irrigation, **intranasal steroids**)
Bacterial	- Symptomatic therapy (as above) - **Antibiotics** (amoxicillin-clavulanate; alt: Doxycycline) - Note: Many with bacterial sinusitis improve without antibiotics, so clinical decision to give
Chronic	- Extended antibiotic therapy (amoxicillin-clavulanate; or per nasal culture data) - **Oral glucocorticoids**, plus long-term intranasal glucocorticoids - Surgery for refractory/severe cases

Complications:

- Orbital/periorbital cellulitis
- CNS (abscess, meningitis, cavernous sinus thrombosis)

Upper Respiratory Infections

Pharyngitis

General: Acute inflammation of the oropharynx. Most commonly due to respiratory viruses (self-limited).

Etiology:

- Viral: Adenovirus, rhinovirus, coronavirus, enterovirus, influenza most common. EBV, HSV, acute HIV.
- Bacterial: **Group A streptococcus**, *Mycoplasma*, diphtheria, *Gonorrhea*, *Chlamydia*

Clinical:

- **Viral**: Sore throat. Associated with cold symptoms (nasal congestion, cough, rhinorrhea, etc.)
- **Bacterial**: Sore throat, associated with fever, tonsillar exudates[A], tender anterior cervical lymphadenopathy
    - Cold symptoms missing (vs viral)

Diagnosis:

<u>Adults</u>

- **Rapid antigen test** preferred (culture only required in rare, high-risk cases)
    - STI testing if at high risk
- **Centor criteria** (below) can be used to help determine who needs testing

(1) Fever
(2) Tonsillar exudates
(3) Tender cervical LA
(4) No cough

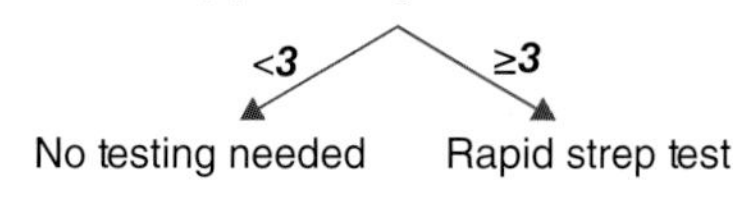

<u>Children</u>

- Rapid antigen test (alt: Culture)
- Test those with signs of bacterial pharyngitis that lack any other viral URI symptoms

Management:

Viral	- Self-limited
GAS	- Penicillin V or amoxicillin (alt: Macrolides, clindamycin, cephalosporin)

Complications:

- Rheumatic fever, poststreptococcal glomerulonephritis (GAS)
- Abscess, recurrent infection

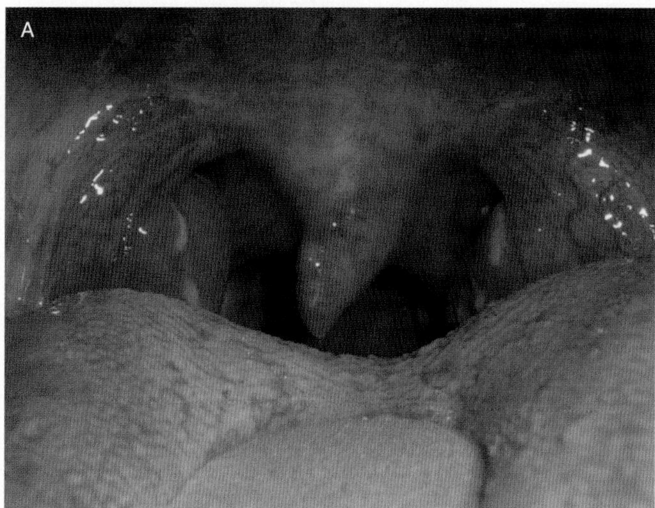

Pediatric Respiratory Disease

Croup

General: Laryngotracheobronchitis, which produces characteristic barking cough

Etiology: Most commonly **parainfluenza virus** (others include RSV, adenovirus, influenza)

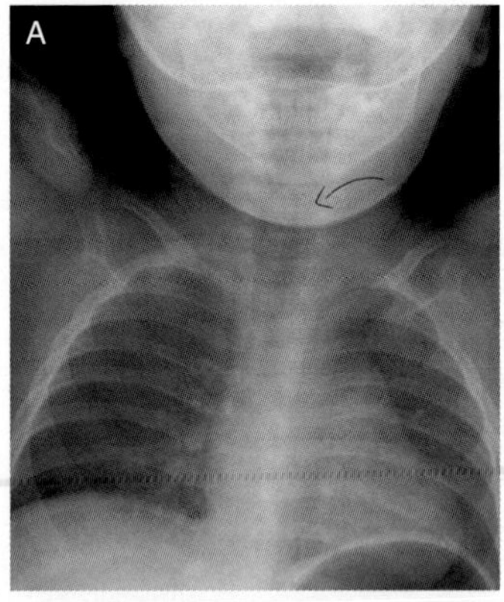

Clinical:

- Starts with congestion/coryza, fever
- Followed by hoarseness, **barking cough**, +/– stridor
- Spasmodic subtype (recurring croup)
  - Recurrent nighttime episodes of barking cough
  - Self-limited, short episodes

Diagnosis: Clinical diagnosis

- XR (may show **steeple sign**[A], referring to tapering of upper trachea)

Management: Corticosteroids PLUS nebulized epinephrine (if severe)

Bronchiolitis

General: Lower respiratory tract infection of the bronchioles. Most common in children < 2 years old.

Etiology: **RSV** is most common (others: Rhinovirus, parainfluenza, metapneumovirus, influenza)

Clinical:

- URI prodrome (mild fever, rhinorrhea, etc.)
- Followed by **respiratory distress** (tachypnea, labored breathing, nasal flaring, retractions)
  - Exam may reveal wheezing, crackles, hypoxemia

Diagnosis: Clinical diagnosis

Management:

- Supportive care, supplemental oxygen (may require NIPPV or mechanical ventilation if severe)
- No evidence for bronchodilators, corticosteroids, or other medical interventions

Prophylaxis: Palivizumab

- Indicated in premature infants (< 29-32 weeks), some bronchopulmonary dysplasia patients, congenital heart disease, immunocompromised

Pertussis

General: *Bordetella pertussis* infection, which causes "whooping cough"

Clinical:

- **Catarrhal** (1-2 weeks): Flu-like prodrome (cough/rhinitis)
- **Paroxysmal** (2-6 weeks): Severe cough with inspiratory whoop, post-tussive emesis
- **Convalescent stage**: Eventual resolution of symptoms

Diagnosis: Culture or PCR for < 4 weeks of symptoms. Serology for > 4 weeks.

Management: Macrolides (Azithromycin). Update Tdap.

- Post-exposure PPX: Macrolide for close contacts

Pediatric Respiratory Disease

Epiglottitis

General: Acute inflammation and edema of the epiglottis and surrounding area

Etiology: ***H. influenzae*** **type B** (rare due to vaccine), group A *Streptococcus, Staphylococcus aureus,* pneumococcus

Clinical:

- Rapidly progressive high fever, toxic appearance, drooling, dysphagia
- Respiratory distress (**tripod or sniffing posture**, stridor)

Diagnosis: Enlarged epiglottis on imaging or direct visualization

Management:

- Airway management
- Antibiotics: Amox-Clav or cephalosporin usually sufficient for *H. influenzae*, but broad spectrum **vanc/ceftriaxone** usually started prior to determining cause
- PPX: Rifampin (young, at risk household contacts of HiB epiglottitis)

Foreign Body Aspiration

General: Most commonly occurs in children between 1-3 y/o

Clinical:

- **Partial obstruction**: Cough, stridor, tachypnea/respiratory distress
    - Extremely acute in onset, often while child playing alone or witnessed choking event
    - Can cause unilateral ↓ breath sounds, focal wheeze
- **Complete obstruction**: Respiratory distress, cyanosis, altered mental status

Diagnosis: CXR: Inspiratory/expiratory films can reveal air trapping. Can consider CT if XR equivocal.

Management:

- Partial: Bronchoscopy
- Complete: Emergency care (back blows in infants, Heimlich in older children)
    - Emergent rigid bronchoscopy

Pediatric Pneumonia (Management)

Situation	Regimen
CAP (outpatient)	- Amoxicillin (typical lobar pneumonia) or macrolide (if suspected atypical pneumonia)
CAP (inpatient)	- Ampicillin or cephalosporin (suspected typical) - Macrolide (suspected atypical) - Combination therapy if severe or requires ICU admission

Pediatric Respiratory Disease

Cystic Fibrosis

General: Chronic multi system disorder from AR inherited mutations of the CFTR gene on chromosome 7. Most commonly due to F508del. Results in abnormal chloride channel, thickened secretions in the lungs, GI tract.

Clinical:

- **Pulmonary** (Productive cough, hyperinflation, obstructive lung disease)
    - Increased risk for bacterial infections (e.g., pneumonia) (*Staph / Pseudomonas* [risk increases as age ↑])
    - Risk for bronchiectasis long term
- **Gastrointestinal**
    - Pancreatic insufficiency/malabsorption (loss of fat soluble vitamins)
        - Fecal elastase for screening
    - Meconium ileus (at birth)
    - Hepatobiliary disease
- **Chronic rhinosinusitis**/Nasal polyps
- **Infertility**
    - Men: Defective sperm transport
    - Women: Abnormal cervical mucus (but still can get pregnant)

Diagnosis: Criteria require symptoms consistent with CF PLUS:

- Lab evidence of CFTR dysfunction
    - **Elevated sweat chloride**
        - Preferred first line. Confirm indeterminate or (+) results with follow-up genetic testing.
    - Genetic testing (confirming two disease-causing mutations)
    - Abnormal nasal potential difference
- Newborn screening (immunoreactive trypsinogen/DNA analysis for CFTR) in all 50 states

Management:

Pulmonary

- Chronic:
    - Hypertonic saline, DNase, chest physiotherapy
    - If reversible airflow obstruction: Inhaled β agonists
    - CFTR modulators (ivacaftor, lumacaftor, tezacaftor)
        - Used in patients with certain mutations, including F508
    - Chronic azithromycin or ibuprofen (anti-inflammatory)
- Acute exacerbations: Antibiotics (cover for *Staph*/*Pseudomonas*)

Gastrointestinal

- Pancreatic enzyme replacement therapy
- Nutritional/vitamin supplementation as necessary

Bronchopulmonary Dysplasia

General: Immature pulmonary system, resulting in long-term oxygen requirement and respiratory support at birth

Risk: **Prematurity**, low birth weight, mechanical ventilation/oxygen toxicity

Clinical: Infant, with the above risk factors, presenting with **respiratory distress** (tachypnea, retractions, rales)

Management:

- Mechanical ventilation (utilizing as low of oxygen and as little pressure as possible)
- No evidence for steroids, bronchodilators, etc.
- In general, lung function should recover months to a few years after birth

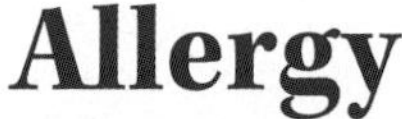

Allergy

Chronic Rhinitis

General: Rhinorrhea, sneezing, congestion. Can be allergic, nonallergic, or mixed.

	Allergic	Nonallergic (Vasomotor)
Gen	- Associated with atopic disorders (eczema, asthma, conjunctivitis)	- Excess fluid leakage from nasal vasculature - Can be triggered by odors, fragrance, smoke, etc.
Clin	- **Prominent nasal itching** - Sneezing, rhinorrhea, congestion - Can be seasonal/related to allergens - Commonly presents in childhood - Possible IgE sensitivity	- **Prominent congestion** - Sneezing, rhinorrhea - Commonly presents in adulthood
Dx	- Clinical - Allergy testing if severe/refractory	- Clinical (diagnosis of exclusion)
Tx	- Intranasal glucocorticoid (first line) - Intranasal antihistamine or oral antihistamine (second generation) are adjuncts	- Intranasal glucocorticoids and/or intranasal antihistamines (azelastine) - Intranasal ipratropium (for pure watery rhinitis)

Anaphylaxis

General: Sudden systemic syndrome caused by massive mast cell release into the bloodstream

Etiology: Common triggers include food reaction, drug, insect sting, or any other allergen

Clinical: Rapid onset (minutes to hours) of:

- **Generalized hives, pruritus**
- Swollen lips/tongue/oropharynx
- Respiratory failure (hypoxemia, dyspnea, bronchospasm, stridor)
- Shock (hypotension, signs of end-organ malperfusion)

Management:

- **Epinephrine** (used in all cases, from mild hives, to life-threatening shock)
    - IM epinephrine for most, IV if patient is severely ill
    - No absolute contraindications to epinephrine
- Fluids (for those in shock)
- Symptomatic: Albuterol, antihistamines

Congenital ENT Lesions/Eye

Congenital ENT Lesions

	General/Clinical	Management
Choanal Atresia	- Blockage of the posterior nasal passage, by bony or membranous abnormality - Associated with **CHARGE, Treacher-Collins** - **Bilateral**: Presents in infancy, with cyclic cyanosis, worse with activities not allowing for mouth breathing (feeding) and better with crying. - Failure in ability to pass catheter through nares - **Unilateral**: Presents later in life with unilateral nasal discharge, obstruction	Dx: CT scan (confirms narrowing of pterygoid plate in posterior nasal cavity) Tx: - Initial: Establish oral airway and feeding tube - Definitive: Endoscopic or surgical correction
Laryngomalacia	- ↑ laxity of supraglottic structures (worse with inspiration) - Infants (~3-9M): **Inspiratory stridor**, noisy respiration, possible poor feeding/respiratory distress if severe - Worse supine, improves when prone	Dx: Flexible fiberoptic laryngoscope Tx: Reassurance for most cases (resolves by 1.5 years) Supraglottoplasty for severe cases
Cystic Hygroma	- Congenital obstruction of the lymphatic system in neck, resulting in lymph accumulation in jugular lymphatic sacs - ↑ risk for fetal aneuploidy	Dx: Prenatal US (fetus) or clinical exam (after birth)
Torus Palatinus	- Bony exostosis of the hard palate[A] - Hard nodule on palate, normal overlying mucosa	Dx: Clinical Tx: Reassurance. Can surgically remove if symptomatic.

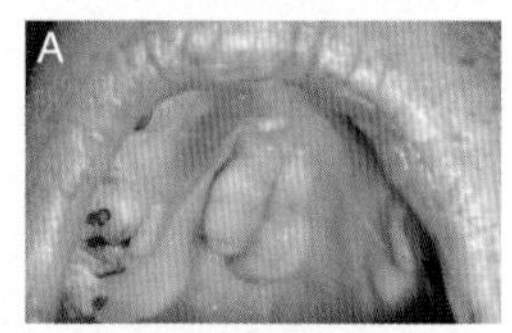

Preseptal (Periorbital) and Orbital Cellulitis

	Preseptal	Orbital
Gen	- Infection of anterior portion of **eyelid** - Risk: Sinusitis, contiguous skin infection (e.g., post bug bite, trauma)	- Infection of **orbit** (fat and ocular muscles) - Risk: Sinusitis, orbital trauma, eye surgery
Clin	- Eyelid erythema, edema, pain - Possible fever, leukocytosis	- Eyelid erythema, edema, tenderness - Possible fever, leukocytosis - **Ophthalmoplegia, painful ocular movements** - Possible proptosis/visual blurring High risk for complications: - Subperiosteal/orbital abscess - Intracranial extension (Cavernous sinus thrombosis, meningitis, abscess) - Blindness
Dx	- CT scan of orbit/sinuses	
Tx	- Oral antibiotics (clindamycin or TMP-SMX)	- IV antibiotics (Vancomycin + 3rd gen cephalosporin or amp-sulbactam) - Surgery for severe/refractory cases

Ear

Otitis Media

	Otitis with Effusion (Serous)	Acute Otitis Media
Gen	- Middle ear effusion without signs of active infection	- Acute infection of the middle ear - **Bulging of the TM[A] (distinguishes AOM from OME)** - Organisms: Pneumococcus, *H. influenzae*
Risk	- Post AOM - Eustachian tube dysfunction (kids) - Barotrauma, allergy (adults)	- Viral URI
Clin	- Generally asymptomatic - Can cause ↓ hearing, pain, tinnitus, "full" feeling	- Ear pain, otorrhea - Nonspecific symptoms in young kids (fever, ear tugging)
Dx	- Pneumatic otoscopy (immobile TM, air-fluid levels, opacification)	- Pneumatic otoscopy (middle ear effusion PLUS bulging TM)
Tx	- Observation for 3 months (most resolve) - No evidence for nose sprays/decongestants Kids: - **Tympanostomy**: If > 3 months, recurrent disease, high risk for developmental delay, or hearing loss	- Antibiotics (amoxicillin, or amox-clav for severe/refractory cases) Indications for antibiotics: - All adults receive treatment - Children - Indicated for most kids < 2 y/o - > 2 y/o that appear toxic, T > 102.2°F, or > 48 hours of symptoms
Cp	- No significant acute complications If chronic (> 3 months): - Conductive hearing loss - Tympanosclerosis, cholesteatoma	Acute complications: - TM perforation, mastoiditis, labyrinthitis - Intracranial infection spread (rare) If chronic (> 6 weeks) - Conductive hearing loss - TM perforation

Ear Infections/Complications

	General/Clinical	Management
Bullous Myringitis	- AOM, complicated by bullae on the tympanic membrane - Causes ↑ pain compared to AOM	- Dx/Tx same as AOM
Hemotympanum	- Blood in middle ear, causing dark opacification of TM - Usually associated with trauma (basilar skull fracture)	
Mastoiditis	- Complication of AOM, with purulence in mastoid cavity - Postauricular erythema, tenderness, swelling - Often also have the fever/ear pain associated with AOM - Complications: Osteomyelitis, CNS spread (meningitis or abscess), facial nerve palsy	Dx: Clinical plus radiographic (CT w/ contrast is best initial imaging test) Tx: - IV Antibiotics (e.g., vancomycin + cefepime) - Myringotomy +/− tympanostomy tube
Otitis Externa (Swimmers Ear)	- Inflammation of the external auditory canal - Risk: Swimming (gram negative like *Pseudomonas*), ear canal trauma, intra-ear devices - Ear pain, itching, and otorrhea	Dx: Clinical (otoscopy shows edematous and erythematous external ear canal) Tx: Clean out ear canal, topical ear drops (antibiotics, steroids, and antiseptic)
Malignant Otitis Externa	- Invasive, necrotizing infection of the ear canal/skull base - Almost always *Pseudomonas* - Risk: Diabetes, immunocompromised - Can spread to bone → osteomyelitis, cranial nerve lesions - Presents as ear pain, otorrhea, facial nerve palsy - Otoscopy shows granulation tissue, erythema	Dx: CT/MRI Tx: IV fluoroquinolone

Oropharyngeal

Salivary Glands

Disorder	Features
Sialolithiasis	- Parotid, submandibular, and sublingual **stone formation** - Occurs with dehydration, anticholinergic drugs, trauma - Presents as **pain/swelling with salivation (while eating)** - Tx: Hydration, compression/massage
Sialadenitis	- **Infection of salivary gland.** Associated with sialolithiasis or poor hygiene. - Can be bacterial (*S. aureus*) or viral (mumps) - Presents with painful swelling, erythema, edema - Tx: Antibiotics, hydration, compression/massage
Sialadenosis	- Benign **noninflammatory, bilateral swelling of salivary glands** (abnormal autonomic innervation) - Associated with liver disease (both alcoholic and nonalcoholic cirrhosis), diabetes, bulimia - Presents as bilateral nontender enlargement of the salivary glands
Malignancy	Subtypes: - Pleomorphic adenoma (benign mixed tumor) - Mucoepidermoid carcinoma (most common salivary malignancy, has mucinous/squamous components) - Warthin tumor (papillary cystadenoma lymphomatosum): Benign cystic tumor with germinal centers - Tx: Superficial or deep parotidectomy

Temporomandibular Joint Disorders

General: Jaw joint pain. Multifactorial etiology, including TMJ trauma and poor cervical spine posture.

Clinical: **Limited jaw mobility**, pain, cracking/popping upon opening mouth

Diagnosis: Clinical

Management:
- Patient education, physical therapy, occlusal bite splints
- NSAIDs, muscle relaxants
- Surgery if refractory

Peritonsillar Cellulitis/Abscess

General: Infectious inflammation in the soft tissues surrounding the palatine tonsil. Can cause distinct pus pocket[A] (abscess) or soft tissue infection (cellulitis). Often a complication of tonsillitis/pharyngitis.

Clinical:
- Severe throat pain, fever
- **Muffled voice**, trismus (spasming of the jaw muscles), pooling of saliva
- Swelling of soft tissues, **deviation of the uvula**, unilateral lymphadenopathy

Diagnosis: Clinical

Management:
- Antibiotics (amp-sulbactam or clindamycin)
- Needle aspiration or I&D
- Severe, recurrent disease → tonsillectomy

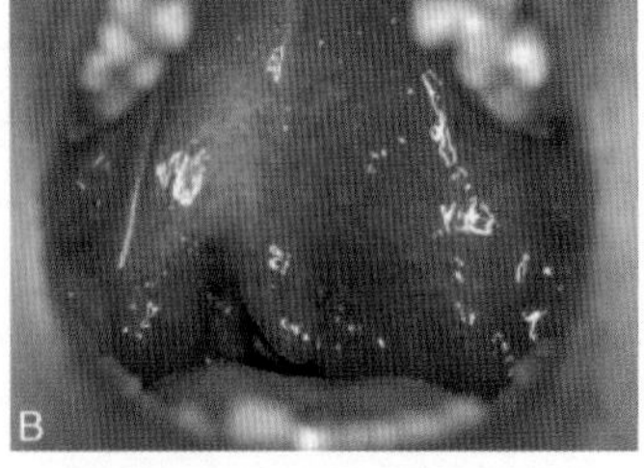

Oropharyngeal

Retropharyngeal Abscess

General: Infection in the retropharynx, with high risk for spread into the danger space that leads into the mediastinum. Occurs after trauma to retropharynx (e.g., fish bone injury), or from spread from local pharyngitis or dental infection.

Clinical: **Neck pain, fever, odynophagia**, drooling, muffled voice

Diagnosis: Neck CT preferred. Classically XR showed widened prevertebral space.

Management:

- Antibiotics (amp-sulbactam or clindamycin)
- Surgical drainage (if abscess is present)

Ludwigs Angina

General: Bilateral cellulitis of the submandibular space. Polymicrobial infection, most often due to an extension of molar dental infection.

Clinical:

- Mouth pain, stiff neck, drooling, dysphagia, fever, **submandibular swelling ("woody" induration)**
- Possible airway compromise (hoarse voice, stridor, respiratory distress)

Diagnosis: Clinical plus CT scan

Management:

- Antibiotics (amp-sulbactam or clindamycin; vancomycin if MRSA)
- Airway management (if necessary)
- Surgical drainage if not improving

Oral Lesion DDx

Candida	- Candidal infection of mucosa, associated with immunocompromised states and inhaled corticosteroids - **Scrapable white plaques**[A]
Leukoplakia	- Premalignant hyperplasia of the squamous epithelium - Associated with classic head/neck cancer risk factors (smoking, EtOH) - White patches or plaques of the oral mucosa
Oral Hairy Leukoplakia	- EBV infection, associated with immunocompromised states - White plaque most commonly covering lateral tongue, not easily scraped off
Aphthous Stomatitis	- **"Canker sores"** - Painful, shallow, round ulcers with gray base - Tx: Self-limited. Symptomatic control with topical steroid gel.

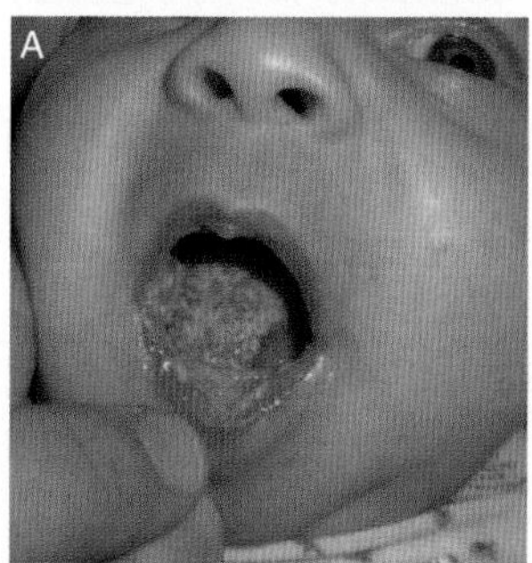

Oropharyngeal/Laryngeal

Head/Neck Cancer

Head/Neck Cancer	- General term for **squamous cell carcinoma**, originating from oropharynx - Associated with **smoking, EtOH use, HPV** - Presentation varies by site: Otalgia, oral lesions, dysphagia/odynophagia, neck lymphadenopathy - Dx: CT head/neck, with **biopsy** for definitive diagnosis *Note: If presents with SCC of neck node → Panendoscopy to find primary source in head/neck - Tx: Surgery/radiation/chemotherapy
Naso-pharyngeal Carcinoma	- Epithelial malignancy of the nasopharynx (usually suqamous in origin) - Associated with **EBV infection**, HPV, and ↑ risk if from southeast Asia - Headache, diplopia, facial numbness, cervical LA - Dx: Endoscopic biopsy + MRI - Tx: Radiation/chemotherapy

Nasal Pathology

Epistaxis	- **Anterior** (Kiesselbach plexus) vs **posterior** bleeds (rare, cause significant hemorrhage) - Risk: Trauma, coagulopathy/platelet disorder, vascular lesions, tumor - Tx: Tamponade maneuvers, topical α_1 adrenergic agonists. Cautery or nasal packing for refractory cases.
Septal Perforation	- Risk: Trauma, cocaine, post rhinoplasty, autoimmune disorder - Presents with whistling noise when breathing, bleeding
Septal Deviation	- Congenital or acquired **displacement of nasal septum**, causing difficulty breathing, congestion, snoring - Tx: Septoplasty
Nasal Fracture	- Tx: Ice, head elevation, with reduction of displaced fractures
Septal Hematoma	- Traumatic complication, high risk for necrosis of septum if not drained

Hoarseness DDx

Etiology:

- **Acute laryngitis** (associated with URI, lasts < 3 weeks, self-limited)
- **Laryngeal cancer** (anyone with > 3 weeks of hoarseness needs laryngoscopy)
- **Benign polyps/nodules**
- **Neurologic** (recurrent laryngeal nerve injury, Parkinson)

Clinical:

- Breathy voice: Incomplete adduction of cords
- Aphonia (lack of voice): Completely abducted cords
- Strained: Large mass on cords

Laryngeal Mass

Nodules	- Benign masses that arise from chronic irritation of vocal cord - Risk: Smoking, GERD, **vocal overuse/abuse**
Papilloma	- Benign papillary vocal cord tumor, associated with HPV 6, 11 - Can present with hoarseness/upper airway obstruction - Juvenile: Rape/abuse can get multiple papillomas - Dx: Laryngoscopy with biopsy
Squamous Cell Carcinoma	- Risk: Tobacco, alcohol - Presents with hoarseness - Dx: Laryngoscopy with biopsy (appears as white plaques) - Tx: Surgery or radiation. Chemotherapy for advanced disease.

Pulmonary Pharm

	Mechanism	Indication	Side Effects/Management
Decongestants and Antihistamines			
1st Gen Antihist Diphenhydramine Dimenhydrinate Chlorpheniramine Meclizine Promethazine Hydroxyzine	- H1 antagonist - Anti M1, 5-HT, α effects	- Allergy - Motion Sickness - Insomnia	- Sedation - Antimuscarinic (urinary retention, dry mouth, constipation, confusion in elderly) - Anti-α (postural hypotension) - Anti-serotonergic (increase appetite, weight gain)
2nd Gen Antihist Loratadine Fexofenadine Desloratadine Cetirizine	- H1 antagonist (more selective than 1st gen)	- Allergy	- All of the above, but much less frequent
Guaifenesin	- Increases volume, ↓ viscosity of sputum	- Expectorant	
Pseudoephedrine Phenylephrine	- α1 agonists	- Decongestant	- Hypertension, tachycardia - Tachyphylaxis: Rebound rhinorrhea if overuse
Pulmonary Hypertension			
Ambrisentan Bosentan	- Endothelin receptor antagonist	- Pulmonary hypertension	- Hepatotoxicity
Sildenafil Tadalafil	- PDE-5 inhibitors	- Pulmonary hypertension	- Headache, flushing, blurry/blue vision - Avoid with nitric oxide donating drugs
Epoprostenol (IV) Iloprost (inhaled)	- Prostacyclin agonist	- Pulmonary hypertension	- Jaw pain, flushing - High output cardiac states (at high doses)
Pulmonary Fibrosis			
Nintedanib Pirfenidone	- TK inhibitor - Anti-inflammatory/ fibrotic	- Idiopathic pulmonary fibrosis	- GI disturbances - Hepatotoxicity
Asthma/COPD			
Albuterol Salmeterol Formoterol Vilanterol	- β2 receptor agonists - Relaxation of smooth muscle in large airways	- Asthma - COPD	- Tachycardia - Tremor, anxiety/agitation, insomnia
Fluticasone Budesonide Mometasone	- Inhaled corticosteroids	- Asthma - COPD	- Oral/esophageal thrush (rinse to avoid)
Ipratropium Tiotropium Glycopyrronium Aclidinium	- Muscarinic antagonist	- Asthma - COPD	- Dry mouth
Montelukast Zafirlukast Zileuton	- Leukotriene receptor antagonists (-ukast) - Lipoxygenase inhibitor (zileuton)	- Asthma - COPD	- GI disturbances, hypersensitivity (anaphylaxis) - Hepatotoxicity (zileuton)
Omalizumab	- Monoclonal antibody against free IgE	- Asthma - Urticaria	- Hypersensitivity (anaphylaxis)
Methylxanthine Theophylline	- Induces bronchodilation via PDE inhibition	- Asthma - COPD	- Narrow therapeutic window, CYP interactions - Cardiotoxic (tachyarrhythmias) - Neurotoxic (seizures) - Nausea, vomiting
Roflumilast	- PDE-4 inhibitor	- COPD	- Weight loss
Methacholine	- M3 agonist	- Induces bronchospasm	
Cromolyn	- Mast cell stabilizer	- Asthma	

Volume

Volume Basics

Fluid Balance:

- **Total body water** (TBW) is estimated at 60% of weight
    - ⅔ of this is intracellular (ICF), ⅓ extracellular (ECF)

- **Normal Intake**: ~2L / day (fluids + solids)
- **Normal Output**: 0.75-1.5 L urine, 0.25 L stool, 0.5-1 L insensible losses

Note: Insensible losses ↑ in patients with sepsis, fever, burns

Intracellular fluid (67%)	Extracellular fluid (33%)
	Plasma (25% ECF)

Fluid Options:

	Indications	Notes
Normal Saline	Volume replacement	Strong anion gradient → Acidosis
Lactated Ringers	Volume replacement	Contains small amounts of K^+
D5 1/2 NS	Maintenance fluid	KCl often added
D5W	Hypernatremia (free water replacement)	
Hypertonic Saline	Severe hyponatremia Elevated ICP	
Mannitol	Elevated ICP	

Maintenance Fluid Calculations:

100/50/20 Rule (Daily Rate)	**4/2/1 Rule (Hourly Rate)**
- 100 mL/kg for first 10 kg - 50 mL/kg for next 10 kg - 20 mL/kg for remainder	- 4 mL/kg for first 10 kg - 2 mL/kg for next 10 kg - 1 mL/kg for remainder

Hypovolemia

Etiology: GI losses (emesis/diarrhea/NG suction), renal losses (DKA, diuretic abuse), poor intake, third spacing (ascites, burns, pancreatitis), sepsis, trauma

Clinical: **Decreased urine output**, dry mucous membranes, poor skin turgor, hypotension

Management:

- For **mild cases**: Oral replacement generally sufficient
- For **severe cases**:
    - Initial bolus of 1-2 L of isotonic crystalloid (NS or LR)
    - Further fluid to maintain MAP > 65 mmHg, urine output > 0.5 mL/kg/hr

Hypervolemia

Etiology: Volume retaining states (HF, CKD, Cirrhosis), iatrogenic fluid administration

Clinical: Weight gain, pitting edema, elevated JVP or CVP, pulmonary edema

Management: Salt/water restriction, diuretics

Sodium

Hyponatremia

General: Sodium < 135 mEq/L
- Mild: 130-135 mEq/L
- Moderate: 120-130 mEq/L
- Severe: < 120 mEq/L

Etiology		Specific Findings
True Hyponatremia (Serum Osm: < 275 mOsm/kg)		
Hypovolemic	Renal Salt Loss (U_{Na} > 40 mEq/L)	- Causes: Diuretics, post-ATN diuresis, low aldosterone (primary adrenal insufficiency)
	Extrarenal salt loss (U_{Na} < 40 mEq/L)	- Causes: Hypovolemia ("nonosmotic ADH release"). Typically due to poor PO intake or GI losses.
Normovolemic	SIADH	[See: SIADH]
	Primary polydipsia	- Abnormal thirst response resulting in excess water intake/abnormal ADH - Associated with psychiatric illness
	Beer potomania	- Excess intake of solute-poor beer
	Tea & toast diet	
	Hypothyroidism	
Hypervolemic	Heart failure Cirrhosis Nephrotic syndrome Renal failure	
Isotonic (Serum Osm: 275-295 mOsm/kg)		
	"Pseudo"- hyponatremia	- Elevated levels of lipids or proteins in serum, which results in abnormal lab calculation of serum sodium - Causes include **hyperlipidemia, monoclonal gammopathy**
Hypertonic Hyponatremia (Serum Osm > 295 mOsm/kg)		
	Hyperglycemia	- **Glucose**
	Exogenous substance	- **Mannitol**, sorbitol

Clinical:
- **Mild symptoms**: Nausea, vomiting, headache, lethargy, confusion
- **Severe symptoms**: Lethargy, coma, seizure, respiratory arrest

Management:

Treatment Based on Symptoms/Sodium Level	
Asymptomatic or Mild symptoms	- Continue to treat underlying cause (see below) - Fluid restriction - Salt tabs (if euvolemic hyponatremia)
Severe (< 120 mEq/L) and/or symptomatic	- Hypertonic saline
Treatment Based on Volume Status	
Hypovolemic	- Restore volume (isotonic fluids)
Euvolemic	- Fluid restriction - Consider salt tabs, urea, or vaptans
Hypervolemic	- Fluid restriction

- Sodium should not be corrected faster than **6-8 mEq/L in 24-hour period**

Sodium

SIADH

General: Inappropriately elevated ADH levels, leading to hyponatremia from impaired clearance of free water

Etiology:

- **Drugs** (cyclophosphamide, chlorpropamide, carbamazepine, SSRI)
- **Paraneoplastic** (small cell lung cancer)
- **CNS disorders** (trauma, stroke, infection)
- **Pulmonary disease** (pneumonia)

Clinical: [See: Hyponatremia] Note that patients are euvolemic.

Diagnosis: Hypotonic hyponatremia, plus $\mathbf{U_{osm} > 100}$ **mOsm/kg** $\mathbf{H_2O}$**,** $\mathbf{U_{Na} > 40}$ **mEq/L**

Management:

- [See: Hyponatremia] for acute management
- For chronic: Fluid restriction, consider salt tabs, urea, or vaptans

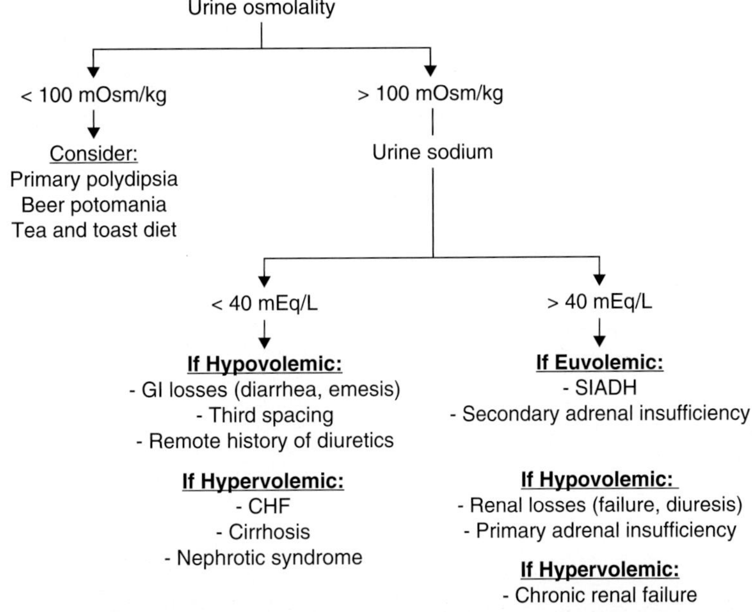

Osmotic Demyelination Syndrome

General: Rapid correction of hyponatremia can lead to irreversible demyelination. More likely to occur with severe and chronic hyponatremia (< 120 mEq/L).

Clinical: Delayed (2-5 days) onset of neurologic symptoms, including dysphagia, dysarthria, paralysis, mental status changes, and other focal neurologic deficits. Can present with locked-in syndrome.

Diagnosis: MRI

Management: Supportive. Can attempt to re-lower sodium.

Sodium

Hypernatremia

General: Sodium > 145 mEq/L. Typically caused by **water depletion** (water losses that are not replaced by patient, due to impaired thirst, lack of available water, or inability to seek water for self).

Etiology:

Etiology	Specific Findings
Renal water loss	- Osmotic diuresis (hyperglycemia)
Extrarenal water loss	- **Poor free water intake** - GI free water losses, insensible water losses (skin/respiratory)
Diabetes Insipidus	[See: Endocrine]
Iatrogenic	- Hypertonic fluids, salt poisoning

Clinical: Altered mental status, weakness, neurologic deficits, seizures, coma

Management:

- Isovolemic/Hypervolemic: D5W or PO water
- Hypovolemic: Free water (D5W or PO) + volume repletion (isotonic crystalloid)

Note: Maximum correction is 12 mEq/L/day (0.5 mEq/L/hr)

Complications:

- **Cerebral edema** (can result in encephalopathy and seizures if severe)
    - Theoretically occurs with overly-rapid correction of hypernatremia

Potassium

Hypokalemia

General: Potassium < 3.5 mEq/L

	Etiology	Specific Findings
Potassium Depletion		
Extrarenal	**Diarrhea, emesis** Laxative abuse	Urine **K < 20 mEq/L**
Renal	Renal tubular acidosis (I/II) **Diuretics** DKA Hyperaldosteronism	Urine **K > 20 mEq/L** Note: Hypovolemia can activate RAAS, with aldosterone promoting K secretion
	Hypomagnesemia	Mg normally inhibits ROMK in distal tubule. Replete Mg before correcting K.
	Bartter	AR defect in Na-K-Cl symporter in thick ascending limb
	Gitelman	AR defect in NaCl absorption in distal tubule
Redistribution		
	- Increased insulin, increased beta-adrenergic activity, metabolic, or respiratory alkalosis	

Clinical: Generally asymptomatic until < 3 mEq/L
- **Muscle weakness**, arrhythmias (PAC, PVC, bradycardia, AV block), ECG changes: Flattened T-waves, U-waves

Management:
- **K > 3.0**: Oral K replacement
- **K < 3.0 or symptomatic**: High dose oral replacement or IV
    - IV K can cause phlebitis at rates > 10 mEq/hr in peripheral veins
- Hyperaldosteronism: Spironolactone/Eplerenone

Hyperkalemia

General: Potassium > 5.0 mEq/L

	Etiology	Specific Findings
Potassium Excess		
Renal (↓ urine K)	Acute/Chronic kidney disease	
	Decreased ECV	- Low distal solute delivery
	Decreased aldosterone	- Hyporeninemic-Hypoaldosteronism (type 4 RTA) - Addisons, **ACEi/ARB use**
	Resistance to aldosterone	- **Potassium sparing diuretics**
Extrarenal	Tissue catabolism	- Rhabdomyolysis
Redistribution		
	- Insulin deficiency, beta-adrenergic blockade, metabolic or respiratory acidosis	
Laboratory Error		
	- Hemolysis, prolonged tourniquet use (can cause movement of K out of cells after venipuncture)	

Clinical: Generally asymptomatic, but > 7 mEq/L can result in:
- Weakness/paralysis
- Cardiac arrhythmias (sinus arrest, AV block)
- ECG: **Peaked T-waves**, lengthened PR/QRS

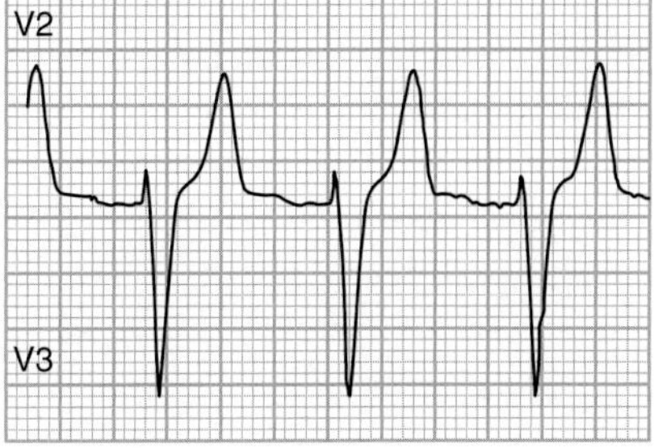

Management:

<u>K > 6.0-6.5 mEq/L or symptomatic/ECG changes</u>
- IV Ca Gluconate + IV Insulin/D5W (2nd line: Sodium bicarbonate or beta-agonists)
- Remove K from body:
    - Diuretics (if renal status is good)
    - K-binding resin (sodium polystyrene or patiromer)
    - Hemodialysis (if severe renal compromise)

<u>K < 6.0 mEq/L</u>: Find and reverse underlying cause

Calcium

Hypocalcemia

General: Calcium < 8.5 mg/dL
- Note: For every 1 g/dL below 4 in albumin, correct Ca by adding 0.8 mg/dL

Etiology	Specific Findings
Low PTH Levels	
Parathyroidectomy	
Hypoparathyroidism	- Autoimmune
Infiltrative parathyroid disease	
Elevated PTH Levels	
Vitamin D deficiency	
Chronic kidney disease	- ↓ Vitamin D production
Pancreatitis	
Tumor lysis syndrome	- Hyperphosphatemia, AKI
Pseudohypoparathyroidism	- [See: Endocrine]
Other	
Hypomagnesemia	
Transfusion	- Citrate binds Ca

Clinical:
- <u>Neuromuscular</u>: Irritability, **tetany**, paresthesias
    - Chvostek sign (tap on facial nerve → Contraction of facial muscle)
    - Trousseau sign (carpal spasm with inflated blood pressure cuff)
    - Hyperactive reflexes
    - **Seizures**
- <u>Cardiac</u>:
    - **Prolonged QT**, possible cardiac arrhythmias (Torsades)

Management:
- Severely Symptomatic or < 7.5 mg/dL: IV calcium
- Symptomatic or > 7.5 mg/dL: Oral calcium
- Hypomagnesemia: Correct Mg first

Calcium

Hypercalcemia

General: Calcium > 10.0 mg/dL

	Etiology	Specific Findings
Endocrine	Primary hyperparathyroid	- [See: Endocrine]
	Tertiary hyperparathyroid	
Malignancy	Bone metastasis	
	Paraneoplastic	- PTHrP production
	Multiple myeloma	
Pharm	Vitamin A/D toxicity	
	Thiazides, lithium	
	Milk-alkali syndrome	- Excessive intake of absorbable alkali (antacids) → Renal vasoconstriction, decreased GFR - Nausea, emesis, polyuria - Dx: Triad of hypercalcemia, alkalosis, AKI
Other	Granulomatous disease	- Excess 1,25 vitamin D production
	Immobilization	
	Genetic	<u>Familial hypocalciuric hypercalcemia</u> - Abnormal CaSR - Low urine Ca, high serum Ca

Clinical:

Note: Generally asymptomatic < 12

- **Stones** (nephrolithiasis, other urinary symptoms including polydipsia)
- **Bones** (bone pain)
- **Groans** (abdominal pain, constipation, anorexia, nausea)
- **Psychiatric overtones** (confusion, fatigue, poor concentration)

Management:

Severe (> 14 mg/dL)	- IV normal saline and calcitonin (acutely) - Bisphosphonate (long-term treatment). Denosumab 2nd line.
Moderate (12-14 mg/dL)	- Treat (as above) if patient is symptomatic
Mild (< 12 mg/dL)	- Treat underlying condition - Avoid exacerbating agents
Other	- Glucocorticoid in lymphoma, MM, granulomatous disease - Dialysis in renal failure

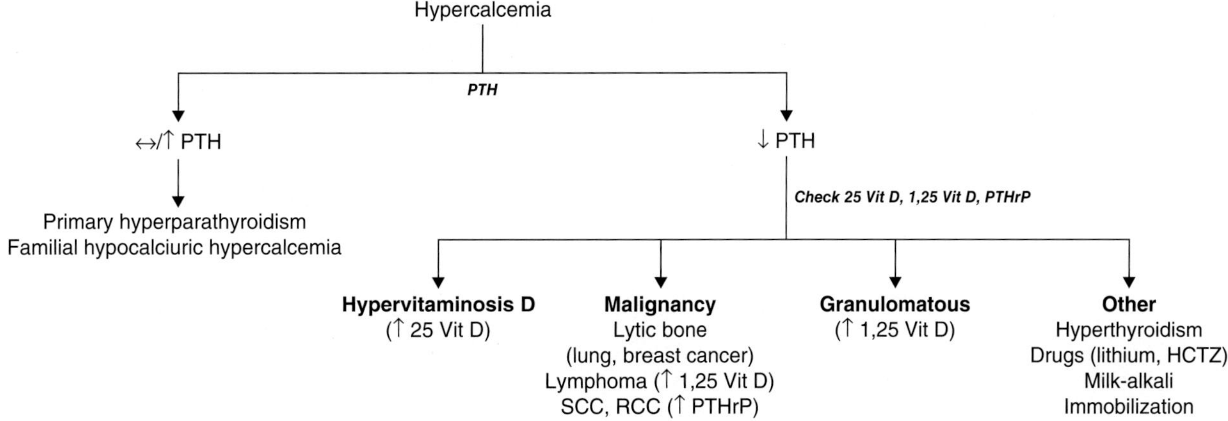

Magnesium/Phosphorus

Magnesium

	Hypomagnesemia	Hypermagnesemia
Gen	< 1.8 mEq/L	> 2.5 mEq/L
Etio	- **GI losses** (diarrhea, malabsorption, PPI use) - **Renal losses** (diuretic use, ATN recovery) - **Malnutrition** (alcoholism) - Genetic disorders (Gitelmans)	- Renal insufficiency - Iatrogenic (Mg infusions, enemas) - Laxative or antacid abuse
Clin	- Neuromuscular excitability - Hypocalcemia, hypokalemia - Cardiac: Prolonged QT, T-wave flattening, Torsades	- **Neuromuscular toxicity** (starts around 4-6 mEq/L) - Loss of DTR, somnolence, muscle weakness/paralysis - **Cardiac effects** (starts around 4-6 mEq/L) - Prolonged PR, QRS, and QT - Complete heart block/cardiac arrest at very high levels - Transient hypocalcemia from PTH receptor blockade
Tx	- Mild/asymptomatic: Oral Mg replacement - Severe/symptomatic: IV Mg replacement	- Stop any magnesium-containing drugs - Correcting underlying cause - Normal saline + loop diuretics - Severe renal failure: Dialysis

Phosphorus

	Hypophosphatemia	Hyperphosphatemia
Gen	< 2.5 mg/dL	> 4.5 mg/dL
Etio	- Decreased intestinal absorption (chronic diarrhea, PPI use, low intake) - Renal excretion (hyperparathyroidism, vitamin D deficiency, DKA) - Refeeding syndrome - Hungry bone syndrome	- Phosphate load (tumor lysis, rhabdo, phosphate laxatives) - **Acute/chronic kidney disease** - ↑ renal phosphate absorption (hypoparathyroidism)
Clin	- ATP Depletion - Metabolic encephalopathy - Impaired myocardial contractility - **Muscular weakness** - Increased bone turnover - Can lead to rickets and osteomalacia	- Ectopic calcification if extremely high - Risk is high if **calcium phosphate product (Ca x Pi) > 70**
Tx	- Oral or IV phosphate replacement	- Low phosphate diet, +/− phosphate binders (sevelamer) - Hemodialysis (severe renal failure)

Acid-Base

Respiratory Acidosis	Metabolic Alkalosis
Alveolar hypoventilation: - COPD, OSA, other lung disease - CNS depression - Neuromuscular weakness - Respiratory muscle fatigue	Saline responsive ($U_{Cl} < 20$) - Vomiting - Laxative/diuretic abuse - GI suctioning - Volume contraction Saline unresponsive ($U_{Cl} > 20$) - 1°/2° Hyperaldosteronism - Cushing - Severe hypokalemia
Metabolic Acidosis	**Respiratory Alkalosis**
Elevated anion gap (MUD PILES) - Methanol - Uremia - Diabetic ketoacidosis - Propylene glycol - Iron or INH - Lactic acidosis - Ethylene glycol - Salicylates Normal anion gap - Renal tubular acidosis - GI loss of HCO_3 (diarrhea, fistula) - Infusion of HCO_3-free Fluids - Acetazolamide - Post-hypocapnia - Renal failure (early)	- Alveolar hyperventilation (anxiety, PE, hypoxemia, high altitude) - Salicylate toxicity (early) - Pregnancy - Sepsis

Y-axis: HCO_3 (10 – 40); X-axis: pH (7.2 – 7.6)

Anion gap

AG = Na − Cl − HCO_3

Expected gap: 2.5 × [albumin]

Urine anion gap

UAG = $[Na^+] + [K^+] - [Cl^-]$

Should be negative with acidosis, but is positive with type I/IV RTAs

Osmolar gap

Osmolar gap = Measured P_{osm} − Calculated P_{osm}

P_{osm} (calculated) = 2[Na] + glucose/18 + BUN/2.8

Osmolar gap ↑:
- Ethylene glycol
- Methanol
- Isopropyl ethanol
- Propylene glycol

Delta/Delta

Delta ratio = Δ anion gap/Δ [HCO_3]

Interpretation:

< 0.4: Normal anion-gap acidosis

< 1: Mixed normal/elevated anion-gap acidosis

1-2: Pure anion-gap acidosis

> 2: Elevated AG acidosis + metabolic alkalosis

Disorder	Primary	Comp	Compensation Calculation
Metabolic acidosis	↓ HCO_3	↓ CO_2	$pCO_2 = 1.5\,[HCO_3] + 8 \pm 2$
Metabolic alkalosis	↑ HCO_3	↑ CO_2	↑ $pCO_2 = 0.7\,[\Delta HCO_3]$
Respiratory acidosis	↑ CO_2	↑ HCO_3	Acute: ↑ HCO_3 1.0 mEq/L for each 10 mmHg CO_2 Chronic: ↑ HCO_3 3.5 mEq/L for each 10 mmHg CO_2
Respiratory alkalosis	↓ CO_2	↓ HCO_3	Acute: ↓ HCO_3 2.0 mEq/L for each 10 mmHg CO_2 Chronic: ↓ HCO_3 4.0 mEq/L for each 10 mmHg CO_2

	Acidosis	Alkalosis
Resp	Hyperventilation	Hypoventilation
CV	Myocardial depression	Myocardial depression
CNS	Increased cerebral blood flow/ICP	Decreased cerebral blood flow/ICP
Hgb	Right-shifts oxyhemoglobin curve	Left-shifts oxyhemoglobin curve
Other		Increased neuromuscular excitability (albumin binds ↑ Ca)

Acute Kidney Injury

General: A rapid decline in renal function, reflected by ↓ **glomerular filtration rate**

RIFLE	Creatinine	GFR	Urine Output
Risk	1.5 fold ↑	↓ 25%	< 0.5 mL/kg/hr for 6 hours
Injury	2.0 fold ↑	↓ 50%	< 0.5 mL/kg/hr for 12 hours
Failure	3.0 fold ↑	↓ 75%	< 0.3 mL/kg/hr for 24 hours or anuria
Loss	- Complete loss of kidney function for > 4 weeks		
ESRD	- Complete loss of kidney function for > 3 months (requiring dialysis)		

KDIGO guideline definition
(1) Abrupt (< 48 hr) increase in Cr by > 0.3 mg/dL
(2) Increase in creatinine 50% from baseline in last week
(3) Reduction in urine output to < 0.5 mL/kg/hr for > 6 hr

Etiology:

	Prerenal (60-70% cases)	Intrinsic Renal (25-40% cases)	Post-renal (5-10% cases)
Etiology	- Hypovolemia - Hypotension - Renal artery stenosis - Hepatorenal - Cardiorenal - NSAID/ACEi	- Acute tubular necrosis - Glomerular disease - AIN - Vascular (PAN, TTP)	- Obstruction (BPH, nephrolithiasis, GU cancer, neurogenic bladder)
BUN/Cr	> 20:1	Varies	Varies
FE_{Na}	< 1%	> 2%	> 2%
U_{Osm} (mOsm/kg)	> 500	< 350	< 350
U_{Na} (mEq/L)	< 20	> 40	> 40

Clinical: Usually asymptomatic. Can cause edema, hypertension, ↓ urine output.
- **Uremia**: Anorexia, vomiting, pericarditis, encephalopathy

Diagnosis: Renal function (as above). Other useful tests include urinalysis, urine sodium excretion, urine volume monitoring.

Management:
- Correct volume status, underlying disorder
- Monitor for below complications, which (if severe) are dialysis indications
- Post-renal: Urinary catheterization

Dialysis Indications: (AEIOU)
- Acidosis
- Electrolyte abnormalities (hyperkalemia)
- Intoxication (ethylene glycol, lithium, etc.)
- Overload (volume)
- Uremia (pericarditis, encephalopathy, platelet dysfunction)

Note: Only initiate dialysis if refractory to medical management of the complication (e.g., fails diuretics for hypervolemia)

Chronic Kidney Disease

General: Decreased kidney function for > 3 months, with GFR < 60 mL/min
- Stage III (Moderate): GFR < 60 mL/min
- Stage IV (Severe): GFR < 30 mL/min
- Stage V (ESRD): GFR < 15 mL/min

Etiology: Most commonly due to **diabetes mellitus or hypertension**, followed by glomerulonephritis, cystic kidney disease

Clinical: CKD is associated with ↑ risk for cardiovascular disease, end-stage renal disease, infection, malignancy, and mortality

System	Findings
Fluids/Lytes	- Volume overload, hyperkalemia, metabolic acidosis
Endocrine	- Vitamin D deficiency/hyperparathyroidism (leads to hypocalcemia, hyperphosphatemia, osteomalacia)
Cardiovascular	- Hypertension, dyslipidemia, accelerated atherosclerosis, uremic pericarditis
Hematologic	- Normocytic anemia (low EPO), uremic platelet dysfunction
Reproductive	- Erectile dysfunction, decreased libido
Neurologic	- Uremic encephalopathy

Management:

Complication	Intervention
Hypertension	- ACEi or ARB preferred
Anemia	- EPO if Hgb < 10 g/dL
Electrolyte Issues	- Low phosphate, potassium diets (for hyperkalemia/phosphatemia)
Acidosis	- Sodium bicarbonate
Hyperparathyroidism	- Calcitriol, vitamin D, or calcimimetics. Phosphate binders (if phosphatemia refractory to dietary control).
Proteinuria	- SGLT-2 inhibitor

Renal replacement therapy: Indicated once **GFR falls < 5 OR GFR 5-15 with AEIOU symptoms**

Renal Replacement

	Hemodialysis	Peritoneal Dialysis
Process	- Blood pumped out of body to artificial semipermeable membrane, with dialysate on other side	- Dialysate is infused into peritoneal space, which acts as membrane for exchange
Access	- Catheter, AV Graft, AV Fistula	- Implanted peritoneal catheter
Timing	~ 3 days/week	- Cycled daily
Pros	- Efficient and emergent	- Convenience, more physiologic
Cons	- Less physiologic, so elevated risk of hypotension - Requires access	- Peritonitis

Transplantation
- More natural renal replacement
- Requires immunosuppressive therapy, risk for acute or chronic rejection

Continuous veno-venous hemofiltration (CVVH)
- Filters blood along highly permeable membrane, removing water and solute
- Short term, continuous form of renal replacement used if critically ill

Calciphylaxis (Calcific Uremic Arteriopathy)

General: Skin ischemia caused by calcification of arterioles in the dermis/adipose tissue. Occurs with longstanding ESRD, likely due to hyperphosphatemia.

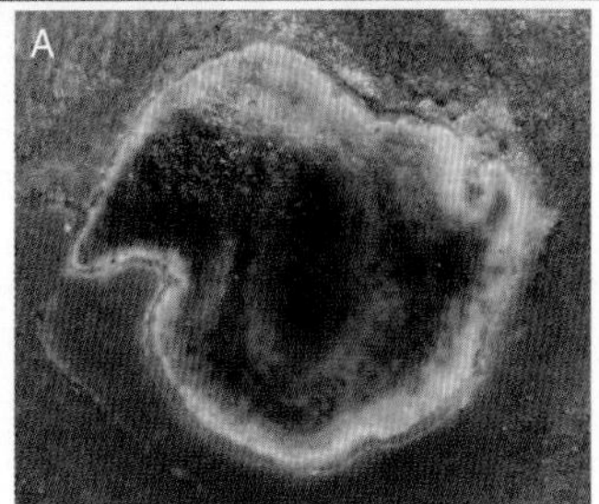

Clinical: Extremely **painful areas of ischemic necrosis** (violaceous nodules/ulcers)[A]
- Lesions occur in areas of high adiposity (distal lower extremities, trunk)

Diagnosis: Clinical (ESRD + clinical appearance). Biopsy if uncertain.

Management: Wound care, phosphate binders, sodium thiosulfate. Overall poor prognosis.

Glomerular Disease

Nephritic Syndrome

General: Glomerular inflammation resulting in the clinical syndrome of **hematuria, proteinuria, and renal failure**

Etiology:

- Post streptococcal glomerulonephritis
- Crescentic glomerulonephritis
    - ANCA + Vasculitis, anti-GBM disease
- Lupus nephritis
- IgA nephropathy

Clinical:

- Hematuria, dysmorphic RBCs
- Proteinuria (< 3.5 g/day)
- Hypertension, edema, azotemia

Management: Depends on underlying etiology

Nephrotic Syndrome

General: Nephrotic syndrome is defined by **protein excretion > 3.5 g/day**, due to a variety of glomerular processes that allow for leakage of protein through glomerular basement membrane and into urine

Etiology:

- Minimal change disease
- Focal segmental glomerulosclerosis (FSGS)
- Membranous nephropathy
- Amyloidosis
- Diabetic nephropathy

Clinical:

- Proteinuria (> 3.5 g/day), hypoalbuminemia (< 3.5 mg/dL), and edema
- Hyperlipidemia (increased liver protein synthesis)
- Hypercoagulability (loss of antithrombin III)
- Increased infection risk (IgG loss in urine)

Management: Treat underlying disease

- Proteinuria: ACEi/ARB
- Edema: Loop diuretics
- Hyperlipidemia: Statin

Nephritic Syndromes

	General/Pathophysiology	Findings	Management
Post-Strep GN	- Occurs ~2 weeks after **group A Strep infection** of skin or respiratory tract - More common in children	Antistreptolysin O ↑, Complement ↓ LM: Glomeruli enlarged/hypercellular IF: Granular appearance EM: Subepithelial humps (IgG/C3)	- Generally self-limited
Rapidly Progressive GN	Type I: Goodpastures or anti-GBM Type II: Progressed lupus/post-strep GN Type III: "pauci-immune" - Granulomatosis with polyangiitis - Microscopic polyangiitis - Eosinophilic granulomatosis w/ polyangiitis	LM/IF: Crescent moon shapes of fibrin Linear immunofluorescence (for anti GBM), granular pattern immunofluorescence (for type II), and no immunofluorescence (for type III)	- Methylprednisolone, Cyclophosphamide +/− Plasmapheresis (for IgG antibodies)
Diffuse Proliferative GN	- Common subtype of **lupus nephritis** (type IV)	LM: Wire-looping of capillaries EM: Subendothelial immune complex deposition	- Steroids + cyclophosphamide or mycophenolate

Glomerular Disease

Nephritic Syndromes (Cont)

	General/Pathophysiology	Findings	Management
IgA Nephropathy	- Gross hematuria days after URT infection, with preserved renal function - Often chronic, recurrent process. Some will progress to ESRD.	IM: Globular IgA deposits in the mesangium	- Steroids (if disease is severe/progressing)
Membrano-proliferative GN (can cause nephritic, nephrotic, or mixed picture)	Type I: Immune-complex mediated: Occurs with viral infection (hepatitis) and autoimmune disease Type II: Complement mediated: Occurs with genetic or acquired overactivation of complement (C3 nephritic factor)	LM: "Tram-track" GBM splitting IF: Continuous, dense ribbon-like deposits along the glomeruli	- Workup for infections if immune-complex mediated
Alports	- X-linked inherited nephritis due to abnormal **type IV collagen**	- ESRD, ocular abnormalities, sensorineural hearing loss - EM: "Split" basement membrane	- Often progresses to ESRD

Nephrotic Syndromes

	General/Pathophysiology	Findings	Management
Minimal Change Disease	- Most common cause of pediatric nephrotic syndrome - Primary: Idiopathic, or associated with recent infection or immunization - Secondary (lymphoma)	LM: Normal glomeruli EM: Effacement of foot processes - **Selective proteinuria (albumin)**	- Prednisone
Focal Segmental Glomerulosclerosis	- Most common cause of nephrotic syndrome in Black patients - Primary (idiopathic) - Secondary (**HIV** ["collapsing subtype"], sickle cell, IFN, heroin, severe obesity)	LM: Segmental sclerosis[A]/hyalinosis IF: Generally negative EM: Effacement of foot process similar to MCD	- Treat underlying - +/− immunosuppressives
Membranous Nephropathy	Primary (idiopathic): Ig against phospholipase A2 receptor (**PLA2R**) <u>Secondary</u>: - Infections (Hep B/C, syphilis) - Drugs (gold, penicillamine, NSAIDs) - Autoimmune (SLE) - Solid malignancy	LM: Diffuse capillary/GBM thickening IF: Granular (IC deposition) EM: Spike and dome appearance with subepithelial deposits	- Treat underlying - ACEi for proteinuria control - Immunosuppressive therapy for idiopathic MN
Amyloid	- Complication of systemic amyloidosis	LM: Congo red stain shows **apple-green birefringence**	- Treat underlying
Diabetic	- Complication of diabetic nephropathy	LM: Mesangial expansion, GBM thickening, "Kimmelstiel-Wilson" nodules[B]	- Treat underlying

Tubulointerstitial Disease

Acute Tubular Necrosis

General: Necrosis of renal tubular epithelium, resulting in renal dysfunction

Etiology:

- **Renal ischemia**: Hypotension from sepsis, hypovolemia
- **Toxins**: Radiocontrast, heme pigments, Ig light chains, crystals
  - Nephrotoxic drugs: Aminoglycosides, cisplatin, amphotericin, acyclovir

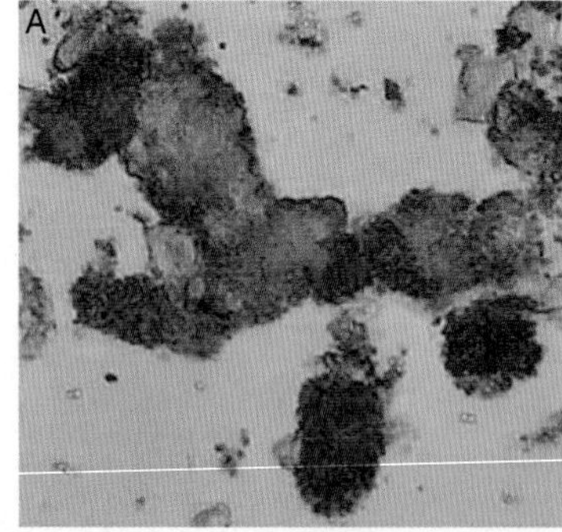

Clinical:

- **Oliguric phase** (days-to-weeks): Oliguria, azotemia, hyperkalemia, acidosis
- **Diuretic phase**: High urine output, with risk for electrolyte depletion (hypokalemia)

Diagnosis:

- Azotemia, plus FeNa > 2% (to differentiate from pure prerenal azotemia)
- Urinalysis (muddy brown granular[A]/epithelial cell casts)
- Limited improvement in kidney function with fluids (versus prerenal)

Management: Supportive care

Rhabdomyolysis

General: Muscle necrosis, with release of nephrotoxic myoglobin

Etiology: Intense exercise, crush injuries, infection, drugs (statins, fibrates)

Clinical: Presents with muscle pain, weakness, and dark urine

Diagnosis: **Elevated CK**, urinalysis (+ blood on UA, no RBCs on microscopy)

Management: Aggressive volume resuscitation, treatment of electrolyte abnormalities, dialysis if severe

Acute Interstitial Nephritis

General: Inflammatory renal interstitial disease, most commonly hypersensitivity to a drug

Etiology:

- **Drugs** (NSAIDs, Penicillin/cephalosporin, PPI, loop diuretics, rifampin, sulfonamides)
- Infection (pyelonephritis, systemic legionella or TB)
- AI (Sjogren, SLE, sarcoid)

Clinical: 1-3 weeks post insult, patients develop **AKI +/– fever, rash, and eosinophilia**

Diagnosis: Clinical. AKI + urinalysis showing WBC, WBC casts, or (rarely) eosinophils.

Management: Remove offending agent, consider steroids

Renal Papillary Necrosis

General: Necrosis of the renal papilla from ischemia

Etiology: Analgesic abuse (**NSAIDs**), sickle cell, pyelonephritis

Clinical: Hematuria, colicky flank pain, passage of sloughed papilla in urine

Management: Supportive. Treat underlying condition.

Tubulointerstitial Disease

Renal Tubular Acidosis

General: Disorder of abnormal renal tubular acid secretion

Type	1	2	4
Location	Distal	Proximal	Hypoaldosteronism
Abnormality	Secretion	Absorption	Generation
HCO_3	< 10 mEq/L	12-20 mEq/L	> 17 mEq/L
K+	Low	Low	High
Urine pH	> 5.5	< 5.5	< 5.5
Urine AG	Positive	Negative	Positive
Causes	- AI Disease (Sjogrens/RA) - Drugs (Amp B, ifosfamide, lithium) - Hypercalciuria	- M-protein disorders (MM, amyloid) - Drugs (acetazolamide, topiramate) - Heavy metals - Fanconi syndrome	- Hyporenin/Hypoaldosteronism (DM) - ACEi/ARB, NSAID use - Aldo resistance (K-sparing diuretics, or trimethoprim)
Tx	- $NaHCO_3$ or other alkali	- $NaHCO_3$ or other alkali - Thiazide	- Fludrocortisone
Other	- Nephrolithiasis (Ca phosphate)		

Other Tubular Abnormalities

Disease	Findings
Hartnup	- AR abnormality in amino acid transport, with decreased resorption of neutral amino acid like tryptophan
Fanconi	- Hereditary or acquired proximal tubule dysfunction, leading to defective transport of glucose, amino acids, sodium, potassium, phosphate, uric acid, bicarbonate - Treat with phosphate, potassium, alkali and salt supplements
Bartter	- Resorptive defect in **thick ascending loop of Henle NaKCl transporter** - Appears like chronic loop diuretic use
Gitelman	- Resorptive defect in **distal convoluted tubule NaCl transporter** - Appears like chronic thiazide diuretic use
Liddle	- Gain of function in ENaC → ↑ Na reabsorption in collecting tubules - Presents like **hyperaldosteronism**, but low aldosterone levels in serum - Tx: Amiloride
Syndrome of Apparent Mineralocorticoid Excess	- Hereditary deficiency of 11b-hydroxysteroid dehydrogenase (unable to convert cortisol to cortisone) - Can acquire from **glycyrrhetinic acid (in licorice)** - Presents as hypertension, hypokalemia, metabolic alkalosis - Treatment: Corticosteroids (down regulate own cortisol production)

Renal Vascular Disease

Renal Artery Stenosis

General: Decreased renal perfusion, leading to elevated RAAS activity and secondary hypertension

	Atherosclerotic Disease	Fibromuscular Dysplasia
Gen	- Most common, seen in those with atherosclerotic risk factors	- Angiopathy of medium sized vessels, resulting in areas of stenosis and aneurysm - Commonly seen in **women of child bearing age**
Clin	- **Secondary hypertension** in someone with high likelihood for vascular disease - Abdominal bruit	- **Renal stenosis** (secondary hypertension, flank pain) - **Carotid Stenosis** (headache, TIA/stroke, carotid bruit, tinnitus) - Vertebral stenosis
Dx	- CTA, MRA, or Duplex US	- CTA, MRA, or Duplex US ("String of Beads")
Tx	- Pharm: ACEi/ARB - Percutaneous transluminal angioplasty - Surgical bypass if all else fails	

Renal Vein Thrombosis

General: Renal venous thrombus, associated with nephrotic syndrome (especially membranous nephropathy)

Clinical: Generally asymptomatic, but can result in pulmonary embolism or worsening renal failure

Diagnosis: CT, MRI, or duplex US

Management: Anticoagulation

Renal Infarction

General: Arterial infarction from cardioembolism, dissection, or hypercoagulability

Clinical: Acute onset flank/abdominal pain, nausea/vomiting

Diagnosis: CT/CTA

Management: Anticoagulation

Cystic Kidney Disease

Autosomal Dominant PKD

General: AD genetic cystic kidney disease, commonly from PKD1 or PKD2 genes

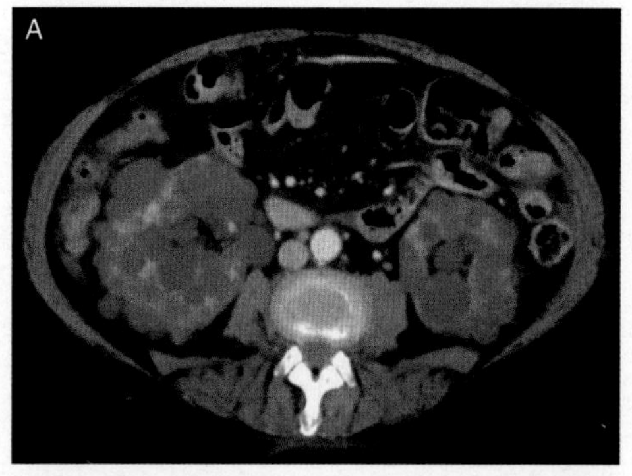

Clinical: **Hypertension, hematuria, renal insufficiency, or flank pain**
- Extrarenal features: Cerebral aneurysms, hepatic/pancreatic cysts, cardiac valvular disorders (MVP), diverticulosis

Diagnosis: Ultrasound, CT[A] (multiple and bilateral renal cysts)

Management:
- BP Control (ACEi/ARB)
- ESRD: Renal replacement (dialysis/transplant)
- Screening for cerebral aneurysms
- Tolvaptan can slow disease progression in some patients

Autosomal Recessive PKD

General: Infantile inherited AR disorder characterized by cystic dilation of the renal collecting ducts

Clinical: (Patients can vary in severity and age of disease onset)
- **Prenatal**: Screening US shows enlarged kidneys
- **Neonates**: Renal dysfunction, +/− pulmonary hypoplasia (Potter syndrome)
- **Children**: Renal dysfunction, + liver disease (biliary dysgenesis, hepatic fibrosis, portal hypertension)

Diagnosis: Ultrasound (enlarged, echogenic kidneys) plus coexisting liver disease
- Genetic testing can confirm

Management: Supportive (no curative therapies)

Simple Renal Cyst

General: Typically benign renal cysts that can be bilateral and multiple. Rarely the cysts can rupture and bleed.

Diagnosis:

Features of Benign Cysts	Features of Malignant Cysts
- Thin walled, nonseptated - Nonenhancing on CT[B]/MRI - Homogenous interior	- Thick walls, irregular, and multilocular - Enhancing on CT[C]/MRI - Heterogeneous interior

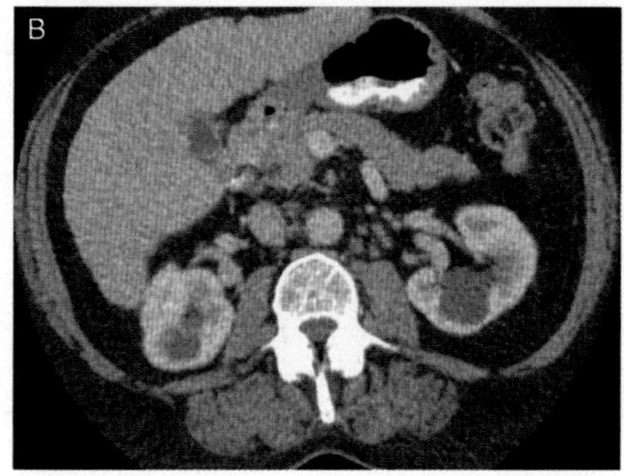

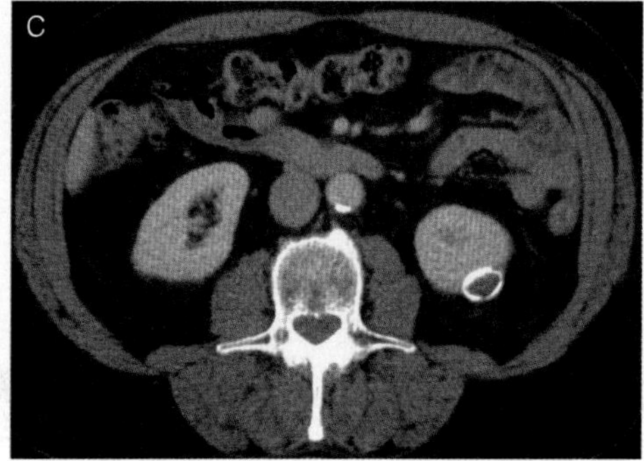

Management:
- Benign: No follow up required
- Suspicious: Requires further workup for malignancy

Nephrolithiasis

Type	Radio	Shape	pH	Cause/Findings
Calcium oxalate (80%)	Dense	Envelope[A]	< 5.5	- Hypercalciuria - Hyperoxaluria (increased oxalate absorption in GI disorders [e.g. IBD, malabsorption], vitamin C abuse, and ethylene glycol)
Calcium phosphate (5%)	Dense		> 5.5	- Hyperparathyroidism, **distal RTA**
Struvite (Ammonium magnesium phosphate) (10%)	Dense	Coffin lid	> 5.5	- UTI from urease producing organisms (***Proteus, Klebsiella***, *Serratia, Enterobacter*) - Common composition for **staghorn calculi**
Uric Acid (10%)	Lucent	Diamond	< 5.5	- Hyperuricemia from gout, liquid tumor/chemotherapy (e.g., leukemia) - Risk factors: Low urine volume, acidic urine, **hot/arid climates**
Cystine (<1%)	Lucent	Hexagonal	< 5.5	- Cystinuria (see genetics)
Drug Stones				- Acyclovir, indinavir, sulfadiazine

Clinical: Flank pain (waxing/waning, radiates to groin), gross or microscopic hematuria, urinary urgency

Diagnosis:

- Noncontrast CT[B]
- Ultrasound (limit radiation in pregnancy, kids)

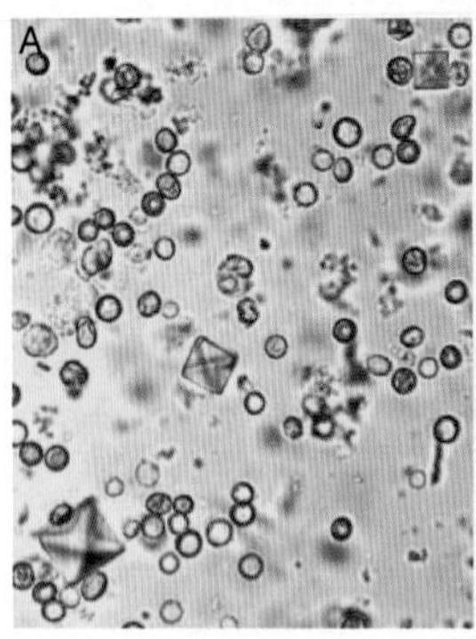

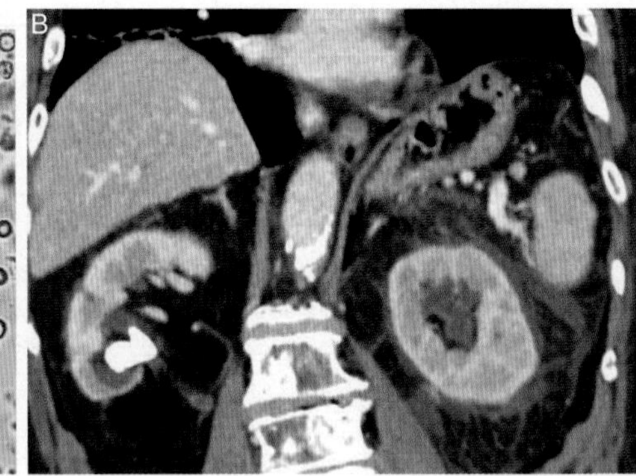

Management:

Scenario	Interventions
≤ 5 mm	- Pain control: NSAIDs or opioids - Fluids
5-10 mm	- Antispasmodics: **Tamsulosin** or nifedipine - Can initially monitor for spontaneous passage, but intervention generally required (see below)
> 10 mm	- Surgical removal. Depending on size/location: (1) Shock wave lithotripsy (2) Ureteroscopy with holmium laser lithotripsy
Staghorn	- Percutaneous nephrolithotomy
Septic patients	- If obstructing stone if found, percutaneous drainage or ureteral stenting is required, plus antibiotics
Prevention	- Increase fluids (> 2 L/day), low sodium diet, low protein diet, high citrate diet, normal calcium diet - Pharm: Thiazides, urine alkalinization (potassium citrate) for Ca stones. Allopurinol for uric acid stones.

Incontinence

Type	General	Clinical	Management
Urge	- **Uninhibited detrusor contraction** - Causes: - Idiopathic (elderly) - Neurologic (CVA, early MS, Parkinson) - Bladder irritation	- Sudden urge with loss of urine - Nocturnal wetting - Dx: Clinical. Urodynamics can confirm (but typically not used).	- **Bladder training, Kegels** - Anticholinergics (Oxybutynin, tolterodine, solifenacin, TCA) - Neurostimulators (sacral nerve modulation, posterior tibial nerve stimulator)
Stress	- Weakness of pelvic floor muscles, leads to proximal urethra below pelvic floor, **transmitting intraabdominal pressure to bladder** - Causes: - Obesity - Vaginal delivery (high parity) - Menopause	- Involuntary loss of urine with ↑ abdominal pressure (sneeze/cough) - Lacks nocturnal urge/symptoms - Dx: Bladder stress test, Q-tip test	- Lifestyle (weight loss, ↓ caffeine) - Kegels - Estrogen replacement (for those post-menopause) - Pessary - Surgery (midurethral sling or colposuspension)
Overflow	- Eventual **overflow from urinary retention**, due to obstruction or lack of normal detrusor muscle contractility - Causes: - Detrusor underactivity - Obstruction (BPH) - Pelvic organ prolapse - Neuropathy (MS, stroke, diabetes)	- Persistent small volume leakage, with small volume voids - Dx: Elevated post-void residual volume	- Catheterization (chronic retention) - Cholinergic (bethanechol) - α-blockers (doxazosin, terazosin) - Surgery may be required for outlet obstruction
Irritative	- Inflammation, from bladder irritant (UTI, malignancy, stone)	- Presents similarly to urge	- Treat underlying
Functional	- Can't get to bathroom		- Bladder training
Fistula	- Fistula formation between vagina and urethra or bladder	- Persistent vaginal leakage of urine - Dx: Dye test, cystourethroscopy	- Surgical repair (must wait 3-6 months after the insulting surgery to correct)

Urinary Tract Infection

Urinary Tract Infection

General: Infection of the lower genitourinary tract, synonymous with cystitis

Risk: Women, sexual activity, urinary catheterization, diabetes, pregnancy

Micro:

(1) ***E. coli* (most common)**
(2) Enterobacteriaceae (*Proteus, Klebsiella*)
(3) *S. saprophyticus*
(4) *Pseudomonas* (if healthcare exposure)

Clinical: **Dysuria, increased frequency/urgency, suprapubic pain**

Diagnosis: Clinical (symptoms above) sufficient for diagnosis
- **Urinalysis** (+ nitrites, leuk esterase) can be supportive
- Culture often not required, but used in those with persistent symptoms/high risk for drug-resistant organism

Management	Criteria	Management
Simple cystitis (uncomplicated)	- Infection confined to bladder in nonpregnant woman or man - Lacks systemic symptoms below	- First line: TMP-SMX, nitrofurantoin, fosfomycin
Complicated	(1) Systemic signs (e.g., Temp > 100°F) (2) Flank pain/CVA tenderness	[See: Next page]
Pregnancy	- [See: OB-GYN]	
Prophylaxis	- Recurrent UTI (≥ 2 UTIs in 6 months or ≥ 3 UTIs in 1 year) - Risks: Frequent sexual activity, spermicide use, post-menopause	- Behavioral modification (post-coital voiding, stop spermicides) - Pharm: Antibiotic prophylaxis. TMP-SMX or other drug can be used. Use can be daily, post-coital, or intermittent self-treatment.

Interstitial Cystitis/Bladder Pain Syndrome

General: Chronic bladder pain and discomfort for > 6 weeks without clear underlying medical cause

Risk: More common in women, psychiatric history

Clinical: Dysuria, increased urinary frequency, dyspareunia, relief with voiding, pelvic pain (with palpation)

Diagnosis: Diagnosis of exclusion. Urinalysis (rule out UTI).

Management:

(1) Behavioral modification (trigger avoidance)
(2) Pharm: Amitriptyline
(3) Analgesics (phenazopyridine, methenamine) for short-term relief
(4) Surgical interventions (bladder hydrodistention)

Urinary Tract Infection

Complicated UTI/Pyelonephritis

General: Infection of the upper urinary tract (extending past the bladder), most commonly from ascending lower urinary tract infection

Micro: *E. coli*, enterobacteriaceae (*Proteus, Klebsiella*), other gram negative (*Pseudomonas*), *Enterococcus*, fungi (*Candida*)

Clinical:

- UTI symptoms, plus **systemic signs (fever, chills, flank pain), CVA tenderness**
- Urinalysis (pyuria/bacteriuria, WBC casts)
- Gram stain and culture positive

Diagnosis:

- Clinical diagnosis (systemic symptoms plus pyuria and bacteriuria)
- Imaging (CT) reserved for cases when patient is not improving

Management:

	General	Empiric Management
Outpatient	- Young, otherwise healthy patients can receive ER care with close follow up	- Fluoroquinolone (ciprofloxacin) OR - IM Dose of ceftriaxone plus TMP-SMX, amox-clav, or cefpodoxime
Inpatient	- Septic/critically ill patients - Urinary hardware/obstruction	- Ceftriaxone (alt: Ciprofloxacin) - Cefepime, piperacillin-tazobactam, or carbapenem (if risk factor for MDRO)

Complications:

Renal/perinephric abscess

- Walled off cavity of necrosis. Can be
  - (1) Renal or
  - (2) Perinephric (perirenal fat to Gerota fascia)
- Presents most commonly as a patient with pyelonephritis who is slow to respond to therapy
- Generally occurs as a complication of pyelonephritis, but can be due to seeding
- Dx: CT or US
- Tx: Antibiotics +/– percutaneous drainage (> 3-5 cm abscesses)

Chronic pyelonephritis

- Chronic interstitial disease due to recurrent/chronic infection
- Causes: Vesicoureteral reflux, chronic urinary obstruction (stone)

Xanthogranulomatous pyelonephritis

- Subtype of chronic pyelonephritis (generally from obstructive stone)
- Massive kidney damage from granulomatous inflammation and foamy macrophages

Renal/Bladder Malignancy

Renal Cell Carcinoma

General: Most common cause of renal cancer (85%), usually composed of **clear cell tumors of proximal tubule epithelium.** Other subtypes include:

- Papillary tumors (proximal tubular cells)
- Oncocytomas (intercalated cell tumors, associated with tuberous sclerosis)

Risk:

- Male, age 50-70, obesity, cigarette smoking, occupational exposures, cytotoxic medications
- Polycystic kidney disease, genetic (including vHL)

Clinical: Variable presentation, including **abdominal mass, flank pain, hematuria**

- Systemic symptoms (fever, night sweats, weight loss) or symptoms from metastases
- Paraneoplastic syndromes:
    - Hypercalcemia (PTHrP or lytic bone lesions), erythrocytosis (excess EPO production)

Diagnosis: Abdominal CT[A] + Biopsy

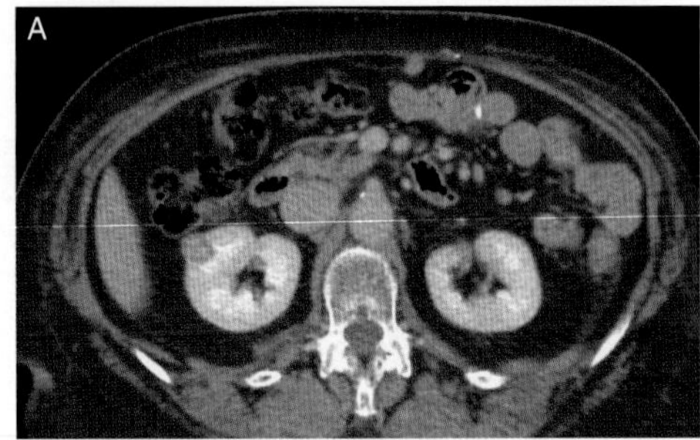

Management:

- Localized: Radical or partial nephrectomy
- Advanced: Targeted immunotherapy +/– surgical nephrectomy/ debulking
    - Immunotherapy includes checkpoint inhibitors (CTLA4 inhibitors, PD-1 inhibitors), anti-VEGF

Von-Hippel Lindau

General: AD defect in vHL gene on chromosome 3, which codes for a tumor suppressor protein

Clinical:

- Hemangioblastomas (retina, brain stem, cerebellum, spine)
- Renal cell carcinomas
- Pheochromocytoma
- Endolymphatic sac tumors of middle ear

Diagnosis: Suspected based on clinical features, but confirmed with genetic testing

Management: Screening (annual eye/retinal exam, abdominal MRI, urine metanephrines, brain/spinal MRI)

Bladder Cancer

Subtype	Risk Factors
Transitional Cell	- Urothelial carcinogens (smoking, cyclophosphamide, phenacetin, aniline dyes) - Jobs at risk for chemical exposure include painters, rubber/textile/leather workers, machinists
Adenocarcinoma	- Urachal remnant - Nonurachal: *Schistosoma* infection, bladder exstrophy
Squamous Cell	- Chronic inflammation (chronic/recurrent UTI, *Schistosoma* infection, radiation, bladder stone)

Clinical: **Painless hematuria** (generally age > 40)

Diagnosis: Cystoscopy + Biopsy

Management:

- No muscle invasion: TURBT (transurethral resection of bladder tumor)
- Muscle invasion: Radical cystectomy, plus neoadjuvant/adjuvant chemo, intravesical BCG or mitomycin

Prostate Malignancy

Prostate Cancer

General: Adenocarcinoma of prostate. 2nd most common cancer in men.

Risk: ↑ Age, Black, family history, genetics (BRCA, lynch)

Clinical:

- Most often asymptomatic, picked up on routine screening
    - **DRE showing nodularity**, irregularity (is indication for biopsy)
    - **PSA** (no clear set criteria or threshold value, but major increases from prior PSA, PSA > 7, or ↑ PSA in conjunction with abnormal exam is indication for biopsy)
- Rarely, advanced disease can cause symptoms (hematuria, dysuria, or bone pain from metastasis)
    - Note: BPH can also cause hematuria/dysuria

Diagnosis: **Transrectal biopsy** (with aid of transrectal US)

- At least 12 samples, add together two worst to calculate Gleason score

Management:

Screening	- Controversial. Currently advise shared decision making with patients (small increased ability to diagnose cancer, balanced with risk of overdiagnosis and unnecessary invasive procedures) - In general, those between 50-70 with > 10 yr life expectancy should consider PSA screening. Other ages unlikely to get benefit, unless at especially high risk.
Initial Eval	- Local Staging (DRE + transrectal US +/– MRI) - Tech-99 bone scan (if symptomatic or high risk for metastasis)
Initial Therapy (local disease)	- Very low/low risk (Gleason ≤ 6) → Active surveillance (consider radiation therapy or prostatectomy) - Intermediate risk (Gleason 7) → RT or prostatectomy - High/Very high risk (Gleason ≥ 8) → RT +/– brachytherapy and androgen deprivation therapy or radical prostatectomy - Surveillance with PSA for all
Lymph Node Involvement/ Disseminated	- Androgen deprivation therapy: Medical (leuprolide) or surgical orchiectomy - Possible chemotherapy

Pediatric Renal Neoplasia

Wilms Tumor

General: Most common childhood renal malignancy. Associated with WT1 mutation on chromosome 11.

Etiology: Can be idiopathic. 10% associated with congenital syndromes (below).

Clinical:

- **Abdominal mass/swelling (usually smooth, rarely cross midline)**
  - Often asymptomatic, discovered on routine health visit
- May be associated with abdominal pain, vomiting, hypertension
- Lung is most common metastatic site

Diagnosis:

- Imaging (US)
- Surgical excision/biopsy for definitive diagnosis

Management:

- Surgical resection
- Chemotherapy and/or radiation therapy (indications depend on stage)

Congenital Syndromes (associated with Wilms)

Beckwith-Wiedemann	- Wilms tumor - Macroglossia - Macrosomia, limb hemihypertrophy - Medial abdominal wall defects (omphalocele) - Hyperinsulinism (hypoglycemia) - Hepatoblastoma (monitor with abdominal US and AFP levels)
WAGR	- Wilms tumor - Aniridia - GU malformation - Retardation
Denys-Drash	- Wilms tumor - Progressive kidney failure - Male pseudohermaphroditism

Pediatric Urology

Congenital Renal Abnormalities

Type	General	Clinical	Management
Potter	- Syndrome due to severe oligohydramnios in utero	- **Pulmonary hypoplasia** - **Limb deformities** (club feet, hip dislocation) - Abnormal facies (flattened ears/nose, recessed chin)	
Horseshoe Kidney	- Fusion of lower poles of the kidneys - Often found in pelvis with abnormal blood supply (**trapped under IMA**)	- Most often asymptomatic - Can result in hydronephrosis, recurrent infection, or stones	- Usually requires no intervention
Renal Agenesis	- Complete lack of kidney one or both kidneys - Ureteric bud fails to develop and induce differentiation of metanephric mesenchyme	- Bilateral renal agenesis is always fatal early in life - Unilateral renal agenesis is often asymptomatic	
Multicystic Dysplastic Kidney	- Congenital cystic renal dysplasia - Nonfunctional kidney consisting of cysts and connective tissue	- Diagnosed on prenatal ultrasound - Often asymptomatic if other kidney normal (which should hypertrophy in response)	- Observation (abnormal kidney will naturally involute)
Ureteropelvic-junction Obstruction	- Blockage where ureter enters kidney, causing hydronephrosis - Caused by ureteral stenosis/compression	- Often discovered due to hydronephrosis - Can present as abdominal mass, UTI - Can also present after large volume intake (binge drinking) - Dx: US, followed by diuretic renography	- Symptomatic patients receive surgical correction
Ectopic Ureter	- Abnormal insertion of ureter into bladder (Note: Girls can also implant into vagina) - Often associated with duplex collecting system	- Associated with pediatric UTI, vesicoureteral reflux, and urinary incontinence - Dx: US (hydroureter/hydronephrosis)	- Surgical correction

Vesicoureteral Reflux

General: Retrograde passage of urine from bladder into upper urinary tract, most commonly due to inadequate closure of the ureterovesical junction. Increased risk for recurrent upper urinary tract infections and CKD.

Etiology:

- **Primary**: Mechanical failure of the ureterovesical junction (most common)
- **Secondary**: Excess bladder pressure (from posterior urethral valve, bladder obstruction)

Clinical: Can be diagnosed prenatally as hydronephrosis

- Also often diagnosed after febrile UTI in infants and young children

Grades

Grade I	- Urine refluxes part way up ureter
Grade II	- Urine refluxes all the way up ureter
Grade III	- Grade II, plus mild dilatation of ureter and blunting of calyces
Grade IV	- Severe dilatation or ureter/blunting of calyces
Grade V	- Massive dilatation or ureter/blunting of calyces, plus loss of renal cortex

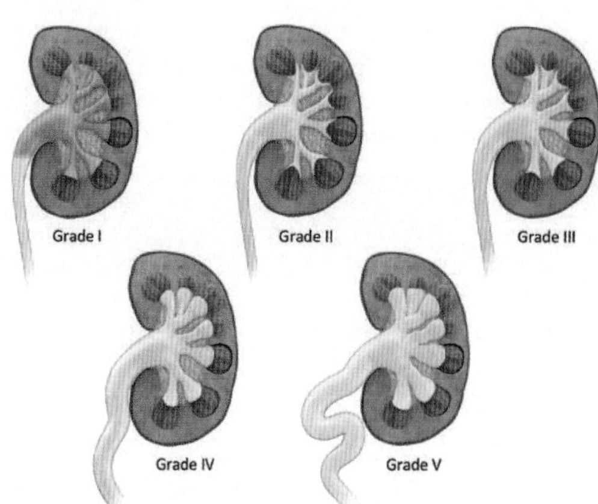

Diagnosis: Voiding cystourethrogram (VCUG)

Management:

- Grade 1/2: Watchful waiting. Antibiotic prophylaxis is an option. 80% have spontaneous resolution.
- Grade 3-5: Antibiotic prophylaxis. Surgery in grade 4-5 and refractory cases.

Pediatric Urology

Pediatric UTI

Clinical: Most commonly presents with fever, abdominal pain, dysuria, incontinence

Diagnosis: Urinalysis/culture (must be clean sample, straight cath often necessary in neonates/infants)
- > 5-10 WBCs/HPF, + leuk esterase or nitrite indicative of UTI
- **> 10,000 CFU on culture of straight cath** (> 100,000 on clean cath)

Management: 1-2 weeks of antibiotics (**2nd/3rd generation cephalosporins** first line)
- Must workup for vesicoureteral reflux with renal/bladder US if < 2 y/o, recurrent UTI, or persistent UTI
- VCUG: Used if positive US results, ≥ 2 y/o febrile UTIs

Posterior Urethral Valves

General: Congenital posterior **urethral obstruction due to membranous folds**

Clinical: Most often identified prenatally on US (hydronephrosis, dilated bladder)
- Postnatally can present as UTI, poor urinary stream, abdominal distension
- ↑ Risk for CKD and bladder dysfunction

Diagnosis: VCUG (dilated posterior urethra with linear defect in the voiding phase). Confirm with cystoscopy.

Management: Postnatal (initial): Urinary catheter for drainage
- After stabilized, **surgical correction (cystoscopy + ablation)**

Hypospadias/Epispadias

Hypospadias	- Congenital anomaly with abnormal ventral opening of male urethra - Often associated with abnormal foreskin/urethral meatus - Tx: Delay circumcision, with surgical closure weeks after birth
Epispadias	- Congenital opening of urethra on dorsal surface of penis - Associated with bladder exstrophy

Cryptorchidism

General: Failure of descent of testicle by 4 months of age. If bilateral, must suspect endocrine or genetic disorder.

Risk: Prematurity, SGA/low birth weight, genetic disorders, neural tube defects

Clinical: **Empty, hypoplastic, poorly rugated scrotum**
- Possible inguinal fullness (indicating testicle in inguinal canal)

Diagnosis: Clinical

Management: **Orchiopexy (before year 1)**
- Indicated after 6 months, as unlikely to spontaneously descend after this point
- Without intervention, high risk for testicular cancer, infertility, torsion, inguinal hernia

Phimosis/Paraphimosis

	Phimosis	Paraphimosis
Gen	- Tight foreskin that cannot be retracted to show glans - Normal (physiologic) in newborns, but should resolve by school age - Pathologic: Truly nonretractable foreskin due to distal scarring of prepuce (from trauma or inflammation)	- Retracted foreskin that cannot be returned to normal position - Usually occurs with forcible retraction of the foreskin
Clin	- Can be associated with irritation, dysuria, painful erections, recurrent infections	- Causes severe pain and swelling, focused on the glans
Tx	- Stretching exercises, topical corticosteroids - Circumcision (definitive)	- Pain control/manual reduction - Surgical correction for severe cases

Pediatric Fluids/Electrolytes

Pediatric Volume

Severity	Symptoms
Mild (3-5%)	- Sticky or slightly dry oral mucosa - Increased thirst - Normal vitals - Normal/slightly decreased urine output
Moderate (6-9%)	- Dry oral mucosa - Increased thirst, irritable - Sunken eyes/fontanelle, reduced skin turgor - Tachycardia, tachypnea, possible hypotension - Decreased urine output
Severe (>10%)	- Very dry oral mucosa - Lethargy, coma - Sunken eyes/fontanelle, reduced skin turgor - Cool skin, acrocyanosis - Tachycardia, tachypnea, hypotension - Anuria

Management:

- Emergent replacement (for moderate/severe dehydration)
    - 20 mL/kg IV bolus of isotonic saline
    - Repeat as necessary until replete
- Secondary fluid repletion (for mild/moderate dehydration, or after emergent replacement if severe)
    - Oral fluid replacement preferred

Proteinuria

General: Protein excretion > 100 mg/m^2 in children

Cause	Features
Transient Proteinuria	- Transient increases in urinary protein excretion - Induced by fever, strenuous exercise, seizures, hypovolemia - No intervention necessary
Orthostatic Proteinuria	- Benign increase in protein excretion when upright - Confirm with early morning urinalysis or P/Cr ratio - Requires no further workup or intervention once diagnosed
Persistent (Pathologic)	- Persistent on multiple occasions, concerning for glomerular or tubular pathology - Workup with 24-hour urine protein, US, and pediatric nephrology referral

Testicular Cancer

Testicular Cancer	
Subtype	**Description/Features**
Germ Cell (Seminomatous)	
Seminoma	- Most common subtype, with good prognosis - Highly sensitive to treatment (chemo/radiotherapy) - "Fried egg cell" histology (large cell, eccentric nucleolus, clear cytoplasm) - Serum biomarkers usually normal
Germ Cell (Nonseminomatous)	
Embryonal	- Malignant subtype with aggressive spread - Modest hCG production
Yolk sac	- Endodermal sinus tumor - Common child subtype, with characteristic **AFP production**
Choriocarcinoma	- Most malignant with rapid hematogenous spread - **β-HCG production**
Teratoma	- Benign (usually in kids) or malignant (usually in adults, associated with mixed-germ cell tumors) - Derived from multiple embryonic layers
Mixed germ cell	- Multiple types of germ cell tumor present
Sex-Cord Stromal	
Leydig	- Produce **androgens or estrogen** (precocious puberty, gynecomastia in kids, or erectile dysfunction, impotence/loss of libido in adults)
Sertoli	- Benign and usually clinically silent
Other	
Lymphoma	- Occurs in older males. Diffuse large B-cell.

General: Generally seen in men between 15 and 35 y/o. Most commonly germ cell tumors.

Risk: Cryptorchidism, infertility, personal/family history of testicular cancer

Clinical: Most common clinical feature of testicular cancer is a **painless testicular mass**

Diagnosis:
- US (solid mass is highly concerning for cancer)
- Further evaluation with β-hCG, AFP, LDH, pelvic CT

Management:
- Radical inguinal orchiectomy (both diagnostic and therapeutic)
- Adjuvant chemotherapy or radiotherapy for higher risk local disease
- Chemotherapy (bleomycin, etoposide, cisplatin) for disseminated disease (lymph node or distant metastasis)

Prostate

Benign Prostatic Hyperplasia

General: Benign enlargement of the prostate from growth of transitional zone (also known as periurethral zone)

Risk: > 50 y/o, Black men

Clinical: Often asymptomatic (especially early on)
- **Storage symptoms** (urgency, incontinence, ↑ frequency, nocturia)
- **Voiding symptoms** (↓ urinary stream, hesitancy, straining to void, dribbling)
- Hematuria (both microscopic and gross) possible
- Diffusely enlarged, firm, nontender prostate on DRE

Diagnosis: Clinical (from history and physical). Check PSA.

Management: Behavioral change (avoid diuretics like caffeine/EtOH, ↓ fluids at bedtime)
- Pharm:
  - Mild to moderate: α1 antagonists (tamsulosin, doxazosin)
  - Severe: α1 antagonists PLUS 5α reductase inhibitor (finasteride)
- Surgery (Indicated if: Renal dysfunction, hydronephrosis, severe urinary retention, recurrent UTI)
  - **Transurethral resection or ablation (TURP)**

Bacterial Prostatitis

	Acute Bacterial Prostatitis	Chronic Bacterial Prostatitis
Gen	- Acute prostate infection, usually affecting younger men - *E. coli, Gonorrhea, Chlamydia*	- Subtle, nonacute prostate infection seen in older men - More common than acute prostatitis - Gram negative rods (e.g., *E. Coli*) most common
Clin	- Fevers, chills, **toxic appearing** - UTI symptoms (dysuria, frequency) - Pelvic/perineal/low back pain - **Exquisitely tender prostate on DRE** - Cloudy urine/pyuria	- **Recurrent UTI with same organism** - Often chronically symptomatic, mild lower UTI symptoms - Prostate may be tender on exam, but is often normal
Dx	- Clinical - Urine gram stain/culture	- Clinical (presumptive dx/treatment) - Urine gram stain/culture after prostatic massage
Tx	- TMP-SMX or fluoroquinolone	- Fluoroquinolone - If no improvement, suspect chronic prostatitis (below)

Chronic Prostatitis/Chronic Pelvic Pain Syndrome

General: Clinical noninfectious syndrome of urologic symptoms and pelvic pain, without clear pathophysiology or etiology

Clinical:
- Pain (in perineum/pelvis/genitalia)
- Voiding difficulty, dysuria
- Pain with ejaculation
- Minimal prostatic tenderness of DRE, sterile urine culture

Diagnosis: Clinical (diagnosis of exclusion)

Management:
- Initial: Tamsulosin + fluoroquinolone
- Chronic: α blockers and 5α reductase inhibitors

Penile/Testicular Pathology

Penile Pathology

Disorder	Clinical Features
Balanitis/ Balanoposthitis	- Infection of head of penis and foreskin, respectively - Usually due to inadequate hygiene in uncircumcised men - Tx: Hygiene, saline irrigation, topical antifungals if severe
Priapism	- **Persistent erection** no associated with sexual stimulation (for at least 4 hours) - Risk for penile ischemia and permanent erectile dysfunction - Causes include ischemic (Low flow: PDE5 inhibitor use, sickle cell, prazosin, trazodone) or nonischemic (high-flow: Fistula between artery/corpus cavernosum, usually after trauma) - Dx: Clinical. Evaluate with US or cavernous aspiration/ABG. - Tx: Ischemic → phenylephrine injection. Nonischemic → observe, with arteriography/ embolization if not improving.
Penile Fracture	- Occurs with erect penis during sex - Snapping sound, with rapid detumescence, and severe pain - Evaluate with US, followed by emergent surgical repair
Carcinoma of the Penis	- Most commonly SCC. Very rare in US/Europe. - Risk: Older men, third-world countries, phimosis, HPV infection - Presents as mass or ulceration, usually at glans, associated with local lymphadenopathy - Dx: Biopsy - Tx: Local excision, +/– lymph node dissection and chemotherapy
Erythroplasia of Queyrat	- Carcinoma in situ on glans, velvety red appearance
Bowen disease	- Carcinoma in situ, on penile shaft epithelium - Presents as single red plaque with crusting and oozing

Scrotum/Testicular Pathology

Disorder	General	Clinical	Management
Varicocele	- Dilation of venous pampiniform plexus - Usually left-sided (nutcracker effect on left renal vein, ↑ pressure) - Right-sided varicocele indicates possible venous thrombosis	- Soft, scrotal mass, "bag of worms" - Becomes less severe when lying down - Can cause aching pain, testicular atrophy, or infertility if severe - US can confirm dilated veins, retrograde flow	- Support/NSAIDs - Gonadal vein ligation or embolization (if severe)
Hydrocele	- Collection of fluid between parietal and visceral layers of tunica vaginalis (from lack of obliteration) - Can also be secondary to neoplasm or inflammation	- Presents as smooth, transilluminating mass - Generally nontender	- No intervention required, unless symptomatic (surgical excision)
Spermatocele	- Cystic sac in the epididymis	- Soft, round mass in head of epididymis	- Supportive
Fourniers	- Necrotizing fasciitis of the scrotum and perineum - Mixed aerobic/anaerobic bacteria	- Causes sudden pain - Skin signs: Tense edema, blistering, crepitus. Odor/purulent discharge. - Systemic signs (fever, weakness, shock)	- IV antibiotics PLUS surgical debridement

Penile/Testicular Pathology

Testicular Torsion

General: Inadequate fixation of the testes to the tunica vaginalis, allowing for twisting of testes around spermatic cord, with ischemia from vascular obstruction

Clinical:

- Acute **severe testicular pain**, can cause nausea, vomiting
- Profound swelling and diffuse tenderness
- **Negative cremasteric reflex**, "high-riding" testis oriented transversely
- Common scenarios include post trauma or physical activity, or waking up in the middle of night (in kids)
- **Prehn sign**: Lifting of testes alleviates pain from epididymitis, not torsion

Diagnosis: Scrotal US

Management: Detorsion and fixation (of both testes)

Appendix Testis Torsion

- Most occurs in school age children
- Presents with gradual onset of pain. Cremasteric reflex is normal.
  - "Blue dot sign" (blue spot seen through scrotum in superior aspect of the testes)
- Dx: Scrotal US
- Tx: NSAIDs, ice, scrotal support

Epididymitis

General: Inflammation of the epididymis. Usually infectious, but can be autoimmune or traumatic.

- < 35: Gonorrhea/Chlamydia most common
- > 35: *E. Coli*, *Pseudomonas*, other gram negatives

Clinical:

- **Localized testicular pain** (tenderness/swelling over epididymis)
- Can spread to testis (orchitis), causing testicular pain
- Dysuria or other urinary symptoms are possible

Diagnosis: Clinical. US to rule out torsion, and obtain urine culture/urinalysis.

Management:

- High-risk for STI: Ceftriaxone/doxycycline
- Low-risk for STI: Fluoroquinolone

Hematuria

General Hematuria

Definitions:

- **Microscopic Hematuria**: ≥ 3 RBC on microscopy
- **Gross Hematuria**: Grossly red urine
- **Pseudohematuria**: Red pigment in urine (from foods like beets, and drugs like rifampin)
- **Other Pigments**: Myoglobin, bilirubin (both can present with dark urine)

Hematuria Throughout	Terminal Hematuria	Initial Hematuria
- Glomerulonephritis - Pyelonephritis - Nephrolithiasis - Upper urinary cancers	- Cystitis - Bladder stones or cancer - BPH/prostate cancer	- Urethra injury (trauma, urethritis)

Hematuria Workup

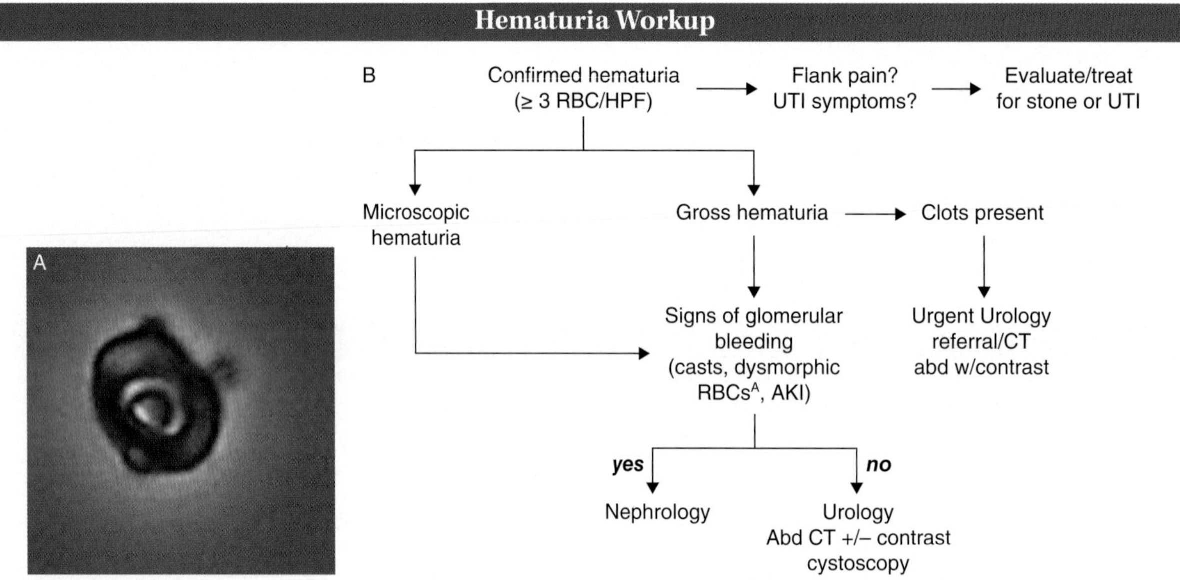

Imaging Options

Test	Indications
CT urography (CT abdomen/pelvis with/without contrast)	- Unexplained hematuria
CT abdomen (w/o contrast)	- Stones, masses
Ultrasound	- Stones, masses in someone with contraindication to radiation
Cystoscopy	- Evaluation of bladder (for mass, bleeding)

Renal Pharm

	Mechanism	Indication	Side Effects/Management
Acetazolamide	- Carbonic anhydrase inhibitor (HCO_3 diuresis)	- Glaucoma - Urinary alkalinization, - Altitude sickness	- Sulfa drug - Proximal RTA - Kidney stones
Loop Diuretics Furosemide Bumetanide Torsemide Ethacrynic acid	- Inhibit Na/K/2Cl transporter of thick ascending limb of the loop of Henle	- Edema - Hypercalcemia	- Sulfa drug (except ethacrynic acid) - Ototoxicity (high doses) - Hypokalemia, hypocalcemia, contraction alkalosis - Nephritis (interstitial) - Gout
Thiazides HCTZ Chlorthalidone Metolazone	- Inhibit NaCl transporter in distal convoluted tubule - Increases distal tubule Ca^{2+} resorption	- Hypertension - Hypercalciuria - Diabetes insipidus	- Sulfa drug - Hypokalemic metabolic alkalosis - Hyponatremia - Hyperglycemia - Hyperlipidemia - Hyperuricemia
K-Sparing Spironolactone Eplerenone Triamterene Amiloride	- Competitive aldosterone antagonists (spirono/ eplerenone) - Na channel blockers in collecting duct	- HF - Cirrhosis - Hyperaldosteronism	- Hyperkalemia - Anti androgen (spirono): Gynecomastia
ACEi Captopril Enalapril Lisinopril	- Inhibits ACE (conversion of ANG to ANG-II) - Also inhibits breakdown of bradykinin	- HTN - CHF - Proteinuria	- Cough - Angioedema - Teratogen - ↑ Creatinine - Hyperkalemia
ARB Losartan Candesartan Valsartan	- Inhibits AR-1 (angiotensin receptor)	- HTN - CHF - Proteinuria	- Teratogen - ↑ Creatinine - Hyperkalemia
Aliskiren	- Direct renin inhibitor	- HTN	- Hyperkalemia, ↑ Creatinine
Urologic Drugs			
Tamsulosin	- $\alpha 1_A$ receptor antagonist	- BPH - Hypertension (second-line agent)	- Hypotension (orthostasis, syncope)
Doxazosin Terazosin Doxazosin	- $\alpha 1$ receptor antagonist		
Finasteride	- 5α-reductase inhibitor	- BPH - Prostate cancer - Male pattern baldness	- Sexual dysfunction
Flutamide	- Androgen receptor antagonist	- Prostate cancer	- Anti-androgen effects (gynecomastia, breast tenderness, sexual dysfunction)
Sildenafil Vardenafil Tadalafil	- Phosphodiesterase 5 inhibitor	- Erectile dysfunction	- Headache, flushing, nausea - Cyanopia (blue vision) - Hypotension (must avoid use with nitrates especially)
Alprostadil	- PGE1 agonist	- Erectile dysfunction (corporal injections or urethral suppositories)	

Hypothalamic Pituitary Axis

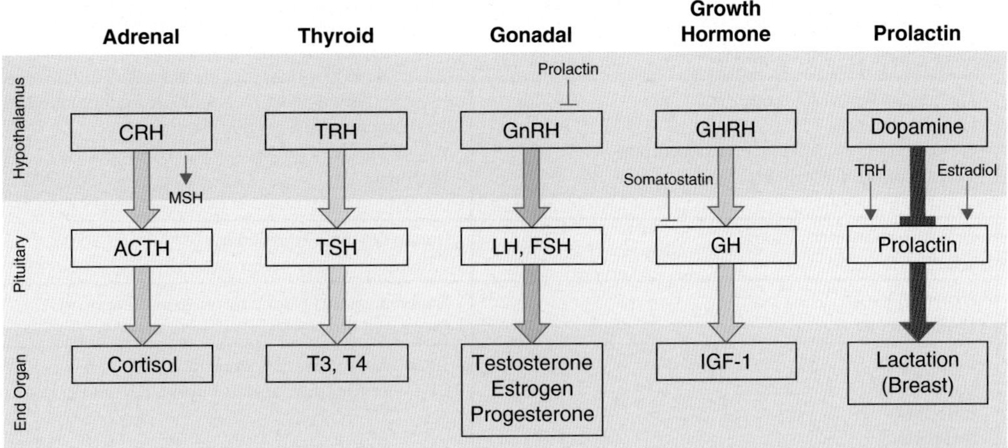

Thyroid Hormone

Functions:

- Bone growth
- CNS maturation
- Increase metabolic rate (Na/K pumps)
- Increased β1 heart receptors (increased CO, contractility, HR, SV)

Regulatory:

- **Wolff-Chaikoff**: Large iodine intake → Decrease T3/T4 level
- **Jod-Basedow**: Excess T3/T4 production after iodine intake in someone with hyperthyroidism

Binding:

- Thyroxine-binding globulin (TBG)
- Increased production due to estrogen (e.g., pregnancy, oral contraceptives)
    - Raises total T4, normal TSH and free T4

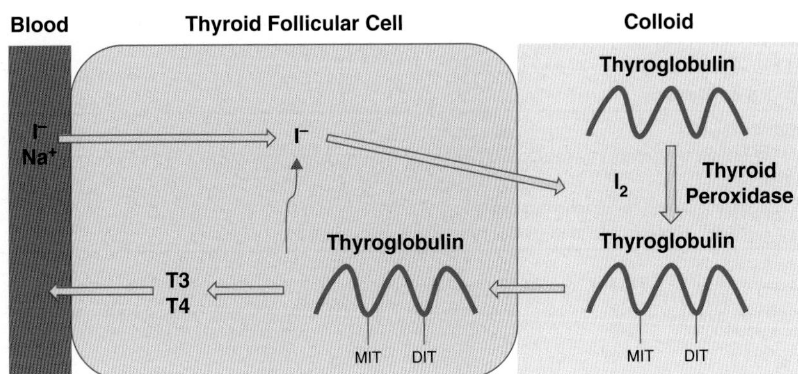

Thyroid Disease

Clinical Features of Hypo/Hyperthyroidism

	Hypothyroidism	Hyperthyroidism
Symptoms	- Fatigue, weakness, lethargy, weight gain - Cold intolerance - Slowed mentation, inability to concentrate - Constipation, menorrhagia	- Hyperactivity, anxiety, insomnia, irritability, palpitations - Tremors, sweating, heat intolerance - Weight loss with normal/increased appetite - Diarrhea
Exam	- Dry skin, hoarseness, edema - ↓ Reflexes	- Goiter, fine hair, stare/lid lag - ↑ Reflexes
Lab	- Hyperlipidemia - Hyponatremia	- Hypercalcemia (↑ bone turnover), osteoporosis - Decreased lipid levels
Other findings	- Bradycardia - Hypertension - Infertility - Myopathy	- Tachyarrhythmias (AF, sinus tach) - CV (↑ contractility, cardiac output, HR, pulse pressure)

Hypothyroidism

Etiology	Clinical	Diagnostic Findings
Chronic Lymphocytic Thyroiditis (Hashimoto)	- Autoimmune lymphocytic thyroid invasion - Presents as gradual loss of thyroid function - Increased risk of non-Hodgkin B cell lymphoma	- Elevated anti-TPO, TG antibody
Painless Thyroiditis	- Variant of Hashimoto - Transient hyper, then (possible) hypothyroid states - Generally resolves to euthyroid	- Low radioiodine uptake
Subacute Thyroiditis (de Quervain)	- Postviral inflammatory process - Transient hyper, then hypothyroid states - Exam: Painful, tender thyroid	- Low radioiodine uptake - Elevated ESR/CRP
Fibrous Thyroiditis (Riedel's)	- Fibrous thyroid infiltration - Signs of thyroid extension (hoarseness, dyspnea, dysphagia) - Exam: Slowly growing, painless, firm goiter	- Associated with IgG4 disorders
Subclinical	- High TSH with normal T3/T4 - Generally asymptomatic	
Euthyroid Sick	- Decreased T3/T4 in the setting of critical illness - TSH can be normal, increased, or decreased. ↑ reverse T3. - Intervention not indicated	
Other	- Postpartum thyroiditis - Iatrogenic (radioiodine therapy, thyroidectomy, drugs [Lithium, Amiodarone]) - Iodine deficiency - Infiltrative disease (sarcoid, hemochromatosis) - Secondary/tertiary hypothyroidism (anterior pituitary & hypothalamic disease)	

Diagnosis: Primary (Overt) Hypothyroidism: **↑ TSH, ↓ free T4**. TPO antibodies.
- Central hypothyroidism: ↓ TSH, ↓ T4

Management:
- Overt: **Levothyroxine** (check TSH in 6 weeks, titrate dose to TSH 0.5-5.0)
- Subclinical: TSH ≥ 10 or symptomatic receive levothyroxine

Myxedema Coma:
- Rare, severe hypothyroidism leading to multiorgan dysfunction
- Clinical: Altered mental status, hypoventilation, hypothermia, hypotension, hyponatremia, bradycardia
- Tx: Levothyroxine/Liothyronine, mechanical ventilation, corticosteroids, fluids

Thyroid Disease

Hyperthyroidism

Etiology	Clinical Findings
Graves	- **Most common** cause of hyperthyroidism - Due to production of **TSH receptor Ig** (specific finding) - Exam: Diffusely enlarged, symmetric nontender thyroid (+/– bruit) - Ophthalmopathy: **Exophthalmos**[A], periorbital edema, diplopia (due to orbital inflammation, GAG buildup) - **Pretibial myxedema** (due to dermal inflammation, GAG buildup)
Multinodular Goiter	- Hyperfunctioning thyroid nodules, with atrophy of remaining thyroid
Thyroid Adenoma	- Rare. Single hyperfunctioning nodule.
Thyroiditis	- All causes of thyroiditis can cause transient hyperthyroidism
Other	- Iatrogenic (Levothyroxine), excess iodine, drugs, central hyperthyroidism (pituitary TSHoma) - Amiodarone (Type 1: Occurs with pre existing thyroid disease. Type II: Destructive thyroiditis.)

Diagnosis: TSH ↓ and T3/T4 ↑ in primary hyperthyroidism
- Acute onset of hyperthyroidism with clinical features of Graves is sufficient for diagnosis
- If unsure, TSH-R Ab, radioactive uptake, and thyroglobulin levels

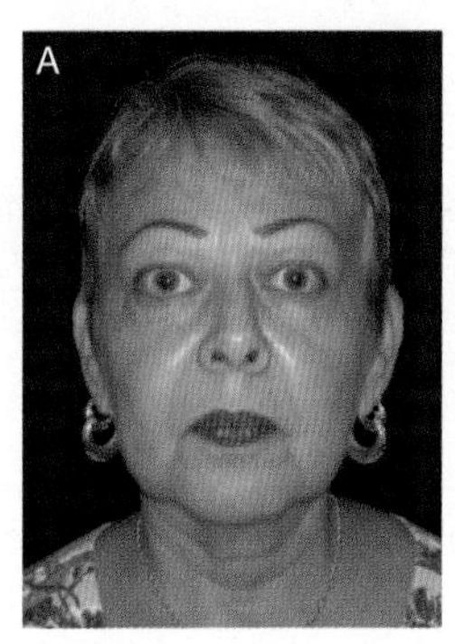

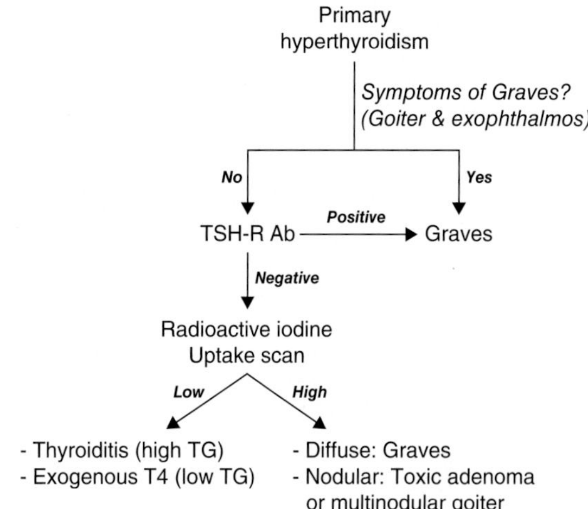

Management: Graves

Acute	Used for initial symptomatic control, prior to definitive therapy: - Beta-blocker (atenolol, metoprolol, propranolol) - Thionamide (methimazole)	
Definitive	**Indication**	**Drawbacks**
Thionamide	- Mildly symptomatic - Older age (limited remaining life)	- Medication side effects (e.g., agranulocytosis)
Radioiodine ablation	- Moderate or severely symptomatic hyperthyroidism	- Permanent hypothyroidism - Worsens orbitopathy
Surgery	- Moderate or severe orbitopathy - Large/obstructive goiter - Cancer	- Permanent hypothyroidism - Hypoparathyroidism - Recurrent laryngeal nerve damage

Note: Toxic adenoma/multinodular goiter follow the same above acute/chronic plan. Radioiodine ablation or surgery are utilized for definitive management.

Thyroid Storm:
- General: Acute, life-threatening complication of thyrotoxicosis. Occurs with chronic untreated hyperthyroidism.
- Precipitated by stressor (sepsis, DKA, trauma, surgery, labor, acute iodine load [contrast])
- Clinical: Hyperpyrexia (up to 106°F), encephalopathy, tachycardia, hypertension, arrhythmia, diarrhea, emesis
- Diagnosis: Clinical features PLUS elevated T3/T4
- Management: Beta-blocker (propranolol), corticosteroids, propylthiouracil, potassium iodine, ICU level care

Thyroid Disease

Thyroid Nodule

General: Cancer is found in ~5-10% of all investigated nodules. Malignancy is suggested by firm, fixed, irregular masses with associated lymphadenopathy. Nodules investigated with algorithm below.

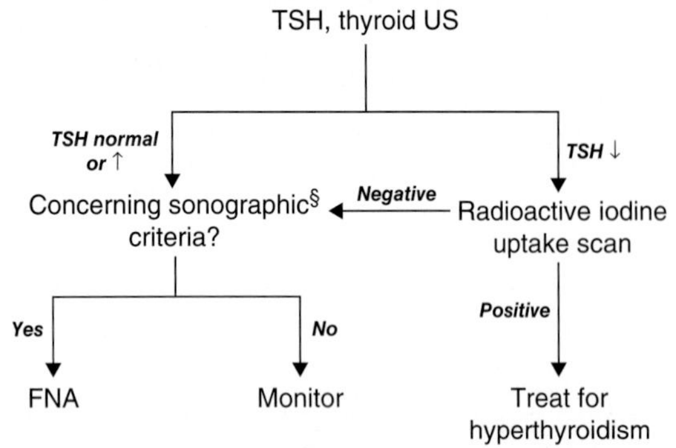

§Sonographic criteria:
- Large nodules (≥ 2 cm)
- Small nodules (≥ 1 cm) with suspicious US features (i.e., micro calcifications, irregular margins, extrathyroidal invasion)

- Purely cystic lesions are almost always benign

FNA Result	Management
Benign	- Reassurance and periodic US monitoring
Indeterminate	- Repeat FNA - If still indeterminate, follow up with molecular testing or diagnostic surgery
Suspicious	- Surgery

Thyroid Malignancy

Subtype	Features	Management
Papillary	- Most common thyroid cancer - Risk: Radiation, family history	- Total thyroidectomy or lobectomy
Follicular	- Well-differentiated tumor of thyroid epithelium - Risk: Radiation, family history - Vascular spread	- Total thyroidectomy or lobectomy
Medullary	- Parafollicular cell tumor with characteristic **calcitonin** production - Risk: Sporadic, or MEN2 associated	- Total thyroidectomy with lymph node dissection
Anaplastic	- Poorly differentiated tumor found more commonly in **elderly** - Poor prognosis	- Chemoradiation + Surgery (for purely local disease)
Lymphoma	- Rare B-cell neoplasm associated with Hashimoto - Presents as rapidly enlarging goiter with extra thyroid compression (dyspnea, dysphagia)	- Chemoradiation

Note: Choice of total vs lobectomy is based on size and lymph node involvement.

Post-surgery management:
- Levothyroxine with TSH monitoring (want it suppressed)
- Radioiodine ablation (for those with regional extension/metastatic disease)

Diabetes Insipidus

Nephrogenic and Central DI

General: Deficient secretion or response to ADH, resulting in polyuria and abnormal water balance

Etiology	Pathophysiology	Causes
Central	- Abnormal neurohypophyseal ADH secretion	- Idiopathic (most likely autoimmune) - Pituitary trauma, surgery, ischemic lesions, infiltrative disease - Congenital (Wolfram syndrome)
Nephrogenic	- Renal tubular ADH resistance	- Drugs (lithium, demeclocycline, foscarnet, amphotericin) - Hypercalcemia - Sjogren syndrome - Congenital (AQP-2 defects)

Clinical: Polyuria (> 3 L/day), polydipsia, nocturia

- Note: Central DI can have impaired thirst mechanism, leading to higher Na^+

Diagnosis:

- High normal or elevated $[Na^+]$ is indicative of DI, but not always present
- Water restriction test (patient water deprived, urine Osm measured)

	Water Deprivation Urine Osm (mOsm/kg)	**+ Desmopressin** Urine Osm (mOsm/kg)
Normal	> 700	No response
Central DI	< 300	> 300 mOsm/kg or > 50-100% increase in Uosm
Nephrogenic DI	< 300	No or minimal response
Polydipsia	> 300-700	No response

Management:

- **Nephrogenic DI**: Sodium restriction, thiazides
- **Central DI**: Sodium restriction, thiazides, desmopressin

Polyuria DDx

Note: Polyuria is defined as > 3 L of urine/day (different than urinary frequency seen with BPH, UTI, etc.)

(1) Nephrogenic or central DI
(2) Primary polydipsia
(3) Solute diuresis
- Glucose
- Sodium (after large volume expansion)
- Urea (azotemia)

(4) Diuretic use
(5) Hypercalcemia

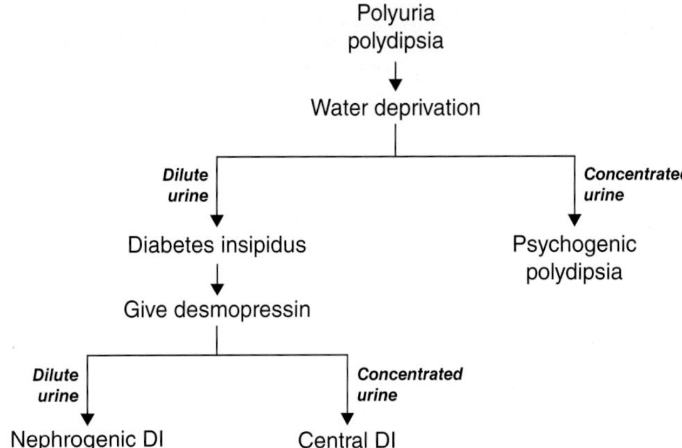

Hyperaldosteronism

Primary Hyperaldosteronism

General: Elevated, unregulated, and inappropriate adrenal aldosterone production

Etiology:

- **Adrenal hyperplasia** (~66%)
- Adrenal adenoma (~33%) ("Conn syndrome")
- Adrenal carcinoma (~1%)

Clinical: **Hypertension, hypokalemia, metabolic alkalosis**, mild hypernatremia

- Euvolemic due to aldosterone escape

Diagnosis:

- ↓ Plasma renin, ↑ plasma aldosterone. **Elevated aldosterone:renin ratio** (> 20).
- If ratio elevated, adrenal suppression test (see below)
    - Patient given sodium load via diet or saline infusion
    - Test is positive if urinary aldosterone is not suppressed

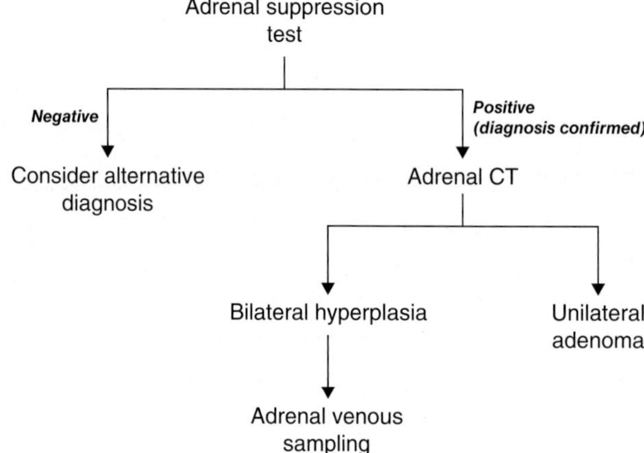

Note: Adrenal venous sampling can help to differentiate unilateral from bilateral disease, as the management differs.

Management:

- Unilateral adenoma/hyperplasia: Adrenalectomy
- Bilateral hyperplasia: Medical therapy (spironolactone or eplerenone)

Secondary Hyperaldosteronism

General: Hyperreninemic hyperaldosteronism (elevated RAAS activity), typically due to limited renal perfusion

Etiology:

- Renal artery stenosis
- Edematous disorders (e.g., HF, cirrhosis, nephrotic syndrome)
- Juxtaglomerular renin secreting tumor (very rare)

Hypercortisolism

Cushing Disease and Syndrome

General: Clinical syndrome of excess effects of cortisol (Cushing syndrome)

Etiology:

- Iatrogenic (taking exogenous glucocorticoids)
- Central pituitary tumor ACTH secretion ("Cushing disease")
- Ectopic non pituitary tumor ACTH production
- Adrenal production (adenoma or carcinoma)

Clinical:

- Appearance: Central obesity, hirsutism, moon facies, "buffalo hump," purple striae, acne, easy bruising
- Hypertension, hyperglycemia
- Menstrual irregularity or hypogonadism
- Proximal muscle weakness/wasting
- Depression, mania, or psychosis
- Skin hyperpigmentation (if ACTH-dependent)
- Immunosuppression: Impairs neutrophils, ↓ eosinophil counts

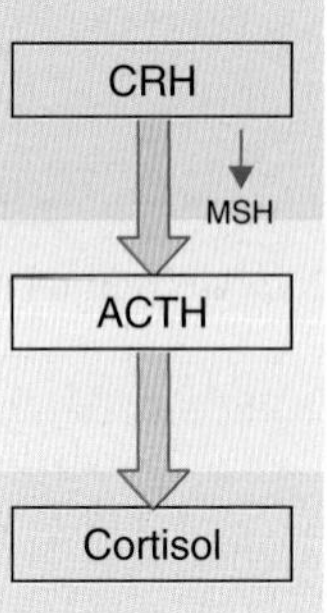

Diagnosis:

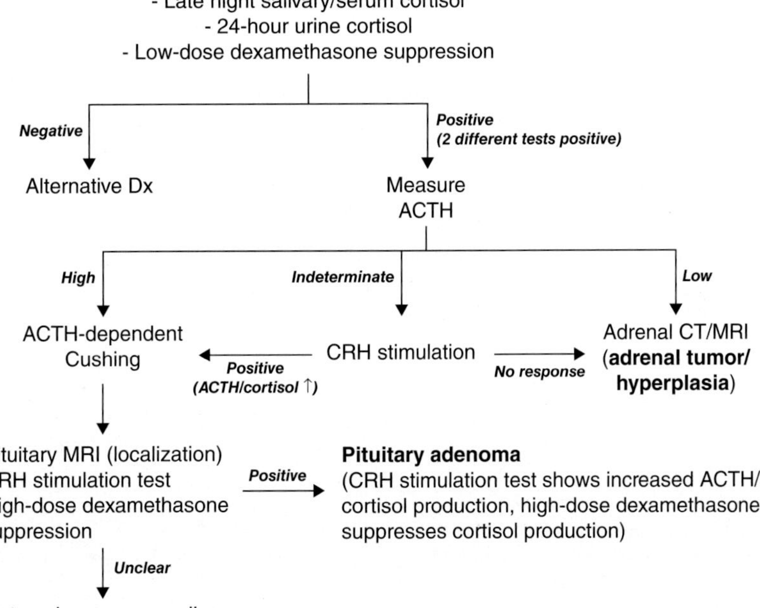

Management:

- Medical therapy: Ketoconazole (typically while awaiting definitive therapy or if surgery is contraindicated)
- Iatrogenic: Taper off steroids
- Pituitary adenoma: Transphenoidal resection
- Ectopic ACTH-secreting tumor: Surgical resection
- Adrenal adenoma or hyperplasia: Unilateral or bilateral adrenalectomy
- Refractory disease (of any cause): Bilateral adrenalectomy

Hypocortisolism

Adrenal Insufficiency and Central Hypocortisolism

General: Loss of adrenal function, causing hypocortisolism, plus hypoaldosteronism in primary disease

	Primary (adrenal)	Secondary/Tertiary (central)
Key Finding	Low cortisol + aldosterone	Low cortisol
ACTH	↑	↓
Na^+	Hyponatremia	Hyponatremia
K^+	Hyperkalemia	Normal
Other	- Hypotension - Hyperpigmentation (↑ MSH→ ↑ melanin)	- Hypotension (less prominent)
Causes	- Autoimmune - Infectious (TB, HIV) - Metastatic cancer - Hemorrhage or infarct	- Chronic steroids - Pituitary or hypothalamic disease

Clinical: Gradual onset of fatigue, weight loss, GI symptoms, orthostasis, syncope

- Acute adrenal crisis
    - Seen in patient with subacute adrenal insufficiency, who undergoes stressor, triggering severe symptoms
    - Presents with shock, with nonspecific symptoms (nausea, vomiting, abdominal pain, weakness)

Diagnosis:

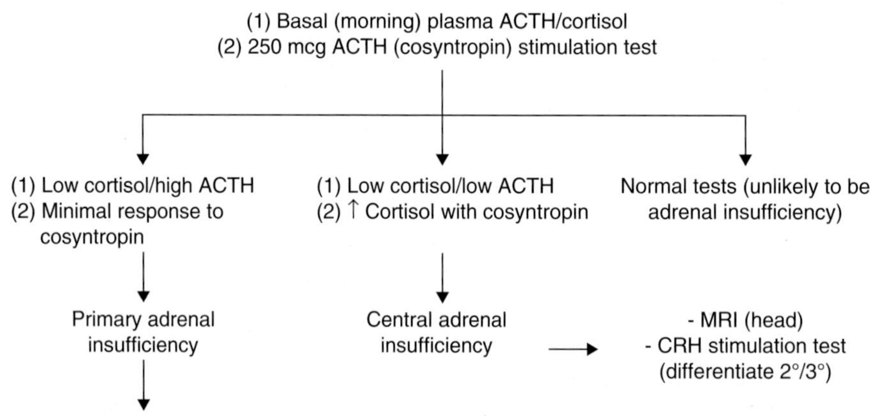

Management:

- Crisis: Fluids/ICU level support. Dexamethasone (not picked up on cortisol assay).
- Chronic:
    - Corticosteroids (dexamethasone, prednisone, or hydrocortisone)
    - Fludrocortisone (in those with primary disease)
    - Stress-dose steroids during minor illnesses or surgery

Pituitary Disorders

Hypopituitarism

General: Decreased secretion of pituitary hormones

Etiology:

- Masses (pituitary adenoma, craniopharyngioma, metastasis)
- Radiation, surgery, infiltrative diseases (e.g., sarcoidosis). Pituitary infarction (Sheehan) or hemorrhage.

Clinical: Presents as a combination of each hormone deficiency

- **Cortisol**: Fatigue, anorexia, weight loss
- **Thyroid**: All typical symptoms of hypothyroidism
- **FSH/LH**:
  - Premenopausal female: Amenorrhea, infertility, hot flashes
  - Postmenopausal female: Asymptomatic
  - Male: Decreased energy, libido, erectile dysfunction
- **GH**: ↓ lean mass, ↑ fat mass
- **Prolactin**: Asymptomatic, unless after giving birth (failure to lactate)

	Diagnosis	Management
ACTH	- Morning cortisol	- Glucocorticoids
TSH	- Free T4 levels (better than TSH, which can be variable)	- Levothyroxine
LH/FSH	- Male: Testosterone (↓), LH (↔) - Female: Estradiol (↓), FSH (↔)	- Testosterone (male) - Estrogen/progestin (female)
GH	- Serum IGF-1, hypoglycemia/arginine stim test	- GH not typically recommended

Specific Etiologies of Hypopituitarism

Sheehan Syndrome:

- Infarction of the pituitary after childbirth, due to severe postpartum hemorrhage
- Clinical presentation ranges from severe hypopituitarism, to subacute disease that presents as failure to lactate or failure for menses to return

Pituitary Apoplexy:

- Sudden hemorrhage into the pituitary, most often into an adenoma
- Presents as sudden onset headache, double vision, and hypopituitarism

Pituitary Adenoma

General: Benign tumor of the anterior pituitary. Macroadenoma (> 10 mm) and microadenoma (< 10 mm).

Etiology: Generally idiopathic, but can be seen associated with MEN1. Subtypes below.

Lactotroph	- Usually cause hyperprolactinemia
Corticotroph	- Usually cause Cushing
Somatotroph	- Usually cause acromegaly
Gonadotroph	- Generally nonfunctioning
Thyrotroph	- Generally nonfunctioning - Rarely produce TSH, leading to hyperthyroidism

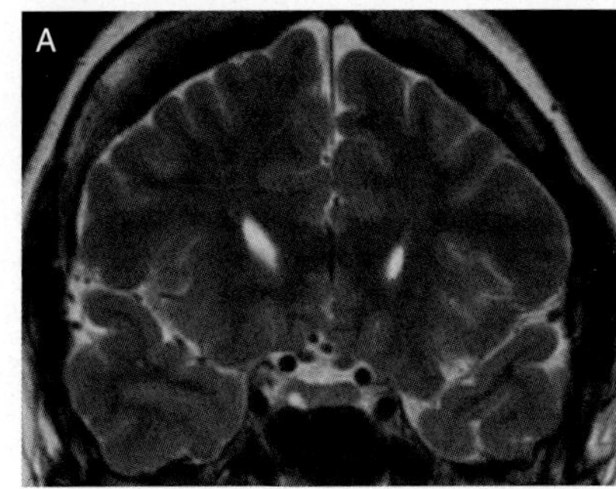

Clinical: Mass effect: Headache and bitemporal hemianopsia. Effects from hormone production.

Diagnosis: Pituitary MRI[A]

Management: Prolactinomas generally treated medically, while others treated surgically (see next page)

Pituitary Disorders

Hyperprolactinemia

General: High prolactin levels

Etiology:

- Prolactinoma
- Drugs (antipsychotics, SSRI)
- ↓ Dopamine inhibition (from mass effect or hypothalamic/stalk lesion)

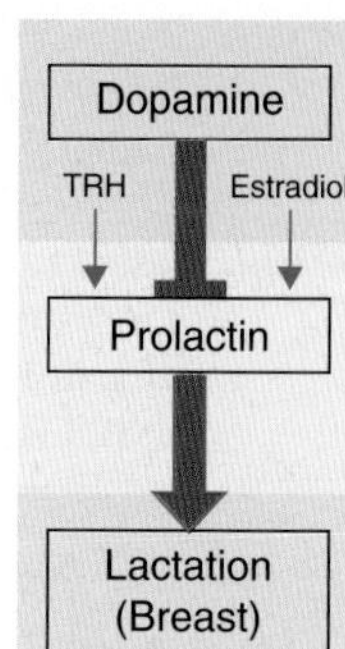

Clinical:

- Male: Decreased energy, libido, erectile dysfunction, gynecomastia
- Premenopausal female: Oligomenorrhea, amenorrhea, infertility, hot flashes, galactorrhea
- Postmenopausal female: Asymptomatic, unless tumor has compressive symptoms

Diagnosis: Serum prolactin level (5-20 is normal, > 200 is indicative of adenoma). MRI to localize.

Management:

- Asymptomatic microprolactinoma: No treatment
- Symptomatic microprolactinoma: Cabergoline
- Macroprolactinoma: Cabergoline. Consider surgical resection if refractory/tumor growing.

Acromegaly

General: Clinical syndrome from excess growth hormone secretion due to GH secreting adenoma

GHRH
Somatostatin
GH
IGF-1

Clinical: Insidious (i.e., > 10 years) onset of tissue overgrowth

- Macrognathia, coarse facies, spaced out teeth, thickened skin. Visceral enlargement: LVH, OSA.
- ↑ colon cancer risk
- Insulin resistance → Diabetes
- Adenoma compressive symptoms (headache, bitemporal hemianopsia)

Diagnosis:

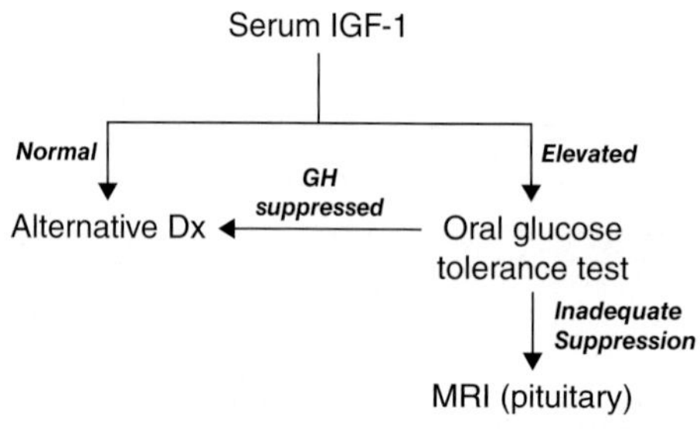

Management:

- Operable: Transsphenoidal resection
- Nonoperable or refractory: Pharmacologic treatment
    - Octreotide (somatostatin analog) +/– Cabergoline
    - Pegvisomant (GH blocker) for refractory disease

Gigantism

General: GH excess that occurs during period of linear growth

Etiology: GH adenoma (often associated with genetic syndromes like McCune-Albright or MEN-1)

Clinical: Rapid linear growth, +/– obesity. Large hands/feet, coarse facies.

Diagnosis: Serum **IGF-1**, with GH suppression test (oral glucose tolerance) for definitive diagnosis

- Brain MRI to identify etiology

Management: Transsphenoidal resection. Radiation/Octreotide if refractory.

Calcium Homeostasis

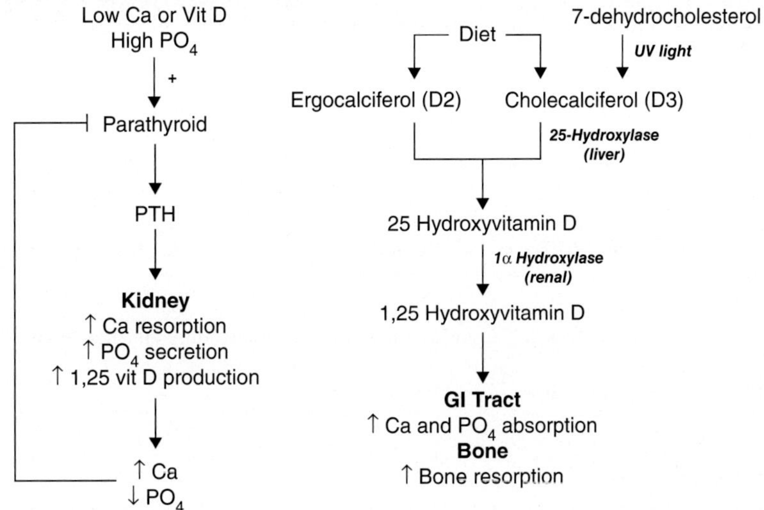

Vitamin D Deficiency

General: Vitamin D deficiency is generally asymptomatic, but can place patients at risk for falls, osteoporosis, and fractures

Etiology:

- Decreased intake or absorption (malabsorption, gastric bypass, dietary)
- Reduced sun exposure (winter time, high latitude)
- Defective hydroxylation (renal failure, cirrhosis, hypoparathyroidism)

Clinical: Generally asymptomatic, but can lead to **osteomalacia** (adults) or **rickets** (kids) if severe. Hypocalcemia and/or hypophosphatemia if moderate.

Osteomalacia	- Bone pain, muscle weakness, "waddling" gait, fractures - Classic radiology findings: Looser pseudofractures, fissures
Rickets[A]	- Abnormal development of growth plates and bones - Presents with parietal and frontal bossing - Enlargement of the costochondral junction ("rachitic rosary") - Lateral bowing of the femur and tibia (bow legs)

Diagnosis: **25-hydroxyvitamin D** level measurement (20 to 50 ng/mL normal)

Management:

Vitamin D	- Vitamin D3 (cholecalciferol) is preferred - If mildly low (10-20 ng/mL): 600-800 IU/day - If very low (< 10 ng/nL): 50K IU weekly for 8 weeks, then ~1000 IU/day
Calcium	- 1000-1200 mg of calcium daily (between diet and supplements)

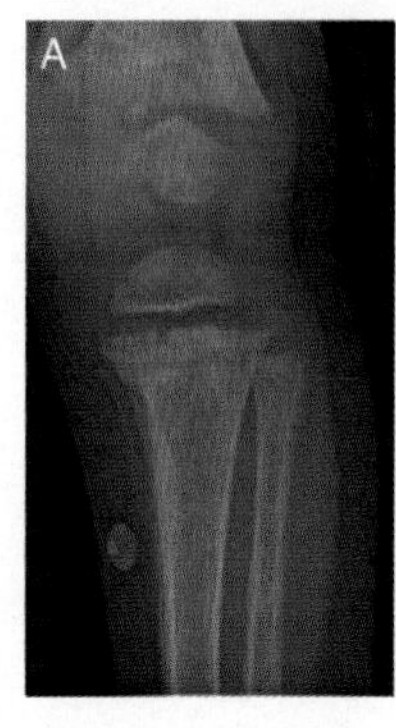

Hypoparathyroidism

Hypoparathyroidism

General: Abnormal PTH secretion due to glandular destruction or abnormal PTH production

Etiology:

- Iatrogenic (surgical parathyroid removal)
- Autoimmune glandular destruction
- Infiltrative disease, radiation
- <u>Genetic disorders</u>:
    - **APS-I** (AR disorder of AIRE. Presents with mucocutaneous candidiasis, AI, hypoparathyroidism.)
    - **DiGeorge**

Clinical: Ranges from asymptomatic to severely symptomatic from hypocalcemia (tetany, spasms, tingling)

Diagnosis: Hypocalcemia PLUS inappropriately low/normal PTH

Management:

<u>Acute</u>: Often post-thyroidectomy
- IV calcium (when symptomatic or Ca < 7.5)
- Otherwise oral calcitriol/vitamin D sufficient

<u>Chronic</u>: Calcitriol and vitamin D
- Recombinant PTH for those with refractory hypocalcemia

Pseudohypoparathyroidism (Type 1A)

General: AD genetic resistance to PTH due to inability to make cAMP when PTH binds its receptor (GNAS mutation). Defect inherited from mother.

Clinical:

- Hypocalcemia and hyperphosphatemia
- "Albright hereditary osteodystrophy": Round face, short stature, short fourth metacarpal, developmental delays

Pseudopseudohypoparathyroidism:

- If abnormal GNAS is inherited from father, the child will have the physical abnormalities of Albright above, but with normal calcium homeostasis.

Hyperparathyroidism

Etiology	Ca	PO_4	PTH	Cause
Primary	↑	↓	↑	- Parathyroid adenoma (most common) - Parathyroid hyperplasia (~15%) - Parathyroid carcinoma (rare)
Secondary	↓	↑/↓	↑	- CKD (↑ PO_4) - Vitamin D deficiency (↓ PO_4) - Calcium malabsorption or renal loss
Tertiary	↑	nl/↑	↑	- Dramatically ↑ PTH secretion, due to parathyroid dysregulation - Rare: Seen with long-term CKD

Clinical:

- Asymptomatic hypercalcemia is most common
- If severe: "Stones, bones, groans, psych overtones" [See: Renal]

Diagnosis:

- Hypercalcemia with PTH inappropriately normal or elevated
- 24-hour urine calcium
    - Differentiates 1° HPT from familial hypocalciuric hypercalcemia
    - Can predict potential renal damage from hypercalciuria
- Localization (only if surgery is to be performed)
    - Sestamibi scintigraphy (MIBI-SPECT), ultrasound, or CT

Management:

Primary	**Surgery:**
	- Indications:
	  - Symptomatic
	  - Age < 50, osteoporosis, CKD (GFR < 60), calcium (> 11.5)
	- Procedure:
	  - Adenoma: Resect single lesion
	  - Hyperplasia: Remove 3.5 glands, or all 4 and implant half of a gland in the arm
	- Complications:
	  - Recurrent laryngeal nerve damage
	  - Post-op hypocalcemia
	
	Pharm: Bisphosphonates or cinacalcet
	  - Indicated if not a surgical candidate, but symptomatic or have side effect like osteoporosis
	  - Observe asymptomatic hypercalcemia

Secondary	- Manage underlying renal disease - Correct vitamin D deficiency and hyperphosphatemia if present (phosphate binders) - Persistently elevated PTH: Calcitriol
Tertiary	- Cinacalcet - Surgery for refractory cases

Hungry Bone Syndrome: Prolonged hypocalcemia after parathyroidectomy for hyperparathyroidism. Caused by sudden shift from ↑ PTH to ↓ PTH, with bone calcium and phosphate absorption.

Male Reproductive Endocrine

Hypogonadism

General: Decreased sperm and testosterone production by the testes

	Findings	Etiology
Primary	↑ LH/FSH ↓↓ Testosterone/Sperm	- Radiation/chemotherapy - Testicular infection, trauma, varicocele - Klinefelter
Secondary	↓/↔ LH/FSH ↓ Testosterone/Sperm	- Pituitary damage (tumors, apoplexy, infiltrative disease, etc.) - Hyperprolactinemia - Kallmann syndrome

Clinical: Decreased libido, energy, muscle mass, body hair. Gynecomastia (usually seen in just primary). Infertility.

Diagnosis:

- **Morning (8-10am) serum total testosterone**. Consider free testosterone levels if concern about SHBG.
- If abnormal, obtain LH, FSH, semen analysis
- Further workup to determine etiology (e.g., karyotype if primary, prolactin and brain MRI if secondary)

Management: Treat underlying condition. Testosterone replacement (transdermal gels/patch preferred method).

- Oral testosterone preparations associated with liver disease

Androgen Abuse

"Positive" Effects	Adverse Effects
- ↑ fat-free mass/muscle strength	- ↓ testicular function (atrophy) - Aggression/behavioral changes - Gynecomastia - Erythrocytosis (↑ HCT) - Hepatotoxicity (17α alk. androgens) - Virilization (women), acne, baldness - ↑ Clotting - ↓ HDL

Synthetic Androgens: Stanozolol, nandrolone, methandienone, trenbolone
Androgen Precursors: Androstenedione, DHEA

Erectile Dysfunction

General: Inability to acquire or sustain a sufficiently rigid and durable erection for sexual intercourse

Risk: ↑ Age, obesity, smoking, comorbid/chronic medical problems. Also associated with atherosclerotic disease, previous pelvic disease/surgery, hypogonadism, drugs (antidepressants, beta-blockers)

Etiology:

- **Psychologic**: Depression, stress.
    - If nighttime erections still occur, it is highly likely that ED is due to psychologic factors.
- **Medical** ("Organic"): Hypogonadism, neurologic (perineal trauma, prostate surgery), atherosclerosis

Management:

- Identify/treat risk factors (testosterone for hypogonadism, lifestyle modifications for vascular disease)
- <u>Pharmacologic</u>:
    - PDE5 inhibitors (sildenafil, tadalafil, etc.) [contraindicated with nitrates]
    - Second line: Alprostadil (intracavernosal), vacuum device
- Penile implants if all else fails

Adrenal Neoplasia

Adrenal Incidentaloma

General: Adrenal mass lesion > 1 cm found on CT or MRI imaging

Etiology: Benign adenoma (+/– functional hormone production), adrenal carcinoma, pheochromocytoma

Diagnosis:

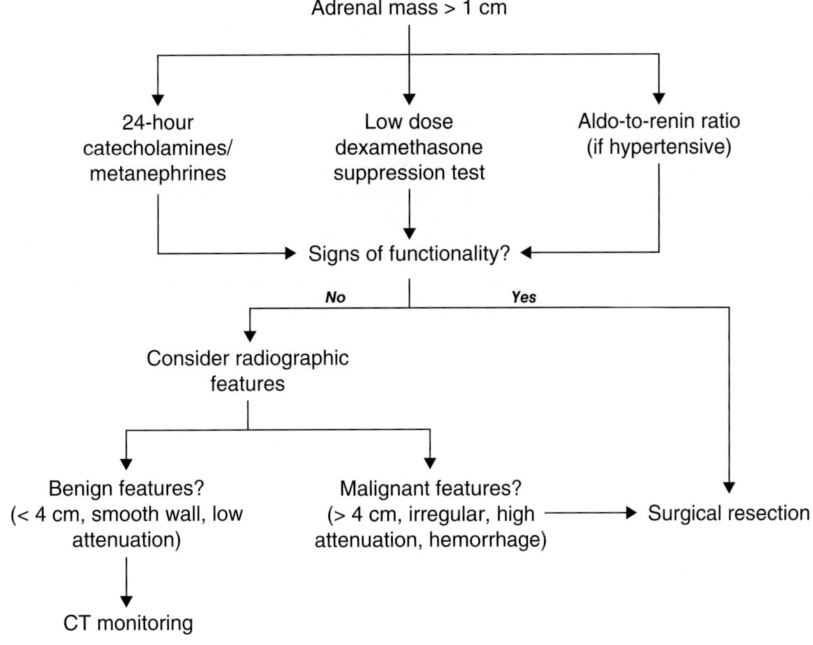

Management:

- Surgically resect: Functional tumors, malignant appearing tumors, > 4 cm benign tumors
- Serial CT/MRI monitoring for those with nonsurgical tumors
    - Consider surgery for those that grow by > 1 cm at follow-up

Adrenal Carcinoma

General: Rare, highly malignant neoplasm of the adrenal cortex. Poor prognosis.

Clinical: Generally found incidentally (see above)

- Can secrete hormones, resulting in Cushing, hyperaldosteronism, or androgens (virilization)

Management: Surgical resection, followed by hormone therapy (mitotane) or chemotherapy

Pheochromocytoma

General: Catecholamine-secreting tumors that arise from chromaffin cells of the adrenal medulla and the sympathetic ganglia. "Rule of 10s": ~10% are bilateral or malignant, ~10% in children, ~10% extra-adrenal

Etiology: Majority are sporadic. Genetic conditions (MEN2, vHL, NF-1).

Clinical: Classic triad: **Episodic headache, sweating, and tachycardia**

- Most common: Sustained/paroxysmal hypertension
- Symptoms can be triggered by surgery (anesthesia) or some drugs

Diagnosis: **24-hour urine fractionated catecholamines/metanephrines** (Alt: Plasma fractionated metanephrines)

- CT/MRI to localize the tumor

Management: Surgical resection (laparoscopic adrenalectomy)

- Preoperative: Alpha-blockade (phenoxybenzamine) followed by beta-blockade (propranolol)

Pancreatic Neuroendocrine Tumors

Tumor	General/Clinical	Diagnosis	Management
Gastrinoma (Zollinger-Ellison)	- Excess **gastrin** secretion → Excess gastric acid secretion - Presents as chronic diarrhea, reflux, abdominal pain - Peptic ulcers (can be distal to duodenum, refractory to PPI)	- Suspect in: Multiple/refractory ulcers, enlarged gastric folds on endoscopy - Serum fasting gastrin level (off PPI): > 1000 → Gastrinoma 100-1000 → Elevated, nonspecific - Secretin stimulation test (secretin ↑↑ gastrin levels in gastrinoma cells) - Localization: CT, MRI	- High-dose PPI - Surgical resection
Insulinoma	- Islet-cell tumor that secretes **insulin** - Presents as fasting hypoglycemia, with neuroglycopenic/hypoglycemic symptoms	- High insulin during period of induced hypoglycemia (72-hour fast) - Localization: CT, MRI	- Surgical resection - Diazoxide (↓ insulin secretion. Used if refractory disease or not undergoing surgery.)
Glucagonoma	- Presents with GI symptoms (diarrhea, weight loss), diabetes - Venous thrombosis, neuropsychiatric disturbance Necrolytic migratory erythema: Erythematous plaques on face, perineum, extremities. Eventually develop central clearing/blistering, with surrounding scaling.	- Elevated fasting plasma glucagon (> 500 pg/mL) - Localization: CT, MRI	- Pharm: - Octreotide - Insulin (if glucose ↑) - Nutritional support - Surgical resection (if local), but most are metastatic (require chemoradiation)
VIPoma	- Presents as: **Watery diarrhea** (secretory, low osmotic gap) - **Hypochlorhydria** (↓ gastric acid) - Flushing, emesis, lethargy - Hypokalemia, hypercalcemia, hyperglycemia	- VIP > 75 pg/mL - Localization: CT, MRI	- Fluid replacement - Octreotide - Surgical resection
Somatostatinoma	- D-cell tumor secreting **somatostatin** - Cholelithiasis (↓ CCK) - Glucose intolerance (↓ insulin) - Steatorrhea (↓ pancreatic enzymes)	- Somatostatin > 30 pg/mL - Localization: CT, MRI	- Surgical resection - Octreotide (if unresectable)

Multiple Endocrine Neoplasia

Patients with diagnosed MEN or with known family history should receive screening for malignancy as below.

MEN1 (AD MEN1 mutation)
- Screen using Ca, PTH, prolactin
- Imaging (controversial, but US, CT, MRI can be used)

MEN2a/2b (AD RET mutations)
- Screen for cancer using plasma metanephrines, serum calcium, calcitonin, thyroid US
- Note: 2b: Generally have associated gastrointestinal issues (chronic constipation/megacolon)

	MEN1	MEN2A	MEN2B
Pituitary (adenomas)	+		
Pancreatic (neuroendocrine tumor)	+		
Parathyroid (adenoma)	+	+	
Thyroid (medullary cancer)		+	+
Pheochromocytoma		+	+
Mucosal/Intestinal neuroma			+
Marfanoid habitus			+

Hypoglycemia

General: Abnormally low plasma glucose concentration, generally < 70 mg/dL OR based on Whipple's triad (symptoms of hypoglycemia, low blood sugar, and resolution of symptoms with normalization of glucose)

Etiology:

- Vast majority of cases occur in diabetics using insulin or secretagogue
- Critical illness
- Hormone deficiency (hypocortisolism)
- Endogenous hyperinsulinemia (see differential table below)

Clinical:

- **Neuroglycopenic symptoms**: Cognitive impairment, psychomotor abnormalities, seizure, coma
- Autonomic symptoms: Tremor, palpitations, diaphoresis, anxiety

Diagnosis: Workup for a nondiabetic, healthy individual with hypoglycemia:

- Check glucose, insulin, C-peptide, proinsulin, and oral hypoglycemic agent screen. Must check during period of symptomatic hypoglycemia, either:
    - Spontaneous or induced (short fast, mixed-meal, or 72-hour fast)

Etiology	Pathophys	Diagnostic Findings
Insulin	- Iatrogenic insulin therapy	↑ Insulin ↓ Proinsulin, C-pep
Insulin Secretagogue	- Sulfonylurea drugs, which stimulate endogenous insulin production	↑ Insulin, C-pep, proinsulin + Secretagogue screen
Insulinoma	- Insulin-producing malignancy	↑ Insulin, C-pep, proinsulin
Autoimmune Hypoglycemia	- Antibodies directed to endogenous insulin or to the insulin receptor	↑ Insulin, C-pep, proinsulin + Insulin autoantibodies
NIPHS*	- Endogenous hyperinsulinemia due to islet hypertrophy and nesidioblastosis - Often postprandial (2-4 hours) - Similar pathophysiology also seen after gastric bypass surgery	↑ Insulin, C-pep, proinsulin
Nonislet Cell Tumor	- Increased insulin-like growth factor-2 (IGF-2) production	- C-pep, insulin, and proinsulin normal

*Noninsulinoma pancreatogenous hypoglycemia syndrome

Diabetes Mellitus

Etiology and Clinical Features of Diabetes Mellitus

	Type 1	Type 2
Path	- Autoimmune B-cell destruction	- Insulin resistance
Inherit	- Multifactorial (increased risk, but still < 10% incidence in child of a type I diabetic)	- Multifactorial (2-3 × increased risk if history in first degree relative)
Risk	- N/A	- Obesity, sedentary lifestyle, smoking, nonwhite
Insulin	- Low or absent	- Normal/elevated early on - Eventual loss of insulin production
Onset	- Childhood (4-14 y/o)	- Generally adult
Clinical	- Polyuria, polydipsia, weight loss - Often presents in DKA	- Asymptomatic (found on routine screening) - Can develop polyuria/polydipsia

Other Causes of Diabetes:

MODY (Mature onset diabetes of the young) [presents in 20s]

Non insulin dependent diabetes from AD mutation in one of the following:

- Glucokinase (↑ glucose required for insulin secretion)
- Hepatic nuclear factor 1-alpha (low insulin secretion)

Pancreatic Diabetes: Chronic pancreatitis, cystic fibrosis, hemochromatosis

Endocrinopathies: Cushing syndrome or exogenous glucocorticoids

Diagnosis: One of the following is sufficient:

- Fasting plasma glucose ≥ 126 mg/dL
- Plasma glucose ≥ 200 mg/dL, 2 hours post oral glucose tolerance test
- Symptoms of hyperglycemia with glucose ≥ 200 mg/dL
- Hemoglobin A1C ≥ 6.5% (typically used for type II DM)

Diabetes Management

	Type 1	Type 2
Goal	A1C < 7	A1C < 7 in average adult, A1C < 8 in elderly or high risk for hypoglycemia

Agent	<u>Multiple daily injections</u>:
	- Once/twice injected long-acting insulin plus pre meal short-acting
	- Multiple different combinations available, but common one is evening long-acting detemir/ Glargine, with premeal lispro/aspart/glulisine
	
	<u>Insulin pump</u>:
	- Continuous infusion of short-acting insulin, with pre-meal bolus
	
	*Multiple daily glucose checks (either via finger stick or continuous glucose monitor)
		<u>Initial therapy</u>:
		- Aggressive lifestyle modifications
		- **Metformin** (started concurrently in most)
		- If severe hyperglycemia (i.e., A1C > 9.5%), consider starting insulin
		
		<u>Failure of one agent</u>:
		- Add additional oral agent (glitazone, sulfonylurea, GLP-1, DPP-4, SGLT-2)
		
		<u>Failure of two agents</u>:
		- Add additional oral agent OR start insulin
		  - Start with basal insulin (glargine/detemir/degludec)
		  - Add premeal rapid acting if fails on basal alone

- Bariatric surgery in BMI ≥ 40 or BMI 35 to 39.9 when hyperglycemia is inadequately controlled with therapy

Inpatient Diabetes Management:

Goal: Preprandial blood sugars < 140 mg/dL, with all glucose checks ideally < 180 mg/dL

Therapy:

- If on home oral meds, can continue if patient is overall well (eating, no contraindications to home med, not critically ill)
- All others → Insulin
  - Basal insulin (detemir or glargine) PLUS prandial insulin (rapid acting lispro/aspart with meals)
  - Correctional insulin (based on a graded scale)

Diabetes Mellitus

Diabetes Complications			
Complication	**Clinical**	**Management**	**Screening**
Macrovascular			
Accelerated Atherosclerosis	- CAD (most common cause of mortality) - PAD - CVA	- ASA/Statin	- Initial lipid screen at time of diagnosis
Microvascular			

Nephropathy	- Efferent arterial glycosylation leads to glomerular hyperfiltration, with eventual GBM and mesangial disease, resulting in albuminuria
	- Long-term damage can lead to glomerulosclerosis and nephrotic syndrome
		- ACEi/ARB
		- BP control < 130/80
		
		- If ongoing proteinuria despite above:
		  - SGLT2 inhibitor
		  - Finerenone
			- Annual urine albumin: Cr

Peripheral Neuropathy	- Peripheral symmetric distal "stocking-glove" sensory neuropathy
	  - Large fiber: Proprioception/pressure
	  - Small fiber: Pain, paresthesia
	- CN III palsy (eye pain, diplopia, ptosis)
		- If painful: Amitriptyline, venlafaxine, duloxetine, or pregabalin	- Annual physical exam, sensory testing

Autonomic Neuropathy	- GU: Neurogenic bladder, erectile dysfunction - GI: Gastroparesis - CV: Postural hypotension, tachycardia, silent ischemia	- Bladder: Urination schedule, or intermittent catheterization - ED: PDE-5 inhibitor - Gastroparesis: If severe, give metochlopromide or erythromycin	
Retinopathy	- Generally nonproliferative, but can progress to proliferative - Hemorrhages, exudates, microaneurysms, venous dilatation	- Photocoagulation for proliferative disease	- Annual slit-lamp exam
Foot	- Wounds (lack of sensation predisposes to injury)	- Frequent self-foot checks	- Annual podiatric check
Infection	- ↑ infection risk/poor wound healing		

*Glycemic control ↓ risk of microvascular complications with type II DM, ↓ risk of micro/macrovascular complications with type I DM

Diabetes Mellitus

Diabetic Ketoacidosis/Hyperosmolar Hyperglycemic State

General: Diabetic states in which insulin deficiency leads to severe hyperglycemia, ketogenesis, and electrolyte/fluid abnormalities. Both states are generally triggered by a precipitating factor (e.g., infection) and/or inadequate insulin therapy. HHS and DKA are on a spectrum.

Criteria	DKA	HHS
Glucose	> 250 mg/dL	> 600 mg/dL, and often > 1000
pH	< 7.30, and near 7.0 if severe	> 7.30
HCO3	< 18 mEq/L	> 18 mEq/L
Ketones	Present in urine and serum	Negative or mild
AG	> 10-12	Normal
Serum Osm	Variable	> 320 mOsm/kg
Pathophys	- More common **type I DM** - Insulin deficiency and glucagon excess, leading to hyperglycemia, and production of ketoacids	- More common **type II DM** - Insulin deficiency and glucagon excess, leading to hyperglycemia, osmotic diuresis, and extreme hyperosmolarity - Enough insulin present to prevent ketone production
Clinical	- Rapid onset of polyuria/polydipsia, abdominal pain, vomiting - Kussmaul respiration - "Fruity" breath (acetone)	- Gradual onset of polyuria/polydipsia and weight loss - Neurologic symptoms (lethargy, mental obtundation, coma)

Management:

Fluids	- Normal saline at ~1 L/hr initially, transitioning to ½ NS once volume status improves - Add 5% dextrose once glucose < 200-250 mg/dL
Insulin	- Initial: IV insulin (bolus plus continuous drip) - Once glucose < 200 mg/dL, can switch to SQ insulin or reduced-dose drip
Potassium	- KCl repletion if ≤ 5.3 mEq/L (and hold insulin if K^+ < 3.3) - Most patients have K^+ depletion from renal loss, but dehydration/insulin deficiency/acidosis has K^+ shifted extracellularly
Other Lytes	- Monitor and replace Mg, Ca - Replace PO_4 if < 1 mg/dL or signs of cardiac dysfunction
HCO_3	- Bicarbonate infusion typically not given, unless pH < 6.9
Monitoring	- Monitor q2-4 hour chemistries, β-hydroxybutyrate until stable

<u>Crisis resolved when</u>:

- DKA: Gap closes, β-hydroxybutyrate normalizes, patient can eat
- HHS: Osm drops < 315 mOsm/kg, mentation normalizes

Pediatric Endocrine

Congenital Neck Mass DDx

Thyroglossal Duct Cyst	- Cystic expansion of remnant of thyroglossal duct tract - Anterior midline neck mass that moves with swallowing or protrusion of the tongue - Often asymptomatic - Can become tender if infected/inflamed - Dx: US or CT - Tx: Antibiotics (if infected), followed by surgical excision
Branchial Cleft Cyst[A]	- Failure of obliteration of a branchial cleft in embryonic development (most commonly 2nd) - Presents as lateral neck mass, usually anterior to the sternocleidomastoid muscle, no movement with swallowing - Dx: US or CT - Tx: Can treated conservatively or surgically excise

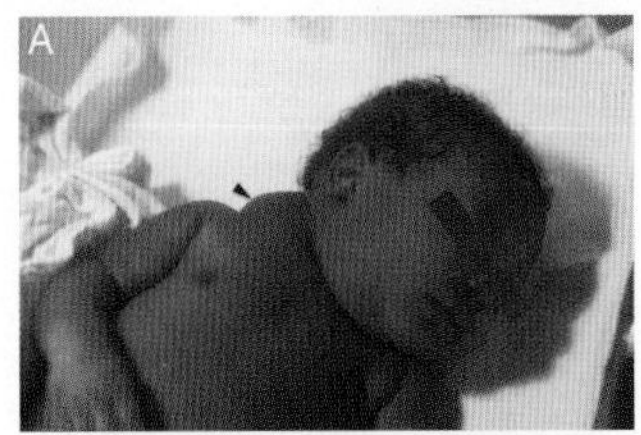

Congenital Hypothyroidism

Etiology:

- Thyroid dysgenesis (most common)
- Defective thyroid hormone synthesis, transport, or ↓ TSH-R sensitivity
- Maternal iodine deficiency or excess iodine exposure

Clinical:

- Usually asymptomatic at birth (maternal T4 crosses over)
- If not picked up with neonatal screens, over the first few months of life:
    - Lethargy, hypotonia
    - Hypothermia, jaundice
    - Poor feeding, constipation
    - Puffy/coarse facies, macroglossia
    - Umbilical hernia, large fontanelles
    - Risk for mental retardation, severe bone/growth delay

Diagnosis: TSH/T4

Management: Levothyroxine (10 mcg/kg then titrate)

Neonatal Thyrotoxicosis

General: Transplacental passage of TSH-R IgG (from maternal Graves, disease), causing excessive release of T4 in the neonate

Clinical:

- Low birth weight, preterm birth, microcephaly
- Warm moist skin, tachycardia
- Poor feeding, irritability, failure to thrive

Diagnosis: ↑ TSH-R IgG in mother

Management:

- Resolves months after birth
- Methimazole, beta-blocker (propranolol)

Pediatric Endocrine

Precocious Puberty

General: Onset of puberty at age > 2 SD lower than normal onset (boys ≤ 9, girls ≤ 8)

Subtype	Definition	Examples
Central	- Early maturation of the hypothalamic-pituitary-gonadal axis	- Idiopathic (constitutional, 90% of cases in girls, ~60% of cases in boys) - CNS lesions
Peripheral	- Sex hormone secretion/exposure (GnRH independent)	- Ovarian cysts/tumors, Leydig tumor, β-HCG secreting mass - Exogenous sex steroids - Congenital adrenal hyperplasia, McCune-Albright - Adrenal tumor
Benign Variants	- Premature isolated thelarche, pubarche, adrenarche - Note: These are isolated findings and do not require intervention	

Clinical:

- Signs of **estrogen** excess: Breast development and possibly vaginal bleeding
- Signs of **androgen** excess: Pubic and/or axillary hair, enlarged clitoris, acne

Diagnosis:

- Basal LH (most important, see algorithm below), FSH, E2/T
- Bone age (within normal limits in benign variants, advanced with central and peripheral etiologies)
- Workup (once precocious puberty diagnosed)
    - Pelvic or testicular US. Head MRI (especially in boys).

Management:

- Central: GnRH agonists (leuprolide)
- Peripheral: Remove underlying cause
    - Surgically excise tumors
    - Remove exogenous sex steroids
    - CAH: Glucocorticoids

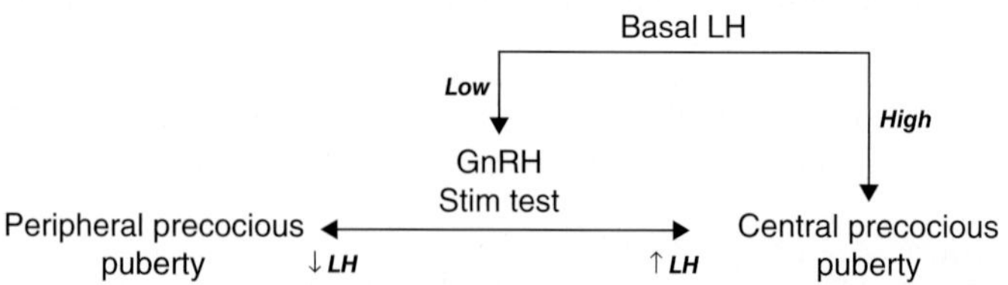

Delayed Puberty

General: Puberty delayed past normal range

- Boys: No testicular enlargement by age 14
- Girls: Absence of breast development by age 12

Etiology:

Primary Hypogonadism	- Lack of gonadal sex hormone production (LH/FSH ↑, T/E2 ↓) - Causes include Turner, Klinefelter, gonadal injury
Secondary Hypogonadism	- Due to failure of GnRH release (causes seen below) - LH/FSH ↓, T/E2 ↓
Constitutional Delay of Puberty	- Most common cause of delayed puberty - Transient, idiopathic delay in GnRH release
GnRH Deficiency	- Occurs with Kallmann syndrome
Others	- Excess exercise or poor nutrition - Chronic illnesses (IBD, hypothyroidism, etc.)

Diagnosis:

- LH, FSH, E2, T levels (help to determine primary vs secondary)
- Workup for underlying cause (TSH, prolactin, imaging)

Management:

- Treat underlying cause if present
- Constitutional delay: Observation. Can consider short-term hormonal (E2 or T) therapy.

Pediatric Endocrine

Congenital Adrenal Neoplasia

Pregnenolone —(**17α-Hydroxylase**)→ 17-OHPregnenolone —(**17, 20 Lyase**)→ DHEA

3β-HSD ↓ (Pregnenolone → Progesterone; 17-OHPregnenolone → 17-OHProgesterone; DHEA → Androstenedione)

Progesterone → 17-OHProgesterone → Androstenedione —(**Aromatase**)→ Estrone

21-Hydroxylase ↓ (Progesterone → 11-Deoxycorticosterone; 17-OHProgesterone → 11-Deoxycortisol)

Androstenedione ↓ Testosterone —(**Aromatase**)→ Estradiol

11β-Hydroxylase ↓ (11-Deoxycorticosterone → Corticosterone; 11-Deoxycortisol → Cortisol)

Testosterone —(**5α-Reductase**)↓ DHT

Aldo Synthase ↓ (Corticosterone → Aldosterone)

Cortisol ↓ Cortisone

Enzyme Deficiency	General/Clinical	Diagnosis/Management
Classic CAH (21-Hydroxylase)	- Adrenal insufficiency (↓ Cortisol) - +/– Salt wasting (from ↓ aldosterone: hypoNa, hyperK, hypotension, dehydration) - Females with ambiguous genitalia - Males with virilization, presenting ~2-4 y/o	Dx: ↑ 17-hydroxyprogesterone Tx: Glucocorticoids + fludrocortisone
Nonclassic CAH (21-Hydroxylase)	- Later onset: School-age or early teens - Can present as precocious puberty (including premature pubarche, accelerated bone growth) or with symptoms of PCOS (hirsutism, menstrual irregularity)	Dx: ↑ 17-hydroxyprogesterone, PLUS exaggerated response to ACTH stimulation test Tx: Glucocorticoids +/– antiandrogens
17α-Hydroxylase	- Mineralocorticoid (DOC) excess (hypertension, ↑ Na, ↓ K) - ↓ Sex hormones (XY: Genital ambiguity, XX: Delayed pubarche, oligomenorrhea)	Dx: ↑ Deoxy/corticosterone, with ↓ cortisol Tx: Glucocorticoids, sex hormones, spironolactone
11β-Hydroxylase	- Mineralocorticoid excess (hypertension, ↑ Na, ↓ K) - ↑ DHEAS/androgens (virilization, precocious puberty, ambiguous genetalia in XX)	Dx: ↑ 11-deoxycortisol, ↓ Cortisol Tx: Glucocorticoids

Neuroblastoma

General: Tumor that arises from primitive sympathetic ganglion cells, most commonly adrenal or paravertebral. Most common neoplasm in infants; more than half of patients present before age 2.

Clinical: Often asymptomatic. Can present with abdominal mass +/– pain, constipation, bone pain, periorbital ecchymosis ("raccoon eyes"), Horner syndrome, back pain

- Paraneoplastic syndromes: **Opsoclonus-Myoclonus**: Rapid, dancing eye movements, rhythmic jerking (myoclonus)

Diagnosis: Imaging (US) to confirm mass. **Urine/serum catecholamines** (↑ VMA/HVA).

- Biopsy confirmatory (small basophilic cells in rosettes)

Management: Surgical resection +/– chemoradiation, immunotherapy

- Prognosis: Highly varied, depends on histology, genetic factors (e.g., NMyc)

Adrenoleukodystrophy

General: Peroxisome disorder resulting in long chain fatty acid accumulation in the body (XR-ABCD1 gene)

Clinical: Neurologic deficits: Intellectual disability/behavioral abnormalities, followed by development of quadriplegia, blindness, and other CNS defects. Sexual dysfunction. Adrenal insufficiency.

Diagnosis: Elevated VLCFA levels. Brain MRI (showing areas of demyelination). Genetic analysis.

Management: HCT. Glucocorticoid replacement.

Pediatric Endocrine

Definitions of Short Stature

General: Short stature is anyone < 2 SD below the mean height (< 3rd percentile)

- Normal variant: < 2 SD, but normal linear growth curve
- Pathologic: < 2 SD, growing with abnormal growth velocity (i.e., < 2 inch/yr)

Mid-parental height

- Can be used to help reassure those with normal variant short stature
- Child should fall +/− 4 inches of the following calculations
- Female MPH= 0.5 × ([Father's height − 5 inch] + mother's height)
- Male MPH= 0.5 × ([Mother's height + 5 inch] + father's height)

Differential of Short Stature

Type	Findings
Normal Variant (see definition above)	
Familial (Genetic)	- Normal bone age/onset of puberty
Constitutional	- Delayed bone age/onset of puberty
Pathologic (see definition above)	
Proportionate	- Normal upper to lower body segment ratio DDx: - Endocrine (hypothyroidism, GH deficiency, Cushing) - Genetic (Turner, Prader-Willi, etc.) - Systemic (e.g., malnutrition, glucocorticoids, severe cardiac/pulmonary/renal disease)
Disproportionate	- Abnormal upper to lower body segment ratio - DDx includes Rickets, skeletal dysplasia (osteogenesis imperfecta, achondroplasia, SHOX mutations)

Common Causes of Dwarfism

Achondroplasia	- Sporadic AD mutation in FGFR3 (failure of longitudinal bone growth/endochondral ossification) - Clinical: Short limbs relative to body, trident hands, large head with frontal bossing, rhizomelia, genu varum - Cervical spinal compression serious potential complication - Mental function, life span, fertility not affected
Laron Dwarfism	- Defective GH receptor (decreased linear growth, increased GH, decreased IGF-1) - Clinical: Short height, small head, characteristic facies with saddle nose and prominent forehead, delayed skeletal maturation, small genitalia - Increased insulin sensitivity (resistant to diabetes and cancer) - Tx: IGF-1

Endocrine Pharm

	Mechanism	Indication	Side Effects/Management
Insulin			
Rapid Insulin Lispro, aspart Glulisine	- 1-hour peak action	- Diabetes mellitus	- Hypoglycemia - Injection site reactions (immediate or long-term lipodystrophy) - Weight gain
Short Insulin Regular	- 2-4-hour peak		
Int. Insulin NPH	- 8-hour peak		
Long Insulin Degludec Detemir, glargine	- 24-hour activity		
Hypoglycemic Agents			
Biguanides Metformin	- ↓ gluconeogenesis - ↑ glycolysis - ↑ peripheral glucose uptake	- Diabetes mellitus (first-line agent)	- GI disturbances (diarrhea, nausea, vomiting) - Lactic acidosis (contraindicated in CKD) - Modest weight loss
Sulfonylurea Glimepiride Glyburide Glipizide	- Stimulates insulin release from pancreatic β-cells	- Diabetes mellitus	- Hypoglycemia - Weight gain - Old agents (e.g., chlorpropamide): SIADH
Thiazolidinedione Pioglitazone Rosiglitazone	- Activator of PPAR (↓ insulin resistance)	- Diabetes mellitus	- Edema (especially in HF) - Hepatotoxicity - Weight gain - Possible ↑ bladder cancer risk
GLP-1 Agonists Dulaglutide Exenatide Liraglutide	- Agonists of the GLP-1 receptor (stimulate insulin release, ↓ glucagon release)	- Diabetes mellitus	- GI upset - Injection site reactions - Weight loss
DPP-4 Inhibitor Linagliptin Saxagliptin Sitagliptin	- Inhibits DPP-4 enzyme that deactivates GLP-1	- Diabetes mellitus	- Nasopharyngitis - Weight neutral
SGLT-2 Inhibitor Canagliflozin Dapagliflozin Empagliflozin	- Inhibit SGLT-2 channel in proximal tubule	- Diabetes mellitus (benefit in patients with CV disease) - Heart failure - Chronic kidney disease	- Glycosuria, dehydration from osmotic diuresis - UTIs/vaginal yeast infections
Meglitinide Nateglinide Repaglinide	- Stimulates insulin release from pancreatic β-cells (like sulfonylureas)	- Diabetes mellitus	- Hypoglycemia - Weight gain
α-glucosidase inh. Acarbose Miglitol	- Inhibits intestinal brush border glucosidases	- Diabetes mellitus	- GI upset (flatulence and diarrhea)

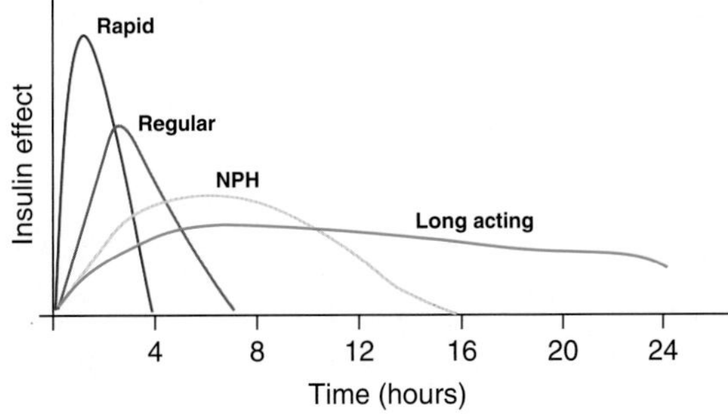

Endocrine Pharm

	Mechanism	Indication	Side Effects/Management
Glucocorticoids			
Beclomethasone Dexamethasone Hydrocortisone Methylprednisolone Prednisone	- Inhibit production of cytokines associated with inflammation (via NF-KB)	- Adrenal insufficiency - Immunosuppression - Autoimmune conditions - Asthma/COPD	- Cushing-type symptoms (with long-term use) - Adrenocortical atrophy - Peptic ulcers - Glucose intolerance - Steroid psychosis - Cataracts - Myopathy
Other Endocrine Meds			
Fludrocortisone	- Aldosterone analog (without glucocorticoid effect)	- Mineralocorticoid replacement	- Sodium/water retention, edema, hypertension
Conivaptan Tolvaptan	- ADH V2 receptor antagonist	- SIADH	- Thirst, dry mouth - Hypotension
Demeclocycline	- ADH antagonist (TCA structure)		
Desmopressin	- ADH agonist	- Diabetes insipidus - Clotting disorders - Bed wetting	- Hyponatremia - Headache, facial flushing
Octreotide	- Somatostatin analog	- Carcinoid syndrome - Pancreatic neuroendocrine tumor - Cirrhosis (variceal bleeds, hepatorenal syndrome)	- Hypothyroidism (suppresses TSH) - Cholelithiasis - Increased insulin resistance
Cinacalcet	- CaSR receptor potentiator	- Hyperparathyroidism	- Hypocalcemia
Thionamides Propylthiouracil Methimazole	- Inhibits thyroperoxidase - PTU also blocks 5-deiodinase	- Hyperthyroidism - Pregnancy (PTU used in 1st trimester, methimazole in 2nd/3rd)	- Rash, itching, hives - Aplastic anemia - Hepatotoxicity - ANCA + vasculitis Agranulocytosis - If fever + sore throat (within 90 days of starting): - Stop drug immediately - Check WBC (< 1 $\rightarrow$ Confirmed agranulocytosis)
Levothyroxine	- Thyroid hormone	- Hypothyroidism	- Hyperthyroid symptoms if dose too high

Esophageal Disease

Gastroesophageal Reflux Disease (GERD)

General: Retrograde flow of gastric contents from decreased lower esophageal tone or anatomic disruption of GE junction

Risk:

- **Smoking, obesity**
- Dietary: Certain foods (chocolate, peppermint, fat), coffee/caffeine, **alcohol**
- Structural abnormalities (hiatal hernia)

Clinical:

- **Heartburn**, regurgitation, dyspepsia (worse lying flat)
- Others: Chest pain, dysphagia, pulmonary symptoms (wheeze/cough)

Diagnosis:

- Initial diagnosis is clinical in those with classic symptoms
- If alarm symptoms, disease > 5 years, cancer risk factors: Endoscopy (evaluates for cancer, Barrett)

Management:

Severity	Definition	Intervention
Mild	- < 2 episodes/week - Mild symptoms	- Lifestyle (weight loss, smoking cessation, raise head of bed) - Avoid dietary triggers (if correlation) - **Low dose H2R antagonist.** Step up therapy if refractory.
Severe	- Esophagitis on endoscopy OR - > 2 episodes/week, severe symptoms	- **Daily PPI therapy** - For refractory, see algorithm below

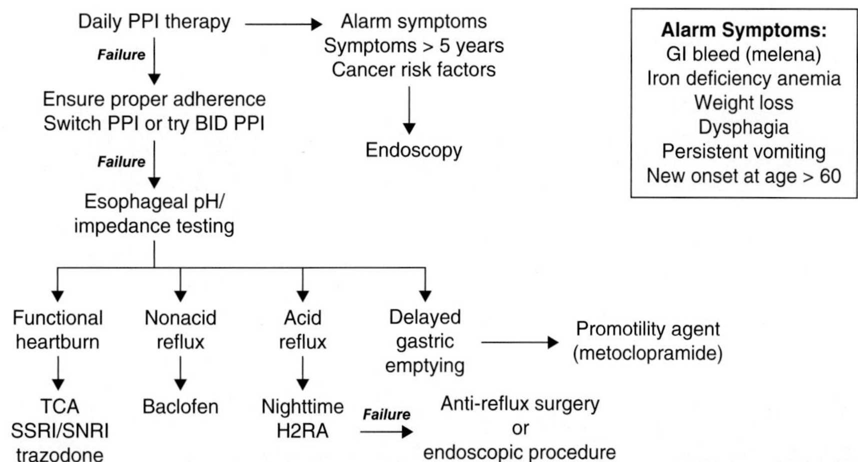

Complications of GERD

Erosive Esophagitis: Erosions and ulcerations of the esophageal mucosa.
Tx: GERD therapy.

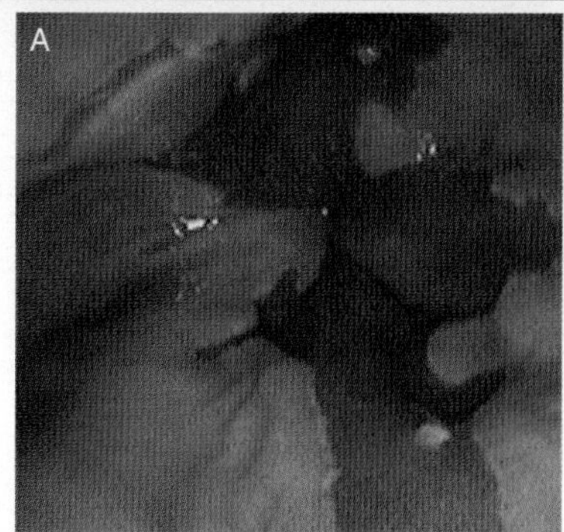

Barrett's: Metaplastic transformation of esophageal epithelium to columnar.
Salmon-colored esophageal mucosa[A].

- Predisposes patient to **esophageal adenocarcinoma**
- Once identified, biopsied to evaluate for dysplasia:
    - No dysplasia: q3-5 year endoscopic surveillance
    - Dysplasia: Endoscopic ablation/resection
    - All continue GERD treatment (i.e., PPI)

Strictures: Fibrous narrowing of the esophageal lumen, often causing dysphagia.
Tx: Endoscopic dilation.

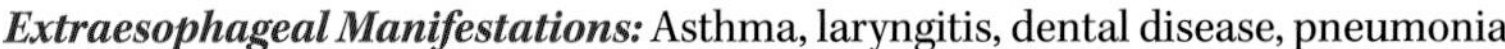

Extraesophageal Manifestations: Asthma, laryngitis, dental disease, pneumonia

Esophageal Disease

Hiatal Hernia

General: Herniation of GI elements through the diaphragmatic esophageal hiatus. Generally a congenital abnormality, but can develop post-surgery or trauma.

Subtype	Definition	Appearance
Sliding	- GE junction displaced above the diaphragm	
Paraesophageal	- Upward displacement of gastric fundus through defect in **phrenoesophageal membrane** - Often occurs **after surgery** - More likely to cause epigastric abdominal pain	

Clinical: Often asymptomatic. High association with GERD. Can also cause nonspecific abdominal pain.

Diagnosis: Generally discovered incidentally with barium swallow, endoscopy, imaging

Management:

- **Sliding**: Manage GERD
- **Paraesophageal**: Surgery in those with gastric complication from the hernia

Esophageal Cancer

	Squamous Cell	Adenocarcinoma
Risk	- Smoking/EtOH Use - Achalasia, strictures - Dietary factors (N-nitroso)	- Barrett/GERD
Location	- Mid-esophagus	- Distal esophagus (GE junction)
Metastasis	- Cervical or mediastinal nodes	- Celiac/gastric nodes

Clinical: **Progressive dysphagia** (initially solids, then liquids). Systemic symptoms (weight loss, anorexia), hematemesis.

Diagnosis: **Endoscopic biopsy**. Metastasis workup (endoscopic US, and CT/PET).

Management:

	Definition	Treatment
Superficial	- Limited to mucosa/submucosa	- Esophagectomy or endoscopic resection
Localized	- Local invasion/node spread	- Surgical resection, chemoradiation
Advanced	- Distant mets or local invasion of trachea, aorta	- Palliative chemoradiation/immunotherapy

Esophageal Disease

Disorder	General	Clinical	Diagnosis	Management
Achalasia	- Degeneration of myenteric ganglion cells → **Failure of LES relaxation** and lower esophagus peristalsis - Can be idiopathic, or associated with Chagas, malignancy, or autoimmune disease	- Dysphagia for **solids and liquids** - Regurgitation or heartburn	- Endoscopy (can't pass scope past LES) - **Manometry** (confirms) - Barium esophagram (if other tests equivocal, "Bird's beak")	- **Pneumatic dilation** or surgical myotomy - Nonsurgical candidates: Botulinum toxin, nitrates, or Ca-channel blockers
Hypertensive Peristalsis (Nutcracker Esophagus)	- Overactive excitatory innervation, resulting in normal timing of peristalsis, but **excess amplitude of contractions**	- Dysphagia for **solids and liquids** - **Chest pain** - Heartburn, regurgitation	- **Manometry** - Endoscopy (normal, rules out other path)	- Treat GERD (PPI) - **Diltiazem** (preferred first-line agent) Alternative options: - Botulinum toxin - Isosorbide dinitrate - Sildenafil
Diffuse-Esophageal Spasm	- Impaired inhibitory esophageal innervation, causing **increased simultaneous contractions** of the esophagus			
Zenker's Diverticulum	- Herniation at **Killian's triangle**, (area of muscular weakness between cricopharyngeus and lower inferior constrictor muscles) - Thought to be due to abnormal esophageal motility	- Oropharyngeal dysphagia - Aspiration/**regurgitation** - **Halitosis**, gurgling, neck mass	- **Barium esophagram** - Endoscopy	- Surgical or endoscopic resection
Esophageal Rings/Webs	- Thin membrane/tissue esophageal obstruction, often from chronic inflammation - **Plummer-Vinson**: Iron deficiency anemia, web, dysphagia, glossitis - **Schatzki Ring**: Most common type of esophageal ring	- Often asymptomatic - Can cause dysphagia, or food impaction	- Barium esophagram - Endoscopy	- Endoscopic dilatation
Mallory-Weiss Tear	- Longitudinal mucosal laceration due to ↑ abdominal pressure - Most commonly due to **vomiting** or iatrogenic (e.g., post endoscopy)	- Hematemesis - Epigastric or back pain	- Clinical symptoms - Endoscopy (to rule out other causes of upper GI bleed)	- PPI - Endoscopy for active bleeds (coag, clip, ligate, epinephrine)
Esophageal Perforation	- **Boerhaave syndrome** → Effort based esophageal rupture - Can result in mediastinal contamination with gastric contents - [Note: Traumatic rupture discussed in surgery/trauma]	- High-grade chest pain - Dysphagia - Subcutaneous emphysema - Pneumomediastinum	- **Contrast esophagram**	- Medical: NPO, PPI, antibiotics, parental nutrition - Surgical Repair (if septic, highly symptomatic)
Eosinophilic Esophagitis	- Immune-mediated esophageal disease with eosinophilic infiltrate and inflammation	- Dysphagia - Chronic GERD - Food impaction	- Endoscopy with biopsy	- Dietary modification - Fluticasone (PO)
Medication Esophagitis	- Tetracycline, KCl, NSAIDs, iron, bisphosphonate	- Odynophagia, dysphagia - Chest pain	- Clinical - Endoscopy if uncertain	- Discontinue medication
Infectious Esophagitis	- Often occurs in immunosuppressed patients Etiology: - **Candida** (white membranes) - **HSV** (round ulcers) - **CMV** (linear ulceration)	- **Odynophagia** - **Dysphagia** - Oral thrush (*Candida*) - Oral ulcers (HSV)	- Upper endoscopy w/ biopsy (if viral) - KOH prep for suspected *Candida*	- *Candida* → Fluconazole - HSV → Val-/acyclovir - CMV → Ganciclovir

Esophageal Disease

Dysphagia Workup

General: Subjective sense of difficulty or abnormal swallowing

Class	Clinical Features	Etiologies
Oropharyngeal	- Difficulty initiating a swallow - Associated with choking, coughing, aspiration and globus sensation	- Variety of neurologic, structural, infectious, and iatrogenic etiologies
Esophageal	- Difficulty swallowing seconds after initial swallow - Sensation of food stuck in esophagus - **Solids/liquids → Motility** - **Solids alone → Structural**	- Motility disorders - Structural lesions (malignancy, strictures) - Esophagitis
Acute-Onset	- Sudden onset inability to swallow food/liquids	- Food impaction

Diagnosis:

Oropharyngeal
- Modified **barium swallow** (investigates oral, pharyngeal, and esophageal phases)

Esophageal dysphagia
- Upper endoscopy (generally first test, to rule out structural lesions)
- Barium swallow
- Manometry

Food impaction
- Upper endoscopy (diagnostic/therapeutic)

Globus Sensation

General: Sensation of lump or food bolus in oropharynx, that is not due to any clear underlying pathology

Risk: Higher occurrence in those with psychiatric disease

Diagnosis: Barium swallow (rule out other disorders)

Management: Reassurance

Gastric Disease

Gastritis/Gastropathy

General: Gastritis and gastropathy refer to states of gastric damage from mucosal barrier dysfunction or mucosal inflammation

	Gastropathy	Gastritis
Pathophys	- Mucosal barrier breakdown, leading to **mucosal damage** (no inflammation)	- **Mucosal inflammation** from an autoimmune or infectious etiology - Inflammation can be either acute or chronic
Histologic Findings	- Foveolar hyperplasia, edema - Lack of inflammatory cells	- <u>Acute</u>: Mucosal damage, **neutrophilic** infiltrate - <u>Chronic</u>: **Lymphocytic** infiltration, with atrophy and metaplasia
Etiology	- Chemicals (**EtOH, bile, NSAIDs**) - Hypoperfusion (sepsis, burns, hypovolemia) - Chemotherapy - Portal hypertension	- ***H. pylori*** infection - **<u>Autoimmune Metaplastic Atrophic Gastritis</u>** - Autoantibody against parietal cells, resulting in gastritis of body/fundus, and pernicious anemia - Dx: Endoscopy with biopsy - Tx: B12, surveillance EGD
Other Findings		- Can lead to atrophy/metaplasia, ↑ cancer risk - Hypochlorhydria, leading to elevated gastrin secretion

Clinical: Epigastric pain, nausea, vomiting, anorexia, weight loss

Diagnosis: Endoscopy with mucosal biopsy
- Macroscopic features (erythema, mucosal erosions, lack of rugal folds) suggestive, biopsy is diagnostic

Management: Treat underlying etiology

Dyspepsia and Epigastric Pain Workup

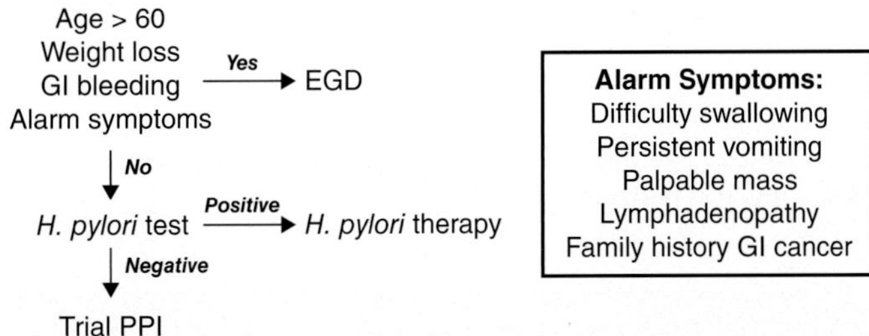

Helicobacter pylori

General: Gram negative gastric bacteria that is associated with gastritis and PUD

Diagnosis:
- If upper endoscopy is indicated: Biopsy with urease testing + culture
- Noninvasive testing: **Stool antigen assay, urea breath test**
    - Serology is avoided (low spec/sens, does not differentiate active from previous infection)

Management:
- **Triple Therapy (First Line)**: Amoxicillin, clarithromycin, PPI
- **Quad Therapy**: Metronidazole, tetracycline, PPI, bismuth (used if local macrolide resistance)
- After treatment, **test for eradication** (same tests as diagnosis)

Gastric Disease

Peptic Ulcer Disease

General: Defect in the gastric or duodenal mucosa that extends through the muscularis mucosa

	Gastric	Duodenal
Etiology	- *H. pylori* - NSAID	- *H. pylori* - NSAID - Zollinger Ellison
Cancer	- Increased risk	- Generally benign
Location	- Type I: **Lesser curvature** (most common) - Type II: Gastric and duodenal - Type III: Prepyloric - Type IV: Near EG junction	- Anterior duodenum more common than posterior, generally 1-2 cm distal to pylorus

Clinical: Epigastric pain, nausea, early satiety, feeling of fullness

Diagnosis: **Endoscopy** (with biopsy of ulcer margin)
- Barium esophagram (suggestive, but not confirmatory like endoscopy)
- Etiology: Assess NSAID history, workup for *H. pylori*

Management:
- Treat underlying cause (**avoid NSAIDs, treat *H. pylori***)
- PPI (regardless of etiology)
- Endoscopic surveillance of gastric ulcers

Complications:

	Clinical	Management
Perforation	- Acute onset severe abdominal pain with signs of peritonitis	- Surgical repair
Bleed	- Either acute or subacute upper GI bleed	- Endoscopic intervention
Outlet Obstruction	- Epigastric fullness, early satiety, weight loss, nausea, vomiting	- Surgical

Stress Ulcers:
- Common among critically-ill patients
- Shock, sepsis, trauma → ↓ mucosal perfusion, loss of protective barrier of mucous
- Prophylactic PPI given to some ICU patients

Misc. Gastric Pathology

Dieulafoy's Lesion: Dilated submucosal blood vessel that, in the absence of ulceration, invades through the gastric mucosa. Rare cause of upper GI bleed.

Menetrier Disease: Rare acquired stomach disease in which gastric hyperplasia results in rugal hypertrophy. Can cause chronic epigastric pain, weight loss, nausea, vomiting. May have increased cancer risk.

Gastric Disease

Gastric Cancer

	Clinical Features	Risk Factors
"Intestinal" Adenocarcinoma	- Well-differentiated, glandular proliferation - Results from **intestinal metaplasia**	- *H. pylori* - Chronic gastritis - Obesity, smoking, EtOH, Diet (N-nitroso) - Family history - Genetic syndrome (BRCA, HNPCC) - Blood type A
"Diffuse" Adenocarcinoma	- Poorly-differentiated proliferation of tumor cells, due to loss of cadherin intercellular adhesions - **Signet ring cells** - Rapidly progressive/poor prognosis	
GIST	- Tumor from interstitial cells of Cajal	- Usually sporadic - Familial syndromes
Lymphoma	- Marginal or diffuse large B-cell lymphoma of the MALT tissue	- ***H. pylori*** - Autoimmune gastritis - IBD/celiac

Clinical: Abdominal pain, weight loss, nausea, early satiety

- **Leser Trelat**: Explosive onset of multiple itchy seborrheic keratoses
- Signature metastatic findings:
  - Krukenberg tumor: Metastasis to the ovary
  - Sister-Mary-Joseph node: Subcutaneous periumbilical lesion
  - Virchow node: Metastasis to supraclavicular node

Diagnosis: **Endoscopy with biopsy**

- Intestinal adeno can look like polypoid mass or ulcer. Diffuse adeno appears diffusely thick/rigid ("linitis plastica").
- Staging: CT, PET, endoscopic US

Management:

Adenocarcinoma	- Partial or total gastrectomy with neoadjuvant/adjuvant chemotherapy - If metastatic: Palliative chemoradiation
GIST	- Local resection +/– imatinib
Lymphoma	- Radiation therapy, rituximab, treat underlying *H. pylori*

Gastroparesis

General: Delayed gastric emptying without mechanical obstruction. Most commonly caused by diabetic neuropathy or after gastric surgery.

Clinical: Presents with nausea, vomiting, early satiety, epigastric pain

Diagnosis: Gastric emptying study

Management: Glycemic control/hydration, prokinetics (metoclopramide), antiemetics

Gastric Outlet Obstruction

General: Mechanical obstruction of the gastric outlet

Etiology: Peptic ulcer disease (causes scar formation), caustic ingestion (stricture), malignancy, gastric bezoar (accumulation of ingestion material, like hair)

Clinical: Nausea/vomiting, epigastric pain, early satiety, abdominal distension

- **Succussion splash**: Hear gastric contents splash > 3 hours after eating

Diagnosis: CT or endoscopy

Management: NPO, NG tube decompression, PPI

- Treat underlying (surgically remove masses, dilate strictures)

Gastric Disease

Bariatric Surgery

Procedure Type	Features
Gastric Band[A]	- Inflatable band placed around upper stomach, creating a small upper pouch of the stomach that holds less food - Allows less food to be consumed and decreases hunger - Can be complicated by band erosion, slippage, and port infection/malfunctioning
Sleeve Gastrectomy[B]	- Removal of 80% of the stomach, leaving a sleeve like pouch - Decreases amount of food able to eat, and alters gut hormones (responsible for hunger, satiety) - Can be complicated by GI bleeding, gastric leaks, and stenosis of the gastric outlet
Roux-en-Y Gastric Bypass[C]	- Stomach is divided into a small upper pouch, and the small bowel is divided 40 cm below the gastric outlet. The small stomach pouch is connected with the distal small bowel. - Weight loss through smaller gastric pouch and diversion of nutrients around a long stretch of small bowel - Can be complicated by gastric remnant distention/rupture, stomal stenosis, marginal ulcers, dumping syndrome
Biliopancreatic Diversion with Duodenal Switch[D]	- Gastrectomy, plus division of the duodenum at the gastric outlet, reconnection of the stomach to distal small bowel, reanastomosis of the bypassed small bowel to the distal small bowel (to deliver bile, pancreatic enzymes) - Weight loss through smaller stomach, diversion of nutrients, and malabsorption due to less time of food being contacted by digestive pancreatic enzymes - Can cause serious protein-calorie malnutrition, and high risk for fat soluble vitamin deficiency

Indications:

(1) BMI $\geq$ 40 kg/m^2 without comorbidity
(2) BMI $\geq$ 35 kg/m^2 with at least one comorbidity
- Includes type II DM, OSA, HTN, HLD, NAFLD/NASH, others

Complications:

- Nutrition:
  - Must supplement and monitor the following: Thiamine, folate, B12, iron, vitamin A/D/E/K, copper, zinc
- Anastomotic leak or obstruction (usually < 30 days postoperative)
- Marginal or gastrojejunal ulcers
- Dumping syndrome
  - Severe diarrhea, nausea, vomiting, and abdominal pain after eating from rapid gastric emptying of certain foods (usually high sugar)

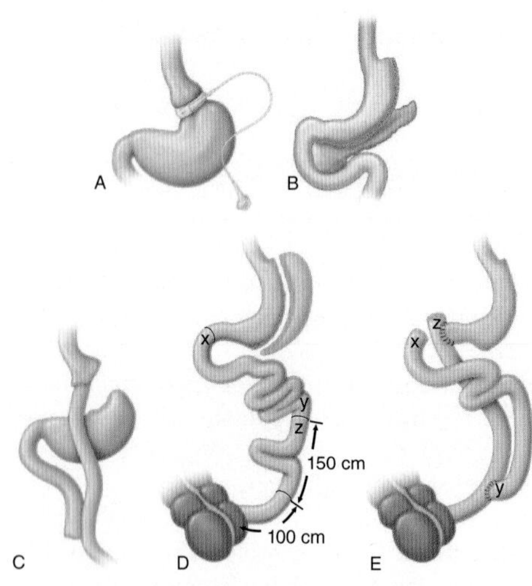

Small Bowel Disease

Malabsorption

General: Impaired nutrient absorption, due to acquired or congenital defects in the absorptive epithelium of the small intestine, or improper digestion of nutrients

Clinical: **Diarrhea with fatty, large-volume, foul-smelling stools** and weight loss. Vitamin and mineral deficiencies.

Diagnosis: Variety of tests for specific etiologies (fecal elastase, hydrogen breath test, etc.)
- Fecal fat malabsorption (Sudan III stain)
- Carbohydrate absorption tests (D-xylose [simple sugar, does not require enzymes to digest] → Detected in urine if absorbed)

Celiac Disease

General: Hypersensitivity to gluten, a protein found in wheat, resulting in small bowel mucosal inflammation

Risk: Family history, **HLA-DQ2/DQ8**

Clinical: **Malabsorption** (diarrhea, weight loss, vitamin/mineral deficiency [**iron**]). Associated with **dermatitis herpetiformis**, autoimmune disorders (type I DM, Hashimoto thyroiditis).

Diagnosis: **tTG-IgA levels** (Alternative test: Deamidated gliadin peptide [DGP] IgG or anti-endomysial IgA)
- Note: ↑ risk of IgA deficiency, so if IgA is low, check tTG or DGP IgG
- Check HLA-DQ2/DQ8 (high NPV)
- Endoscopy with duodenal biopsy: Villous atrophy, crypt hyperplasia, intraepithelial lymphocytosis

Management: Gluten-free diet. Ensure proper vitamin and mineral levels (i.e., iron).

Etiologies of Malabsorption

	General	Clinical	Diagnosis	Treatment
Pancreatic Insufficiency	- Loss of **exocrine pancreas function** - Causes: Chronic pancreatitis, cystic fibrosis, duct obstruction, small bowel resection (↓ secretin/CCK production), advanced hemochromatosis	- Steatorrhea, malabsorption	- ↑ Fecal fat - ↓ **Fecal elastase** - ↓ Duodenal pH	- Pancreatic enzyme replacement - Supplementation of fat soluble vitamins
Lactose Intolerance	- **Lactase deficiency**, resulting in lactose transit to colon, with production of hydrogen gas and fatty acids - Primary: Congenital or acquired nonpersistence of enzyme - Secondary: Lactase loss after GI disease (e.g., gastroenteritis)	- Abdominal pain, bloating, flatulence - High volume, watery diarrhea	- **Hydrogen breath test** (diagnostic) Other signs: - Stool: Osm gap > 125 - pH < 6	- ↓ Dietary lactose - Lactase enzymes
Whipple Disease	- SI overgrowth of ***T. whipplei***, resulting in buildup of macrophages with PAS+ intracellular material	- **Chronic diarrhea, abd pain** - **Arthralgias, weight loss** - Cardiac (myocarditis) - Neurologic dysfunction	- Endoscopy with biopsy (classic macrophages, PCR for bacterial DNA)	- Antibiotics (penicillin or ceftriaxone, followed by 1 year of TMP-SMX)
Tropical Sprue	- Chronic diarrheal disease with unclear etiology - Occurs in those that have spent ≥ 1 month in endemic area (band of countries ~30° latitude, including India, Haiti, DR, PR)	- Chronic diarrhea and malabsorption, in someone with consistent travel history	- Endoscopy with biopsy	- Tetracycline and folate
SIBO (Small Intestinal Bacterial Overgrowth)	- Overgrowth of colonic bacteria in the SI, resulting in enterocyte damage and malabsorption - Risks: Motility disorders, structural issues (adhesions, IBD)	- Watery diarrhea, bloating, flatulence, abdominal pain	- **Carbohydrate breath test**, jejunal culture (> 10^3 CFU) Note: Low levels of many vitamins possible, but ↑ folate/vitamin K	- Antibiotics (rifaximin)

Small Bowel Disease

Acute Mesenteric Ischemia

General: Sudden onset intestinal hypoperfusion, in the **superior mesenteric artery**

Etiology:

- **Arterial Embolization** (AFib, valvular disease)
- Arterial thrombosis (over an atherosclerotic plaque)
- Venous thrombosis (rare)

Clinical:

- Classic presentation is acute, **severe abdominal pain disproportionate to physical findings**
- Peritonitis, sepsis, and shock if severe ischemia/perforation

Diagnosis:

- **CT Angiography**
- Laparotomy for those hemodynamically unstable

Management:

Type	Indication	Intervention
Surgical	- Peritonitis, sepsis, pneumatosis intestinalis	- Mesenteric embolectomy or bypass - Bowel resection for necrotic bowel
Endovascular	- Stable - No advanced intestinal ischemia	- Pharm thrombectomy - Balloon angioplasty/stent
Medical	- All patients	- NPO, fluids - Antibiotics, PPI - Heparin

Chronic Mesenteric Ischemia

General: Atherosclerotic disease of mesenteric vessels (celiac artery, superior and inferior mesenteric arteries), resulting in hypoperfusion

Clinical: **Postprandial dull pain**. Weight loss or nutritional deficiency.

Diagnosis: CT angiography

Management: Endovascular revascularization (for those with severe symptoms)

Small Bowel Disease

Appendicitis

General: Inflammation of the appendix, a common cause of acute abdomen. Secondary to obstruction (fecalith, lymph node hyperplasia, tumors, etc.), leading to distension, vascular compromise, and eventual bacterial invasion.

Risk: Age (most common in 2nd/3rd generations of life)

Clinical:

- **Abdominal pain**: Periumbilical (visceral), followed by RLQ (peritoneal) at McBurney point
- Nausea, vomiting, anorexia
- Variety of signs:
    - Rovsing: RLQ pain with LLQ palpation
    - Iliopsoas: RLQ pain with active right hip flexion
    - Obturator: RLQ pain with internal rotation of the hip

	Diagnosis	Management
Child	- Purely clinical (if classic), can go to surgery - US preferred imaging test	- Laparoscopic appendectomy - Antibiotics (enteric coverage, e.g., CTX/metronidazole)
Adult	- CT with contrast preferred	- Laparoscopic appendectomy - Antibiotics (enteric coverage, e.g., CTX/metronidazole)
Pregnant	- US	- Laparoscopic appendectomy - Antibiotics

Note: Some evidence points toward purely antibiotic management of appendicitis, but this is not widely accepted in the United States at this time, as many of these patients require surgery within a few years.

Complications:

Perforation:

- Perforation of the appendix, generally contained in a phlegmon or abscess

Tx:

- Unstable (peritoneal signs, septic, etc.): Emergent appendectomy
- Stable: IV antibiotics, percutaneous drainage of abscess or appendectomy

Small Bowel Disease

Small Bowel Obstruction

General: Obstruction of normal flow in the small bowel. Subtypes:

Complete: No passage of stool or gas

- Compromised blood supply can result in ischemia or necrosis

Partial: Some gas still passes, much lower risk for strangulation

Etiology:

- **Adhesions** (prior GI surgery or inflammation)
- Bowel (hernias)
- Cancer
- IBD (strictures)
- Intussusception, volvulus, gallstone ileus
- SMA syndrome (intermittent obstruction of the 3rd portion of the duodenum between the SMA/aorta)

Clinical:

- **Abdominal pain, bilious emesis, nausea/vomiting**
  - Borborygmi (high tympanic bowel sounds) initially as peristalsis is frequent
  - Followed by decreased bowel sounds as distension increases and peristalsis declines

Diagnosis:

- Abdominal XR (dilated loops, air-fluid levels)
- **CT[A] with oral + IV contrast**

Management:

- Stable patients undergo trial of nonoperative management, including NPO, NG tube decompression, IVF, and PO water-soluble contrast
- Surgery indicated for any with peritoneal signs, hemodynamic instability, or evidence of bowel ischemia/necrosis

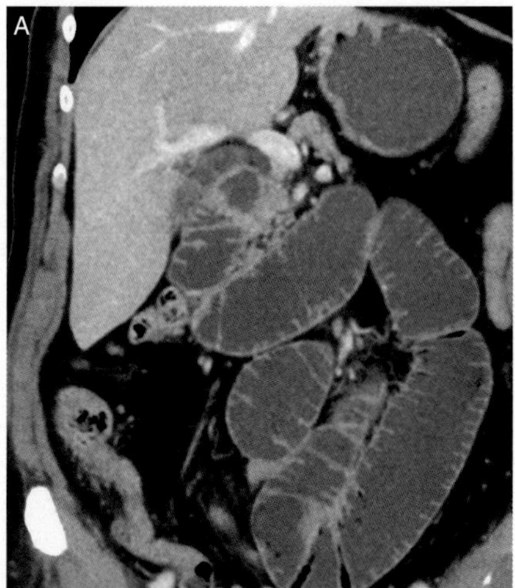

Paralytic Ileus

General: Decreased or absent peristalsis, resulting in obstipation and intolerance of oral intake

Etiology: Commonly occurs post-operatively (2-3 days is normal). Risk factors include narcotics, electrolyte abnormalities.

Clinical: Abdominal pain/distension, nausea/vomiting, failure to pass flatus, inability to tolerate oral diet

Diagnosis: Clinical. Plain abdominal XR shows dilated bowel loops.

Management: Supportive care (IVF, pain control without narcotics, dietary restriction)

Small Bowel Disease

Hernias

General: Protrusion of bowel through a weak spot in the abdominal fascia. Can be reducible (able to be pushed back inside the abdominal wall) and irreducible.

Subtype	Definition	Risk
Indirect Inguinal	- Protrusion of hernia sac through **internal inguinal ring**, lateral to the inferior epigastric artery	- Congenital defect (patent processus vaginalis)
Direct Inguinal	- Protrusion of hernia sac through **Hesselbach triangle**, medial to the inferior epigastric artery	- Acquired abdominal wall defect (chronic straining)
Femoral	- Peritoneal hernia sac passing through the **femoral canal**	- More common in women
Ventral	- Anterior abdominal wall hernia - Includes incisional, umbilical, epigastric, Spigelian	- Prior surgery for incisional - Obesity or ascites for umbilical

Clinical: Physical bulge in abdominal wall, with varying degrees of pain and discomfort

Diagnosis: Generally a clinical diagnosis. US/CT can be used to confirm.

Management:

	Definition	Management
Strangulated	- Necrotic tissue from ischemia	- **Emergency surgery**
Incarcerated	- Compromised blood supply, without necrotic bowel - Richter's hernia is special subtype with incarceration of part of the bowel wall	- **Urgent surgery** (especially if SBO or not reducible) - Can attempt to reduce (but surgery is generally preferred)
Minimal Symptoms	- No evidence of incarceration or strangulation	- **Elective surgery** OR - Watchful monitoring

Small Bowel Disease

Subtypes of Small Intestinal Cancer	
Neuroendocrine (Carcinoid)	- Secrete serotonin and other bioactive products
Adenocarcinoma	- Rare. Generally seen in someone with chronic inflammation (e.g., Crohn).
Lymphoma	- Primary GI lymphoma most often associated with autoimmune conditions, IBD
GIST	- Malignant mesenchymal tumors (sarcomas)

Carcinoid Tumor

General: Well-differentiated neuroendocrine tumors arising from **enterochromaffin cells**. Most commonly found in small bowel, but can be found in the lungs and stomach.

Clinical: Vague symptoms, generally relating to the impacted organ

Diagnosis: Often discovered incidentally (imaging like CT). Confirmed with biopsy.

Management: Surgical resection

Carcinoid Syndrome

General: Carcinoid tumor that **metastasizes to liver**, allowing for systemic serotonin release (normally degraded by MAO in liver)

Clinical:

- GI: **Diarrhea**, abdominal pain
- Pulmonary: Bronchospasm/wheeze
- Skin: **Flushing**, telangiectasias
- CV: Right-sided valvular lesions (fibrosis, collagen deposition)

Diagnosis:

- **Elevated urinary 5-HIAA**
- CT/MRI to localize

Management:

- Octreotide
- Hepatic resection (of metastasis)

Small Bowel Disease

Overview of Functional GI Disorders

General: Disorders of the GI tract producing symptoms (pain, nausea, etc.) without any clear anatomical or biochemical basis

Disorders include functional abdominal pain (commonly in children), heartburn, dyspepsia, diarrhea

Irritable Bowel Syndrome (IBS)

General: Functional GI disorder characterized by chronic abdominal pain and altered bowel habits. Unclear pathophysiology, but theories include gut visceral hypersensitivity, motility disorder, abnormal immune system functioning, altered microbiome.

Risk: Associated with **psychiatric disorders**

Clinical: **Periodic cramping pain**, constipation, and/or diarrhea
- Patients can have predominantly diarrhea, constipation, or mixed features
- Defecation can make better or worse

Diagnosis: ROME IV Criteria
- **Recurrent abdominal pain** (≥ 1 day/week), for the last three months PLUS two of the following:
  - (1) Related to defecation
  - (2) Change in stool frequency
  - (3) Change in stool appearance

Management:
- Initial: Dietary and lifestyle modification
  - Exclude gas-producing foods, lactose, gluten (low **FODMAP** diet)
  - Psyllium if constipation predominant
  - Physical exercise
- **Refractory IBS-C** (constipation):
  - Polyethylene glycol, lubiprostone, linaclotide
- **Refractory IBS-D** (diarrhea):
  - Loperamide
- **Refractory Abdominal Pain**:
  - Dicylcomine/hyoscyamine or TCA
  - If bloating/no constipation: Rifaximin

Cyclic Vomiting Syndrome

General: Recurrent episodes of vomiting with intervening periods of normal health. Association with migraine headaches, chronic cannabis use.

Clinical:
- Up to a week long episode of **daily morning vomiting**
- Intermittent (months long) periods of normal health

Management:
- Abortive: Anti-migraine therapy (sumatriptan) if identified in prodromal phase (prior to significant symptoms)
- Acute (ER) Care: IV fluids, antiemetics (e.g., ondansetron), diphenhydramine, lorazepam
- Preventative: TCA (amitriptyline)

Inflammatory Bowel Disease

<table>
<tr><th></th><th>Crohn Disease</th><th>Ulcerative Colitis</th></tr>
<tr><td>Gen</td><td>- Areas of transmural inflammation found throughout the GI tract
- Terminal ileum involvement is classic, but can involve anywhere from mouth to anus, with "skip lesions"</td><td>- Recurring episodes of mucosal inflammation[A] in the colon (spares rest of GI tract)</td></tr>
<tr><td>Path</td><td>- Microscopy: Transmural inflammation, noncaseating granulomas
- Cobblestone mucosa, creeping fat, bowel wall thickening ("string sign"), linear ulcers and fissures</td><td>- Microscopy: Inflammation, crypt abscess, architectural distortion
- Friable mucosal pseudopolyps, loss of haustra ("lead pipe")</td></tr>
<tr><td>Risk</td><td colspan="2">- Peak age is bimodal (15-40, 50-80 y/o)
- More common in Caucasians
- Family history
- Smoking (↑ Crohn risk, ↓ UC risk [quitting smoking ↑ risk for UC flare])</td></tr>
<tr><td rowspan="2">Clin</td><td>- Diarrhea (usually nonbloody)
- Abdominal pain (often RLQ)
- Malabsorption, weight loss

- Complications include abscess, fistula, strictures</td><td>- Hematochezia or bloody diarrhea
- Abdominal pain
- Tenesmus

- Greatly increased colon cancer risk
- Associated with primary sclerosing cholangitis</td></tr>
<tr><td colspan="2"><u>Extraintestinal manifestations</u>:
- Skin: Rash (pyoderma gangrenosum, erythema nodosum)
- Eye: Uveitis, episcleritis
- Joints: Arthritis, spondylitis, sacroiliitis</td></tr>
<tr><td rowspan="2">Dx</td><td>- Colonoscopy (for colon/ileum)
- Capsule or CT/MR enterography (for small intestine)</td><td>- Colonoscopy</td></tr>
<tr><td colspan="2">- For flares: Must exclude other causes of intestinal inflammation (e.g., check C. Diff antigen, stool culture, O&P)
- Monitor ESR, CRP, fecal calprotectin</td></tr>
<tr><td rowspan="2">Tx</td><td><u>Initial induction of remission</u>:
- Steroids (Budesonide or Prednisone) +/− early initiation of anti-TNF

<u>Maintenance of remission</u>:
- anti-TNF and/or thiopurine</td><td><u>Initial Induction of Remission</u>:
- Oral/Topical 5-ASA
- Steroid course if severe

<u>Maintenance of Remission</u>:
- Oral/Topical 5-ASA
- anti-TNF and/or thiopurine used for moderate-severe disease

<u>Surgical (Colectomy)</u>:
- Severe, debilitating, refractory disease, increased colon cancer risk, or severe complication (megacolon, hemorrhage)</td></tr>
<tr><td colspan="2"><u>Drug options</u>:
- 5-ASA: Sulfasalazine or mesalamine
- Thiopurines: 6-Mercaptopurine, azathioprine
- Anti-TNF: Adalimumab, infliximab
- Other biologics: Ustekinumab, vedolizumab, risankizumab</td></tr>
</table>

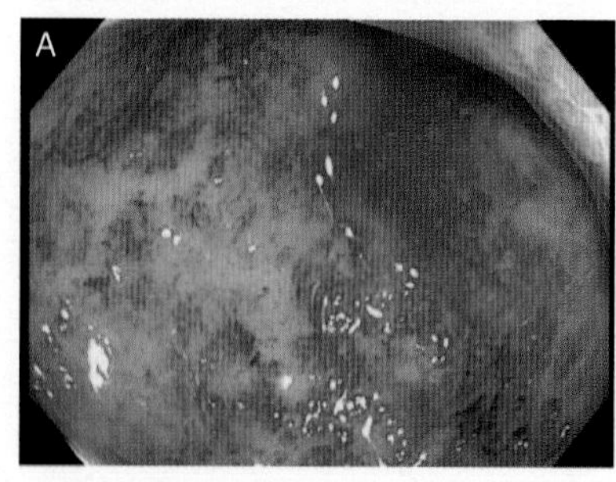

Colorectal Disease

Colon Cancer

General: Majority of tumors are endoluminal adenocarcinoma, typically arising from adenomatous polyps. Molecular pathway involves the loss of APC, KRAS, and p53 (adenoma-carcinoma sequence) or microsatellite instability.

Risk: Age > 50, prior history of colon cancer, history of adenomatous polyps, IBD, family history, genetic conditions

Clinical: Often asymptomatic (found on normal screening), but can present as abdominal pain, **hematochezia**, partial bowel obstruction, **iron deficiency anemia**, thin stools
- Right-sided: Iron-deficiency anemia, weight loss
- Left-sided: Hematochezia, change in stool "caliber"

Diagnosis: Colonoscopy (with biopsy)

Management:
- **Localized disease**: Colonic resection (partial colectomy)
    - Adjuvant chemotherapy for node-positive disease
- **Metastatic disease**: Palliative chemothcrapy
    - Some patients with limited metastasis can have aggressive surgery with chemotherapy (attempt at cure)
- Follow patients in remission with annual CT, colonoscopy, and CEA level

Colon Cancer Screening/Polyps

	Features	Malignancy Potential
Hyperplastic	- Simple glandular hyperplasia - ~ 90% of polyps found	- None (**benign**)
Adenoma	- Tubular (most common) - Tubulovillous - Villous: Greatest risk of malignancy	Increasing risk with: - Villous - Larger size (> 1 cm) - Sessile polyp - Cellular dysplasia - Higher number
Hamartoma	- Normal mucosa cells, with distorted architecture - Most common juvenile polyp - Associated with Peutz-Jeghers - Cause painless rectal bleeding	- Sporadic hamartomas are rarely malignant - If associated with genetic syndrome → ↑ cancer risk

Screening Methodology

Colonoscopy	- q10 years
Flex sigmoidoscopy	- q5-10 years + annual FIT
CT colonography	- q5 years
FIT (fecal immunochemical test)-DNA	- q1-3 years
FOBT (fecal occult blood testing)	- q1 year

Colorectal Disease

Colorectal Cancer Screening

Population	Timing of Onset	Freq	Notes
General	- **45-75 y/o** > 75 depends on preference, life expectancy	10 yr	- Frequency can be increased to 3-5 years if the patient is found to have adenomatous polyps (exact timing depends on type and quantity of the polyps)
Family Hx	- 40 y/o, or - 10 years prior to relative's cancer diagnosis	5 yr	- 1° relative < 60 y/o OR - Two 1° relatives with colon cancer at any age
IBD	- 8 years post diagnosis	1-3 yr	
FAP	- 10-15 years old	1 yr	
HNPCC	- 20-25, or prior to first family colon cancer diagnosis	1-2 yr	

Hereditary Conditions

Syndrome	Characteristics
FAP (Familial Adenomatous Polyposis)	- AD defect in the **APC gene** - > 100 pancolonic adenomatous polyps arise starting around puberty, in addition to upper GI (duodenal) cancer - Management: **Colectomy** (once polyps are found), with upper endoscopy monitoring for duodenal adenomas Subtypes (FAP + the following): - **Gardner**: Osteoma, dental issues, desmoid tumor, hypertrophy of retinal pigment epithelium, cutaneous lesions (cysts, fibromas) - **Turcot**: Brain tumors (medulloblastoma or glioma)
HNPCC (Lynch or Hereditary Nonpolyposis Colon Cancer)	- AD **DNA mismatch repair gene defect** (MSH/MLH), causing **microsatellite instability** - Greatly **increased colon** and **endometrial cancer risk** - Also at risk for ovarian, stomach, small bowel and other cancers - Amsterdam Criteria: Suspect in those with 3 relatives, 2 generations, 1 diagnosed < 50 y/o, and 1 first degree relative - Colon screening (see above), endometrial/upper GI screening
Peutz-Jeghers	- AD defect in STK11 gene - Mucocutaneous macules (lips, hands, feet), **gastrointestinal hamartomatous polyps** (which can bleed, obstruct, become malignant) - ↑ risk of cancer (gastric, small intestinal, colon, pancreatic, breast) - Management: Early onset screening for cancer (colonoscopy, mammography, and pancreatic MRI)
Juvenile Polyposis	- Genetic syndrome of childhood onset of gastrointestinal polyposis (hamartomas), with increased CRC risk - Early onset colonoscopy screening is indicated

Colorectal Disease

Diverticulosis

General: False outpouching of the colonic mucosal layers, commonly occuring where the vasa recta penetrate the colonic muscularis. Most commonly found in the sigmoid colon. Increased intraluminal pressure (e.g., constipation) predisposes this condition.

Risk: Diet (low fiber, high fat/meat), obesity

Clinical: Asymptomatic, but very common cause of GI bleed (**painless hematochezia**)

Diagnosis: Often incidentally identified on colonoscopy, CT scan

Management:

- Asymptomatic: Monitor
- Bleeds: Resuscitation, colonoscopy (with intervention on active bleeders)

Diverticulitis

General: Inflammation and/or infection of a colonic diverticulum

Risk: Diverticular disease risk listed above. Note: Nuts/seeds not associated.

Clinical: **LLQ abdominal pain**, diarrhea/constipation, **fever**

Diagnosis: **CT[A] (with oral/IV contrast)**: Look for bowel wall thickening, inflamed pericolic fat, phlegmons/abscesses.

Note: Colonoscopy/enema are contraindicated during active inflammation

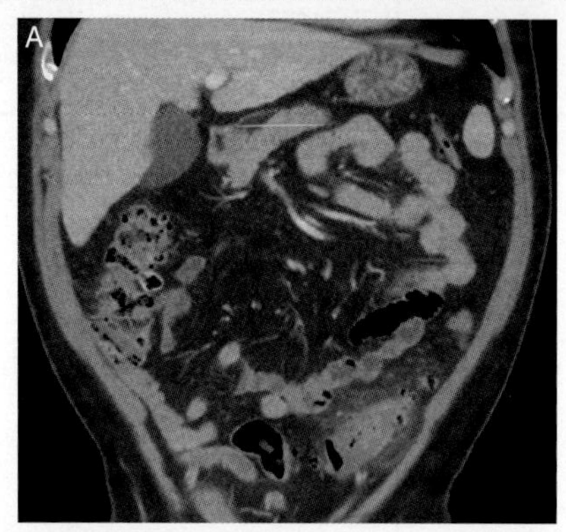

Management:

Type	Indication	Therapy
Outpatient Medical	- Uncomplicated disease (no complications seen below)	Antibiotics: - Cipro/metronidazole - TMP-SMX/metronidazole - Amox-clavulanate
Inpatient Medical	- Uncomplicated disease, but high risk due to comorbidities (e.g., old age) or sepsis	- IV pain control, fluids, NPO - IV antibiotics (enteric coverage, such as ceftriazone/metronidazole)
Complications		
Frank Perforation	- Microperforations medically treated, but large perforations need surgical correction	- Emergent surgery
Fistula		- Surgery
Obstruction		
Abscess	> 4 cm	- Percutaneous drainage - Surgery if refractory
	< 4 cm	- IV antibiotics

Follow-up: Colonoscopy ~ 6 weeks after episode resolves

- If complicated disease, > 2 episodes, or smoldering symptoms → elective colectomy

Colorectal Disease

	General	Clinical/Diagnosis	Management
Ischemic Colitis	- Malperfusion of large bowel, resulting in colonic ischemia - Can be transient to full-blown necrosis - Impacts "watershed" areas - Risk: Aortic instrumentation, cardiac bypass, **any cause of hypotension**	- Mild to severe abdominal pain - **Hematochezia** Dx: - Clinical, colonoscopy can confirm - Impacts **splenic flexure**	- Medical: Antibiotics, NPO, NG tube - If necrosis: Surgical resection
Sigmoid Volvulus	- Sigmoid colon twisting about its mesentery, causing obstruction - Occurs in elderly (mean age 70) - Risk: Long sigmoid, narrow mesentery	- Progressive abdominal pain, nausea, bloating, and constipation Dx: - Abd XR: **Coffee bean sign**[A] - CT (preferred confirmatory test)	- **Endoscopic detorsion + rectal tube** - Surgery if signs of necrosis or endoscopy fails - Elective sigmoid resection (high risk for recurrence)
Angio-dysplasia	- Sporadic, aberrant blood vessels that have a tendency to bleed - Risk: Old age, CKD, von Willebrand, aortic stenosis (Heyde syndrome)	- Generally asymptomatic, unless bleeding Dx: - Colonoscopy	- GI bleed: Endoscopic intervention
Large Bowel Obstruction	- Causes: Cancer, volvulus, inflammation (IBD, diverticulitis), stricture (prior surgical anastomosis)	- Acute or subacute presentation of **pain, bloating, obstipation** Dx: - Abdominal XR or CT	- Supportive: IVF, NPO, gastric decompression - Surgical intervention often required
Ogilvies Syndrome	- Acute **nonstructural obstruction** of colonic flow - Occurs in acutely ill and hospitalized patients - Associated with opiates	- Abdominal distension - Pain, nausea, emesis, constipation Dx: - Abdominal CT (rule out mechanical obstruction)	- Initially conservative/supportive measures (IVF, stop offending medications) - **Neostigmine** - **Colonoscopic decompression**

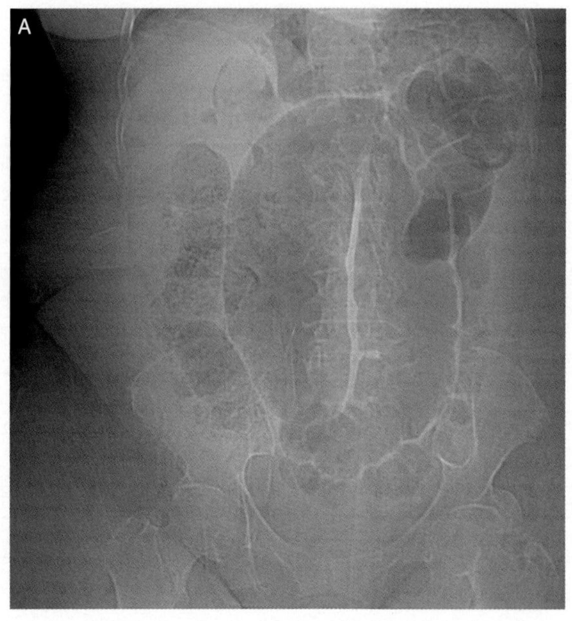

Approach to GI Bleeds

Location	Clinical	Etiology
Upper GI (Proximal to Ligament of Treitz)	- **Hematemesis** - Coffee ground emesis - **Melena** - Brisk upper bleed can present as hematochezia	- PUD - Esophagitis/gastritis - Esophageal varices - Portal hypertensive gastropathy - Cancer
Lower GI (Distal to Ligament of Treitz)	- **Hematochezia** - Maroon stool	- Diverticulosis - Angiodysplasia - Malignancy - Colitis (infectious, ischemic, IBD, radiation) - Anal bleeding (hemorrhoid, fissure)

Initial Management:

- Two 16 gauge IVs with IVF (crystalloid)
- CBC, type and screen
- NPO
- Blood product transfusions:
    - Blood (if Hgb < 7, Hgb < 8 with underlying CAD, or Hgb < 10 with hemodynamic instability or rapid bleed)
    - Platelets (if count is < 50k)
    - FFP or prothrombin complex (for coagulopathy)
- Pharm therapy:
    - **IV high dose PPI**
    - Octreotide/IV antibiotics if likely variceal bleed

Localization of bleed:

- Endoscopy (either EGD or colonoscopy, based on algorithm below)
- Arteriography with IR embolization (used in rapid bleeds when acute intervention required)

- If cause of bleeding not identified:
    - Push enteroscopy (examines for small bowel bleeding)
    - Capsule enterography (examines for small bowel bleeding)
    - Tagged RBC scan (for slow, occult bleeding)
    - CT angiography (can pick up faster, active bleeding)

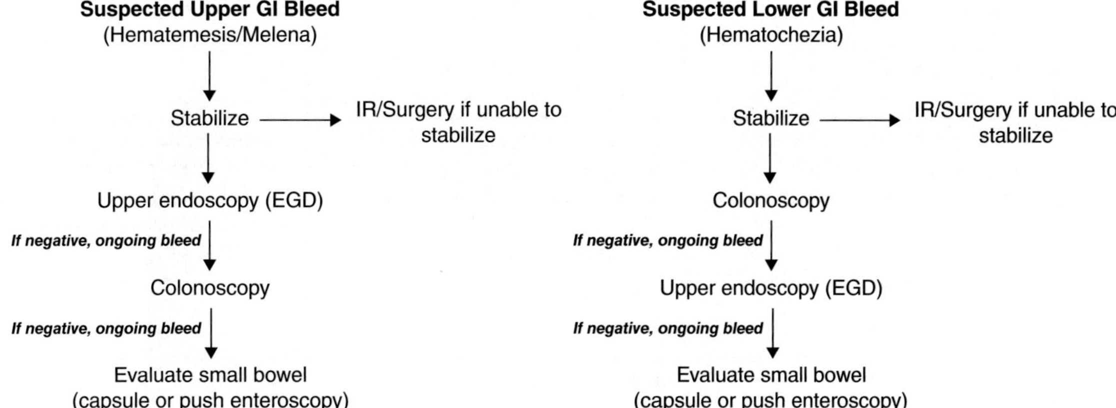

Colorectal Disease

Hemorrhoids

General: Dilated submucosal veins in the anal mucosa

Risk: Constipation, hard stools

	Internal	External
Gen	- Dilated vein of superior (internal) hemorrhoidal plexus - Above dentate line	- Dilated vein of inferior (external) hemorrhoidal plexus - Distal to dentate line
Clin	- **Painless bleeding with bowel movement** - Irritation, pruritus, but no pain	- **Pain, irritation, pruritus** - Severe pain if thrombosed
Dx	- Rectal exam, anoscopy	
Tx	- All: Dietary modification, high fiber diet - Supportive: Topical analgesics, topical steroids, sitz bath - Refractory: Rubber band ligation or sclerotherapy	- All: Dietary modification, high fiber diet - Supportive: Topical analgesics, topical steroids, sitz bath - Refractory or thrombosed: Surgical hemorrhoidectomy

Other Anal Lesions

	General	Clinical/Diagnosis	Treatment
Anal Fissure	- Tear in the lining of the anal canal distal to the dentate line - Most commonly in the posterior midline, possibly with associated skin tag	- **Anal pain**, worse after defecation - Bloody stools - Dx: Rectal exam (visualize, or reproduce pain)	- Supportive: High fiber diet, stool softener, sitz, topical analgesic - Nifedipine or nitroglycerine (relaxes anal sphincter) - Refractory: Botulinum toxin injection or lateral internal sphincterotomy
Perianal Abscess	- Infected **anal crypt gland**, likely due to obstruction - Perianal: Simple abscess of the superficial anus - Perirectal: Deep abscess (ischiorectal, supralevator, intersphincteric)	- Severe pain in anal or rectal area, +/− fever - Dx: Clinical exam (perianal erythema, fluctuant mass) - Deeper abscesses may require imaging (CT/MRI)	- I&D, plus antibiotics (amox-clav or ciprofloxacin) - Complication: Anal fistula (requires fistulotomy)
Pilonidal Cyst	- Soft tissue disorder of the upper gluteal cleft, in which debris plugs hair follicles, resulting in possible infection - Risk: Obesity, trauma, prolonged sitting	- Can be asymptomatic, but acute flares present as tender mass with possible pus or bleeding - Dx: Clinical exam	- Asymptomatic: Supportive, encourage perineal hygiene - Acute Infection: I&D + antibiotics - Chronic: Excision of sinus tracts and skin pores
Anal Cancer	- Cancer of the anal mucosa, most commonly SCC - Risk: Men who have sex with men, HPV (16, 18), HIV	- Rectal bleed, +/− palpable mass - Dx: Biopsy. CT/MRI for staging.	- Chemoradiotherapy (5-fluorouracil/mitomycin + radiation therapy)

Biliary Disease

Cholelithiasis

Type	Risk Factors
Cholesterol	- Excess estrogen (female, pregnancy, OCP) - Obesity, rapid weight loss - Cirrhosis, Crohn disease, cystic fibrosis, fibrates - Native Americans
Bilirubin ("black pigment")	- Hemolysis, cirrhosis, recurrent biliary tree infections
Mixed ("brown pigment")	- Bacterial or parasitic infection of the biliary system

Clinical: Can cause biliary colic (colicky RUQ pain that generally occurs after meals)
- Many cases asymptomatic and can be detected on routine imaging workups

Diagnosis: **RUQ US**

Management:
- Asymptomatic: Reassurance, monitor
- **Biliary colic: Elective cholecystectomy**

Cholecystitis

General: Stones obstructing the biliary duct, resulting in gallbladder distension, with eventual ischemia, bacterial invasion, and necrosis. Organisms are typical enteric:
- *E. Coli, Bacteroides, Enterobacter, Enterococcus, Klebsiella*

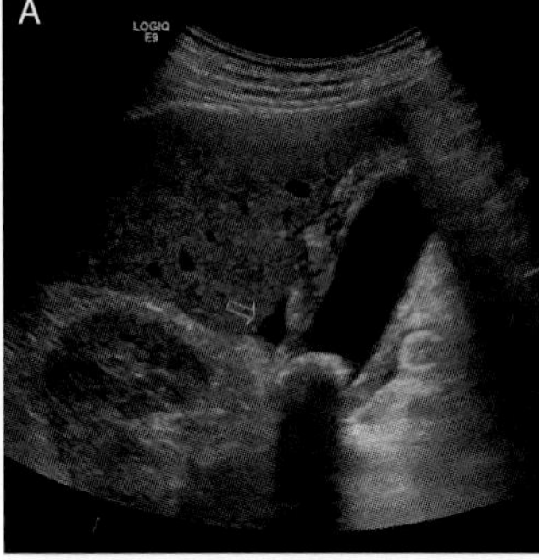

Clinical: Constant RUQ pain, with fever and leukocytosis. + **Murphy sign.**

Diagnosis:
- **RUQ US**[A] (thickened wall, pericholecystic fluid, sonographic murphy, stones)
- HIDA scan (second line, if RUQ US is not diagnostic)

Management:
- Initial: Fluids, pain control
- Antibiotics (ceftriaxone-metronidazole or amp-sulbactam)
- Surgery:
  - **Emergent laparoscopic cholecystectomy** (usually done during hospitalization)
  - Percutaneous cholecystostomy (if high surgical risk, critically ill)

Complications:
- Gallbladder gangrene, perforation, abscess
- Emphysematous cholecystitis (air in gallbladder wall from gas-producing bacterial organism. Worse prognosis, need for emergent surgery higher)

Surgical complications:
- Postcholecystectomy syndrome: RUQ pain or dyspepsia that continues after surgery. Typically due to residual stone, biliary dysfunction, or other GI pathology.
- CBD injury: Blood/bile leakage into the peritoneal space. Dx with US or CT. Presents as fever, pain, bilious ascites. Requires T-tube repair or Roux-en-Y hepaticojejunostomy.

Biliary Disease

	General	Clinical/Diagnosis	Treatment
Acalculous Cholecystitis	- Biliary stasis, resulting in ischemia, infection, and necrosis - Risk: **Critically ill**, hospitalized	- Sepsis - Jaundice - RUQ pain - Dx: RUQ US (CT is alternative)	- Antibiotics - Percutaneous cholecystostomy
Choledoco-lithiasis	- Stone in the common bile duct - Presents as **obstructive jaundice** (↑ bilirubin, LFTs, alk phos)	- RUQ pain - Nausea, vomiting - Dx: RUQ US	- ERCP - Followed by cholecystectomy
Cholangitis	- Stone in CBD, with ascending infection - Can also be caused by strictures, parasitic infections, and biliary instrumentation	- **Charcot**: RUQ pain, fever, jaundice - **Reynaud pentad**: Hypotension and altered mental status - Dx: RUQ US (CT is alternative)	- Antibiotics, IVF, supportive care - **ERCP** (emergent) - Followed by cholecystectomy
Biliary Dyskinesia	- Sphincter of Oddi spasm/dysfunction - Dilated biliary system without evidence of stones	- RUQ pain (mimics cholecystitis) - Dx: HIDA scan, sphincter manometry	- Endoscopic sphincterotomy
Gallstone Ileus	- Stone passes through enteric fistula, lodges in ileum	- Intermittent obstructive symptoms (nausea/emesis), with eventual **small-bowel obstruction** - Dx: CT (pneumobilia, obstructing stone)	- Enterolithotomy - Cholecystectomy (and fistula repair)
Chronic Cholecystitis	- Fibrosis, inflammation of gallbladder from chronic cholelithiasis/cystitis - Leads to calcified **"Porcelain" gallbladder**	- Can have symptoms of gallbladder disease (RUQ pain) - Dx: CT	- Cholecystectomy (↑ risk of gallbladder cancer)

Biliary Cysts

General: Cystic dilatation of the biliary tree. Associated with cholangiocarcinoma, as well as rupture, stricture, cholangitis, and stone formation. Variety of subtypes, but type I cysts (most common) are single, extrahepatic dilations of the bile duct.

Clinical: Abdominal pain, jaundice, nausea, vomiting, pruritus. Palpable mass.

Diagnosis: US, CT, MRCP

Management: Surgical excision (reduces malignancy risk) +/– Roux-en-Y hepaticojejunostomy

Cholangiocarcinoma

General: Adenocarcinoma arising from **bile duct epithelial cells**

Risk: Majority occur without underlying risk factor, but **chronic biliary inflammation** ↑ risk (primary sclerosing cholangitis, cystic liver/biliary disease, Chinese liver fluke)

Clinical: Jaundice (+ pruritus/dark urine), RUQ pain, systemic signs (weight loss, fever)

Diagnosis: CT, MRI, MRCP, or EUS

Management: Chemotherapy, radiotherapy, with surgery for purely local disease. Prognosis is generally poor.

Gallbladder Cancer

General: Adenocarcinoma of the gallbladder

Risk: Chronic gallbladder inflammation (**gallstones**, chronic infection, biliary cysts)

Clinical: Nonspecific/vague presentation. May present as biliary obstruction (jaundice, biliary colic, weight loss, RUQ mass).

Diagnosis: US, MRI/MRCP

Management: Cholecystectomy, adjuvant chemotherapy/radiation. Poor prognosis.

Biliary Disease

Bilirubin Metabolism (Overview)

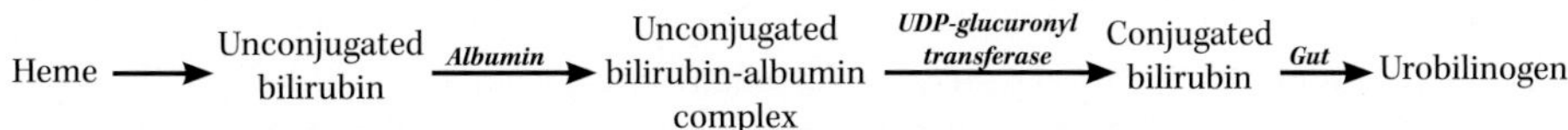

Jaundice occurs when total bilirubin is > 2 mg/dL

	Unconjugated Hyperbilirubinemia	Conjugated Hyperbilirubinemia
Features	- Water insoluble, neurotoxic - Elevated **urobilinogen excretion**	- Water soluble, nontoxic - **Excreted in urine (dark urine)**
Etiology	- Hemolysis - Decreased conjugation (Gilbert, Crigler-Najjar) - Cirrhosis - Impaired hepatic bilirubin uptake	- Extrahepatic biliary obstruction (stones, malignancy, stricture) - Decreased intrahepatic secretion (cirrhosis, PBC/PSC, Dubin-Johnson/Rotor)
Clinical	- Elevated risk of pigmented stones	- **Dark urine** with pale stools - Pruritus (elevated serum bile salts) - **Steatorrhea**: Impaired fat digestion - Elevated urine bilirubin

Genetic Causes of Hyperbilirubinemia

Gilbert	- Inherited disorder of bilirubin glucuronidation (UDP-glucuronyltransferase) - **Mild unconjugated hyperbilirubinemia/jaundice**, exacerbated by periods of stress (fasting, illness, surgery)

Crigler-Najjar	- Type 1: Complete absence of UDP glucuronyltransferase in hepatic tissue
	  - High risk of **kernicterus.** Requires phototherapy daily.
	- Type 2: Reduced UDP glucuronosyltransferase activity. Not as severe as type 1.
	  - Managed with daily phenobarbital

Dubin-Johnson	- Defective excretion of conjugated bilirubin from hepatocytes into bile - Mild icterus, conjugated hyperbilirubinemia. Liver is grossly **black.**
Rotor	- Defect in hepatic conjugated bilirubin storage, which leaks into the plasma - Mild icterus, conjugated hyperbilirubinemia

Biliary Pathology

	General	Clinical	Diagnosis	Treatment
Primary Sclerosing Cholangitis	- Chronic, progressive fibrosis, and stricturing of intra/extra hepatic bile ducts - Strong association with **ulcerative colitis**, P-ANCA, human leukocyte antigen DRw52a	- **Pruritus, jaundice**, dark urine, light stool - Hepatosplenomegaly - Cholestatic LFT pattern (increased bili/Alk Phos) ***Complications:*** - Cholangiocarcinoma (PSC) - Hepatocellular carcinoma - Cirrhosis - Malabsorption - Osteoporosis	- **MRCP/ERCP (usually diagnostic)**	- Strictures: Endoscopic stent and dilatation - Liver transplant (for cirrhosis) - Screen for cholangiocarcinoma
Primary Biliary Cholangitis	- **Autoimmune** intrahepatic bile duct destruction - Commonly seen in middle age women (with comorbid autoimmune disease) - Associated with **osteoporosis**		- US (to rule out extra hepatic obstruction) - **AMA antibodies** - Liver biopsy (definitive)	- **Ursodeoxycholic acid** - Liver transplant
Secondary Biliary Cirrhosis	- Extrahepatic biliary obstruction, causing bile stasis - Caused by cancer, strictures, or gallstones		- US, CT, MRI, MRCP, ERCP depending on etiology	- Treat underlying

Pancreatic Disease

Acute Pancreatitis

General: Inflammation of the pancreas from inappropriately activated pancreatic digestive enzymes, causing autodigestion. Subtypes:

- Interstitial Edematous (~85%): Enlarged pancreas with inflammatory edema
- Necrotizing (~15%): More severe, areas of pancreatic necrosis

Etiology:

- **Gallstones**
- **Ethanol**
- Hypertriglyceridemia
- Tumors (obstructing outflow)
- Hypercalcemia
- Post-instrumentation (ERCP)
- Trauma
- Infections (Mumps, *Mycoplasma,* Coxsackie, HIV, others)
- Toxins (brown recluse, certain scorpions)
- Drugs
- Hereditary (SPINK, PRSS1 gene mutations)

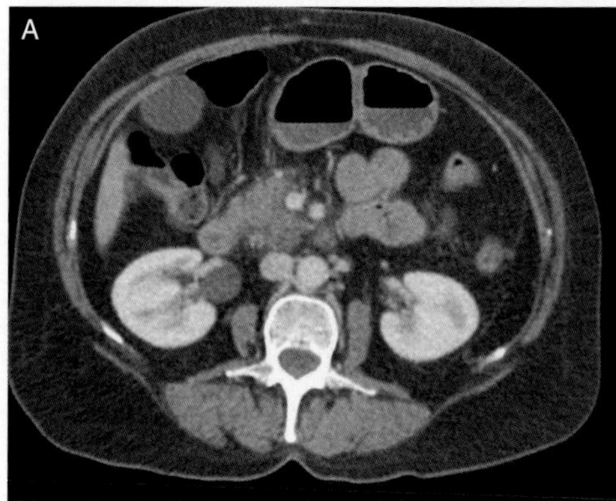

Clinical:

- **Severe epigastric pain**, may radiate to back. **Nausea, vomiting**, fever, tachypnea, tachycardia.
- Associated (rare) clinical signs
    - Grey-Turner (flank hemorrhage)
    - Cullens (blue discoloration at umbilicus)

Diagnosis: (2/3 of the following)

(1) **Epigastric pain**
(2) Elevation of amylase/**lipase ≥ 3x** the upper limit of normal
(3) **Characteristic imaging findings**: CT[A]/MRI can reveal edema and areas of necrosis

* Multiple criteria (Ranson's, APACHE) can be used to prognosticate

Management:

- IV fluids (moderate resuscitation), pain control, electrolyte correction, NPO (early feeding if mild)
- Nutritional support
- Provide ICU level care for those with severe disease
- CT to look for complication if septic, severe pancreatitis, or deterioration after > 72 hours

Complications of Acute Pancreatitis

Systemic	- ARDS, DIC, sepsis	
Acute Peripancreatic Fluid Collection	- Acute fluid collection within 7-10 days	- Usually asymptomatic, resolves spontaneously
Necrosis	- Necrotic pancreatic tissue with **high risk for infection** - Can occur acutely, and become walled-off late in course	- Can diagnose infection with CT or CT guided FNA - Treat with broad spectrum antibiotics +/– necrosectomy (debridement of pancreatic necrosis, reserved for severe cases)
Pancreatic Pseudocyst	- Encapsulated collection of fluid with a well-defined wall - Usually occurs > 4 weeks after acute episode	- Asymptomatic: Monitor - Symptomatic or Enlarging: Endoscopic or surgical drainage
Abdominal Compartment Syndrome	- Intra-abdominal pressure > 20 mmHg, causing organ failure - Screen in ICU using bladder pressure	- Surgical decompression

Pancreatic Disease

Chronic Pancreatitis

General: Progressive and chronic disease of fibrosis and inflammation of the pancreas, resulting in structural damage, and impaired exocrine and endocrine function

Risk: Chronic alcohol use, cystic fibrosis, malignancy, stones/obstructions

Clinical: **Chronic, recurrent epigastric pain**, nausea, vomiting. Weight loss, malabsorption.

Diagnosis: Imaging (CT, XR showing **pancreatic calcifications**)
- Secretin stimulation test, fecal elastase

Management:
- Small volume meals, quit alcohol/tobacco use, pain control, PPI
- Pancreatic enzyme supplementation (Lipase)
- Surgery (if all else refractory): Pancreaticojejunostomy and/or pancreatic resection

Complications:
- Pancreatic insufficiency: Malabsorption, steatorrhea
- Splenic vein thrombosis
- Pseudocyst, duct stricture, duodenal obstruction
- Diabetes mellitus (usually late in disease course)
- **Pancreatic adenocarcinoma**

Pancreatic Adenocarcinoma

General: Adenocarcinoma of the pancreatic exocrine ducts

Risk: Age > 50, smoking, diabetes, males, chronic pancreatitis

Clinical: **Jaundice**, weight loss, possible vague abdominal pain
- Migratory thrombophlebitis (Trousseau syndrome)
- Palpable gallbladder (Courvoisier sign)

Diagnosis: RUQ US. MRCP/CT are second line if US not diagnostic. Biopsy for definitive diagnosis.
- CT for staging/disease extent (FNA or during surgery)

Management:
- Surgery (only if no mets or local vascular invasion)
  - Head tumor: Pancreaticoduodenectomy (Whipple)
  - Tail tumor: Distal pancreatectomy + splenectomy
- Chemotherapy
- Monitor CA-19-9 or CEA for prognosis/recurrence
- Palliative care for complications: Abdominal pain, biliary obstruction, gastric outlet obstruction

Other Pancreatic Masses

<u>Benign masses</u>
- Serous or mucinous cystadenomas
- Treatment: Surveillance or resection

<u>Intraductal papillary mucinous neoplasm</u>
- Produce mucin that obstructs ducts, causing recurrent pancreatitis
- Diagnosis with CT
- Treatment: Resection

<u>Periampullary cancers</u>
- Cancer that obstructs the ampulla of vater, which can arise from the ampulla itself, pancreas, or duodenum
- Clinical: Obstructive jaundice, possible GI bleed
- Diagnosis: CT, with ERCP/biopsy for definitive diagnosis
- Treatment: Pancreaticoduodenectomy

Cirrhosis

Cirrhosis Overview

General: Chronic liver disease characterized by hepatic fibrosis, distortion of architecture, and formation of regenerative nodules

Etiology: Most common in the US include **alcohol use, hepatitis C, and nonalcoholic fatty liver disease**, but many other causes (hemochromatosis, autoimmune hepatitis, others covered on the following pages)

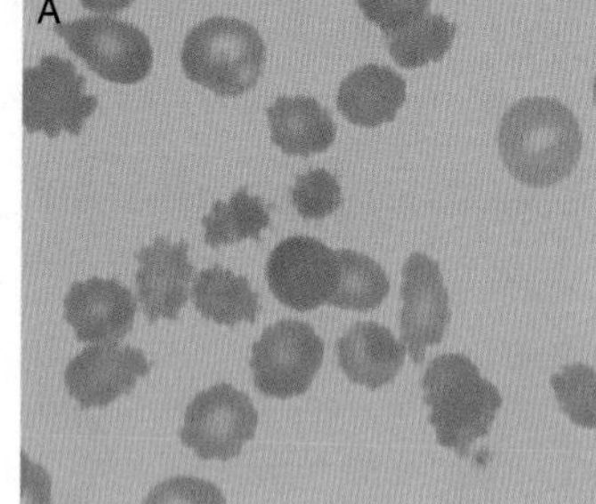

Clinical:

- **Constitutional**: Anorexia, weight loss, fatigue
- **Portal Hypertension**: Ascites, hepatosplenomegaly, variceal bleeding
- **Neurologic**: Hepatic encephalopathy, asterixis
- **Skin**: Jaundice, palmar erythema, spider angiomas, terry nails
- **Heme**: Thrombocytopenia, anemia (macrocytosis, burr/spur cells[A]), coagulopathy
- **Reproductive**: Testicular atrophy, gynecomastia
- Poor synthetic function: ↓ albumin, ↑ INR, ↑ bilirubin

Diagnosis: **Stigmata of liver disease + lab/imaging evidence + evidence of decompensation** (e.g., ascites, HE, SBP)

- RUQ US is typically used to evaluate liver/extrahepatic manifestations
- Hepascore/Elastography (used to evaluate degree of hepatic fibrosis, risk stratify potential to develop cirrhosis)
    - **Hepascore** (serologic scoring system of fibrosis)
    - **Elastography** (US that measures "stiffness" of liver)
- Biopsy (definitive diagnosis, but not always necessary)

Management:

- Slow progression of disease by treating underlying cause (i.e., alcohol abstinence, treat hepatitis, etc.)
- Protect the liver: Vaccination (Hep A/B), avoid hepatotoxic drugs
- Manage the complications seen on the following pages
- Monitor for HCC (AFP + liver US q6 months)
- Consider liver transplantation

Classifications: Scoring systems to monitor severity of disease include Child Pugh (below) and MELD score

Child Pugh	1	2	3	
Ascites	Absent	Mild	Moderate	**Class A (5-6 points)** **Class B (7-9 points)** **Class C (10-15 points)**
Bilirubin	< 2	2-3	> 4	
Albumin	> 3.5	2.8-3.5	< 2.8	
PT (INR)	< 1.7	1.7-2.3	> 2.3	
Encephalopathy	None	Grade 1 or 2	Grade 3 or 4	

Ascites (from Portal Hypertension)

General: Accumulation of fluid in the peritoneal cavity due to **portal hypertension** (increased hydrostatic pressure) and hypoalbuminemia (reduced oncotic pressure)

Clinical: Abdominal distension, fluid wave, shifting dullness

Diagnosis: RUQ US, with paracentesis showing SAAG > 1.1

Management:

- Salt restriction (< 2000 mg)
- Combination **furosemide-spironolactone therapy**
- For tense ascites: Large volume paracentesis (+/− supplemental albumin)
- Refractory: TIPS procedure or transplant

Cirrhosis

Spontaneous Bacterial Peritonitis

General: Ascitic fluid infection without an evident intra-abdominal surgical source. Thought to be due to bowel translocation. Organisms include *E. Coli, Klebsiella, Strep, Staph.*

Clinical: **Abdominal pain, fever (> 100°F)**, altered mental status

Diagnosis: Paracentesis (**PMN > 250 /mm³**, SAAG > 1.1, some with positive ascites culture/gram stain)

Management: Antibiotics (**3rd Generation cephalosporin or fluoroquinolone**)
- Albumin (for preload/renal perfusion). Watch for and manage renal failure (common complication).
- Prophylaxis: Ciprofloxacin or TMP-SMX. Indicated if high-risk (hx of SBP, current GI bleed, low ascitic protein < 1.5).

Hepatic Encephalopathy

General: Reversible neuropsychiatric abnormalities from toxic effect of ammonia and other substances on CNS function

Risk: Precipitated by GI bleeding, infection (SBP), hypokalemia, metabolic alkalosis, renal failure, hypovolemia, hypoxemia

Clinical: Decreased mental function (may be subtle or overt, depending on severity)
- Neuromuscular abnormalities: Hyperreflexia, rigidity, bradykinesia, myoclonus, and **asterixis**

Diagnosis: Clinical diagnosis of exclusion. Ammonia levels frequently elevated but not helpful/diagnostic.

Management: Supportive care, treat underlying cause, give **lactulose +/− rifaximin**
- Prophylaxis: Lactulose and/or Rifaximin therapy for recurrent episodes

Hepatorenal Syndrome

General: Progressive renal failure in advanced liver disease, secondary to renal hypoperfusion (increased vasodilatory molecules, with subsequent RAAS activation, and worsening renal perfusion)

Risk: Advanced cirrhosis. Often precipitated by GI bleed, vomiting, overdiuresis.

Clinical: Azotemia, oliguria, hyponatremia, hypotension

Diagnosis: Elevated BUN/Cr, with FeNa < 1 % and no other cause. **No response to fluids** (differentiates from prerenal).

Management: **Midodrine, octreotide, albumin**
- Norepinephrine used if in ICU. Terlipressin in Europe. Transplant is only definitive therapy.

Variceal Bleeding

General: Portal hypertension results in venous variceal formation between portal and systemic venous systems

Esophagus	High risk for bleeding	Left gastric ↔ azygous
Rectum	Anorectal varices	Superior ↔ inferior rectal
Umbilicus	Caput medusae	Paraumbilical ↔ epigastric

Esophageal Variceal Bleeds

Clinical: Upper GI bleed (hematemesis, melena)

Diagnosis: Urgent endoscopy

Management:

Acute	- Initial resuscitation with IV access, IVF, antibiotics, and octreotide. Balloon tamponade if severe bleeding. - Urgent upper endoscopy (with variceal ligation or sclerotherapy) - Severe rebleeding: Endoscopy preferred, but TIPS or surgery if refractory
Prophylaxis	- Most cirrhotics should undergo screening for varices (upper endoscopy) - Smaller, lower risk varices receive **beta-blocker** (nadolol) for prophylaxis - Larger, higher risk varices receive **endoscopic variceal ligation**

Acute Liver Failure

Interpretation of LFTs

AST/ALT	< 500	~500s - 1000s	> 10000
Etiology	- Cirrhosis - Chronic viral hepatitis - Chronic alcohol use - NAFL/NASH	- Acute viral hepatitis - Autoimmune hepatitis - DILI (drug-induced liver injury)	- Severe shock liver - Acetaminophen toxicity

Hepatocellular pattern: AST/ALT predominantly elevated
Cholestatic pattern: Alk phos, bilirubin predominantly elevated

Alkaline Phosphatase:
- Can come from liver or other parts of body (e.g., bone, intestines, etc.)
    - Can differentiate with **GGT**
- True hepatic elevation indicates cholestasis. Differential includes:
    - Biliary epithelial damage (cirrhosis, hepatitis)
    - Intrahepatic cholestasis
    - Biliary obstruction

Acute Liver Failure

General: Severe acute liver injury with encephalopathy and impaired synthetic function in someone without prior liver disease

Etiology:
- Viral (hepatitis A, B, D, E, CMV, HSV)
- Drug/toxin (most commonly acetaminophen, EtOH)
- Ischemia (shock liver)
- Vascular (Budd-Chiari)
- Autoimmune hepatitis

Clinical:
- Fatigue, weakness, lethargy, confusion
- Jaundice, hepatomegaly, RUQ pain, and thrombocytopenia

Diagnosis:
- Clinical diagnosis with the combination of:
    - **Hepatic encephalopathy**
    - **INR ≥ 1.5**
    - **Elevated AST/ALT (often marked elevation > 1,000)**
- Other findings: Elevated bilirubin, thrombocytopenia
- RUQUS (to rule out Budd-Chiari)

Management:
- ICU level supportive care, treat underlying cause, monitor for cerebral edema
- **IV N-acetylcysteine**
- Liver transplant in those unlikely to recover

Budd-Chiari

General: Hepatic venous outflow obstruction, either due to clot (primary) or infiltrative lesion (secondary)
- **Primary**: Hypercoagulable state, OCP use, myeloproliferative disorder (e.g., polycythemia vera)
- **Secondary**: Malignancy, benign liver lesions, or structural abnormality

Clinical:
- Presentation ranges from acute liver failure to chronic liver disease
- Symptoms include abdominal pain, ascites, jaundice, hepatomegaly

Diagnosis: RUQUS (with Doppler)

Management: **Anticoagulation**. Thrombolytic therapy, angioplasty with stenting if refractory.

Liver Disease

	General	Clinical	Diagnosis	Treatment
Non-Alcoholic Fatty Liver	- Hepatic steatosis without history of alcohol use - NAFL: Steatosis - NASH: Steatosis + inflammation	- Asymptomatic or mild RUQ discomfort - **Associated with metabolic syndrome (obesity, HTN, insulin resistance, HLD)**	- Steatosis (on US/CT imaging or biopsy) - History (absence of EtOH use, but features of metabolic syndrome)	- Lifestyle modification (weight loss, control of comorbidities)
Alcoholic Steatosis	- Accumulation of fatty acids in liver - Occurs with chronic EtOH use - Risk to progress to cirrhosis	- Asymptomatic - **Elevated AST/ALT, with AST:ALT > 2**	- CT or US	- Alcohol abstinence
Alcoholic Hepatitis	- Acute hepatic inflammation from **EtOH abuse (often after binge)**	- **RUQ tenderness** - **Fever** - Jaundice - AST:ALT > 2, ↑ GGT	- Clinical (history of EtOH use, with other causes of hepatitis ruled out)	- Supportive care - **Prednisolone** (if discriminant function > 32) - Alcohol abstinence
Autoimmune Hepatitis	- Chronic autoimmune hepatitis	- Variable, ranging from asymptomatic to acute liver failure	- + ANA/**Anti- SM Ab** - Liver biopsy	- **Steroids** - Immunosuppressants (azathioprine or 6-MP)
Congestive Hepatopathy	- Any cause of right heart failure, resulting in elevated central venous/hepatic venous pressure	- Evidence of LFT elevation and right heart failure - Generally asymptomatic	- RUQ US with Doppler	- Treat CHF
Wilson Disease	- Impaired copper excretion in bile (AR mutation in **ATP7B gene**) - Mean age onset 12 to 23 years	- **Acute or chronic hepatitis** - Yellow corneal rings (**Kayser–Fleischer**[A]) - Renal injury - CNS (psychiatric changes, Parkinsonism, chorea) - Hemolysis	↓ **Serum ceruloplasmin** ↑ Urinary copper - Slit lamp exam - Biopsy/genetics if above are equivocal	- Low copper diet - D-penicillamine or Trientine
Hereditary Hemochromatosis	- AR disorder of iron absorption (**HFE gene** on chromosome 6), which causes increased iron absorption, with buildup of storage in tissues - Most commonly C282Y mutation - Secondary hemochromatosis can occur from iron overload due to chronic blood transfusions	- Asymptomatic until ~age 40 (women delayed due to menses) - GI: **Transaminitis**, eventual cirrhosis. ↑ HCC risk. - Skin: Hyperpigmentation - MSK: Arthralgias, chondrocalcinosis - Endocrine: Diabetes mellitus, hypogonadism, hypothyroidism - CV: Cardiomyopathy, conduction issues - Infection risk (*Vibrio vulnificus, Yersinia enterocolitica, Listeria*)	- **Elevated ferritin/ transferrin saturation** - Genetic testing (used for definitive diagnosis), liver biopsy	- Asymptomatic patients with ferritin < 500 ng/mL are typically monitored - Phlebotomy if symptomatic or ↑ ferritin - Avoid EtOH, Fe, vitamin C, uncooked seafood - Screen for HCC - Iron chelation (only required if contraindication to phlebotomy)

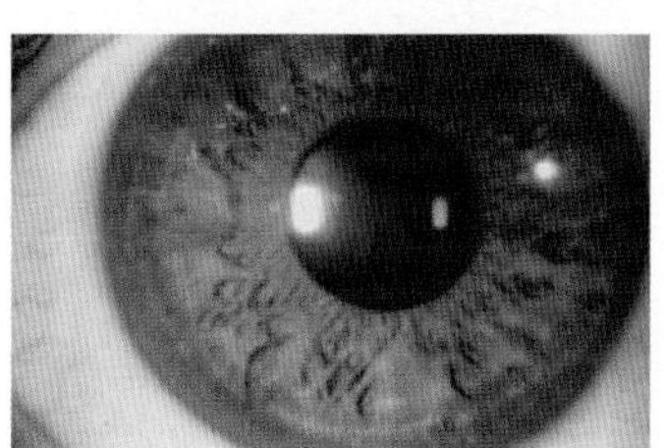

Viral Hepatitis

	General	Clinical	Diagnosis	Treatment
Hepatitis A	- Picornavirus (ss-RNA) - **Fecal-oral spread** - Risk: Travel to endemic areas, MSM, drug use	**Acute Hepatitis** - Initial signs of RUQ pain, fever, anorexia, nausea - Hepatosplenomegaly, jaundice (~1 month, self-limited) - Never chronic, fulminant disease is rare	- LFT elevation (can be > 1000 IU/L) - Bilirubin elevation - Confirmed via serology **(Hep A IgM)**	- Supportive care - PPX: Hep A Vax (use prior to travel, or if high risk)
Hepatitis B	- Hepadnavirus (ds-DNA) - Spread via sexual contact, blood	See below		
Hepatitis C	- Flavivirus ssRNA - Transmitted by **blood** (IVDU, transfusions prior to 1992) - Rarely sexual transmission	<u>Acute</u> - Asymptomatic or symptoms of acute hepatitis <u>Chronic</u> (> 50% develop) - Generally asymptomatic - Eventually leads to cirrhosis	- **HCV RNA** - Anti-HCV Ab (ELISA)	- Antivirals (see below)
Hepatitis D	- Incomplete ssRNA - Requires hepatitis B infection - Often spread with Hep B (via sex/blood)	- Acute hepatitis (more likely to be severe/result in liver failure compared to hep B alone)	- Serum HDAg and/or HDV RNA	- Peg-interferon
Hepatitis E	- Hepevirus (ss-RNA) - Enteric transmission	- Acute Hepatitis [See: Hep A] - Acute liver failure more likely in **pregnant women**	- HEV IgM/ HEV RNA	- Supportive care

Hepatitis B

	HBsAg	HBeAg	Anti-HBc IgM	Anti-HBc IgG	Anti-HBs	Anti-HBe	HBV DNA
Acute Early HBV	↑	↑	↑				↑↑
Acute Window			↑				↑
Acute Recovery				↑	↑	↑	
Chronic	↑			↑			
Acute on Chronic	↑	↑	↑	↑			↑
Vaccine					↑		
Cleared Infection				↑	↑		

Clinical:

- <u>Acute infection</u>
  - Many are asymptomatic or anicteric, but ~30% get symptoms
  - Symptomatic patients suffer from prodrome of **arthralgia, rash, followed by acute hepatitis**
  - Fulminant disease is rare
- <u>Chronic infection</u> (~5% adults, but 50% of young kids, and 90% of neonates)

Management:

- Acute: Supportive, monitor serology for clearance
- Chronic: Antivirals (tenofovir or entecavir)

Hepatitis C (Management)

Check the HCV genotype (which directs therapy)

- Genotype 1 (most common): Glecaprevir-pibrentasvir, ledipasvir-sofosbuvir, or sofosbuvir-velpatasvir
- Genotype 2-3: Glecaprevir-pibrentasvir

*In General: Regimens are a combination of a NS3/4A protease inhibitor with NS5A inhibitor (both proteins are required for RNA replication). Antivirals now standard of care (interferon/ribavirin almost entirely out).

Class	Drug Options
Protease (NS3/4A) inhibitors	- Boceprevir, glecaprevir, paritaprevir, simeprevir, telaprevir
NS5A inhibitors	- Daclatasvir, ledipasvir, pibrentasvir, velpatasvir
NS5B inhibitors	- Dasabuvir, sofosbuvir

Liver Malignancies

Hepatocellular Carcinoma

General: Most common primary liver tumor, associated with chronic liver disease

Risk: **Cirrhosis** (of any cause)
- Increased risk with chronic hepatitis B/C, hereditary hemochromatosis
- Toxins (aflatoxin, alcohol, smoking)

Clinical: **Generally asymptomatic, identified on screening**
- Can present as decompensated cirrhosis
- Other symptoms possible (weight loss, abdominal pain, palpable mass)
- Paraneoplastic syndromes:
    - Hypoglycemia (high metabolic demand, IGF-II secretion)
    - Erythrocytosis (EPO secretion)

Diagnosis:
- **Most commonly diagnosed with US** (screening or incidental finding)
    - CT/MRI can be used to better characterize
- AFP (used as screening test)
- Biopsy if diagnosis uncertain

Management:
- Surgery (resection)
    - Often not possible due to underlying cirrhosis/invasion of tumor
- Ablation, TACE (transarterial chemoembolization), radiotherapy
    - Used for local unresectable disease
- Extrahepatic metastasis:
    - Systemic therapy (sorafenib)

Other Liver Masses

Hepatic Adenoma	- Benign epithelial liver tumors found in young woman - Associated with estrogen (OCP use, pregnancy), anabolic steroids - Generally asymptomatic, but can present with RUQ fullness - May rupture leading to sudden-onset symptoms - Dx: US/CT/MRI - Tx: Surgically resect if > 5 cm or symptomatic. Others can be monitored.
Cavernous Hemangioma	- Common benign liver lesion, most often occurs in women (30-50 y/o) - Generally asymptomatic, but can cause RUQ pain/mass - Dx: US/CT/MRI (often discovered incidentally) - Tx: Surgically resect if > 5 cm or symptomatic. Others can be monitored.
Focal Nodular Hyperplasia	- Benign liver mass without malignant potential - Occurs in reproductive age women (no OCP correlation) - Dx: US/CT/MRI (central scar, hyperattenuation on arterial phase CT) - Tx: Reassurance
Angiosarcoma	- High-grade malignant vascular neoplasm - Associated with vinyl chloride, arsenic, thorium, anabolic steroids
Metastasis	- Most commonly GI (colon, stomach, pancreas), breast, lung - Presents as multiple liver nodules

Liver Masses

Liver Cysts

Etiology	Characteristics
Simple Cyst	- **Simple, uniform, clear fluid containing cystic lesions** - Generally asymptomatic, but can cause RUQ fullness if large - US and CT[A] (w/ contrast) can help characterize - Tx: Conservative monitoring if asymptomatic. Rarely larger cysts drained + injected with sclerosing agent.
Polycystic Liver	- Multiple liver cysts seen in patients with ADPKD
Hydatid Liver Cyst	- Acquired from ***Echinococcus granulosus***, a dog tapeworm - Humans ingest eggs → Hatch and migrate to liver - Generally asymptomatic, but as cyst grows can cause mild **RUQ pain, nausea, hepatomegaly** - Dx: US/CT/MRI (see cyst with internal septa and calcifications). Serologic (ELISA) testing. - Tx: Albendazole, plus drainage of lesions > 5 cm

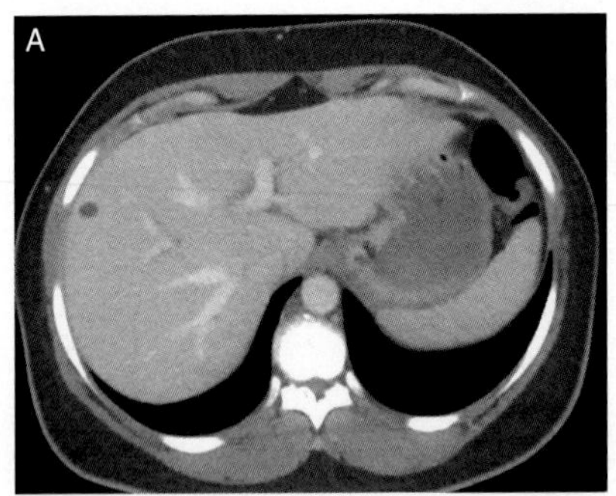

Liver Abscess

Etiology	Characteristics

Pyogenic	- Bacterial liver abscess, seen in patients with spread from bacterial peritonitis or bacteremia
	- Clinically presents as **abdominal pain, fever**, and other nonspecific findings (nausea, emesis, etc.)
	- Diagnosis: US/CT, followed by aspiration gram stain/culture
	- Management:
	  - **Antibiotics**: Ceftriaxone plus metronidazole or beta-lactam/inhibitor
	  - **Drainage**: Percutaneous needle, catheter, or surgical drainage

Amebic	- Caused by intestinal amebiasis (Entamoeba histolytica), which invades the portal vein - Presents as weeks of RUQ pain, fever, emesis - Possible **concurrent or prior history of dysentery** - Dx: US/CT/MRI. Plus serology (ELISA IgG). - Tx: Metronidazole + paromomycin (for intraluminal cysts) *Surgical aspiration dangerous due to rupture risk

Diarrhea

Acute Diarrhea

General: Most cases of acute diarrhea are viral, but bacterial causes can result in more severe disease requiring hospitalization
- "**Dysentery**" is diarrhea plus visible blood and mucous

Clinical: **> 3 loose**, watery bowel movements per day for **< 14 days**

Diagnosis: Clinical diagnosis
- Further workup (stool cultures) if:
    - Severe illness (hospitalized, hypovolemia, severe abdominal pain, profuse diarrhea)
    - Blood/mucous in stool or fevers > 100.4°F
    - High-risk (age > 70, immunocompromised)
- Consider *C. diff*, Ova/Parasite testing if indicated by clinical scenario

Management:
- Supportive (fluids, ondansetron, loperamide, etc.) for most
- Antibiotics (azithromycin or fluoroquinolone) if high-risk, including:
    - Fever, volume depletion, bloody or mucoid stools

DDx of Infectious Diarrhea

Bug	Source	Clinical Clues
Watery Diarrhea		
Norovirus	- Fecal-oral (food or water)	- Outbreaks in health care, restaurants, schools, military
Rotavirus	- Fecal-oral (food or water)	- Daycare, young children
ETEC	- Fecal-oral (food or water)	- Travel to endemic areas (usually resource-limited areas)
Clostridium perfringens	- Infected meats and poultry	
Staph aureus	- Spoiled mayo, dairy	
Bacillus cereus	- Reheated rice	
Listeria	- Processed meats, cheeses	- Immunocompromised, pregnancy
Giardia	- Fecally contaminated water	- Travel, hiking, camping, pools
Cryptosporidium	- Infected fruit/vegetables	- Immunocompromised
Inflammatory Diarrhea		
Salmonella	- Meats, eggs, fish, produce	- Animal contact (especially petting zoos, reptiles)
Shigella	- Raw vegetables	- Daycare, resource-limited settings
Campylobacter	- Meats, unpasteurized milk	- Animal contact (puppies/kittens) - Resource-limited settings
EHEC	- Meats, unpasteurized milk	- Daycare, nursing homes
Yersinia	- Pork	
Vibrio	- Raw shellfish	- Cirrhosis
Entamoeba	- Fecally contaminated food or water	- Resource-limited settings

Diarrhea

Clostridioides difficile Infection

General: Nosocomial infection from overgrowth of *C. difficile*, most commonly after alteration of normal gut flora. Produce toxins (A/B) which cause mucosal inflammation and injury. NAP1/BI/027 hypervirulent strain gaining increased recognition for outbreaks.

Risk: **Recent antibiotic therapy**, increased age, chronic PPI
- Commonly implicated: Fluoroquinolone, penicillin/cephalosporins, and clindamycin

Clinical:
- *C. diff* colitis: Diarrhea (**> 3 watery stools/day**), LLQ abdominal pain, fever, leukocytosis
- Fulminant colitis: Above, plus severe pain, distension, hypovolemia

Diagnosis: (Preferred lab test varies between institutions)
- **ELISA or PCR for GDH, toxin A/B**
- Endoscopy generally not required (but can find classic pseudomembranes)

Management:

Class	Criteria (No Consensus)	Treatment
Nonsevere	- Otherwise healthy patients	- Oral **vancomycin or fidaxomicin**
Severe	- WBC > 15 K - Cr ≥ 1.5 × baseline	- Oral vancomycin or fidaxomicin For refractory/recurrent: - Prolonged taper of vancomycin or fidaxomicin - Bezlotoxumab (toxin B monoclonal antibody) - Fecal transplant
Fulminant	- Hypotension, shock, megacolon	- Vancomycin (PO) + metronidazole (IV) - Colectomy

Toxic Megacolon

General: Nonobstructive colonic dilatation and systemic toxicity. Can lead to perforation.

Etiology: Complication of **IBD** or **infectious colitis**

Clinical: Severe, bloody diarrhea and systemic toxicity (see criteria below)

Diagnosis:
- Radiographic **colonic distension** (plain XR)[A] PLUS **3 of the following**:
  - HR > 120, Temp > 38°C, Anemia, Neutrophils > 10.5K, hypotension

Management:
- Supportive (fluids, NPO, antibiotics, NG decompression)
- If supportive care fails → Subtotal colectomy

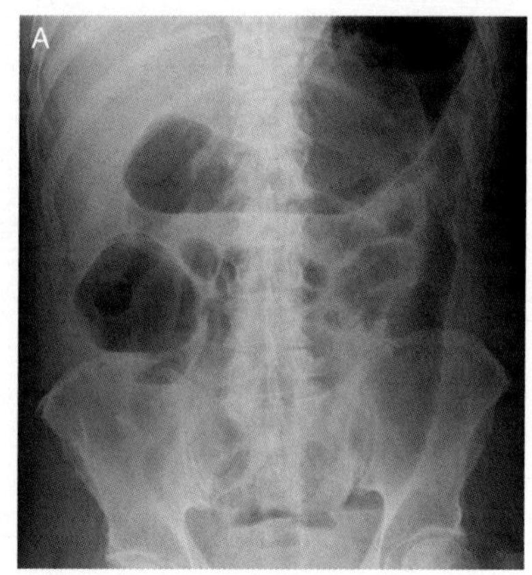

Diarrhea

Chronic Diarrhea

Clinical: ≥ 3 loose or watery stools daily lasting ≥ 4 weeks

Etiology	Clinical	Workup
Secretory (stool osmotic gap < 50 mOsm/kg)		
Microscopic Colitis	- Chronic inflammatory disease of colon resulting in chronic, **watery secretory diarrhea** - Diagnosis: Biopsy (collagenous and lymphocytic subtypes) - Treatment: Budesonide	- Exclude infection (stool culture, O/P) - Exclude structural causes (CT, colonoscopy) - Cholestyramine trial (to rule out bile acid malabsorption) - Plasma peptides (gastrin, VIP) - Urine 5-HIAA
Neuroendocrine Tumor	- Includes VIPoma and gastrinoma	
Bile Acid Malabsorption	- Associated with diseases of the terminal ileum (Crohn) or surgical removal of the ileum	
Postsurgical (post-cholecystectomy)	- Excess bile acids entering GI tract, irritating colon, resulting in secretory diarrhea - Improves with bile acid resins	
Nonosmotic Laxatives	- Senna, docusate	
Osmotic (stool osmotic gap > 125 mOsm/kg)		
Lactose Intolerance	- Carbohydrate malabsorption leading to osmotic diarrhea	- Stool osmotic gap - Fasting (should correct issue if truly osmotic)
Osmotic Laxatives	- PEG, lactulose	
Inflammatory		
IBD	- See IBD section - **Fecal calprotectin** can suggest diagnosis, confirm with colonoscopy with biopsy	- Stool culture, O/P - Fecal WBCs - Fecal calprotectin
Chronic Infection	- *C. difficile, Campylobacter, Giardia, Cryptosporidium,* etc.	
Malabsorption		
Chronic Pancreatitis	- All present with greasy, floating stools	- Quantitative stool fat - Fecal elastase
SIBO		
Celiac Sprue		
Functional		
IBS	- Chronic crampy abdominal pain and diarrhea	- Diagnosis of exclusion
Medications		
Drug Side Effects	- Antibiotics, SSRIs, PPIs	

Constipation

Constipation

Etiology:

- **Primary** (functional): From slow transit, dyssynergic defecation, or IBS
- **Secondary**:
  - Mechanical (mass, cancer, stricture, etc.)
  - Drugs (opiates, antihypertensives)
  - Lifestyle (low fiber, dehydration)
  - Neurologic (spinal cord injury, MS, Parkinsonism)

Clinical: Defined by ≥ 2 of the following

- Hard lumpy stools
- Sensation of incomplete evacuation
- Need to use digital maneuvers
- Straining with bowel movements
- Decrease in stool frequency

Management:

- Lifestyle modification: Defecate when motility the highest (after meals, mornings), increase dietary fiber
- Laxatives (see below)
- Refractory IBS-C: Linaclotide, lubiprostone, prucalopride

Class	Examples
Bulk Forming	- Psyllium - Methylcellulose
Osmotic	- Polyethylene glycol - Lactulose - Magnesium sulfate, citrate
Stimulant	- Bisacodyl - Senna
Surfactant (softener)	- Docusate
Severe Constipation	
Suppositories	- Bisacodyl
Enema	- Warm water - Saline - Mineral oil - Sodium phosphate (can cause hypovolemia)
Manual Disimpaction	

Neonatal/Congenital GI

Meconium

General: Meconium is normally passed within 24 hours after birth. If passed in the uterus, risk for fetal meconium aspiration. If passed > 24 hours, concerning for one of the following conditions:

	Meconium Ileus	Hirschsprung
Gen	- Obstruction from inspissated meconium in the ileum - Highly associated with **cystic fibrosis**	- Megacolon due to lack of ganglion cells in distal segment of colon (failed neural crest migration) Etiology: - Syndromic: **Trisomy 21**, Bardet-Biedl, Smith-Lemli-Opitz - Other cases idiopathic
Clin	- Delayed meconium - Abdominal distension - Feeding intolerance, biliary vomiting	- Delayed meconium (> 48 hours), signs of complete bowel obstruction (abdominal distension, vomiting) - Often with other congenital issues (GU/CV anomalies, hearing/visual defects) (+) Squirt sign: Rectal exam relieves obstruction with rapid emptying
Dx	- XR (to rule out dangerous pathology), followed by contrast enema (generally shows **microcolon** throughout colon, meconium pellets in ileum)	- Contrast enema (shows **transition zone**[A]: Change from the normal caliber rectum [aganglionic segment] to the proximal dilated colon) - Rectal suction biopsy (full thickness): Confirmatory
Tx	- Gastrografin enema (diagnostic/therapeutic)	- Colonic resection with anastomosis

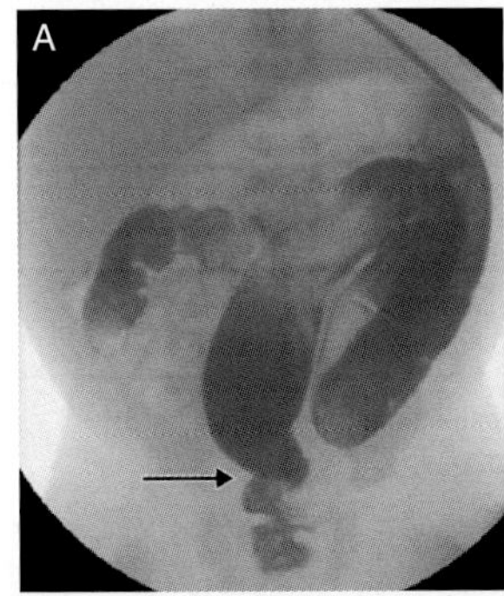

Necrotizing Enterocolitis

General: **Ischemic necrosis of GI mucosa**, with transmural inflammation, infection with gas-producing organisms, and dissection of gas

Risk: **Preterm, low birth weight**, antibiotics, early exposure to nonhuman milk
- If term, associated with congenital heart disease, sepsis, hypotension

Clinical:
- Feeding intolerance, **abdominal distension, hematochezia**
- Lethargy, respiratory failure, other hemodynamic changes all possible
- XR: **Pneumatosis intestinalis**, pneumoperitoneum, or sentinel loops

Diagnosis: Clinical (based on findings above)

Management:
- Supportive: NPO, GI decompression, parenteral nutrition, fluid/electrolytes
- Broad spectrum IV antibiotics (amp + gentamicin + metronidazole)
- Surgery (bowel resection): Indicated if perforation or deteriorating clinical condition

Neonatal/Congenital GI

Bilious Emesis DDx/Workup

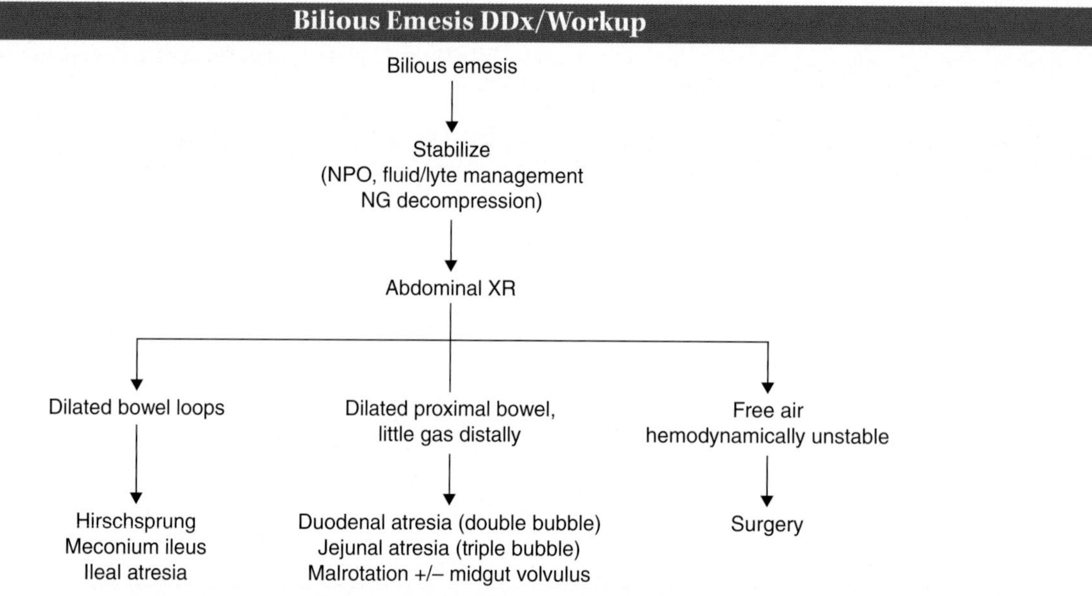

Intestinal Atresia

General: Congenital obstruction of the normally hollow GI tract. Can occur anywhere, but most frequently occurs at level of the duodenum.

	Duodenal	Jejunal/Ileal
Gen	- Failure of duodenum to recannulate during embryogenesis	- Vascular disruption, leading to ischemic necrosis, with "apple peel" appearance
Risk	- Trisomy 21, other chromosomal abnormalities	- Cystic fibrosis, malrotation
Clin	- Emesis (+/– bilious), abdominal distension	- Bilious emesis, distension
Dx	- XR: **Double-bubble**[A] (dilated stomach/proximal duodenum) - Upper GI series (rule out annular pancreas, malrotation, other similarly presenting pathologies)	- XR: Multiple **dilated bowel loops, air-fluid levels** - "Triple bubble" sign in jejunal atresia - Upper GI series/contrast enema
Tx	- Surgery within few days of birth (duodenoduodenostomy)	- Surgery (resection/anastomosis)

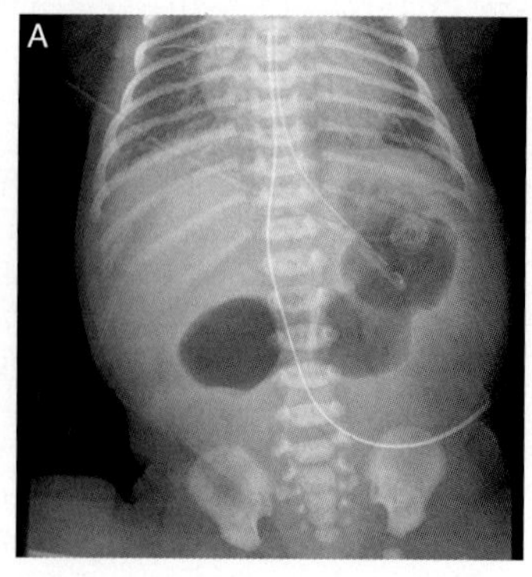

Neonatal/Congenital GI

Malrotation/Midgut Volvulus

General: Failure of the embryonic gut to complete normal rotation, with resulting improper positioning of bowel, and formation of fibrous adhesions ("Ladd's bands"). Often insidious until development of volvulus.

Risk: Often idiopathic, but can be associated with abdominal wall defects, intestinal atresia, diaphragmatic hernia, and other congenital GI malformations

Clinical:

- Highly variable and can present during infancy or early childhood
- Mild, nonspecific symptoms include vomiting, abdominal pain, failure to thrive
- Duodenal obstruction possible (from Ladd band adhesions)

- **Midgut volvulus**
  - Bowel twists along SMA, causing ischemia/necrosis
  - Presents with vomiting, severe abdominal pain, distension
  - Complicated by hematemesis/hematochezia, peritonitis, shock
  - Urgent surgery indicated if above complications present

Diagnosis:

- XR (initial, to rule out perforation)
- **Upper GI series**: Misplaced/corkscrew/obstructed duodenum

Management:

Malrotation	- Elective surgical correction (controversial, some recommend supportive care/observation)
Volvulus	- NG decompression, broad-spectrum antibiotics - Emergent surgery (**Ladd procedure**: Remove adhesions, put viable small bowel on right and colon on left)

Biliary Atresia

General: Idiopathic, progressive, fibro-obliterative degeneration of the extrahepatic biliary system

Clinical:

- Initially normal, but development of **conjugated hyperbilirubinemia 1-8 weeks after birth**
- Jaundice, acholic stools/dark urine, hepatomegaly

Diagnosis:

- Abdominal US (gallbladder often abnormally shaped)
- Hepatobiliary scintigraphy (tracer excretion rules out biliary atresia)
- Intraoperative cholangiogram (definitive diagnosis)

Management: Hepatoportoenterostomy (**Kasai procedure**)

- Postoperative ursodeoxycholic acid

Neonatal/Congenital GI

Esophageal Atresia/Tracheoesophageal Fistula

General: Esophageal narrowing, which most often occurs with fistula formation between esophagus/trachea. Can occur as part of VACTERL series of abnormalities.

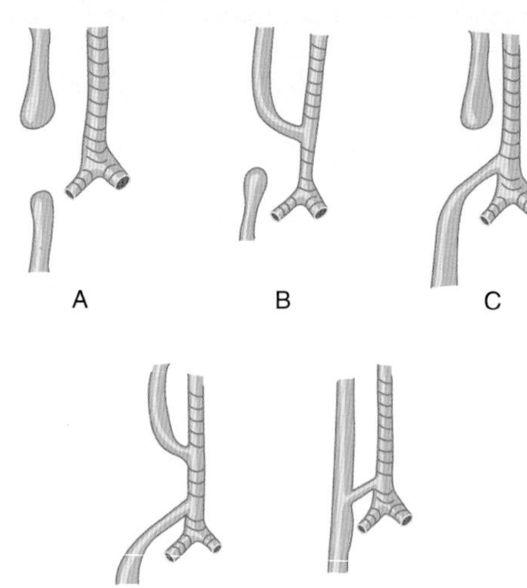

Subtypes:

A: Pure esophageal atresia
B: Esophageal atresia with proximal TEF (rare)
C: Esophageal atresia with distal TEF (most common)
E: **Pure TEF ("H-type")**

Clinical:

- Polyhydramnios (if any degree of esophageal atresia)
- Excess secretions, drooling, choking, respiratory distress
- Air in stomach with TEF
- Cyanosis from laryngospasm

Diagnosis:

- Place NG tube → CXR
    - EA: Tube curled in chest
    - TEF: Air in stomach
- Contrast esophagram if unsure
- Screen for other VACTERL abnormalities

Management: Surgical (TEF ligation, with esophageal anastomosis)

Anorectal Malformations

General: Heterogenous group of disorders, ranging from stenosis of the anus, to completely imperforate anus with blind rectal pouch. Associated with VACTERL malformations.

Clinical:

- Failure to pass meconium
- Usually obvious on first physical examination

Diagnosis: Clinical, but pelvic XR can be used as an aid in uncertain cases

Management: Surgery (perineal anoplasty or colostomy)

Neonatal/Congenital GI

Congenital Diaphragmatic Hernia

General: Congenital diaphragm defect in which abdominal contents herniate into the chest, compressing lung tissue, resulting in varying degrees of pulmonary hypoplasia. Defects most commonly left sided and posterior.

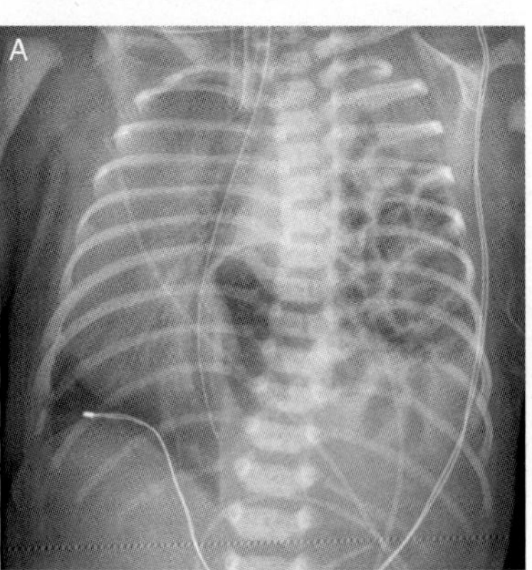

Clinical:

- Respiratory distress soon after birth
- Decreased left sided breath sounds, barrel-shaped chest

Diagnosis:

- In utero: US
- After birth: CXR[A] (with **abdominal contents in chest**)

Management:

- Initial supportive care/stabilization
    - Intubation, NG decompression, fluid/electrolyte management
- Surgery: Surgical reduction + primary or patch repair
    - Delayed until medically stabilized (hope for some lung maturity)

Hypertrophic Pyloric Stenosis

General: Hypertrophy of the pylorus, resulting in stenosis of the gastric outlet

Risk: Family history, erythromycin use during pregnancy

Clinical:

- **Projectile, nonbilious vomiting** in healthy 4–8 week-old male
- "**Olive-shaped**" mass RUQ
    - Possible retrograde peristaltic stomach waves
- Hypochloremic, hypokalemic metabolic alkalosis, dehydration

Diagnosis: Abdominal US

- Long, thick pylorus. Causes "doughnut sign."

Management:

- Volume resuscitation/electrolyte replacement
    - Medical stabilization vital before surgery
- Surgery: **Pyloromyotomy** (Ramstedt)
    - Mild vomiting/regurgitation common after surgery, but patients should start feeds

Neonatal/Congenital GI

	General	Clinical	Management
Omphalocele	- **Midline abdominal wall defect** - Associated with trisomy 13/18/21, Turner, and other chromosomal abnormalities	- Membranous herniation sac containing abdominal contents[A], most commonly at the site of cord insertion (cord inserts into membrane) - Diagnosed on prenatal US - Liver herniation/damage feared complication	- Prenatal: Careful observation, C-section, dressing at birth Surgical Closure - Small (2-3 cm) can be reduced and closed soon after birth - Larger (> 5 cm) should be placed in silo, allowed to naturally reduce, then surgically close
Gastroschisis	- **Full-thickness abdominal wall defect** - ↑ risk for inflammation, bowel wall thickening, NEC	- Evisceration of bowel contents - Located periumbilically, usually on right, with normal cord insertion - ↑ Maternal AFP during pregnancy - Diagnosed on prenatal US	- Careful fetal monitoring during pregnancy. Deliver if signs of bowel ischemia/necrosis. - At birth: Sterile dressing, antibiotics, gastric decompression - Primary surgical closure (use silo if too large to reduce initially)
Bladder Exstrophy	- Embryological defect in abdominal wall development, resulting in outside exposure of bladder	- Exposure of bladder and urethra on the surface of the lower abdomen - Diagnosis made on prenatal US (or apparent at birth on exam)	- Properly dress opening at birth - Surgical repair weeks after birth
Umbilical Hernia	- Herniation through fascial opening that allows passage of umbilical vessels - Associated with hypothyroidism, prematurity, Beckwith-Wiedemann, Ehlers-Danlos	- Reducible paraumbilical sac - Usually asymptomatic - Very rarely rupture/strangulate	- Monitor (most spontaneously close) - Consider closing if > 5 years old or symptomatic - Surgical reduction if incarcerated or strangulated

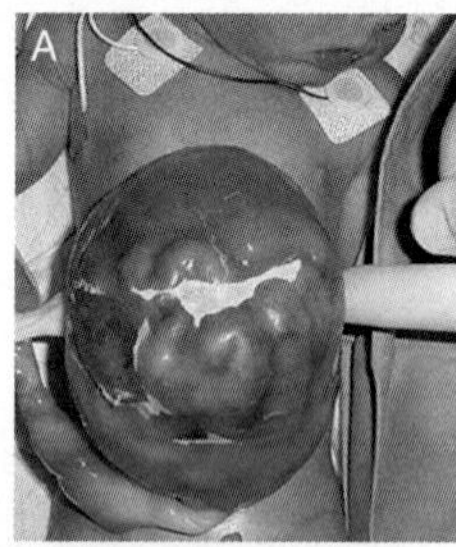

Meckel Diverticulum

General: True diverticulum (all bowel wall layers) of the small intestine, due to failure of obliteration of **Vitelline duct**

- Can contain heterotopic gastric (most common) or pancreatic tissue. HCl secretion can result in bleeding.
- Rule of 2s
    - 2% prevalence, 2:1 boy:girls
    - 2 feet from ileocecal valve
    - 2 inches long
    - 2% get complications, usually before 2 y/o

Clinical: Most often asymptomatic

- **Painless hematochezia** is most common presentation
- Intussusception, volvulus, obstruction all possible

Diagnosis: **Technetium-99 Scan ("Meckel Scan")**

- Other: Mesenteric arteriography (used especially during acute GI bleeds)

Management:

- Symptomatic: Surgery (diverticulectomy or small bowel resection)
- Asymptomatic (incidentally found): Controversial. Can either monitor or remove electively.

Neonatal/Congenital GI

Intussusception

General: Telescoping of a part of the intestine into itself. Common pediatric issue (< 2 y/o), with decreased frequency at older ages.

Risk: Usually idiopathic, but can be associated with certain **lead points**, including mesenteric lymphadenopathy (postviral or rotavirus vax), Meckel's diverticulum, or tumor/mass

Clinical: **Waxing/waning, cramping, severe abdominal pain**. 15-min episodes, followed by asymptomatic periods.
- Palpable mass, "currant jelly" stools (uncommon but pathognomonic)

Diagnosis: Abdominal US ("Bull's Eye" or "**Target sign**")

Management:
- Reduction with air enema (alt: Water-soluble contrast enema)
- Surgery: If evidence of perforation or refractory to multiple attempts at nonoperative reduction

Pancreatic Malformations

Annular Pancreas	- Ring of pancreatic tissue surrounding the descending duodenum - Caused by failure of the ventral bud to rotate with the duodenum - Risk for pancreatic duct obstruction (pancreatitis) and duodenal obstruction - Dx: GI series or abdominal CT - Tx: Duodenoduodenostomy (bypass the annulus, do NOT resect)
Pancreatic Divisum	- Failure of fusion of the ventral and dorsal ducts - Usually asymptomatic. Possible ↑ risk for pancreatitis. - Diagnose with abdominal imaging (CT or MRCP) - If severely symptomatic, can consider endoscopic sphincterotomy

Short Bowel Syndrome

General: Shortened small intestine, resulting in malabsorption/malnutrition and abnormal bowel function

Etiology: Any congenital lesion that requires **small bowel resection** (gastroschisis, volvulus, or intestinal atresia)

Clinical: Diarrhea, malabsorption, failure to thrive

Management: Long-term TPN

Food Protein-Induced Enterocolitis Syndrome (FPIES)

General: Infantile food hypersensitivity, most commonly induced by **protein in milk or soy** (but rarely solid food)

Clinical: Starts weeks after birth, either with repetitive vomiting, diarrhea, dehydration, or weight loss/failure to thrive

Diagnosis: Clinical, plus confirmed improvement after withdrawal of suspected trigger

Management: Dietary elimination of triggering substance, generally resolves by 3 y/o

Gastroesophageal Reflux

General: Normal spit-up caused by short esophagus, immature gastroesophageal sphincter. Note: Not called "disease" because no pathologic consequences, such as weight loss, esophagitis, etc.

Clinical: Frequent regurgitation events after feeding. No red flag features (failure to thrive, GI bleeding, forceful vomiting).

Management: Education/reassurance
- Frequent small volume feeds, upright position for 20-30 min after
- Thickening formula/breast milk if symptoms bothersome
- Should resolve spontaneously by 1 y/o. PPIs only indicated if esophagitis.

GI Pharm

	Mechanism	Indication	Side Effects/Management
Anti-ulcer			
PPIs Omeprazole Lansoprazole Esomeprazole Pantoprazole Dexlansoprazole	- Irreversible inhibition of the H+/K+ ATPase	- GERD - Gastritis/PUD - Esophagitis - *H. pylori* eradication	- Short-term: Well tolerated, possible diarrhea - Long-term: - Hypomagnesemia, other nutrient malabsorption - Increased risk of *C. Difficile* infection, pneumonia - ↓ Calcium absorption, ↑ fracture risk
H_2 Antagonist Cimetidine Ranitidine Famotidine	- Competitive antagonist of the H_2 receptor, resulting in decreased stomach acid	- GERD - Gastritis/PUD - Esophagitis	- Cimetidine (CYP450 inhibitor, anti-androgen, headache, mental status changes) - Others are well tolerated
Bismuth	- Binds to ulcers, may suppress *H. pylori* growth	- Quadruple therapy (*H. Pylori*) - Diarrhea	- Blackens stool
Sucralfate	- Binds to areas of mucosal damage and promotes healing	- GERD, PUD (second-line agent)	- Can bind other drugs
Al hydroxide	- Neutralize gastric acid and reduce acid delivery to the duodenum	- GERD (used for short-term symptomatic management of mild disease)	- Hypophosphatemia, constipation
Ca carbonate			- Hypercalcemia, Milk-alkali syndrome
Mg hydroxide			- Diarrhea
Antiemetics			
Ondansetron	- 5-HT3 antagonist	- Antiemetic	- Headache, constipation - QT Prolonging
Metoclopramide Prochlorperazine Droperidol	- D2 antagonist	- Antiemetic - Gastroparesis (metoclopramide)	- QT prolonging - Dystonia, Parkinsonism
Aprepitant Fosaprepitant	- NK1 antagonists	- Antiemetic	- CYP inhibitor
Laxatives/Motility			
Lubiprostone	- Chloride channel activator that increases intestinal fluid secretion	- Constipation predominant IBS	
Linaclotide Plecanatide	- Guanylate cyclase agonists that stimulates intestinal fluid secretion	- Constipation predominant IBS	
Methylnaltrexone Naloxegol	- Mu receptor antagonist, limited blood brain barrier penetrance	- Constipation associated with opiate use	
Prucalopride	- 5-HT_4 receptor agonist (pro motility)	- Chronic constipation	
Anti-diarrheal			
Loperamide Diphenoxylate	- Mu-receptor opiate agonists	- Diarrhea	- QT prolonging
Other			
Ursodiol	- Nontoxic bile acid (increases bile secretion)	- Primary biliary cirrhosis - Gallstone prevention	

Anemia

Anemia Overview

Definition: Hgb < 12 g/dL in women, < 13.5 g/dL in men

Clinical: Varies from asymptomatic to vague symptoms (weakness, fatigue, dyspnea, skin, or conjunctival pallor)

Diagnostic Tests:

- **MCV** (average volume of RBC, see below)
- **MCH** (mean corpuscular hemoglobin)
- **MCHC** (mean corpuscular hemoglobin concentration)
- **Reticulocyte Count**: Correction = Retic % × (Pts hematocrit/normal hematocrit)
    - < 2% → inadequate bone marrow response
- Blood smear (look for morphologic abnormalities)
    - Hypochromia[A]: Iron deficiency
    - Spherocytes: Spherocytosis, autoimmune hemolytic anemia
    - Targets: Thalassemia
    - Dacrocytes (tear-drop): Marrow fibrosis
    - Acanthocytes: Liver disease
    - Schistocytes: Hemolysis

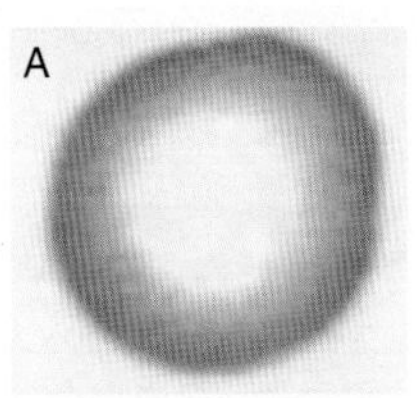

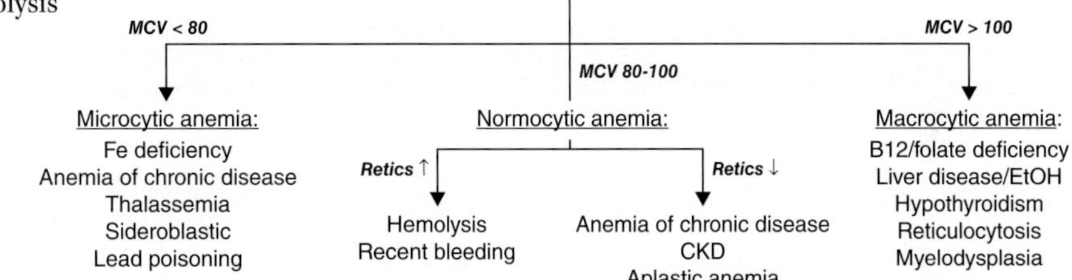

Evaluation of Iron Studies

	Serum Fe	Ferritin	TIBC	% Sat	Smear
Fe Deficiency	↓	↓	↑	↓	Hypochromic cells
Chronic Disease	↓	↔/↑	↓	↓	
Thalassemia	↔/↑	↔/↑	↔	↔/↑	Target cells
Sideroblastic	↑	↑	↔	↔	Ringed sideroblasts

Workup for Anemia

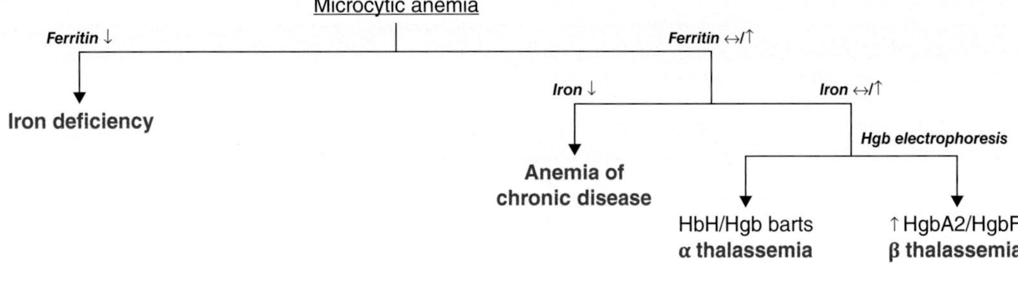

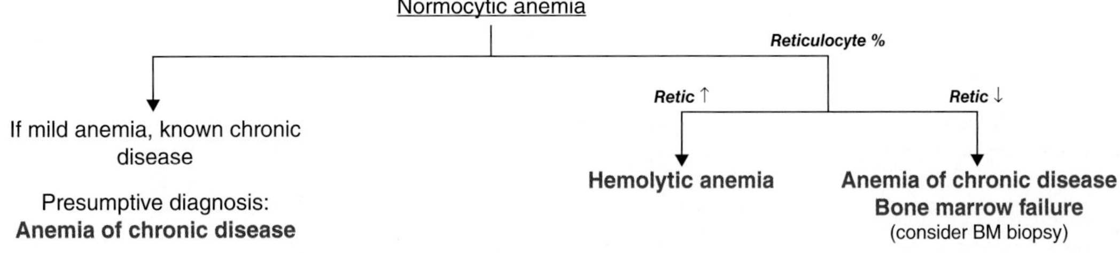

Microcytic Anemia

Microcytic Anemia

	General/Etiology	Clinical/Diagnosis	Management
Fe Deficiency	- Chronic blood loss - ↓ Fe absorption (i.e., Celiac, bariatric surgery, gastritis) - Redistribution (post EPO) - Poor diet (mostly kids) - ↑ utilization (pregnancy)	- Symptoms of anemia - Pica, ice-craving - Associated with restless leg Dx: - ↑ RDW, ↓ MCV/MCH/MCHC - **Ferritin (< 30 ng/mL)** - ↓ transferrin saturation (< 20%) - ↑ soluble transferrin receptor	- PO iron supplements (watch for GI side effects) - IV iron (now utilized with increased frequency)
Sideroblastic	Acquired: - EtOH, isoniazid, B6 deficiency - Myelodysplastic syndromes Genetic: - Most commonly XL-SA from mutation in ALA-synthase (part of heme synthesis)	- Symptoms of anemia Dx: - Bone marrow biopsy (ringed sideroblasts)	- Acquired: Correct underlying etiology - Genetic: Vitamin B6, manage anemia/iron overload

Alpha-Thalassemia

General: Abnormality in the alpha globin gene on chromosome 16

Gene	Name	Clinical
aa/a-	Trait or minima	- Silent carrier, normal H/H
aa/-- or a-/a-	Minor	- Mild, asymptomatic anemia
a-/--	HbH (β4 tetramers form, causing hemolysis)	- Hemolytic anemia, with ineffective RBC production - Indirect hyperbilirubinemia, splenomegaly - Skeletal abnormalities
--/--	Barts (γ4 tetramers)	- Fetal hydrops/incompatible with life

Diagnosis: Suspected with hypochromic, microcytic anemia, with abnormal smears (target cells[A], poikilocytosis)
- Confirmed with hemoglobin analysis and/or genetic testing

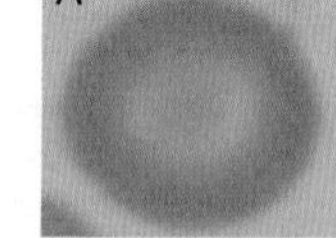

Management: Folate supplementation
- HbH disease can have moderate to severe anemia that requires transfusions
- Splenectomy, stem cell transplant if severe

Beta-Thalassemia

General: Abnormality in the beta globin gene on chromosome 11

Gene	Name	Clinical
β / β°	Minor (trait/carrier)	- Mild microcytic anemia
β+/β+ or β°/β+	Intermedia (nontransfusion dependent)	- Moderate microcytic anemia
β°/β° or β°/β+	Major (transfusion dependent)	- Severe anemia - Skeletal deformities (bossing, premature fusion, osteopenia, marrow expansion) - Hepatosplenomegaly, iron overload, growth abnormalities

*Presentation delayed until ~6 months due to fetal hemoglobin (vs alpha thal)

Diagnosis: Suspected with hypochromic, microcytic anemia, with abnormal smears
- Confirmed with hemoglobin analysis and/or genetic testing. $HgA_2 > 4$ %.

Management: Folate supplementation
- For major: Chronic transfusions (watch for secondary iron overload)
  - Luspatercept, splenectomy and stem cell transplant can be considered

Macrocytic Anemia

B12/Folate Deficiency

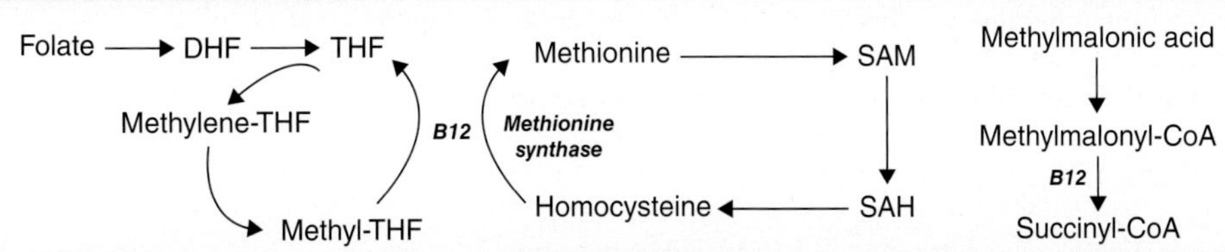

	Folate	B12
Source	- Many meat and vegetables - Fortified in food (first world)	- Meat products (meat, eggs, dairy)
Absorp	- Jejunum	- B12 is protein-bound in food - Haptocorrin (in saliva) binds B12 in stomach - Pancreatic proteases cleave haptocorrin off in duodenum - Intrinsic factor (IF) binds in duodenum - B12-IF absorbed in ileum
Cause	- Malnutrition (EtOH, elderly) - Increased use (pregnancy, hemolysis) - Malabsorption (celiac, bypass) - Drug side effect (methotrexate, TMP)	- Pernicious anemia (autoantibodies to IF/parietal cells) - Poor diet (year-long stores, but can develop with alcoholism or strict vegans) - Crohn disease, ileum resection - Bariatric surgery - Fish tapeworm

Clinical	- Megaloblastic[A] anemia	- Megaloblastic anemia
		- Subacute combined degeneration
		  - Neuropathy (lower extremity weakness, ataxia)
		  - Neuropsychiatric changes

Diagnosis	- Serum folate level (< 4 ng/mL)	- Serum B12 level (< 200-300 pg/mL) - If equivocal, use MMA/homocysteine (Both ↑ in B12 deficiency, just homocysteine in folate deficiency)
Treatment	- Oral folate	- Oral B12 - IV/IM B12 for severe disease

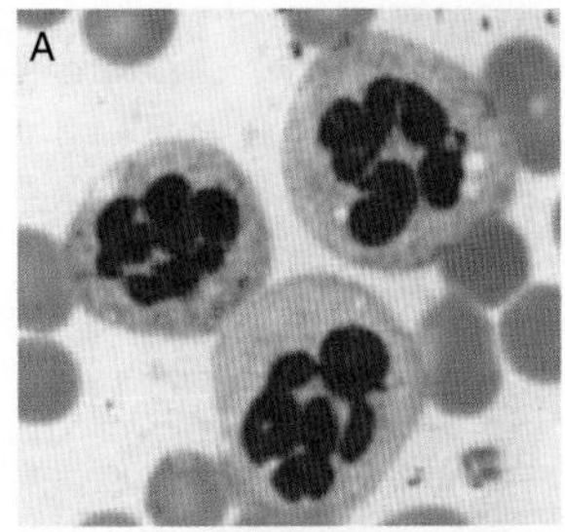

Other Causes of Macrocytosis

- EtOH
- Liver disease
- Hypothyroidism
- Reticulocytosis
- Drug-induced (methotrexate, phenytoin, many chemotherapeutics)
- Myelodysplasia
    - Note: Isolated macrocytosis without anemia is often a sign of MDS

Normocytic Anemia

Anemia of Chronic Disease (Inflammation)

General: Chronic anemia from inflammation (results in the ↑ of acute phase reactant hepcidin)

Etiology: Malignancy, infection, autoimmune disease, other chronic conditions

Clinical: General mild (Hgb > 8-10 g/dL) and asymptomatic

Diagnosis: Normocytic or slightly microcytic anemia, low reticulocyte count
- Normal/↑ ferritin, ↓ serum Fe

Management: Treat underlying condition

Anemia as a Complication of CKD

General: Normocytic anemia from the lack of EPO production from the peritubular capillaries

Management: EPO: Generally given to CKD patients with Hgb < 10. Hgb goal is 10-11.5 g/dL. Ensure iron replete.

Aplastic Anemia

General: Pancytopenia secondary to bone marrow hypoplasia from loss of hematopoietic stem cells

Etiology: Often idiopathic
- Radiation
- Drugs (carbamazepine, phenytoin, methimazole, cytotoxic chemotherapy)
- Virus (EBV, CMV, HIV, parvovirus [RBC only], hepatitis A-E)
- Autoimmune disease (SLE), Fanconi anemia

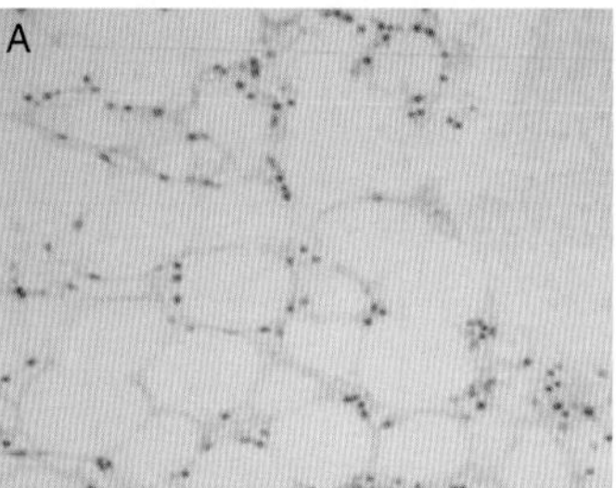

Clinical: Symptoms from **pancytopenia** (bleeding, bruising, infection, anemia)

Diagnosis: Confirmation with bone marrow biopsy (hypocellular marrow[A])
- If likely reversible cause is present, can correct and monitor prior to biopsy

Management:
- Stop offending agent, transfuse RBC/platelet as necessary
- Bone marrow stimulation (i.e., GM-CSF)
- If severe: HCT (if < 50 y/o and otherwise healthy) or immunosuppression (if not qualified for HCT)

Hemolysis (Overview)

General: Premature destruction of RBCs, resulting in normocytic anemia with elevated reticulocyte count

Etiology:

Extrinsic	Intrinsic
- Autoimmune hemolytic anemia - Microangiopathic hemolytic anemia (TTP/HUS/DIC) - Mechanical (mechanical valve, AS) - RBC infections (malaria, babesia)	- Sickle cell - Spherocytosis - PNH - G6PD deficiency

Clinical:

	Intravascular	Extravascular
Pathophys	- Vascular RBC destruction	- Splenic destruction of RBC
LDH	↑	↑
Haptoglobin	↓↓	↓/↔
Indirect bili	↑	↑
Urine	Hemoglobinuria ↑ Urobilinogen	↑ Urobilinogen

Note: Features often overlap as often have components of both intravascular and extravascular hemolysis.

Normocytic Anemia

Autoimmune Hemolytic Anemia		
	IgG ("warm")	IgM ("cold")
Etio	- SLE - CLL, lymphoma - Drug (penicillins, methyldopa)	- Infection (mycoplasma, EBV) - Lymphoproliferative disorders
Clin	- Various degrees of hemolytic anemia - Spherocytes on smear	- Various degrees of hemolytic anemia - Livedo reticularis - Acrocyanosis
Dx	- Direct Coombs (positive for **IgG +/– C3**)	- Direct Coombs (positive for **C3 or IgM**)
Tx	- Corticosteroids (first-line) - Rituximab, other immunosuppression - Splenectomy if refractory	- Avoidance of cold (mild disease) - Rituximab

Genetic Hemolytic Anemia			
	General	Clinical/Diagnosis	Treatment
Hereditary Spherocytosis	- AD defects in RBC structural proteins (ankyrin, spectrin, band-3) - Causes **spherocytosis** and **chronic extravascular hemolysis**	- Hemolytic anemia - Jaundice - Splenomegaly - ↑ MCHC, reticulocytes, RDW - Spherocytes on smear - Dx: Eosin-5-maleimide binding test (confirmatory) - Osmotic fragility no longer used	- Folate - Transfusions as necessary - Splenectomy
G6PD Deficiency	- XR disorder in the glucose-6 phosphate dehydrogenase enzyme - Hemolysis precipitated by oxidant stress (infection, drugs [sulfonamides, primaquine], fava beans)	- Episodic hemolytic anemia - Blood smear with "bite cells" and Heinz bodies - Dx: **G6PD enzyme assay** (fluorescent spot test screen, followed by quantitative NADPH calculation) Note: Can be negative during acute episode	- Avoidance of triggers - Transfuse as necessary during episodes
Paroxysmal Nocturnal Hemoglobinuria	- Acquired defect in the GPI molecule (a phospholipid anchor for surface proteins) - Results in lack of **CD55** (blocks splenic extravascular hemolysis) and **CD59** (blocks complement) on RBCs	- Chronic hemolysis with normocytic anemia - Pancytopenia - Thrombosis - Smooth muscle dystonia (abdominal pain, erectile dysfunction, pulm HTN) - Renal insufficiency - Dx: **Flow cytometry (for CD55/59)**	- Eculizumab (complement inhibitor) - HCT

Normocytic Anemia

Sickle Cell Anemia

General: AR condition in Hgb beta chain, which results in HbS replacing HbA. Point mutation (Glutamic acid → valine) which promotes Hgb polymerization, especially under conditions of stress (acidemia, hypoxia, dehydration, infection).

Clinical: Chronic hemolytic anemia
- Variety of complications (see next page)

Diagnosis:
- **Hgb analysis** (via HPLC, gel electrophoresis, or isoelectric focusing)
    - Provides information about Hgb distribution (see chart below)
- Prenatal diagnosis made by genetic testing

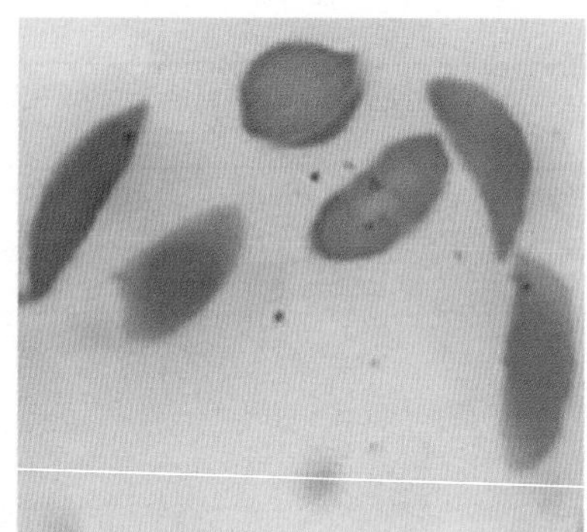

Management:
- Avoid crisis precipitators (stay hydrated, avoid high altitudes, etc.)
- Vaccinations (including pneumococcal, flu, HIB, meningococcal)
- Folate supplementation
- Antibiotic PPX (until at least age 5): Penicillin (alt: Erythromycin)
- Selective use of RBC transfusion (monitor for iron overload)
- Severe, refractory disease: Consider HCT

Pharm:
- Hydroxyurea (↑ HgbF) is recommended in most children and adults that suffer from recurrent occlusive crises
- L-glutamine, crizanlizumab, voxelotor

Sickle Cell Trait

General: Carrier of one mutated Hgb beta gene. Patients have significant amounts of both HgbA and HgbS.

Clinical: Generally asymptomatic, but the following complications can occur:
- Hematuria (due to renal papillary infarcts)
- Hyposthenuria (abnormal urinary concentration, leading to polyuria)
- Renal medullary carcinoma
- Splenic infarct (especially at high altitude)

Hemoglobin Distribution (> 5 y/o)

Disorder	Hgb	HgbA	HgbA2	HgbF	HgbS	HgbC
Normal	AA	95%	3%	< 2%	–	–
Sickle Cell Disease	SS	0	3%	5-15%	> 85%	–
Sickle Trait	AS	> 50%	3%	< 2%	30-40%	
HgbSC Disease	SC	0%	3%	< 5%	45%	45%
β-Thalassemia Minor	Aβ	90%	> 3.5%	< 2%	–	–
β-Thalassemia Major	ββ	0%	> 3.5%	> 90%	–	–
Sickle-Beta Thal	Sβ	0%	> 3.5%	10-15%	> 80%	–

Normocytic Anemia

Complications of Sickle Cell

	Clinical	Management
Pain Crisis (Vaso-Occlusive Episode)	- Acute episode of severe pain due to vaso-occlusion - Can occur anywhere in body, but dactylitis is common (especially in kids) - Often preceded by trigger - Purely clinical diagnosis	- Hydration (oral or IV) - Opioid pain medication
Splenic Sequestration Crisis	- Splenic occlusion, seen in kids without complete splenic fibrosis - Traps large volumes of blood in the spleen - Presents as LUQ pain, splenomegaly, worsening anemia, hypovolemic shock	- Transfusion - Elective splenectomy after episode has resolved
Aplastic Crisis	- Acute drop in reticulocyte %, leading to worsening anemia - Most commonly due to parvo B19	- Supportive transfusions
Acute Chest Syndrome	- New pulmonary infiltrate, along with fever/respiratory symptoms - Multifactorial etiology, but likely due to some combination of ischemia, infarction, atelectasis, and infection	- Fluids, pain control - Broad spectrum antibiotics (to cover for pneumonia, which often can't be ruled out) - Bronchodilator treatments - Transfusions as needed

Other Complications:

GI	- Bilirubin gallstones
ID	- ↑ infection risk (due to hyposplenism, progressive splenic autoinfarction) - ↑ risk of infection with encapsulated organisms
MSK	- Avascular necrosis (chronic, progressive pain compared to acute pain episodes) - Osteomyelitis (*Salmonella*) - Chronic leg ulcers
Renal	- Renal insufficiency, hematuria
GU	- Priapism
CNS	- Stroke (cerebral thrombosis) - Can screen with transcranial doppler

Disorders of Heme Synthesis

Lead Poisoning

General: Exposure to lead, leading to systemic toxicity, including abnormal heme synthesis (via inhibition of ferrochelatase and ALA-dehydratase)

	Children	Adults
Etio	- Absorption primarily GI - Sources include paint, food/water, breast milk (if mom has ↑ lead)	- Absorption from lungs (predominant) and GI tract - Sources include gas, paint, gun powder, moonshine
Clin	- Neurologic/behavioral changes - Encephalopathy/hearing loss at high levels - Abdominal pain, renal insufficiency	- Abdominal pain - Neurologic (poor concentration, memory issues) - Anemia (+/− basophilic stippling) - Nephropathy
Dx	- Measure blood lead level (> 5 mcg/dL abnormal)	
Tx	< 45 mcg/dL: Confirm level, removal from exposure, family education 45-70 mcg/dL: Above, plus chelation with succimer > 70 mcg/dL: Succimer + EDTA	< 50 mcg/dL: Remove exposure 50-80 mcg/dL: Remove exposure, consider chelation > 80 mcg/dL: Chelation

Chelation agents: DMSA (succimer) generally preferred. CaNa2EDTA/penicillamine are alternative agents. EDTA and dimercaprol used if child has encephalopathy.

Porphyria

	Acute Intermittent Porphyria	Porphyria Cutanea Tarda
Gen	↓ porphobilinogen deaminase activity (AD inherited) - Episodes triggered by stress, fasts, EtOH, smoking, estrogen, certain drugs	↓ uroporphyrinogen decarboxylase activity - Associated with HIV, Hep C, smoking, EtOH, estrogen use
Clin	- Neurologic dysfunction (peripheral neuropathy, weakness, seizures) - Autonomic dysfunction (tachycardia, tremors, sweating) - Abdominal pain - Dark urine	- Blisters, bullae to photoexposed skin - Scarring, with pigmentation changes - Transaminitis
Dx	- Urinary porphobilinogen	- Increased plasma/urine porphyrin
Tx	- Supportive care during episodes - Hemin administration - Avoid triggers	- Phlebotomy or low-dose hydroxychloroquine

Thrombocytopenia

Overview of Thrombocytopenia

General: Platelet count < 150K/mm^3. Generally asymptomatic, but severe (< 50K) have elevated risk for bleeding. Can be due to increased destruction, decreased production, or sequestration.

Etiology:

Autoimmune	- ITP, SLE, RA
Consumption	- HUS/TTP, DIC, HIT
Production	- Bone marrow failure (presents as pancytopenia), myelodysplasia, B12/folate deficiency
Drug induced	- NSAIDs, sulfa drugs, IIb/IIIa inhibitors, heparin, quinine, EtOH
Infection	- HIV, Hep C, EBV
Genetic	- Bernard soulier (AR defect in GPIb-IX) - Glanzmann thrombasthenia (AR defect in GPIIb-IIIa)
Sequestration	- Seen with hypersplenism, portal hypertension
Pseudo	- Pseudothrombocytopenia (platelet clumping, resulting in abnormal test)
Special scenarios: - Malignancy (bone marrow invasion or DIC) - Pregnancy (gestational thrombocytopenia, preeclampsia, HELLP) - Liver failure (↓ TPO, splenic sequestration)	

Clinical: **Superficial bleeding** (petechiae, purpura, mucosal bleeding), epistaxis, menorrhagia

Management:

- Generally want platelets > 50K prior to surgical procedure
- Platelet transfusion: Active bleeding with count < 50K OR any person < 10K

Immune Thrombocytopenic Purpura

General: Auto-antibody formation against host platelet glycoproteins, resulting in removal of platelets by splenic macrophages. The disorder tends to be acute and self-limited in children, but chronic and relapsing in adults.

Etiology:

- Primary: Idiopathic, generally occurs after viral infection
- Secondary: CLL, SLE, HIV, hep C, CMV

Clinical: Generally asymptomatic, but can develop bleeding (purpura, petechiae, and mucosal bleeding like epistaxis)

Diagnosis: Isolated thrombocytopenia with otherwise normal smear[A]

- **Primary ITP**: Diagnosis of exclusion
- **Secondary ITP**: Thrombocytopenia in someone with associated condition

Management:

Adult	
Acute	
Platelets > 30K	- Observe
Platelets < 30K or severe bleeding	- Glucocorticoids and/or IVIG
Chronic	
Refractory to initial therapy	- Rituximab, romiplostim or eltrombopag, splenectomy
Children	
Life-threatening/severe-bleeding OR desire for rapid rise in platelets	- Steroids, IVIG +/− platelet transfusion
Asymptomatic or minimal symptoms	- Monitor

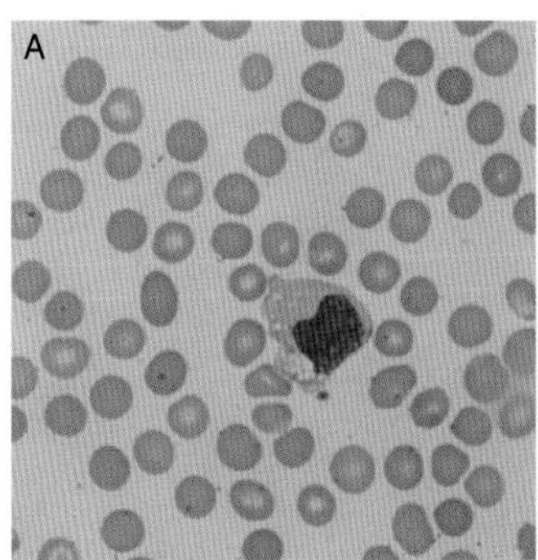

Thrombocytopenia

Thrombotic Microangiopathy

	Thrombotic Thrombocytopenic Purpura	Hemolytic Uremic Syndrome
Gen	- Deficiency or autoantibody to ADAMTS13, which normally cleaves VWF multimers	- Released toxin promotes thrombogenesis over the endothelium
Etio	- Often idiopathic, can be related to SLE, HIV, drugs, and pregnancy - Rarely hereditary	- Shiga-toxin *E. coli* [O157:H7] (90%) - Acquired complement deficiency, pneumococcus rarer causes
Clin	- Microangiopathic hemolytic anemia (MAHA) - Thrombocytopenia - Neurologic dysfunction (HA, confusion, focal deficits) - AKI less common	- Microangiopathic hemolytic anemia (MAHA) - Thrombocytopenia - AKI - STEC: Prodrome of bloody diarrhea and abdominal pain
Dx	- Clinical diagnosis (hemolysis, thrombocytopenia, etc.) - ADAMS T13 activity assay	- Clinical diagnosis (classic prodrome followed by above triad)
Tx	- Urgent plasma exchange w/ FFP - Glucocorticoids	- Supportive care (fluids, electrolyte management) - Transfusions - Dialysis for severe renal failure

Disseminated Intravascular Coagulation (DIC)

General: Abnormal activation of the coagulation pathway, leading to microthrombi throughout the vasculature, with consumption of platelets, coagulation factors, and fibrin

Etiology: Sepsis, malignancy, trauma, OB complications (amniotic fluid embolism)

Clinical:
- Bleeding/oozing from catheter sites
- **Thrombocytopenia, prolonged PT/PTT, prolonged bleeding time**
- Low fibrinogen, elevated D-dimer. Schistocytes on peripheral smear.

	ITP	TTP	HUS	DIC
↓ ***Platelets***	+	+	+	+
MAHA	–	+	+	+
↑ ***PT/PTT***	–	–	–	+

Diagnosis: Clinical PLUS laboratory diagnosis (no single definitive test)

Management:
- Supportive care (fluids, hemodynamic support). Treat/manage underlying cause.
- Manage active bleeding with transfusions (FFP, platelets, pRBC)

Heparin-Induced Thrombocytopenia (HIT)

General: Immune-mediated complication of heparin, due to autoantibodies against platelet factor-4 (in type 2)
- **Type 1**: Transient drop in platelet count, self-limited (can continue heparin)
- **Type 2**: More severe form, with the clinical manifestations seen below

Clinical: "4 Ts"
- **Timing**: > 5 days from exposure (can be sooner with previous heparin use)
- **Thrombocytopenia**: Platelet reduction > 50% from baseline
- **Thrombosis**: Arterial or venous thrombosis
- Other causes not apparent
- Necrotic skin lesions at injection sites

Diagnosis: ELISA immunoassay for PF4-heparin antibody (sensitive test)
- If positive, serotonin release assay to confirm (specific test)

Management: Stop heparin products if suspicion for HIT. Start direct thrombin inhibitor (e.g., argatroban).

Coagulopathy

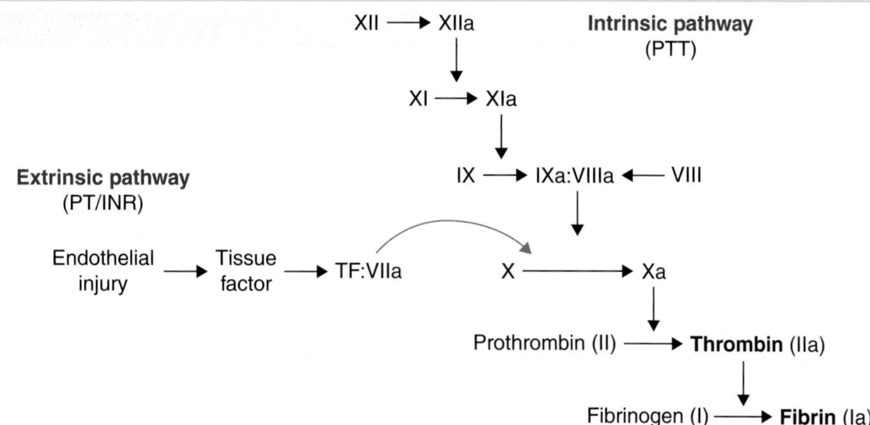

Hemophilia A/B

General: Inherited XR disorder in factor VIII (A) or factor IX (B). Female carriers generally asymptomatic, but can have mild symptoms.

Clinical:

- **Prolonged bleeding** (after trauma or surgery)
- **Hemarthrosis**, leading to chronic arthropathy
- Mucosal bleeding (GI bleeds), intracranial bleeds
- Hematoma formation (intramuscular, retroperitoneal)
- Prolonged PTT (normal platelets, bleeding time, PT)

Diagnosis: Factor VIII or IX activity assay (< 40% of expected)

Management:

	Indication	Intervention
Acute	- Bleeding - Surgical procedure	- Desmopressin (mild disease) - Factor concentrate infusions - Antifibrinolytic therapy for mucosal bleeding (TXA)
Chronic PPX	- High risk (< 1% factor activity) - Recurrent bleeding	- Emicizumab (hemophilia A) - Factor infusions
Hemarthrosis		- Analgesia, immobilization, ice - Arthrocentesis - Factor infusion

Acquired Coagulation Inhibitors

General: Antibodies that inhibit activity/increase clearance of clotting factor. Factor VIII most common. Acquired, associated with malignancy, postpartum period, autoimmune disorders, and long-term exogenous factor exposure (hemophilia).

Clinical: Presents like hemophilia (bleeding, ↑ PTT)

Diagnosis: Mixing study

Management: Steroids (improve some cases)

Coagulopathy

von Willebrand Disease

General: AD disorder characterized by deficiency or defect of vWF. Most common inherited coagulopathy. Subtypes:
- Type 1 (most common): Decreased levels of vWF
- Type 2 (less common): Dysfunctional vWF
- Type 3 (least common): Absent vWF (most severe form)

Clinical:
- Superficial bleeding (mucosal/cutaneous bleeds, epistaxis, easy bruising)
- Menorrhagia
- Bleeding time prolonged, normal or mildly increased PTT

Diagnosis: Screen with: vWF:Ag assay, vWF activity assay (ristocetin cofactor), or factor VIII activity assay

Management: Therapy only indicated when patients develop bleeding/hemostatic stress
- Mild bleed, minor surgery: Desmopressin
- Major bleed, surgery: vWF replacement therapy
- Other options: Antifibrinolytics, topical agents

Supratherapeutic INR (Warfarin Toxicity/Vitamin K Deficiency)

General: Vitamin K is required for the γ-carboxylation of clotting factors II, VII, IX, X, C, and S

Etiology:
- Warfarin
- Liver failure (not true deficiency, rather lack of factor synthesis)
- Malabsorption (CF, pancreatic insufficiency)
- Malnutrition
- Antibiotic use

Clinical: Elevated risk for severe hemorrhage
- PT/INR prolonged (more sens/spec). PTT can be mildly prolonged.

Management:

Indication	Intervention
Active bleeding (w/ INR > 2) or Surgery (emergent reversal)	- Prothrombin complex (first-line) or FFP
INR > 10	- Hold warfarin, give vitamin K
INR > 4.5	- Hold warfarin, consider vitamin K

Thrombophilia

Differential Diagnosis of Hypercoagulability

General: Risk for thrombus formation is increased in those with features of Virchow triad:
(1) Endothelial damage, (2) Hypercoagulability, (3) Stasis

Etiology	Findings
Acquired	
- Surgery (inflammation from surgery, immobilization, endothelial damage) - Immobilization (hospitalization, long flights) - Malignancy - Hormonal (OCPs, pregnancy, tamoxifen) - Nephrotic syndrome - Other syndromes: Antiphospholipid syndrome, PNH, myeloproliferative neoplasms	
Genetic	
Factor V Leiden	- Most common inherited coagulopathy among Caucasians - Mutated factor V that is resistant to cleavage by protein C
Antithrombin Deficiency	- Can be inherited or acquired (from cirrhosis, nephrotic, DIC) - Lack of antithrombin results in unregulated thrombin activity, heparin resistance
Protein C/S Deficiency	- Unregulated protein V/VIII activity - Associated with warfarin skin necrosis (protein C deficiency)
Prothrombin Mutation	- G20210A mutation, resulting in ↑ prothrombin production

Diagnosis: Protein activity assay (C/S, antithrombin deficiency) or genetic testing
- Testing indicated if strong family history, recurrent thromboses, thromboses in odd locations

Management: If recurrent thrombotic episodes, patients require chronic anticoagulation (warfarin/LMWH/DOAC)

Antiphospholipid Syndrome

General: Prothrombotic state induced by the presence of an antiphospholipid antibody

Risk: Autoimmune predisposition, especially SLE

Clinical:
- **Venous thrombosis** (DVT/PE) and arterial thrombosis (CVA)
- **Pregnancy complications** (recurrent abortions)
- Thrombocytopenia and prolonged PTT
- Derm: Livedo reticularis, superficial venous thrombosis, skin ulcers

Diagnosis: (At least 1 of clinical and lab criteria below)

Clinical	Laboratory
(1) Vascular thrombosis (arterial/ venous) (2) Pregnancy morbidity - ≥ 3 straight abortions prior to week 10 - Premature birth (< 34 weeks) with pre-eclampsia - Unexplained fetal demise > 10 weeks	(1) Lupus anticoagulant (dilute russell venom viper test, mixing study) (2) Anti-cardiolipin (ELISA IgM/IgG) (3) Anti-β-2 glycoprotein (ELISA IgM/IgG)

Management:
- Acute thromboembolism: Anticoagulation
- Chronic PPX: Warfarin +/– Aspirin (indicated if history of arterial thrombus)

Oncology Basics

Cancer Definitions

Neoplastic Progression	
Dysplasia	- Abnormal growth of cells with abnormal shape/orientation
Carcinoma in situ	- Neoplastic cells, but contained within basement membrane
Carcinoma	- Neoplastic cells invade basement membrane of normal tissue
Metastasis	- Spread to distant organ

Nomenclature	
Carcinoma	- Malignancy of epithelial cell origin Adenocarcinoma: Glandular epithelium Angiocarcinoma: Endothelial cells
Sarcoma	- Malignancy of connective tissue origin Liposarcoma: Adipose Chondrosarcoma: Cartilage Osteosarcoma: Bone Myosarcoma: Muscle
Leukemia	- Leukocyte malignancy found in blood and bone marrow
Lymphoma	- Leukocyte malignancy found in lymphoid tissue

Grade/Stage	
Grade	- Pathologic description of differentiation
Stage	- Classifying cancer based on extent of invasion/spread

Cancer Therapy

Cancer Therapy	
Surgery	- Often part of treatment for nonhematologic malignancies
Radiation	- Ionizing radiation to disrupt DNA and result in death of cells
Chemotherapy	- Cytotoxic drugs which inhibits growth of all rapidly dividing cells
Targeted therapy	- Drugs that target deregulated proteins specific to cancer cells
Immunotherapy	- Using own immune system's cells, cytokines, etc to target cancer

Hematopoiesis

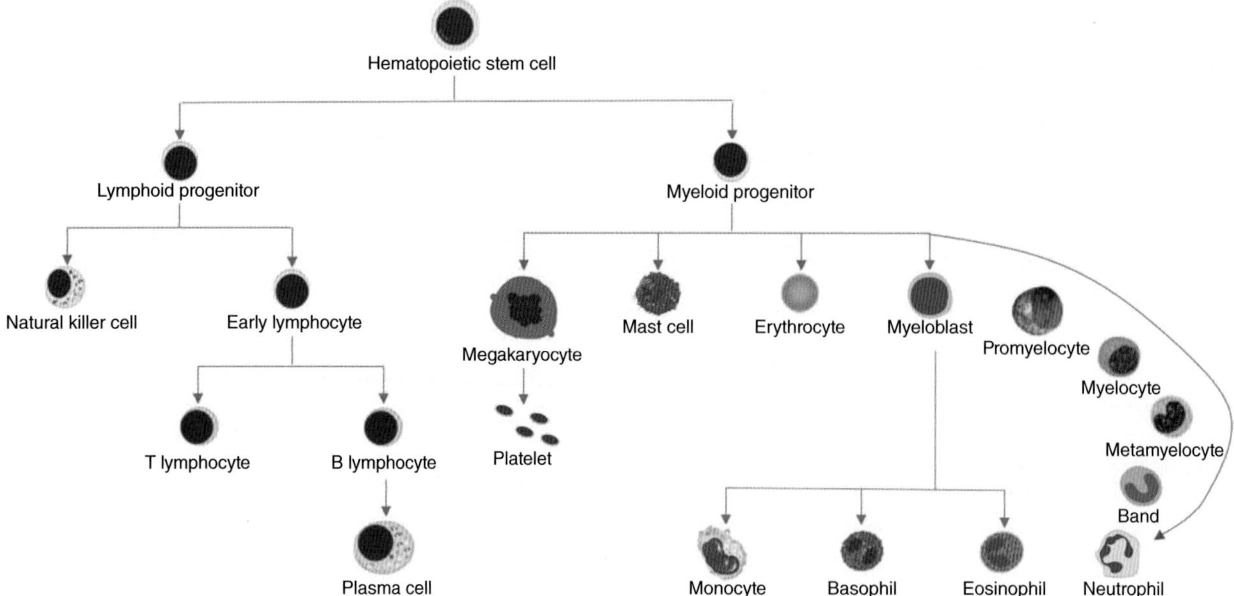

Oncologic Emergencies

	General	Clinical	Management
Tumor Lysis Syndrome	- Massive tumor cell lysis, with release of intracellular contents - Can occur with the initiation of cytotoxic chemo or spontaneously (especially with aggressive leukemia/lymphoma)	- Electrolyte abnormalities (↑ PO_4, uric acid, K, but ↓ Ca) - AKI (deposition of uric acid or CaPhos crystals)	Acute episode: - Supportive care (aggressive fluids/lytes repletion, telemetry), rasburicase Prophylaxis: - IV fluid hydration - Hypouricemic drug (allopurinol)
Febrile Neutropenia	- Patients undergoing cytotoxic chemotherapy can develop neutropenia and the translocation of GI flora across the compromised GI mucosa, resulting in severe infection	- Fever (temp > 100.4°F) [may be only sign due to blunted neutrophil response] - Neutropenia (ANC < 1500, but especially at risk if ANC < 500)	- Infectious workup (cultures, etc.) - Empiric antibiotics: Gram-negative coverage (e.g., cefepime) +/− gram-positive coverage
Hypercalcemia	- Either from osteolytic mets, PTHrP production, or vitamin D production	- Bones, stones, groans, psychiatric overtones - [See: Hypercalcemia]	- Acute: Hypercalcemia management - Prophylaxis: Bisphosphonates
Hyperviscosity	- Most commonly occurs with high protein disorders (Waldenström's macroglobulinemia, multiple myeloma)	- Visual blurring, headache - Vertigo, nystagmus, diplopia - Ataxia - Can measure serum viscosity to confirm	- Plasmapheresis
SVC Syndrome	- Obstruction of SVC, resulting in facial/upper extremity edema	- Edema - Severe manifestations include CNS edema and laryngeal edema	- Endovenous stenting or radiation therapy (for emergencies) - Chronic: Treat underlying malignancy
Spinal Cord Compression	- Tumor compressing the dural sac	- Back pain, focal neurologic deficits (weakness, incontinence, sensory loss) - Dx: MRI	- Corticosteroids, surgery
Other Complications			
Cachexia	- Multifactorial weight loss from muscle catabolism, systemic inflammation, and poor caloric intake		- Tx: Progesterone or corticosteroids (increase appetite)

Plasma Cell Dyscrasias

Monoclonal Gammopathy of Uncertain Significance (MGUS)

General: Asymptomatic, premalignant clonal plasma cell proliferative disorder. Risk to progress to:
- Multiple myeloma (if IgA/IgG producing)
- Waldenström macroglobulinemia (if IgM producing)

Clinical: Asymptomatic, no end-organ damage like that seen with myeloma

Diagnosis: **Serum/Urine protein electrophoresis** (monoclonal Ig at < 3 g/dL)
- Serum FLC (free light chain) and immunoglobulin

Note: Patients must have no clinical symptoms consistent with MM or WM, and < 10% clonal plasma cells on bone marrow biopsy (if performed)

Management: Monitor patients (progress to malignancy at ~1% per year)
- Annual serum and urine M-protein, CBC, calcium, etc.

Multiple Myeloma and Waldenström Macroglobulinemia

	Multiple Myeloma	Waldenström Macroglobulinemia
Gen	- Plasma cell neoplasm with monoclonal Ig production	- Clonal lymphoplasmacytic proliferation with IgM production
Clin	"**CRAB**" Features - Hypercalcemia - Renal Failure (bence jones protein) - Anemia (BM infiltrate/renal failure) - Bone (osteolytic lesions[A] with ↑ fracture risk) - Increased infection risk (due to monoclonal Ig)	- Weakness, fatigue, weight loss - Lymphadenopathy, hepatomegaly or splenomegaly - **Hyperviscosity** (CNS symptoms: blurred vision, HA, stroke) - Neuropathy (paresthesia, weakness) - Anemia - Bleeding
Dx	- SPEP: **Non-IgM** serum monoclonal protein **≥ 3 g/dL** - ≥ 10% clonal plasma cells in bone marrow aspirate - Free light chain analysis (abnormal kappa:lambda ratio)	- SPEP: **IgM** serum monoclonal protein **≥ 3 g/dL** - ≥ 10% clonal lymphoplasmacytic cells in bone marrow aspirate
Tx	- Chemotherapy for induction (such as bortezomib, lenalidomide, dexamethasone) - HCT (if eligible) - Bisphosphonates for bone lesions	- Asymptomatic: Monitor - Symptomatic: Chemotherapy (rituximab, dexamethasone, Bendamustine common in regimens) - Hyperviscosity: Plasmapheresis

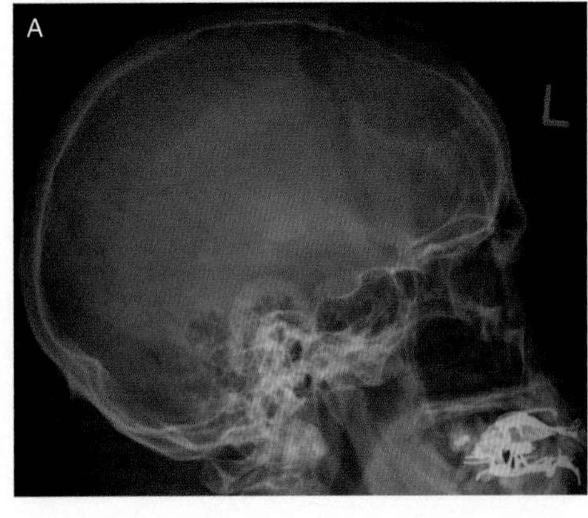

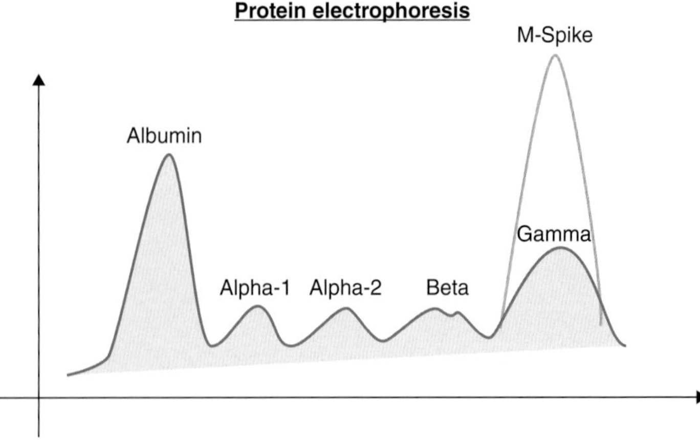

Myeloproliferative Disorders

Differential Diagnosis for Polycythemia

	Etiology	RBC Mass	EPO	Other Findings
Primary	- Polycythemia vera	↑	↓	- Hypervolemia
Appropriate absolute	- Lung disease, cyanotic heart defects - High altitude	↑	↑	- Hypoxemia
Inappropriate absolute	- Ectopic EPO production (malignancy)	↑	↑	
Relative	- Volume loss	↔	↔	- Hypovolemia

Myeloproliferative Neoplasms

General: Group of myeloid neoplasms that have terminal myeloid cell expansion in the peripheral blood. Often associated with JAK-2 gene mutations.

Clinical: Depending on the disorder, various degrees of erythrocytosis, leukocytosis, thrombocytosis, bone marrow hypercellularity/fibrosis, and splenomegaly

	General	Clinical	Management
Essential Thrombocytosis	- Excessive clonal platelet production, often due to JAK2 mutation	- Unexplained, persistent thrombocytosis - Vasomotor symptoms (syncope, headache, dizziness, erythromelalgia) - Thrombosis/hemorrhage risk	***Diagnosis:*** - Thrombocytosis > 450K/mm^3 - Bone marrow biopsy (proliferation of enlarged, mature megakaryocytes) - Classic mutation or clear clonal marker ***Treatment:*** - Aspirin or anticoagulation - Cytoreduction (hydroxyurea)

Polycythemia Vera	- Acquired disorder characterized by primary polycythemia, most commonly associated with JAK2 V617F mutation in myeloid progenitor	- Elevated hemoglobin (↓ EPO level)
		- Thrombocytosis, leukocytosis possible
		- Hyperviscosity
		  - Erythromelalgia (burning cyanosis in hands/feet)
		  - Blurry vision
		- Aquagenic pruritus
		- Thrombosis (Budd-Chiari, portal/splenic thrombosis)
		- Can progress to AML or myelofibrosis
			Diagnosis:
			- ↑ Hgb
			- Bone marrow biopsy (hyper-cellular)
			- JAK2 or other classic mutation
			
			Treatment:
			- Phlebotomy (goal Hct < 45%)
			- Aspirin
			- If refractory: Cytoreductive therapy (hydroxyurea or others)

Myelofibrosis	- Clonal myeloid proliferation, resulting in fibroblast hyperactivity and fibrosis of the bone marrow - Can be primary or secondary (due to "burnout" of myeloproliferative disorder like PV or essential thrombocytosis)	- Systemic symptoms (fatigue, fever, weight loss) - Splenomegaly (key finding in disease), hepatomegaly - Extramedullary hematopoiesis - Anemia (teardrop RBCs on smear) - WBC/platelet counts are variable	***Diagnosis:*** - Bone marrow biopsy (fibrotic marrow) ***Treatment:*** - Hydroxyurea for mild disease - Ruxolitinib (JAK 2 inhibitor) - HCT for severe disease

Leukemia

Acute Lymphoblastic Leukemia

General: Neoplasm of early lymphocytic precursors. Subtypes:

B-cell ALL	- Markers: CD10+, 19+, 22+, TdT+ - t(12;21) common mutation, favorable prognosis - t(9;22) BCR-ABL also possible (can use TK inhibitors)
T-cell ALL	- CD 2-8 +

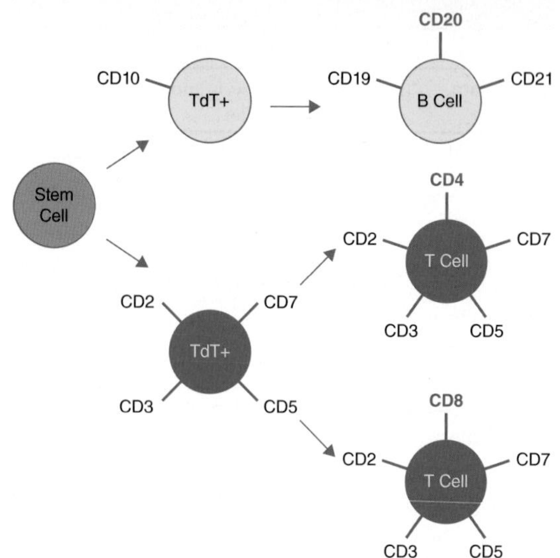

Risk: Most common malignancy in kids (usually 2-5 y/o), Down syndrome
- Second peak in those ~60 y/o

Clinical: Systemic symptoms (fevers, chills, fatigue, lymphadenopathy, splenomegaly, bone pain)
- Cytopenias (bleeding, recurrent infections)
- T-cell can present with mediastinal mass in teenager, with possible dysphagia, stridor, SVC syndrome

Diagnosis: Bone marrow biopsy (> **25% lymphoblasts** diagnostic)
- Specialized immunophenotype and cytogenetic testing

Management: Induction Chemotherapy: Cytotoxic regimens
- Common 1st line: Vincristine, corticosteroids, asparaginase
- Localized chemotherapy for CNS/Testes ("sanctuary sites")
- HCT for high risk patients

Hairy Cell Leukemia

General: Clonal B-cell neoplasm, almost universally from BRAF (serine/threonine kinase) mutation

Clinical: Cytopenias (anemia, thrombocytopenia, neutropenia)
- Significant splenomegaly, often causing abdominal pain
- Circulating mononuclear cells with hairy appearance[B]

Diagnosis: Bone marrow biopsy: Hypercellularity with **hairy cell infiltrate**. + TRAP stain (historically used).
- "Dry-Tap" from bone marrow fibrosis
- Flow cytometry: Mature B cell markers

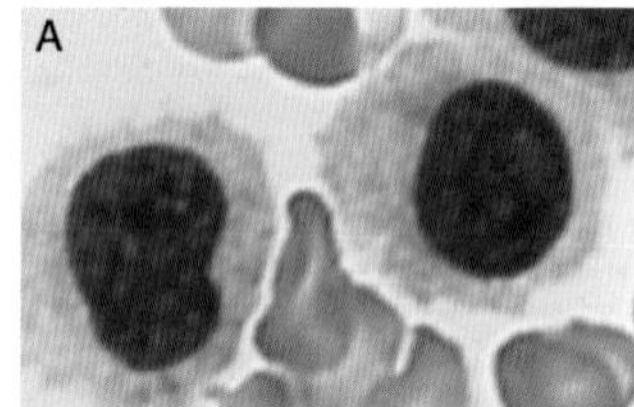

Management:
- Asymptomatic: Monitor
- Symptomatic: Cladribine (or pentostatin), +/– rituximab

Chronic Lymphocytic Leukemia

General: Chronic lymphoproliferative disorder with production of mature malfunctioning lymphocytes. Same disorder as small lymphocytic lymphoma.

Risk: Generally idiopathic, occurring in elderly (age > 70)

Clinical: Generally asymptomatic, and found on routine labs. Can have painless, waxing/waning cervical lymphadenopathy.
- Bloodwork shows lymphocytosis, with possible cytopenias
- Smear reveals mature lymphocytes with possible "smudge cells"

Diagnosis: Flow cytometry: Clonal population of CD19, CD20, CD23, or CD5 + cells
- Bone marrow biopsy: Not required for diagnosis, but shows > 30% lymphocytes

Management: Asymptomatic: Monitor. Symptomatic, advanced stage: Localized radiation, systemic chemotherapy.

Complications:
- Infection (hyper or hypogammaglobulinemia, but the Ig produced not useful for fighting infection)
- Autoimmune hemolytic anemia
- Progression to diffuse large B-cell lymphoma (Richter transformation)

Leukemia

Myelodysplasia

General: Malignant hematopoietic stem cell disorder caused by myeloid dysplasia, resulting in ineffective red and white cell production. Risk to progress to AML.

Risk: Old age, prior chemotherapy/radiation exposure

Clinical: Pancytopenia (can present as macrocytic anemia, thrombocytopenia, and/or leukopenia [↑ infection risk])
- Blood smear shows dysplasia in RBC/WBC lineages.

Diagnosis: Bone marrow aspirate (significant dysplasia [> 10%], blasts < 20% [> 20% would be leukemia])

Management: Symptomatic cytopenias treated with blood product transfer
- Depending on risk, these patients can be simply monitored, started on chemotherapy, or undergo HCT

Acute Myeloid Leukemia

General: Clonal expansion of malignant hematopoietic precursor cells of myeloid lineage. Median age 65 (can occur earlier).

Risk: Associated with prior chemo/radiation, myelodysplasia, Down syndrome

A

Clinical: Weakness, fatigue, other nonspecific symptoms
- Anemia, thrombocytopenia, neutropenia (dyspnea, bleeds, infections). High risk for DIC.

Diagnosis: **> 20% blasts** in peripheral blood and/or bone marrow biopsy
- Flow cytometry: Confirms myeloid lineage
    - Other signs: Auer rods[A] + myeloperoxidase

Management: (for AML other than promyelocytic)
- Intensive induction chemotherapy: Daunorubicin plus cytarabine
    - Followed by consolidation, maintenance chemotherapy
- Allogeneic HCT for high risk patients

Acute promyelocytic leukemia	- PML-RARA translocation t(15;17) - Highly associated with DIC - Responds to ATRA, arsenic +/− anthracycline-based chemo

Chronic Myeloid Leukemia

General: Myeloproliferative neoplasm of maturing granulocytes (neutrophils) with fairly normal differentiation. Most commonly due to fusion of BCR (on chromosome 22) and ABL1 (on chromosome 9).

Clinical: Multiple phases.
- <u>Chronic</u>:
    - Asymptomatic or nonspecific symptoms (fatigue, night sweats)
    - Hepatosplenomegaly
    - Leukocytosis (> 100K), thrombocytosis, anemia all possible
- <u>Accelerated</u>: Increasing leukocytosis, often difficult to control
- <u>Blast crisis</u>: Phase of blast and promyelocyte production (AML, rarely ALL)

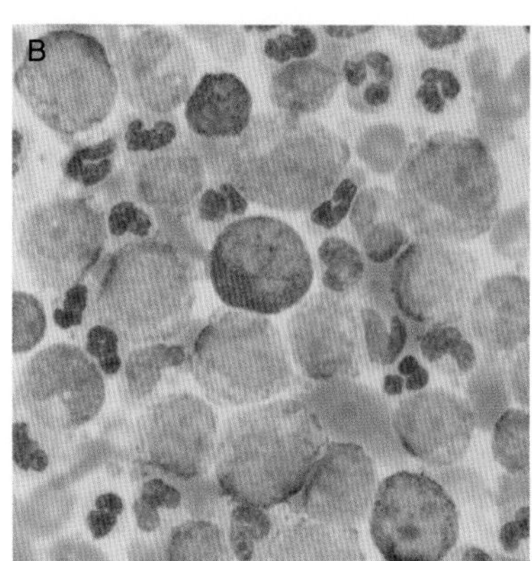

Diagnosis:
- Peripheral smear: Myelocyte lineage proliferation[B]
    - Increased amounts of immature myelocytes ("myelocyte bulge")
    - Low leukocyte alkaline phosphatase activity
    - Eosinophilia/basophilia possible
- Bone marrow biopsy (similar to smear above: granulocyte hyperplasia)
- Confirmation of t(9;22) via cytogenetics

Management: Chronic: Tyrosine kinase inhibitor (TKI) imatinib or nilotinib
- Accelerating/blast: TKI plus HCT

Lymphoma

Hodgkin Lymphoma

General: B-cell lymphoma. Subtypes below:

Subtype	Pathologic Findings
Nodular sclerosing	- Nodular growth pattern, with fibrous bands
Mixed cellularity	- Reed–Sternberg cells, pleomorphic background, eosinophilia
Lymphocyte rich	- Few Reed–Sternberg cells and many B cells
Lymphocyte deplete	- Paucity of inflammatory cells, poor prognosis

Risk: Bimodal age distribution (15-30, 65 y/o), EBV, immunosuppression

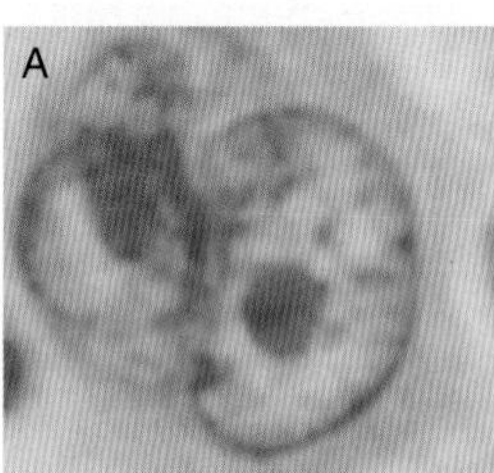

Clinical:
- Painless lymphadenopathy (often cervical)
- B-symptoms sometimes present (fever, night sweats, weight loss)
- Possible mediastinal mass on X-ray or CT imaging

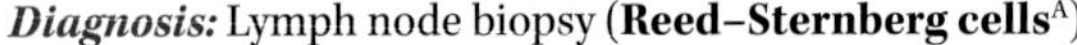

Diagnosis: Lymph node biopsy (**Reed–Sternberg cells**[A])
- Large cell with two or more nuclei ("owl's eyes"), CD 15, 30+
- Inflammatory infiltrate around RS cells (plasma cells, eosinophils, fibroblasts, and lymphocytes)

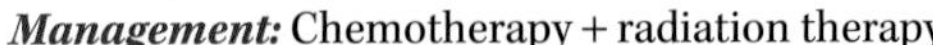

Management: Chemotherapy + radiation therapy
- ABVD regimen (doxorubicin, bleomycin, vinblastine, dacarbazine)

Non-Hodgkin Lymphoma

General: Heterogeneous group of lymphoid malignancies from B or T cell lineages

Risk: Prior radiation/chemotherapy, immunosuppression, viruses (HIV, HTLV-1, EBV)

Clinical:
- **Indolent** (Follicular, CLL/SLL, marginal zone)
    - Present as slow growing lymphadenopathy, hepatosplenomegaly, cytopenias
- **Aggressive** (DLBCL, Burkitt)
    - Present with B symptoms (fever, night sweats, weight loss), mass/lymphadenopathy, ↑ LDH

Diagnosis: Excisional biopsy (with histology, immunologic/molecular assessment)

Management:
- Dependent on underlying subtype, but the majority are treated with combined systemic, cytotoxic chemotherapy
- Rituximab (anti-CD-20 monoclonal antibody) is added to many regimens for B-cell lymphomas

Lymphoma

Subtype	Clinical Features and Management
B-Cell Non-Hodgkin Lymphomas	
Burkitt	- Highly aggressive B cell neoplasm, commonly in adolescents - Either endemic (typically seen in Africa, associated with EBV), sporadic, or immunodeficiency-associated - **Endemic**: Presents as rapidly enlarging facial or bone lesions - **Sporadic**: Presents as abdominal mass, often with tumor lysis - Dx: Biopsy ("starry sky[A]" pattern, t(8,14) C-myc/heavy chain Ig)
Diffuse Large B-Cell	- Most common NHL subtype - Presents as rapidly enlarging mass in neck/abdomen, +/− B symptoms - Dx: Biopsy (diffuse proliferation of mature B-cells, obliterate follicles)
Follicular	- Germinal-center B-cell proliferation - Presents as indolent, waxing/waning painless peripheral lymphadenopathy - Can progress to DLBCL - Dx: Biopsy (nodular growth pattern, often expressing BCL2, t(14;18))
Mantle Cell	- Aggressive, mature B-cell lymphoma - Presents as lymphadenopathy, often with extranodal disease at the time of presentation, with possible B-symptoms - Dx: Biopsy (often has t(11;14), overexpression of cyclin D1)

Marginal Zone	- Can be nodal or extranodal (from chronic inflammatory disorders)
	  - Salivary glands in Sjogren
	  - Thyroid gland in Hashimoto thyroiditis
	  - Stomach in chronic *H. pylori* infection (MALToma)
	- Presents with nonspecific/variable symptoms, typically based on the organ that is affected

T-Cell Lymphoma	
Peripheral T-Cell	- Variety of different T-cell-based lymphomas - Dx: Biopsy (w/ CD2-8 + cells)
Adult T-Cell Leukemia-Lymphoma	- Associated with HTLV-1 - Presents with lymphadenopathy, hepatosplenomegaly, lytic bone lesions, and skin lesions
Cutaneous T-Cell Lymphoma	- Skin disorders of malignant CD4+ T-cells - Presents as skin plaques and lesions - Localized disease: **Mycosis fungoides** - Diffuse systemic disease: **Sezary syndrome** - Dx: Biopsy (CD4 cells with cerebriform nuclei)

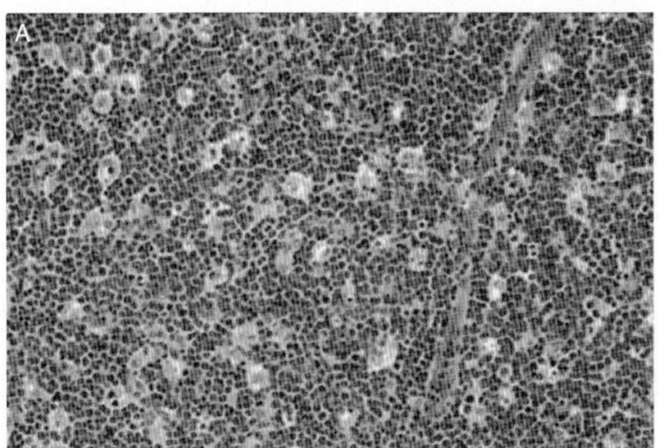

Misc Hematology

Langerhans Cell Histiocytosis

General: Rare disease of histiocytic infiltration of tissues, most commonly bone. Occurs commonly in age 1-3.

Clinical:

- Lytic bone lesions ("Eosinophilic Granuloma")
  - Can present as pathologic fracture
- Skin lesions: Can present as rash or ulcerative lesions
- Lung cysts/nodules (can lead to spontaneous pneumothorax)
- CNS: Diabetes insipidus

Diagnosis: Biopsy of lesion (CD1a+, or Birbeck granules on EM)

Management: Chemotherapy

Mastocytosis

General: Rare, excessive mast cell proliferation/accumulation in dermal tissue (cutaneous) or extradermal tissue (systemic). Generally due to activating mutation in KIT gene.

Clinical:

- Dermal: Flushing, pruritus, urticaria pigmentosa (tan macules)
  - Can be episodic, mimicking anaphylaxis
- Systemic:
  - GI: Steatorrhea, malabsorption, hepatosplenomegaly
  - Skeletal lesions (lytic or sclerotic)
  - Heme: Bone marrow invasion (mild anemia, other cytopenias)

Diagnosis: Tryptase level (elevated if systemic)
- Biopsy (bone marrow if systemic, skin if cutaneous)

Management: Epinephrine pens (many experience anaphylaxis), antihistamines and other therapy for allergic mediators
- For advanced disease: HCT or midostaurin (kinase inhibitor)

Cryoglobulinemia

General: Proteins that precipitate from serum and plasma when cooled

	Type 1	Type II/III
Path	- Monoclonal Ig	- Mixed monoclonal Ig or polyclonal Ig
Risk	- Lymphoproliferative disease (e.g., multiple myeloma)	- HCV - SLE and connective tissue diseases - Other infections (HBV, HIV)
Clin	- **Hyperviscosity** (blurry vision, HA or focal neuro deficits) - Thrombosis - Reynaud - Livedo reticularis or purpura	- **Immune-complex vasculitis** - Palpable purpura - Arthralgias - LA and HSM - Renal disease (glomerulonephritis, usually years later)
Dx	- Normal complement - Test for cryoglobulins	- ↓ C4 Levels, CH50 - Test for cryoglobulins - Biopsy (can confirm vasculitis)
Tx	- Treat underlying malignancy - Manage hyperviscosity	- Glucocorticoids PLUS - Cyclophosphamide or rituximab - Plasma exchange (if severe)

Amyloidosis

Primary and Secondary Amyloidosis

General: Extracellular tissue deposition of conformationally abnormal protein fibrils, most commonly in beta-pleated sheets

Etiology	Clinical Features
Primary AL	
Ig Light Chain	- Caused by plasma cell dyscrasias
Secondary AL	
AA	- Secondary to chronic inflammation (RA, IBD, vasculitis, chronic infection [osteomyelitis/TB], lymphoma) Familial Mediterranean fever - Chronic hereditary serosal inflammation - Recurrent attacks of fever and serosal inflammation - Increased risk for AA amyloid - Tx: Colchicine
Dialysis	- β2 microglobulin from ESRD patients - Tx: Change renal replacement methodology
Heritable	- Variety of different inherited mutated proteins Examples: - Mutated transthyretin (causing cardiomyopathy)
Senile	- Transthyretin (wild-type) deposition most commonly in heart - Results in restrictive cardiomyopathy - Dx: Cardiac MRI or Tc-99 pyrophosphate nuclear scan - Tx: Tafamidis
Organ-Specific	Examples: - Alzheimer (Beta-amyloid)

Clinical: Variable multisystem infiltration
- Derm: Waxy skin, easy bruising, nodules
- MSK: Enlarged tongue, muscles, arthropathy
- GI: Hepatomegaly, splenomegaly
- CV: Restrictive cardiomyopathy
- CNS: Neuropathy, dementia
- Renal: Insufficiency, proteinuria, nephrotic syndrome
- Heme: Increased hemorrhage risk

Diagnosis: Tissue biopsy (either fat pad or of specific organ)
- Hyaline material, stains with Congo red, apple green birefringence under polarized light

Management: Treat underlying condition (i.e., plasma cell dyscrasia or inflammation)

Blood Product Transfusions

Blood Product Transfusion	
Product	**Indication**
Packed RBCs	- Transfuse to maintain hemoglobin at > 7 g/dL - Transfuse when Hgb < 8 g/dL in acute coronary syndrome - Transfuse when Hgb < 10 g/dL in symptomatic anemia
Platelets	- Bleeding with a platelet count < 50,000 - Any patient < 10,000 (Exceptions: Platelet-consuming disorder)
FFP	- Elevated INR (> 2) with major bleeding or for surgery
Prothrombin Complex	- Recombinant four-factor concentrate (factors II, VII, IX, and X) - Similar indications to FFP, and now preferred
Cryoprecipitate	- Contains fibrinogen, factors VIII, XIII, and VWF - Now used less commonly, but can be used in disorders of fibrinogen or with DIC

Specialty RBC Treatments	
Irradiated	- Radiation to disrupt donor T lymphocytes (prevents graft vs host disease) - Indications: Bone marrow transplant/immunosuppressed
Leukoreduced	- Eliminates leukocyte debris and cytokines, prevent CMV transmission - Most hospitals leukoreduce all blood - Indications: Prevent CMV in immunosuppressed, chronically transfused, transplant recipients
Washed	- Removes any residual plasma/plasma proteins from RBC - Indications: IgA deficiency, recurrent allergic reaction to transfusion

Bone Marrow Stimulating Agents	
Neutrophils	- Filgrastim
Platelets	- Romiplostim, eltrombopag
Red Blood Cells	- Erythropoietin, epoetin alfa, darbepoetin alfa

Transfusions Reaction			
	Mechanism	**Clinical**	**Treatment**
Acute Hemolytic	- ABO incompatibility - Immediate onset	- Fever, flank pain, renal failure, DIC - Positive direct Coombs test - ↑ plasma hemoglobin/hemoglobinuria	- Stop transfusion - IV Fluids - Supportive
Delayed Hemolytic	- Revival of Ig against minor RBC Ag that was at low levels (so missed on screen) - 3-10 days onset	- Low-grade hemolysis/mild fever - Positive direct Coombs	- Generally self-limited
Febrile Nonhemolytic	- Cytokine accumulation in stored blood - Risk reduced with leukoreduction - Hours after transfusion	- Fevers, chills, headache, flushing	- Stop transfusion - Antipyretics
Anaphylactic	- Associated with IgA deficiency - Immediate onset	- Acute onset shock, urticaria, edema, and respiratory distress	- Stop transfusion - Epinephrine
Allergic (Urticarial)	- IgE/mast cell activation - Hours after transfusion	- Urticarial rash, pruritus, flushing - Angioedema	- Diphenhydramine - *Can administer remainder of product*
TRALI (transfusion-related acute lung injury)	- Antibodies to human leukocyte antigens, which result in inflammatory activation and pulmonary capillary leakage - Hours after transfusion	- Acute hypoxemic respiratory failure - Noncardiogenic pulmonary edema	- Stop transfusion - O_2/ventilatory support
TACO (transfusion-associated circulatory overload)	- Volume overload from infusion	- Acute dyspnea and signs of volume overload, pulmonary edema	- Supplemental O_2 - Fluid diuresis

Transplant

General Principles

General: Organs that can be transplanted include heart, kidney, liver, lungs
- Bone marrow transplants are a special type of transplant, in which the transplanted cells are used to replace recipient's marrow

Subtypes:
- Autograft: Transplant of graft from same person
- Allograft: Transplant of an organ or tissue between two humans
- Xenograft: Transplant of organ or tissue between two different species

Management:
- Require chronic immunosuppression to prevent graft rejection
    - Options include steroids, tacrolimus, mycophenolate, others
- Infection prophylaxis
    - PCP (TMP-SMX, atovaquone, others)
    - HSV (acyclovir)
    - CMV (High risk: Valganciclovir)
    - Fungal (required for some)

Transplant Rejection

Type	Clinical Findings	Management
Hyperacute (within hours)	- ABO/ lymphocytotoxic mismatch (rarely seen clinically) - Results in immediate vascular thrombosis	- Explant tissue
Acute (weeks to months)	- CD8 cells activated against donor MHC - Graft vasculitis and lymphocytic infiltration	- Corticosteroids - Should not occur if proper immunosuppression is initiated
Chronic (years)	- CD4 cells respond to recipient APCs presenting donor peptides - Results in proliferation of vascular smooth muscle, atrophy, interstitial fibrosis	- Poor prognosis - Retransplant
Graft vs Host	- Immune cells from donor recognize the recipient as foreign, initiating an immune reaction - Utilized for its antileukemia/lymphoma effect, but too much can result in the systemic issues below: - Skin: Maculopapular rash - Liver: ↑ bilirubin, hepatomegaly - GI: Diarrhea - Lung: Bronchiolitis obliterans	- Corticosteroids

Immunology

Hypersensitivity Reactions

	Clinical Features	Examples
Type I	- Anaphylaxis/atopy - IgE response to antigen (e.g., food, sting, drug) - Rare IgE-independent causes	- Atopic dermatitis - Asthma - Urticaria - Anaphylaxis
Type II	- Cytotoxic reaction of IgM or IgG against antigen	- Myasthenia gravis - Graves - Many others
Type III	- Immune complex formation - Serum sickness (fever, skin rash, arthralgias weeks after exposure to Ag) - Arthus reaction (local inflammatory reaction to injected antigen)	- SLE - Post-Strep GN - Acute hepatitis B
Type IV	- Delayed T-Cell mediated reaction to antigen	- Contact dermatitis - Multiple sclerosis - Transplant rejection

Complement Disorders

Disorder	Clinical Features
Hereditary Angioedema	- Deficiency of C1 esterase inhibitor, resulting in elevated bradykinin levels - Presents as recurrent episodes of angioedema (without pruritus or urticaria) - No response to steroids or antihistamines - Dx: Low C4 levels and C1INH - Tx: Replace serum C1INH, Icatibant (bradykinin inhibitor) for acute episodes
C1 Deficiency	- C1q, C1r, C1s deficiency most common complement deficiency - Associated with increased SLE risk, recurrent infections
C3 Deficiency	- Severe/recurrent infections with encapsulated bacteria - Presents very early in life
C5-C9 Deficiency	- Increased risk of meningococcal infection

Immunodeficiencies

	Mechanism	Clinical	Diagnosis/Treatment
B-Cell Disorders			
Bruton's Agammaglobulinemia	- X-linked disorder in BTK, which prevents B-cell maturation	- Recurrent bacterial and enteroviral infections after age ~6 months (not before then because maternal IgG) - Scanty lymph nodes and tonsils	Dx: ↓ Ig/B-cells, with molecular defect in BTK Tx: IVIG
Selective IgA Deficiency	- Selective deficiency of serum IgA	- Generally asymptomatic - Complications can include increased risk for autoimmune disease, atopic reaction, anaphylaxis to blood products	Dx: ↓ IgA, normal IgM/IgG Tx: Education/monitoring
Common Variable Immunodeficiency	- Impaired B-cell differentiation, defective production of Ig - Can present in ages 20-40 - Increased risk for autoimmune disease	- Bacterial sinopulmonary infection - Pulm: Bronchiectasis, pneumonia - GI: Chronic diarrhea - ↑ risk for non-Hodgkin lymphoma	Dx: ↓ IgA, IgM, IgG Tx: IVIG

Immunology

	Mechanism	Clinical	Diagnosis/Treatment
T-Cell Disorders			
DiGeorge	- Deletion of 22q11, resulting in thymic and parathyroid abnormalities	- Conotruncal cardiac anomalies - Hypoplastic thymus/parathyroid (↓Ca) - Recurrent viral/fungal infections - Facial abnormalities (cleft palate)	Dx: ↓ CD 3 + T-cells, confirmed 22q11 mutation Tx: Surgical correction of structural abnormalities, HCT for severe immunodeficiency
Hyperimmunoglobulin E (Job Syndrome)	- AD STAT3 mutation, causing impaired neutrophils chemotaxis	- Recurrent skin and pulmonary infections - Eczematous dermatitis	Dx: ↑ IgE, eosinophilia Tx: PPX antibiotics
Chronic Mucocutaneous Candidiasis	- Heterogeneous group of genetic defects (including AIRE) resulting in chronic *Candida*	- Chronic skin/mucosal candidiasis - Endocrine: Hypoparathyroidism, adrenal insufficiency, etc.	Dx: Clinical Tx: Antifungals
Combined T- and B-Cell Disorders			
Severe Combined Immunodeficiency	Several causes: - Defective IL-2R gamma chain (XR) - ADA deficiency (AR) - Many others	- Recurrent severe infections, diarrhea, and failure to thrive in infants - Often leads to early death	Dx: ↓ T-cells, genetic analysis Tx: IVIG, infection prophylaxis, HCT, or ADA enzyme replacement
Ataxia-Telangiectasia	- AR defect in DNA double strand break repair (ATM gene)	- Progressive cerebellar ataxia/atrophy - Immunodeficiency (↓ IgA, IgM, IgG) - Telangiectasia - ↑ AFP	Dx: ATM gene analysis Tx: Supportive care. Poor prognosis.
Wiskott-Aldrich	- X-Linked disorder of WASP, responsible for actin cytoskeleton rearrangement	- Recurrent bacterial, viral, fungal infections - Thrombocytopenia - Eczema - ↑ Risk for autoimmune disease, malignancy	Dx: Genetic analysis, ↓/↔ IgG and IgM. ↑ IgA and IgE. Tx: IVIG/antibiotics, platelet transfusions for active bleeds, HCT only definitive therapy
Hyper IgM Syndrome	- Defective class-switch recombination, most often from CD40 ligand deficiency	- Recurrent sinopulmonary and GI infections	Dx: ↑ IgM. ↓ IgA, IgG, IgE. Flow cytometry for CD40L, genetic testing confirms. Tx: IVIG/prophylactic antibiotics
Phagocyte Disorders			
Chronic Granulomatous Disease	- X-linked defect in phagocyte NADPH oxidase	- Recurrent bacterial and fungal infections (PNA, soft tissue, adenitis, osteomyelitis) - Common organisms: *Staphylococcus aureus, Pseudomonas, Burkholderia, Serratia, Nocardia, Aspergillus*	Dx: Dihydrorhodamine 123 test Tx: Chronic PPX with TMP-SMX, itraconazole - IFN-g injections if severe - HCT for definitive cure
Chediak-Higashi	- AR defect in vesicle trafficking proteins, resulting abnormal neutrophil digestion and neurologic dysfunction	- Recurrent pyogenic infections - Hypopigmentation - Neurologic deficits (neuropathy, ataxia) - Accelerated phase: Lymphohistiocytic infiltration of all organ systems (fatal)	Dx: Smear (characteristic granules in leuks/platelets) Tx: HCT
Leukocyte Adhesion Deficiency (Type I)	- Defect in beta-2 integrin (CD18), impairs chemotaxis/migration	- Recurrent bacterial infections - Absent pus - Impaired wound healing - Omphalitis is classic presentation	Dx: Absent CD18 on flow cytometry Tx: HCT if severe
Leukocyte Adhesion Deficiency (Type II)	- Defect in fucosylation of macromolecules on leukocytes, preventing binding to selectin molecules (impaired chemotaxis)	- Less severe and fewer infections than those with LAD type I	Dx: Flow cytometry (absent CD15 [Sialyl-Lewis X]) Tx: Prophylactic antibiotics, fucose supplementation

Hematology Pharm

	Mechanism	Indication	Side Effects/Management
Antiplatelet			
Aspirin	- Irreversible inhibition of COX - ↓ prostaglandin and TXA_2 synthesis	- Analgesia, antipyretic - Anti-inflammatory - ASCVD PPX	- Bleeding - Gastritis, GI bleeds - Reye syndrome (kids)
Clopidogrel Prasugrel Ticagrelor	- ADP receptor ($P2Y_{12}$) inhibitor (↓ GPIIb/IIIa activation)	- Acute coronary syndrome - Vascular stenting	- Bleeding - Dyspnea (ticagrelor)
Cilostazol Dipyridamole	- Phosphodiesterase inhibitor (↓ platelet aggregation)	- Claudication (cilostazol) - Coronary vasodilation, CVA (dipyridamole)	- Headache, flushing, heat intolerance, palpitations
Abciximab Eptifibatide Tirofiban	- Direct GPIIb/IIIa inhibitor	- Acute coronary syndrome - Vascular stenting	- Bleeding - Thrombocytopenia
Anticoagulants			
Heparin Enoxaparin Fondaparinux	- ↓ activity of thrombin and factor Xa	- DVT/PE treatment and prophylaxis - AF, ACS	- Bleeding - HIT
Apixaban Rivaroxaban	- Factor Xa inhibitor	- DVT/PE - Atrial fibrillation	- Bleeding - Dabigatran reversed with idarucizumab
Bivalirudin Dabigatran	- Direct thrombin inhibitor		
Warfarin	- Inhibits γ-carboxylation of vitamin K-dependent clotting factors (II/VII/IX/X C, S)	- DVT/PE - Atrial fibrillation	- Bleeding - Teratogenic - Skin/tissue necrosis (seen with protein C deficiency)
Fibrinolytics			
Alteplase Reteplase	- Tissue plasminogen activator (tPA) (plasminogen to plasmin)	- Ischemic stroke - PE - STEMI	- Extremely high risk for bleeding - Long list of contraindications [See: Neuro]

Oncology Pharm

	Mechanism	Side Effects (Selected)
Nucleotide Analogs		
Azacitidine	- Purine or pyrimidine analogs that inhibit DNA synthesis	- Myelosuppression - Hepatotoxicity
Azathioprine		
Cladribine		
Cytarabine		
Gemcitabine		
Mercaptopurine		
5-fluorouracil	- Inhibition of thymidylate synthase, ↓ DNA production	- Myelosuppression
Methotrexate	- Folic acid analog, inhibiting dihydrofolate reductase, ↓ DNA production	- Myelosuppression (reversible with Leucovorin) - Hepatotoxicity, stomatitis, pneumonitis/fibrosis
Alkylating Agents		***Myelosuppression (all)**
Busulfan	- Cross link DNA (triggers cellular apoptosis)	- Pulmonary fibrosis, hyperpigmentation
Cyclophosphamide		- Hemorrhagic cystitis (reversed with Mesna), bladder cancer
Dacarbazine		- Severe nausea
Nitrosoureas		- Neurotoxicity
Anthracyclines		
Daunorubicin Doxorubicin	- Intercalates DNA, preventing DNA replication	- Myelosuppression - Cardiotoxicity (dilated CM)
Taxanes		
Paclitaxel, docetaxel	- Microtubule inhibitor (hyperstabilize mitotic spindles)	- Myelosuppression, neuropathy
Topoisomerase Inhibitors		
Topotecan	- Topoisomerase I inhibitor	- Myelosuppression, severe GI side effects
Etoposide	- Topoisomerase II inhibitor	
Peptide Antibiotics		
Actinomycin	- Inhibits RNA transcription	- Myelosuppression, alopecia
Bleomycin	- Induces DNA strand breaks	- Pulmonary fibrosis
Platinum Agents		
Carboplatin, cisplatin	- DNA cross linker, inhibiting replication	- Myelosuppression - Neuropathy/ototoxicity, nephrotoxicity
Vinca Alkaloids		
Vincristine Vinblastine	- Inhibit microtubule proliferation	- Peripheral neuropathy
Targeted Therapy (Selected)		
Bortezomib	- Proteasome inhibitor	
Imatinib	- Inhibit the BCR-ABL tyrosine kinase	- Hepatotoxicity
Ruxolitinib	- JAK inhibitor	

Immunology Pharm

<table>
<tr><th></th><th>Mechanism</th><th>Indication</th><th>Side Effects/Management</th></tr>
<tr><td colspan="4">Immunosuppressants</td></tr>
<tr><td>Cyclosporine</td><td rowspan="2">- Calcineurin inhibitor (↓ IL-2 production, prevent T-cell activation)</td><td rowspan="2">- Transplant rejection ppx</td><td rowspan="2">
<table>
<tr><th>Side Effect</th><th>Cyclosporine</th><th>Tacrolimus</th></tr>
<tr><td>Nephrotoxicity</td><td>++</td><td>+</td></tr>
<tr><td>Hypertension</td><td>++</td><td>+</td></tr>
<tr><td>NODAT (new-onset diabetes)</td><td>+</td><td>+</td></tr>
<tr><td>Thrombotic microangiopathy</td><td>+</td><td>+</td></tr>
<tr><td>Neurotoxicity</td><td>–</td><td>+</td></tr>
<tr><td>GI side Effects</td><td>–</td><td>+</td></tr>
<tr><td>Alopecia</td><td>–</td><td>+</td></tr>
<tr><td>Gingival hyperplasia</td><td>+</td><td>–</td></tr>
<tr><td>Hirsutism</td><td>+</td><td>–</td></tr>
<tr><td>Hyperlipidemia</td><td>+</td><td>–</td></tr>
</table>
</td></tr>
<tr><td>Tacrolimus</td></tr>
<tr><td>Sirolimus</td><td>- mTOR inhibitor</td><td>- Transplant rejection ppx</td><td>- Pancytopenia
- NODAT (new-onset diabetes)
- Hyperlipidemia</td></tr>
<tr><td>Mycophenolate Mofetil (MMF)</td><td>- Inosine monophosphate dehydrogenase inhibitor, blocking purine synthesis</td><td>- Transplant rejection ppx</td><td>- Pancytopenia (especially anemia and leukopenia)
- GI side effects (nausea, vomiting, diarrhea, gastritis, GI bleed, GI ulcerations)</td></tr>
<tr><td>Azathioprine</td><td>- Inhibitor of purine synthesis, preventing proliferation of B/T cells</td><td>- Transplant rejection ppx
- Autoimmune conditions</td><td>- Pancytopenia</td></tr>
<tr><td colspan="4">Monoclonal Antibodies (Selected)</td></tr>
<tr><td>Belimumab</td><td>- B-cell activating factor</td><td>- SLE</td><td></td></tr>
<tr><td>Bevacizumab</td><td>- VEGF</td><td>- Cancer</td><td>- ↑ risk of bleeding</td></tr>
<tr><td>Cetuximab</td><td>- EGFR</td><td>- Cancer (CRC, head/neck)</td><td></td></tr>
<tr><td>Daratumumab</td><td>- CD 38</td><td>- MS</td><td></td></tr>
<tr><td>Dupilumab</td><td>- IL-4Rα</td><td>- Atopic dermatitis, asthma</td><td></td></tr>
<tr><td>Eculizumab</td><td>- C5</td><td>- PNH, atypical HUS</td><td>- Infection (meningococcus)</td></tr>
<tr><td>Natalizumab</td><td>- Integrin α_4</td><td>- MS, Crohn</td><td>- Progressive multifocal leukoencephalopathy (PML)</td></tr>
<tr><td>Nivolumab</td><td>- PD-1</td><td>- Cancer</td><td></td></tr>
<tr><td>Ocrelizumab</td><td>- CD 20</td><td>- MS</td><td></td></tr>
<tr><td>Pembrolizumab</td><td>- PD-1</td><td>- Cancer (melanoma)</td><td>- Pneumonitis, endocrine issues</td></tr>
<tr><td>Risankizumab</td><td>- IL-23A</td><td>- Crohn, psoriasis</td><td></td></tr>
<tr><td>Rituximab</td><td>- CD-20</td><td>- Lymphoma, leukemia</td><td>- Opportunistic infections, PML</td></tr>
<tr><td>Secukinumab</td><td>- IL-17A</td><td>- Uveitis</td><td></td></tr>
<tr><td>Trastuzumab</td><td>- HER-2</td><td>- Breast cancer</td><td>- Cardiotoxicity</td></tr>
<tr><td>Ustekinumab</td><td>- IL-12, 23</td><td>- MS, psoriasis</td><td></td></tr>
<tr><td>Vedolizumab</td><td>- Integrin α4 β7</td><td>- IBD</td><td></td></tr>
</table>

Arthritis

Differential Diagnosis for Joint Pain

	Monoarticular	Polyarticular
Noninflammatory	- Osteoarthritis - Trauma - Malignancy - Avascular necrosis - Charcot joint - Internal derangement	- Osteoarthritis
Inflammatory	- Gout/pseudogout - Septic arthritis	- Infection (viral, Lyme) - Rheumatoid arthritis - Spondyloarthropathy - SLE

Arthrocentesis

Indications:

- Signs of joint inflammation (septic arthritis or gouty arthritis)
- Relief of moderate or large sized effusion

Interpretation:

	Color	WBC	PMN	Other Findings
Normal	Clear	< 200	< 25%	
Noninflammatory	Clear/yellow	< 2000	< 25%	
Inflammatory	Cloudy/yellow	> 2000	> 50%	- Crystals seen with gout
Septic	Turbid purulent	> 20,000	> 75%	- Culture often positive
Hemorrhagic	Bloody	Variable	50-75%	

Charcot Joint

General: Progressive degeneration of a bony joint due to repetitive trauma in the setting of loss of sensation from neuropathy

Etiology: Diabetic neuropathy, vitamin B12 deficiency, tertiary syphilis, any cause of peripheral neuropathy or spinal cord injury with sensory deficit

Clinical:

- Insidious onset of erythema and swelling of joint (most often foot/ankle)
- Lack of sensation in same extremity
- Deformity of joint
- Degenerative joint disease or fractures on x-ray

Management:

- Manage underlying condition
- Acute inflammation: Casting (off-loading) and immobilization
- Chronic: Mechanical devices (braces) to protect and support from further damage

Arthritis

	Osteoarthritis	Rheumatoid Arthritis
Gen	- Degeneration of cartilage, hypertrophy of bone at articular margins	- Chronic inflammatory autoimmune arthritis involving the synovium
Risk	- Age - Obesity - Excessive joint loading - Trauma (major injuries or micro-trauma over time)	- Family history/genetics (HLA-DR4) - Smoking - Females
Clin	- Insidious onset of joint pain - Morning stiffness < 30 min - Limited ROM - Joint crepitus - Most commonly affects weight bearing joints (hips, knees, lumbar spine) and finger IP joints - Bouchard/Heberden nodes (PIP/DIP) - XR[A] (joint space narrowing, osteophytes, subchondral cysts) - Can support, but not diagnostic	- Insidious joint pain, stiffness, and swelling - Morning stiffness > 1 hour, improves with activity - Typically symmetric joint involvement - MCP, PIP joints common early in disease (spares DIP) - Ulnar deviation[B], swan neck deformities (chronic disease) - Cervical instability (C1/C2): Spine subluxation, spinal cord compression - XR (joint space narrowing, bony erosions) <u>Extra-articular manifestations</u>: - **Skin**: Rheumatoid nodules - **Ocular**: Scleritis - **Pulm**: ILD - **Heme**: Anemia of chronic inflammation **Felty's**: Splenomegaly, neutropenia, RA
Dx	- Clinical diagnosis	<u>Clinical criteria</u>: > 3 joint involvement, > 6 weeks + RF or anti-citrullinated peptide Ab ↑ ESR/CRP
Tx	<u>Nonpharmacologic</u> - Weight loss - PT (strengthening exercises) - Canes/crutches, braces <u>Pharmacologic</u> - Topical NSAID, capsaicin - Oral NSAIDs <u>Intraarticular injections</u> - Steroids: Every 3-4 months, but effect is short term - Hyaluronic acid: Poor evidence <u>Surgery</u> - Total joint replacement (reserved for severe disease)	<u>Initial treatment</u> - Initiate DMARD (see options below) - Bridge with NSAIDs or steroids <u>Flares</u> - Steroids <u>Refractory Cases</u> - Add additional DMARD agents, or consider adding biologic <u>Classic DMARD options</u> - Methotrexate (first line) - Alternatives: Leflunomide, hydroxychloroquine, sulfasalazine <u>Biologic/targeted DMARD</u> - TNF-α inhibitors, Il-6 antagonists, JAK inhibitors

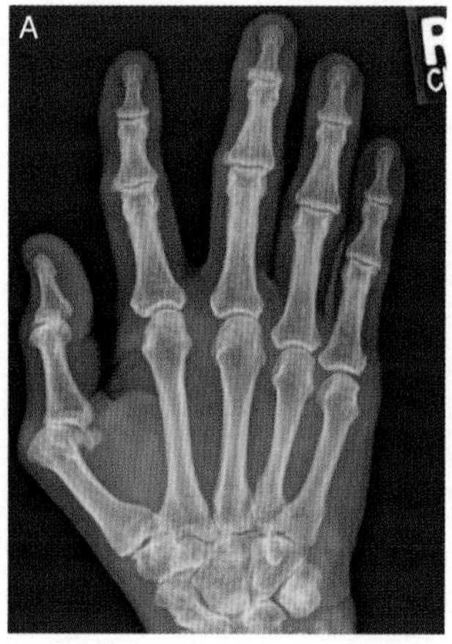

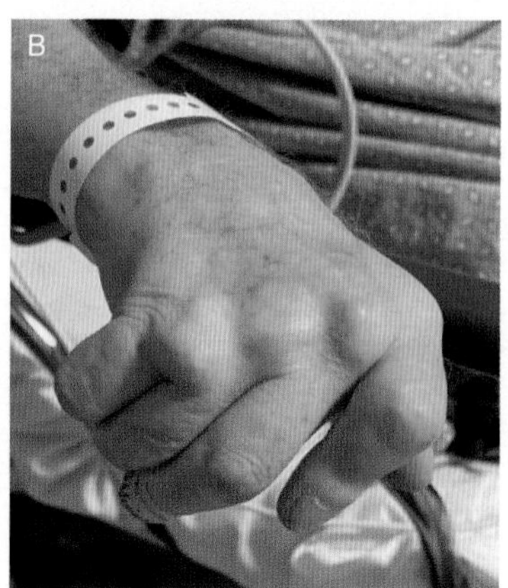

Arthritis

Juvenile Idiopathic Arthritis (JIA)

General: Childhood-onset inflammatory arthritis (JIA is a heterogeneous entity that likely includes multiple distinct disorders)
* Previously called Still's disease or juvenile rheumatoid arthritis

Subtype	Clinical Findings
Oligoarticular	- Symmetric arthritis for > 6 weeks - Arthritis with < 4 joints involved
Polyarticular	- Symmetric arthritis for > 6 weeks - Arthritis with ≥ 5 joints involved
Systemic	- Arthritis (as above) - Daily high spiking fever ("quotidian fever" pattern) - Rash (salmon pink, macular rash)

Diagnosis: Purely clinical diagnosis of exclusion
- The following labs can be associated (but not specific)
    - ↑ ESR/CRP
    - ↑ ferritin
    - Hypergammaglobulinemia
    - Thrombocytosis, leukocytosis, anemia

Management:
- NSAIDs
- Glucocorticoids (intraarticular or oral)
- Biologics (anti Il-1 agents, anti Il-6, anti-TNFα)

Adult-Onset Still's Disease

General: Inflammatory polyarthritis that presents similarly to systemic JIA but occurs in adults

Clinical:
- Polyarthritis
- Daily high spiking fever
- Salmon pink macular rash[A]
- Other nonspecific findings: LA, splenomegaly, leukocytosis

Diagnosis: Diagnosis of exclusion
- Ferritin often extremely elevated
- ANA/RF generally not positive

Management:
- NSAIDs
- Corticosteroids
- Methotrexate, or other DMARD or biologic agent

Crystal Arthropathy

Gout

General: Inflammatory monoarticular arthritis caused by the crystallization of monosodium urate in joints

Etiology/Risk:

Decreased Uric Acid Excretion	- > 90% of those with gout - Associated with renal disease, diuretic/NSAID use, EtOH use
Increased Uric Acid Production	- Chemotherapy - Hematologic malignancy - Chronic hemolysis
Genetic Enzyme Defects	- Lesch–Nyhan (HGPRT deficiency) - PRPP synthetase overactivity (Von Gierke)

Clinical:

- **Asymptomatic Hyperuricemia**
  - Typically years before first episode
  - Not all with hyperuricemia develop gout, but high levels ↑ risk
- **Acute Flare**: Acute, painful monoarthropathy with edema and erythema
  - Podagra (1st MTP) is classic
- **Intercritical Periods**: Asymptomatic time between gout flares
  - > 50% have recurrence in a year, < 10% never have flare again
- **Tophaceous Gout**: Chronic pain in joint
  - From packed uric acid crystals causing joint inflammation
  - Can visualize tophi (nodules of uric acid collection)

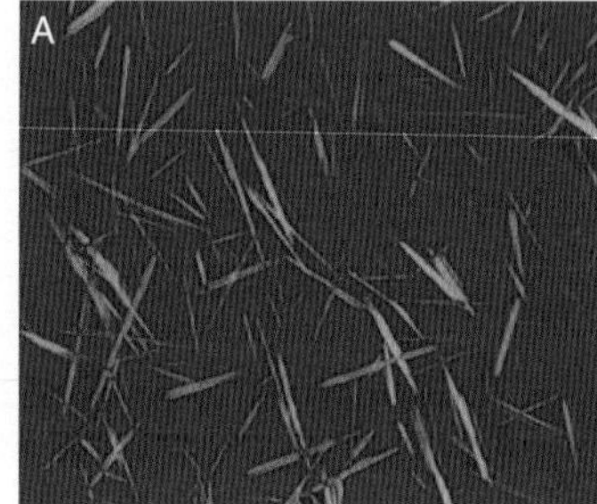

Diagnosis:

- Arthrocentesis (during acute flare)
  - Needle-shaped, negatively birefringent urate crystals[A]
  - Yellow → Parallel, Blue → Perpendicular
- Imaging can reveal articular destruction in advanced, chronic disease

Management:

Acute	- Oral glucocorticoids - NSAIDs (Naproxen/indomethacin) - Colchicine (both NSAID and colchicine contraindicated with CKD) - Intra-articular steroid injection (if only 1 or 2 joints affected) - IL-1 inhibitors (anakinra or canakinumab) for refractory cases
Chronic	Urate lowering medication (indicated for recurrent gout flares or tophi/chronic gouty arthritis) - Allopurinol (alt: Febuxostat, probenecid) - Uric acid goal is < 6 mg/dL - Colchicine used concurrently for first few months to prevent flares
Lifestyle	- Weight loss - Reduce dietary animal/seafood protein consumption - Reduce EtOH intake

Crystal Arthropathy

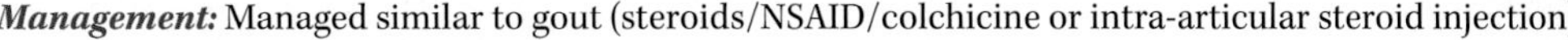

Calcium Pyrophosphate Deposition Disease (CPPD, Pseudogout)

General: Calcium pyrophosphate crystal deposition, causing inflammatory arthritis

Risk:

- Majority idiopathic
- Hyperparathyroidism
- Hemochromatosis
- Joint trauma/osteoarthritis

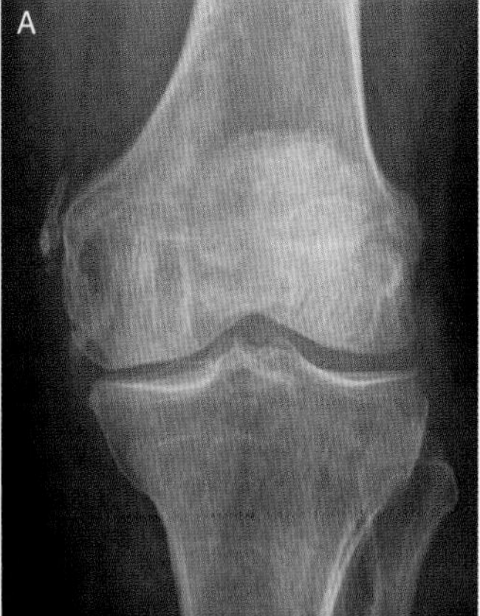

Clinical:

- Often asymptomatic up until flare
- **Acute flare**: Acute/subacute arthritis of single extremity joint
    - Large joints (knees) most commonly affected
- Can result in polyarticular inflammatory arthritis (looks like RA)

Diagnosis:

- Weakly positively birefringent rod-shaped and rhomboidal crystals
    - Inflammatory synovial fluid findings
- Joint XR: **Chondrocalcinosis**[A] (cartilage calcification)

Management: Managed similar to gout (steroids/NSAID/colchicine or intra-articular steroid injection)

Reynaud Phenomenon

General: Abnormal vascular reactivity in distal extremities, characterized by exaggerated vasoconstriction in response to cold temperatures or stress

Clinical: Classic attack includes acute onset coldness in the distal extremity, followed by pallor[B] ("white attack"), ischemia/cyanosis ("blue attack"), and eventual reperfusion (back to pink/red)

	Primary	Secondary
Etio	- Idiopathic	- Connective tissue disease (SLE, RA, scleroderma) - Drugs (amphetamines, others) - Cryoglobulinemia, cold agglutinin disease - Trauma (use of vibrating tools)
Clin	- Minimal systemic symptoms - No tissue injury - ESR/CRP, ANA typically normal	- Symptoms of underlying autoimmune disease - Distal extremity ulcerations and tissue damage + Nailfold capillary microscopy
Tx	- Avoid triggers - Calcium channel blockers	- Treat underlying condition - Calcium channel blockers (alt: Sildenafil) - Aspirin (for ulcerations)

Connective Tissue Disease

Systemic Lupus Erythematosus

General: Autoimmune disorder characterized by autoantibody formation against intracellular proteins/material (DNA), which results in immune complex formation and subsequent multiorgan inflammatory damage

Risk: Middle-aged, Black, Hispanic, female sex

Clinical:

- Constitutional symptoms (fatigue, fever, and weight loss)
- Dermatologic/mucous membrane
    - **Malar* "butterfly" rash** (erythematous rash over cheeks/nose)
    - Discoid* lesions (erythematous raised patches with scaling)
    - Photosensitivity, oral or nasopharyngeal ulcers*, alopecia*
- Polyarthritis*
- Serositis* (pleuritis, pericarditis)
- Vascular disease (vasculitis, Raynaud, VTE)
- Renal* (**lupus nephritis** [DPGN, membranous nephropathy], proteinuria)
- Hematologic (hemolytic anemia*, leukopenia*, thrombocytopenia*)
- Immunologic dysfunction (impaired immune response, ↑ infection risk)
- Neuropsychiatric* dysfunction
- Ophthalmologic (scleritis)
- Cardiovascular (Libman-Sacks endocarditis: Thrombi on both sides of valve)

Diagnosis:

- **ANA*** (initial screening test of choice, sensitive but not specific)
- **Anti-dsDNA*, Anti-Smith*** (specific)
- Positive direct Coombs*
- Antiphospholipid*, low complement* (low C3, C4, or CH50)

SLICC diagnostic criteria: ≥ 4/17 of the above (starred) features, with at least one clinical and one lab feature

Management: Lifestyle management: Sun protection, proper immunizations, pregnancy and contraception counseling

Severity	Definition	Intervention
Mild	- Skin, joint, and mucosal involvement	- Hydroxychloroquine +/− course of NSAIDs/low-dose steroids
Moderate	- Significant symptoms, but no evidence of organ failure	- Hydroxychloroquine + short course of prednisone
Severe	- Severe/life-threatening organ involvement	- High dose IV methylprednisolone - Immunosuppression (azathioprine, mycophenolate, cyclophosphamide, or rituximab)

Mixed Connective Tissue Disease

General: Overlap syndrome of SLE, systemic sclerosis, and polymyositis

Clinical:

- Raynaud
- Myositis, sclerodactyly
- Polyarthritis
- Pulmonary hypertension (major cause of death) and interstitial fibrosis
- GI dysmotility
- Lack of renal, CNS disease

Diagnosis: Anti-U1 ribonucleoprotein (RNP) antibodies is characteristic

Management: Glucocorticoids

Connective Tissue Disease

Systemic Sclerosis (Scleroderma)

General: Autoimmune condition characterized by immune activation, vascular damage, and **systemic tissue fibrosis** (collagen deposition). Most commonly impacts middle-aged (30-50 y/o) women.

	Limited	Diffuse

Clin	- Cutaneous fibrosis, usually of distal extremities
	  - Morphea: Fibrotic plaques
	  - Linear fibrotic bands
	  - Sclerodactyly
	
	- Some have **CREST syndrome**
	Calcinosis of fingers
	Raynaud phenomenon
	Esophageal dysmotility
	Sclerodactyly
	Telangiectasia
		- Cutaneous fibrosis more widespread (versus limited)
		- Raynaud, telangiectasias
		
		<u>Organ involvement</u>:
		- GI: Esophageal dysmotility, reflux, dysphagia, dyspepsia
		- Pulm: Interstitial fibrosis and pulmonary hypertension
		- CV: Myocardial fibrosis, pericarditis
		- Renal: HTN, **scleroderma renal crisis** (MAHA, oliguria, thrombocytopenia)

Dx	Clinical features plus autoantibodies:
	  - ANA (positive in most)
	  - Anti-topoisomerase I (anti scl-70, most commonly diffuse)
	  - Anti-centromere (most commonly limited)
	  - Anti-RNA polymerase III (associated with severe systemic disease)	

Tx	- No effective cure, manage problems of each individual organ system - Immunosuppression (methotrexate, mycophenolate, cyclophosphamide) used for systemic or severe skin disease	

Skin	- Topical/intralesional steroids, or other topical agents
Raynaud's	- Calcium channel blockers
Arthritis	- NSAIDs
Renal	- ACEi
GI	- PPI
Pulm	- Immunosuppression for fibrosis, vasodilators for PAH

Sjogren Syndrome

General: Autoimmune lymphocytic infiltration and destruction of lacrimal and salivary glands. Can be primary or secondary to other autoimmune disease (SLE, RA).

Clinical:

- Dry eyes (**keratoconjunctivitis sicca**): Burning/red eyes, blurred vision
  - Can be confirmed objectively via Schirmer test
- Dry mouth (**xerostomia**): Tooth decay, parotid enlargement
- Extraglandular manifestations: Reynaud, arthritis, vasculitis, interstitial lung disease, interstitial nephritis, RTA

Diagnosis:

- Autoantibody: **Ro/La (SS-A/B)** positive
  - Can cross placenta, causing neonatal lupus and heart block
- ANA and RF often also positive
- Lip biopsy is highly specific (lymphocytic glandular infiltrate)

Management:

Mouth	- Behavioral modification (good oral hygiene, regular oral hydration) - Artificial saliva or pilocarpine can be used if necessary
Eyes	- Artificial tears
Systemic	- DMARDs (hydroxychloroquine, methotrexate), steroids, or other systemic agents

Seroneg Spondyloarthropathy

	General/Clinical (*All associated with HLA B27)	Diagnosis	Management
Psoriatic Arthritis	- Inflammatory polyarthritis seen in up to 30% of people with psoriasis - **Asymmetric and polyarticular arthritis**, generally years after skin findings - Finger edema, "**sausage digits**" (dactylitis) - Onycholysis (separation of nail) and nail pitting	- Clinical diagnosis - XR (joints show erosive changes and new bone formation) - "**Pencil in cup**" DIP deformity	- Mild arthritis (without evidence of joint damage) → NSAIDs - Refractory arthritis, or evidence of joint damage → DMARD (methotrexate, leflunomide) - Biologics often required (TNFα inhibitors) if severe
Ankylosing Spondylitis	- Inflammatory arthritis of the spine, typically presenting in young adult males - **Bilateral sacroiliitis** - **Impaired spinal mobility** (loss of lordosis, restricted chest mobility) - Peripheral arthritis, dactylitis, enthesitis - Extra-articular: Uveitis, IBD, psoriasis, aortitis/aortic root disease	- Clinical diagnosis - Lumbar imaging (XR/MRI) - Erosions, ankylosis, or sclerosis - "**Bamboo spine**" - No labs specific (ESR/CRP generally elevated)	- **NSAIDs**, + regular exercise/PT - Refractory: TNFα inhibitors *DMARDs not effective
Reactive Arthritis	- Inflammatory arthritis associated with recent extra-articular infection Presents weeks after infection with: - **Asymmetric arthritis**, enthesitis, dactylitis - Eye: Conjunctivitis or uveitis - Oral ulcers - Keratoderma blennorrhagica (scaly foot rash) - Circinate balanitis (ulcerative genital lesions)	- Clinical diagnosis - Associated with recent GI/GU infection with the following: *Salmonella, Shigella, Campylobacter, Chlamydia, Yersinia*	- **NSAIDs** - Refractory: Intra-articular/oral steroids
IBD Associated Arthritis	- Peripheral arthritis, spondylitis, or sacroiliitis associated with IBD (UC/Crohn)	- Clinical diagnosis	- Treat IBD (helps arthritis) - NSAIDs

Sarcoidosis

General: Chronic granulomatous inflammation characterized by the presence of noncaseating granulomas in different organs. Most commonly affects young adult, Black females.

Clinical:

Pulm	- Most common clinical manifestation (> 90%) - Cough, dyspnea, chest pain, bilateral hilar lymphadenopathy and interstitial infiltrates (restrictive lung disease)
Derm	- Papules, nodules, plaques, and atrophic or ulcerative lesions
MSK	- Acute and/or chronic polyarthritis
Ophtho	- Anterior or posterior uveitis
CNS	- Central DI, cranial mononeuropathy, other focal defects
CV	- Restrive or dilated cardiomyopathy, pericarditis, conduction disease
Misc Findings	- Peripheral lymphadenopathy, splenomegaly - Elevated serum ACE levels - Hypervitaminosis D (↑ 1α hydroxylase activity) → Hypercalcemia - ↑ CD4/CD8 ratio in bronchoalveolar lavage
Lofgren Syndrome	- Hilar LA, fever, polyarthritis, and erythema nodosum

Diagnosis:

- CXR: **Bilateral hilar adenopathy**[A] (+/− pulmonary infiltrate) [CT can be used for higher resolution]
- Biopsy of lesion (noncaseating granulomas). Use most accessible (cutaneous lesions, superficial lymph node).
    - If not available, use lung lesion (via bronchoscopy/endobronchial biopsy)

Management:

- Pulmonary disease:
    - **Asymptomatic**: Observe/monitor. Often spontaneous remission.
    - **Symptomatic**: Corticosteroids
- Derm: Topical/intralesional/systemic corticosteroids
- Arthropathy: NSAIDs, corticosteroids

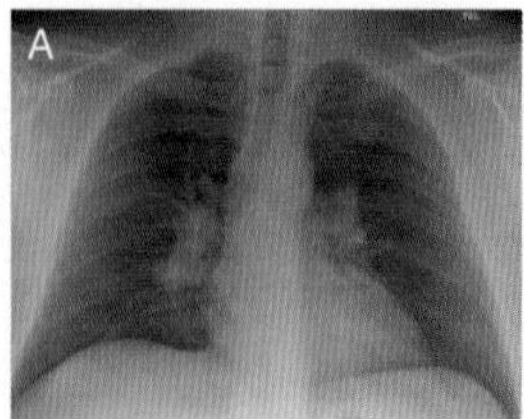

Myopathy

Myopathy Differential Diagnosis

	Clinical	Abnormal Labs
Inflammatory myopathy (DM/PM)	- Proximal muscle weakness	↑ ESR/CRP, ↑ CK
Inclusion body myositis	- Muscle weakness and atrophy without pain	Normal ESR, ↔/↑ CK
Glucocorticoid induced	- Proximal muscle weakness without pain or tenderness	
Statin induced	- Muscle pain/tenderness	↑ CK
Hypothyroidism	- Proximal muscle pain, tenderness, and weakness	↑ CK, ↑ TSH
Myasthenia gravis	- Progressive weakness with activity	Anti-AchR antibodies
Polymyalgia rheumatica	- Proximal muscle pain and stiffness, without weakness	↑ ESR/CRP
Others: - Muscular dystrophy (including adult onset types like limb-girdle) - Myotonic dystrophy - Inherited metabolic myopathy - Infiltrative disorders (amyloid, sarcoid, trichinellosis)		

Inclusion Body Myositis

General: Rare, sporadic, adult-onset disorder of muscle weakness

Clinical:

- Insidious onset (years long) of muscle weakness. More often distal (compared to polymyositis).
- Muscle atrophy
- Dysphagia, facial muscle involvement possible
- Normal or modest CK elevations

Diagnosis: Clinical features above PLUS

- Muscle biopsy (shows CD8 infiltration as in polymyositis, but with inclusions on electron microscopy)

Management: Physical, speech, occupational therapy. Poor response to any pharmacologic agents.

Polymyalgia Rheumatica

General: Common inflammatory rheumatologic condition of unclear etiology

Risk: Almost exclusively in those **> 50 y/o**, associated with temporal arteritis, HLA-DR4

Clinical:

- **Symmetrical pain and morning stiffness in the shoulders**, hip, neck, torso
  - Decreased range of motion on exam, but no weakness
- Constitutional symptoms may be present (fever, weight loss). **ESR/CRP elevated.**

Diagnosis: Clinical diagnosis

- Suspected with > 2 weeks of pain/morning stiffness, elevated ESR/CRP, and response to glucocorticoids

Management:

- Glucocorticoids (start at initial episode, then slowly taper as long as patient remains asymptomatic)
  - Disease is self-limited. Steroids can often be stopped in 1-2 years.

Myopathy

Polymyositis/Dermatomyositis

	Polymyositis	Dermatomyositis
Gen	- Immune-mediated myocyte injury - Endomysial CD8 T cells (surround and invade myofiber fascicles)	- Immune-mediated myocyte injury - Unclear pathophysiology, but CD4+ T cells are visualized perifascicularly and perivascularly *Associated with occult malignancy (including lung, breast, ovary, GI, kidney)
Clin	- **Proximal, symmetric muscle weakness** - Neck flexors, deltoids, hips commonly affected - Dysphagia/aspiration (upper esophageal muscle weakness) - Muscle atrophy in advanced disease Extramuscular: - Interstitial lung disease - Myocarditis	- Muscle weakness (similar to polymyositis) Skin findings: - Gottron papules[A] (papular, erythematous scaly lesions over the knuckles) - Heliotrope rash (periorbital rash) - Photodistributed erythema ("shawl sign") Extramuscular: - Interstitial lung disease - Myocarditis
Dx	- ↑ CK, LDH, Aldolase, AST/ALT - Autoantibodies: - **Anti Jo-1 (anti t-RNA synthetase)** - Anti-SRP - Anti Mi-2 - Electromyography (often abnormal but not specific) - Muscle biopsy A * Diagnosis can be made with classic muscle weakness, elevated muscle enzymes, and classic rash (for DM). Biopsy and myography may be required in those with partial features.	
Tx	- **Glucocorticoids** (for acute episode) PLUS DMARD for chronic management (e.g., azathioprine, MTX, or IVIG)	

Fibromyalgia

General: Chronic pain caused by CNS/PNS hyperirritability

Risk: Most common in middle aged women (20-55 y/o)

Clinical:

- Chronic, diffuse musculoskeletal pain (for > 3 months)
    - Exam demonstrates tenderness in specific anatomic locations
- Fatigue, abnormal sleep patterns
- Cognitive and psychiatric disturbances, headache, paresthesias

Diagnosis: Clinical diagnosis of exclusion

- Labs (ESR, CRP, CBC, TSH, etc.) all normal
- Current guidelines focus on symptoms (widespread pain index and symptom severity scale) for diagnosis rather than tender point count

Management:

- **Nonpharm**: Patient education, regular exercise
- **Pharm**: Indicated if nonpharm measures do not sufficiently relieve symptoms
    - TCA (**amitriptyline**)
    - SNRI (milnacipran/duloxetine), pregabalin
- Severe, refractory cases: Combine drugs, try CBT (with biofeedback training)

Vasculitis

	General/Clinical	Diagnosis	Management
Large Vessel Vasculitis			
Giant Cell "Temporal" Arteritis	- Chronic inflammatory response of large/medium vessels - Classically **temporal arterial involvement**, but can also involve carotid and aorta - Seen almost exclusively in > 50 y/o Clinical: - Constitutional symptoms (fever, malaise) - **Severe HA** - **Visual impairment** (25-50%) (Optic neuritis, amaurosis fugax, anterior ischemic optic neuropathy, can lead to **blindness**) - Jaw pain with chewing (intermittent claudication of jaw/tongue) - Tenderness over temples, possible nodules - Arm claudication with possible bruits, decreased pulses	- **ESR/CRP ↑↑↑** - **Temporal artery biopsy** gold standard (for confirmation) *High association with PMR, aortic aneurysm/dissection	Acute: - High dose prednisone early (40-60 oral, unless visual symptoms → 1000 mg IV methylpred) - Do not wait for lab/biopsy results to initiate treatment Chronic: - Taper steroids - ESR to monitor effectiveness of therapy - Ultimately is self-limited and rarely refractory, but can use MTX or **Tocilizumab** (Il-6 inhibitor)
Takayasu	- Granulomatous vasculitis of **aortic arch** and major branches, potentially leading to stenosis - Risk: Young adult (20-40 y/o), Asian, female Clinical: - Constitutional (fever, weight loss) - Arterial-occlusive disease in UE (claudication) - Pain, bruits over involved vessels - Absent pulses in carotid, radial, ulnar - MI/stroke - Aortic aneurysms, regurgitation	- **MRA (or CTA)** - ESR/CRP often elevated	- Glucocorticoids - Other immunosuppressives (MTX, azathioprine, mycophenolate, tocilizumab) in refractory cases - Severe stenosis may require angioplasty/stenting
Medium Vessel Vasculitis			
Polyarteritis Nodosa	- Medium vessel vasculitis of adults - Risk: Often idiopathic, but increased risk with **Hepatitis B/C**, hairy cell leukemia Clinical: - Constitutional: Fever, fatigue, weight loss - Derm: Livedo reticularis, tender nodules, purpura - GI: Abdominal pain (mesenteric artery involvement) - Renal: **Insufficiency, HTN** (renal artery stenosis) - CNS: **Mononeuritis multiplex**	- **Biopsy** (inflammation of fibrinoid necrosis of medium vessels) - Mesenteric angiography (see multiple aneurysms and irregular constrictions)	- Glucocorticoids +/− Cyclophosphamide (if severe)
Kawasaki's	- Seen in 1-5 year olds, especially Asian Clinical Criteria: - **Fever (> 5 days)** - Bilateral nonexudative conjunctivitis - Erythema of the lips/tongue/oral mucosa - Rash (polymorphous) - Extremity edema, erythema - Cervical lymphadenopathy Others: Leukocytosis, thrombocytosis, ↑ ESR	- Clinical diagnosis (fever > 5 days, plus 4 more of the clinical signs, plus no other possible underlying etiology) * Risk for **coronary artery aneurysms** (can thrombose/ rupture)	- **IVIG plus Aspirin** - ECHO (at time of diagnosis, and at weeks ~2 and 6, to rule out coronary involvement)
Buerger's Disease (Thromboangiitis obliterans)	- Small and medium vessel vasculitis that occurs in **middle-aged male smokers** - Inflammatory thrombotic vessel occlusions - Clinical: Superficial thrombophlebitis, migratory phlebitis, ischemic ulceration	- Clinical diagnosis (age < 45, hx of tobacco use, extremity ischemia) - Angiography used to image vessels	- **Smoking cessation** - Iloprost, calcium channel blockers, and pneumatic compression (improve pain)

Vasculitis

	General/Clinical	Diagnosis	Management
Small Vessel Vasculitis			
Granulomatosis w/ Polyangiitis [GPA] (Wegener)	- Small vessel necrotizing vasculitis, granulomatous inflammation - Risk: Older, white men Clinical: - Constitutional: Fever, anorexia, and weight loss - Upper resp: **Sinusitis, otitis**, discharge, ulcers - Lower resp: Nodules, infiltrates, hemoptysis - Renal: Pauci-immune **rapidly progressive GN** - Derm: Ulcers, purpura - Eye: Conjunctivitis, scleritis, uveitis	- **c-ANCA**/PR3-ANCA (but other is possible) - Biopsy (definitive diagnosis)	- Glucocorticoids PLUS - Cyclophosphamide or rituximab - Avacopan (C5a receptor inh.) - Plasma exchange (in severe renal or pulmonary disease)
Microscopic Polyangiitis	- Vasculitis without granuloma formation - Clinical: Very similar to GPA, but with decreased likelihood for upper respiratory disease	- **p-ANCA**/MPO-ANCA (but other is possible) - Biopsy (definitive diagnosis)	
Eosinophilic Granulomatosis w/ Polyangiitis [EGPA] (Churg Strauss)	- Vasculitis with allergic features Clinical: - Chronic rhinosinusitis - **Asthma** (pulmonary infiltrates/fibrosis) - Peripheral neuropathy (mononeuritis multiplex) - Skin (**palpable purpura**, nodules) - Cardiac, renal disease	- **ANCA positive** (~50%) - Peripheral **eosinophilia** - CT chest (pulm infiltrates, ground glass, nodules) - Biopsy (generally lung or skin) for definitive diagnosis	- Glucocorticoids +/− other immunosuppression (cyclophosphamide, azathioprine)
Henoch-Schonlein Purpura	- **IgA vasculitis**, most common **childhood** vasculitis Clinical: (Often occurs within days of **viral URI**) - Skin: Palpable purpura - Arthralgias - Abdominal pain - Renal (hematuria, IgA nephropathy)	- Clinical - Biopsy (often not required)	- **Supportive care** (fluids, NSAIDs for pain control, rest) as disease usually self-limited - Glucocorticoids if high-risk

Behcet's Disease

General: Syndrome of recurrent ulcers due to systemic vasculitis of all sized vessels

Risk: Young adults of Middle-Eastern (e.g., Turkish) and Eastern Asian descent

Clinical: Recurrent **aphthous ulcers, urogenital ulcers**, uveitis, vascular disease/thrombosis
- Derm: Acne-like eruptions, pustules, erythema nodosum, pseudofolliculitis
  - Pathergy (erythematous papular response to local skin injury)

Diagnosis: Clinical diagnosis (recurrent ulcers, plus some of the other above features and positive pathergy test)

Management: Topical steroids for ulcers, colchicine for chronic prevention of ulcers
- System immunosuppression for organ system involvement

Hypersensitivity Vasculitis

General: Also known as cutaneous leukocytoclastic vasculitis or cutaneous small vessel vasculitis. Small vessel vasculitis that characteristically results in purpura.

Risk: Idiopathic often, but can be caused by drugs, infection, or autoimmune disease

Clinical: **Nonblanching, palpable purpura**[A]. Rash can cause pain or pruritus. Postinflammatory hyperpigmentation.
- Systemic symptoms (fever, myalgias, arthralgias)
- *No organ system involvement

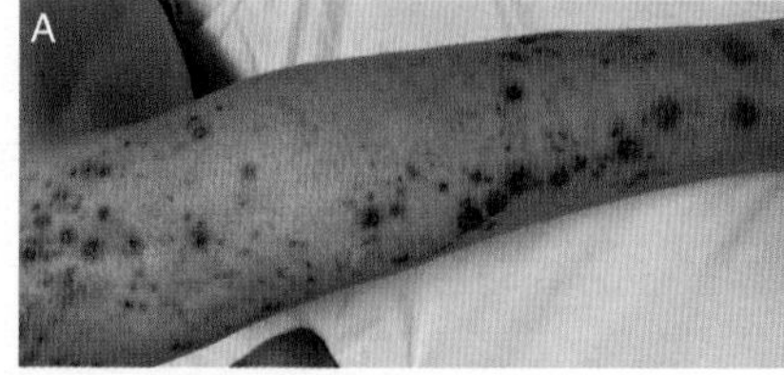

Management:
- Treat underlying (remove drug, treat infection if present)
- Generally self-limited (just manage symptoms like pain/itching)
- Glucocorticoids if severe

Bones

Osteoporosis

General: Disorder of low bone mass, abnormal bone structure, and fragility, resulting in decreased bone strength/increased fracture risk. Can be:

- Primary:
    - Post-menopausal osteoporosis (type I): Estrogen deficiency
    - Senile osteoporosis (type II): Age-related bone loss (men and women)
- Secondary:
    - Drugs (glucocorticoids, heparin, cyclosporine, phenytoin)
    - Endocrine (Cushing, hyperthyroidism, hyperparathyroidism, hypogonadism)
    - Nutritional (vit D/Ca deficiency, malabsorption)

Risk:

- Modifiable: Smoking, EtOH, sedentary, low dietary Ca
- Nonmodifiable: ↑ Age, low weight, post-menopause, white or Asian

Clinical:

- Asymptomatic until fracture occurs
- All clinical manifestations (pain, deformity, loss of height, disability) associated with fracture
    - Vertebral fracture[A] (most common, often asymptomatic, can lose height)
    - Hip and distal radius fracture (Colles) also common

Diagnosis: History of fragility fracture OR DEXA Scan

Normal	T score between −1 and 1
Osteopenia	T score between −1 and −2.5
Osteoporosis	T score between < −2.5
Severe Osteoporosis	T score < −3.5 OR < −2.5 plus fragility fracture

Management:

- Lifestyle (exercise, smoking cessation, prevent falls, ↓ EtOH)
- Vitamin D (800 IU/day) and calcium (1200 mg/day)

Pharmacologic

- Indicated if: Osteoporosis (DEXA < -2.5) OR osteopenia plus high risk (↑ FRAX score > 20%)
- Agents:
    - Bisphosphonate (alendronate, risedronate)
    - Second line: Denosumab or teriparatide

Screening: DEXA scan screening q3-5 years

- All women > 65, women < 65 with risk factors
- Only men with clinical manifestations of osteoporosis or risk factors

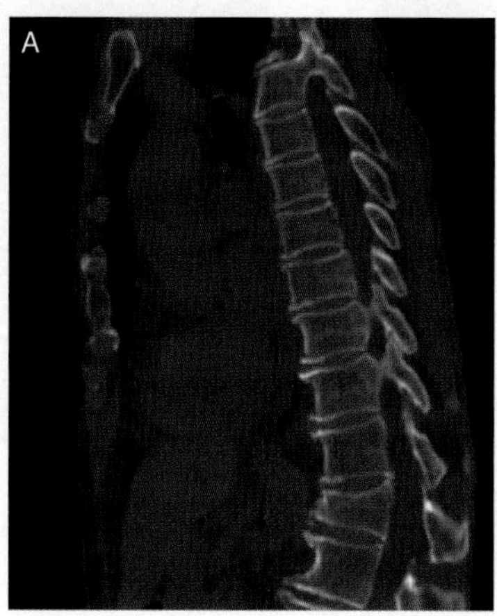

Bones

	General/Clinical	Diagnosis	Management
Osteomalacia	- Defective mineralization of osteoid - Most commonly caused by vitamin D deficiency Ricket's (kids) - Bow legs, bead-like costochondral junctions, craniotabes (soft skull), frontal bossing Osteomalacia (adults) - Bone pain, muscle weakness, cramps, difficulty walking	↓ Ca, PO_4, 25-vit D ↑ PTH, Alk phos XR: Thin cortex, decreased density, pseudofractures	- Vitamin D if deficient (50K IU for 6-8 weeks, followed by standard 800 IU supplement)
Osteopetrosis	- Increased bone density from failure of proper osteoclastic bone resorption - AR (defect in carbonic anhydrase) is severe childhood form, while AD disease affects adults - Cranial nerve impingement from skull sclerosis	- XR[A]: Sclerotic bone, or "bone within bone" appearance	- Bone marrow transplant (if genetically based)
Paget (Osteitis Deformans)	- Disorder of excessive bone remodeling, from osteoclastic dysfunction Clinical - Most often asymptomatic - Bone pain and deformities - Skull (HA, hearing loss) & spinal (radiculopathy) - Increased risk for bone tumors (osteosarcoma)	↑ Alk phos. Normal Ca/PO_4. ↑ Urine hydroxyproline, PINP - XR[B]: Osteolytic and/or sclerotic lesions - Bone scintigraphy: Assess extent of disease	- Bisphosphonates
Osteonecrosis (Avascular Necrosis)	- Death of bone marrow due to disruption of vasculature - Most commonly hip (medial circumflex femoral artery) - Risk: Trauma, corticosteroids, sickle cell, SLE, Legg-Calve-Perthes, SCFE - Presents as joint pain	- XR: Density changes, sclerosis, cysts, "crescent sign" (subchondral collapse) - MRI (provides much higher sensitivity)	- Try to spare joint for as long as possible (bisphosphonates or joint sparing procedures) - Joint replacement if severe

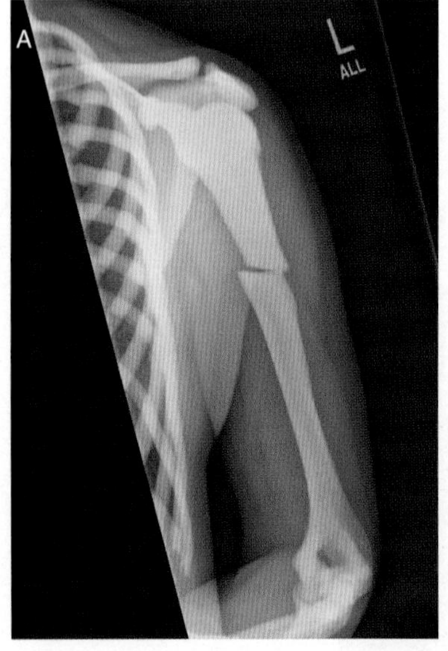

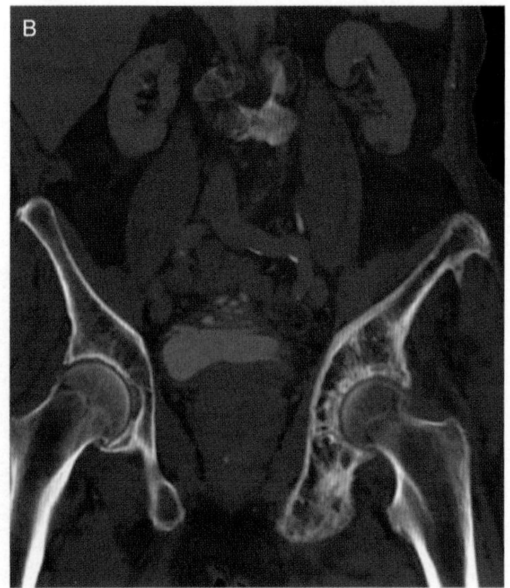

Bone and Joint Infections

Septic Arthritis

General: Bacterial infection of a joint, most commonly due to:

- **Hematogenous spread**
- **Contiguous spread** from another locus of infection (osteomyelitis)
- **Direct inoculation** (trauma, surgery, bites)

Etiology: Organisms include *Staphylococcus aureus and Streptococci*, and gram negatives (if immunocompromised)

- Prosthetic joints: *S. aureus* and gram negatives (< 3 months post surgery), *Staph epidermidis* and *Enterococcus* (3-12 months post surgery), *S. aureus* and beta-hemolytic *Streptococci* (> 12 months post surgery).

Risk: Pre-existing arthritis (especially RA, but also OA, gout, and diabetic arthropathy), immunocompromised, IV drug use

Clinical:

- Monoarticular, severely painful arthritis. Erythema, edema, swelling of joint.
- Constitutional (fever, chills, malaise)

Diagnosis:

- Arthrocentesis (definitive)
    - Gram stain, culture, cell counts
    - Septic fluid counts (> 20K WBC, > 75% neutrophils)
- Imaging (can rule in/out bone infection, help examine tough-to-tap joints)

Management:

- **Antibiotic Therapy** (based on initial gram stain). Generally ~4 weeks required.
    - Gram stain (+) bacteria: Vancomycin
    - Gram stain (−) bacteria: Third-gen cephalosporin (or cefepime if concern for *Pseudomonas*)
    - Gram stain not revealing: Vancomycin (+ ceftriaxone if immunocompromised)
    - Adjust to culture results

- **Drainage** (needle, arthroscopic, or open): Indicated in most cases

Gonococcal Arthritis

General: Arthritis secondary to disseminated gonococcal infection

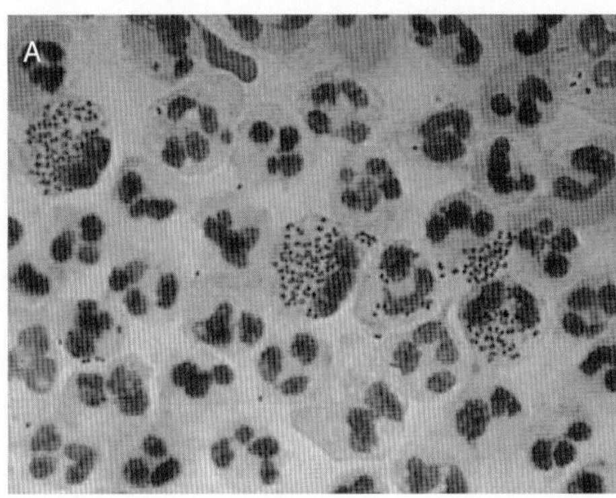

Clinical:

- Purulent monoarthritis or migratory, asymmetric polyarthritis
- Tenosynovitis
- Skin lesions (erythematous papules/pustules)

Diagnosis:

- Arthrocentesis (with gram stain[A]/fluid analysis, NAAT)
- GU gonorrhea NAAT

Management:

- Ceftriaxone + azithromycin/doxycycline

Bone and Joint Infections

Transient Synovitis

General: Self-limited inflammatory joint pain, most commonly after viral URI infection. Common cause of hip pain in children.

Clinical:

- Joint pain
- Systemic symptoms (low grade fever, malaise, etc.)

Diagnosis: Clinical diagnosis (must rule out septic arthritis, but can follow clinically if T < 101.4°F, WBC < 12K, ESR < 20)

Management: NSAIDs

Osteomyelitis

General: Bacterial infection of bone, most commonly due to:

- Hematogenous spread
    - Most common cause of osteomyelitis in children
- Contiguous spread from another locus of infection (e.g., soft tissue infection)
- Direct inoculation (trauma, like open fractures)

Micro: Most commonly *Staphylococcus aureus, Streptococcus*, gram negatives

- Puncture wound: *Staph, Pseudomonas*
- Prosthetic joint: Coagulase-negative *Staphylococci*
- Diabetic foot ulcer: Polymicrobial organisms
- IV drug abuse/Immunocompromise: Fungal species, *Pseudomonas*
- Sickle cell disease: *Salmonella*

Risk: IV drug use, open fractures, diabetes mellitus (i.e., ulcers), bacteremia

Clinical:

- Gradual onset of local pain with possible erythema, swelling at site
- Constitutional symptoms (fever, malaise) may be present. ESR ↑.
- Can become chronic with waxing/waning pain

Diagnosis:

- Imaging
    - XR: Periosteal thickening or elevation
    - MRI: Most sensitive
    - If hardware present: PET scan or triple phase bone scan
- Bone biopsy is definitive (may not need if + blood cx, image findings)

Management:

- Empiric antibiotics (vancomycin and ceftriaxone)
    - Tailor to specific organism/sensitivities once available
- Surgical debridement often required (depending on response to antibiotics)

Bone and Soft Tissue Malignancy

	General/Clinical	Diagnosis/Management
Osteochondroma	- Benign bony exostosis with cartilaginous cap, seen in children and young adults - Most common at end of long bone (i.e., femur) - Presents as painless mass (but can rarely cause pain, deformity)	XR Tx: Observation. Resect if remains symptomatic. *Small chance of progression to osteochondrosarcoma
Giant Cell Tumor	- Benign, locally aggressive bone tumor most commonly seen in young adults - Presents as a lytic lesion in the epiphysis of long bones (most commonly distal femur) - Clinically presents as pain, swelling, decreased ROM of joint, pathologic fracture	XR: Soap bubble appearance (eccentric, locally aggressive lesions), CT/MRI used for better definition Biopsy: Multinucleated giant cells Tx: Surgery
Osteoid Osteoma	- Benign bone-forming tumor, seen most commonly in teens, with characteristic prostaglandin-producing central nidus - Presents as progressive night time pain, most commonly in long bone (femur) or spine	XR: Well-defined round lesion Tx: NSAIDs for pain. Surgical resection if symptomatic.
Osteosarcoma	- Malignant, primary tumor of bone, with bimodal onset of presentation (10-20 y/o, and > 65) - Associated with hereditary retinoblastoma, Li-Fraumeni syndrome, Paget's, other bone lesions - Presents with local bone pain with onset over months	XR[A] (sunburst, Codman triangle [elevated periosteum]) Biopsy (for definitive diagnosis) Tx: Chemotherapy and surgical resection
Ewing Sarcoma	- Malignant, anaplastic small cell tumor, found in long bones - Seen most commonly in boys < 15 y/o - Presents with subacute presentation of localized pain and swelling	XR (moth eaten appearance, onion skin periosteal reaction) Biopsy (for definitive diagnosis) Tx: Chemoradiation (neoadjuvant) + surgery

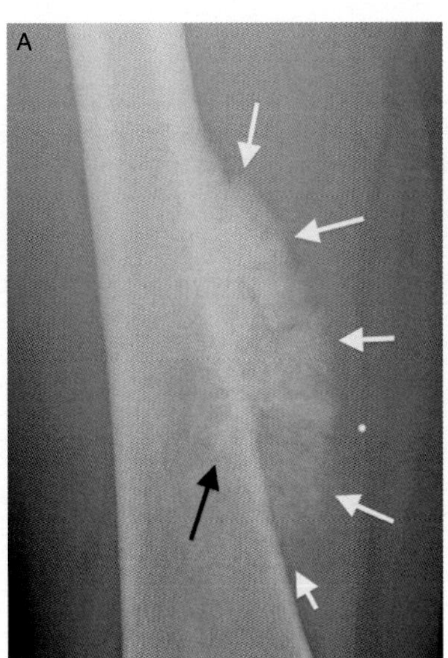

Musculoskeletal: Back

Overview of Low Back Pain

General: 85% of back pain cases are due to idiopathic, nonspecific, musculoskeletal pain that is self-limited in nature

- **Acute** (< 4 weeks)
- **Subacute** (4-12 weeks)
- **Chronic** (> 12 weeks)

Etiology:

- Mechanical:
    - Strain, spondylosis, osteoarthritis, spondylolisthesis, disc herniation, spinal stenosis, compression fracture, kyphosis/scoliosis
- Nonmechanical:
    - Neoplasia, infection (osteomyelitis, epidural abscess), rheumatic disease (ankylosing spondylitis)
- Visceral:
    - Kidney pain (PKD), AAA, pancreatitis, PID

Diagnosis:

- Imaging not generally indicated within 4 weeks
    - **Exceptions**: Image patients with **red flag features** (severe neurologic deficits, cancer history, constitutional symptoms, osteoporosis, IV drug use)
- After 4-6 weeks of conservative therapy, consider further workup
    - Plain XR (if nonspecific)
    - CT/MRI (if concerned about radiculopathy or spinal stenosis)

Management:

Acute	- Moderate activity levels - Trial of heat, massage, acupuncture, or spinal manipulation (if desired) - NSAIDs/acetaminophen - Adjuncts (for refractory cases): Muscle relaxants, short opioid course
Subacute	- Similar to acute - Consider physical therapy and/or exercise therapy at this time
Chronic	- Treat underlying disease (surgery if necessary) - Intermittent NSAID/acetaminophen use (can consider adding muscle relaxant, opiate, or duloxetine in severe cases) - Exercise/physical therapy

Lumbosacral Radiculopathy

General: Compression of spinal nerve root, most commonly due to **disc herniation**. Herniated discs usually occur posterolaterally, affecting nerve root below level of disc herniation.

L3-L4	- Weakness of knee extension, weak patellar reflexes
L4-L5	- Weak dorsiflexion, difficulty heel walking, **lateral leg**/dorsal foot sensory loss/pain
L5-S1	- Weakness of plantarflexion, difficulty toe walking, decreased Achilles reflex, **pain down back of leg**

Musculoskeletal: Back

	General/Clinical	Diagnosis/Management
Lumbar Strain	- Common cause of acute low back pain. Due to stretching injury to muscles/tendons/ligaments. - Presents as **paraspinal muscle tenderness**, spasms	Dx: Clinical Tx: Conservative (see prior page). Self-limited.
Disc Herniation	- "Slipped disc." Protrusion of **inner nucleus pulposus** through outer fibrous ring - Herniation often caused by trauma - Presents as **acute lumbosacral radiculopathy** (including sciatica), +/– back pain. Exacerbated by ↑ pressure/valsalva.	Dx: Clinical. Imaging indicated if severe neurologic deficit or signs of infection or malignancy. Tx: Conservative (see prior page). Surgery if refractory (only required in ~ 10% of cases).
Spinal Stenosis	- Narrowing of spinal canal from **degenerative spinal disease** - Causes: Osteophytes (OA), ligamentum flavum hypertrophy, disc bulging, or spondylolisthesis - Presents with pain, **neurogenic claudication** (numbness/ paresthesias in legs) - Worse with walking, relieved with sitting/leaning forward (+ leg raise test in ~ 10%)	Dx: MRI confirms diagnosis Tx: Conservative (if not severe/not progressive). Consider surgery if conservative therapy fails.
Spondylolisthesis	- **Anterior or posterior translation of vertebral body** compared to adjacent vertebral body - Causes spinal stenosis (and its associated symptoms)	Dx: MRI Tx: Conservative initially. Surgical fusion if fails.
Compression Fractures	- Most commonly seen with **osteoporosis**, but also chronic steroid use, infection, spinal metastasis, Paget disease - Presents as **acute back pain**, often post minor trauma in person with osteoporosis or risk factors - **Severe pain with palpation of site** - Note: Can be chronic, which do not present with pain, but rather progressive kyphosis/loss of stature	Dx: XR (often mid or lower thoracic spine) Tx: Conservative (pain control, activity modification, etc.). If pain extremely severe, or neurologic symptoms, consider surgery (kyphoplasty or vertebroplasty).

Epidural Abscess

General: Abscess formation in the epidural space, from bacterial hematogenous spread, direct extension, or iatrogenic inoculation. *S. aureus* responsible for most cases.

Risk: IV drug use, spinal procedures

Clinical: Classic triad: **Fever, back pain, neurologic findings** (motor/sensory deficits, bowel/bladder dysfunction)
- ↑ ESR

Diagnosis: **Spinal MRI (with contrast)**. Blood culture or aspiration (for organism identification).

Management: Broad antibiotics (vancomycin + 3rd/4th generation cephalosporin)
- Urgent surgical decompression/drainage (in most cases)

Vertebral Osteomyelitis/Discitis

General: Infection of vertebrae or disc, from hematogenous spread, direct extension, or iatrogenic inoculation. *S. aureus* most common.

Clinical: **Back pain, tenderness upon palpation of spine, fever**, ↑ ESR/CRP

Diagnosis: MRI (confirms diagnosis)
- Tissue biopsy/culture

Management: Antibiotics (vancomycin + 3rd/4th generation cephalosporin)
- Surgery not usually necessary (unless complication, like abscess)

Musculoskeletal: Back

Spinal Cord Compression

General: External compression of the spinal cord from vertebrae/abscess/neoplasm

Risk: Direct spinal cord injury (trauma), infection (abscess), malignancy

Clinical: Progressive, lower back pain, pain worse lying down, with neurologic deficits
- Lower extremity weakness, ↓ DTR, decreased rectal tone
- Long term: Eventual (+) Babinski, ↑ DTR

Diagnosis: MRI

Management: IV glucocorticoids for acute cases. Often require neurosurgical intervention.

Cauda Equina/Conus Medullaris Syndrome

	Cauda Equina Syndrome	Conus Medullaris Syndrome
Gen	- Compression of one of the cauda equina nerve roots	- Compression of the lower end of the spinal cord (conus)
Risk	- Herniated disc, spondylosis, spinal trauma, infection (abscess)	
Clin	- **Gradual** low back pain with bilateral lower extremity radiation (radicular pain) - Sensory loss (“**saddle**” distribution) - **Asymmetric** weakness - **Hyporeflexia** - Erectile dysfunction rare - Possible bladder/bowel dysfunction (late in disease)	- **Acute**, severe back pain (radicular pain less common) - Sensory loss (**perianal**) - **Symmetric** motor weakness (mild/less marked compared to cauda equina) - **Hyperreflexia** - Erectile dysfunction common - Possible bowel/bladder dysfunction(early in disease)
Dx	- Emergent MRI	
Tx	- Urgent surgical decompression	

Cervical Back Pain

Etiology	Features
Nonspecific Pain (cervical sprain)	- Most common cause of acute neck pain - Nonspecific paraspinal muscle tenderness - Treated similarly to general low back pain
Osteoarthritis (spondylosis)	- Common cause of chronic neck pain - Can result in myelopathy/radiculopathy
Cervical Radiculopathy	- Compression of spinal nerve leads to arm pain, numbness, weakness. Unilateral neck pain. - Dx: MRI - Tx: Conservative initially (NSAIDs, PT). Surgery if refractory.
Cervical Myelopathy	- Cervical spinal cord compression, most commonly from stenosis - Presents with gait disturbance, loss of motor function, and possible bowel/bladder findings - Dx: MRI - Tx: Surgical

Atlanto-axial Instability

General: Excessive laxity of the posterior cervical ligament, allowing for increased susceptibility to movement at the C1-C2 junction, with potential spinal cord injury

Risk: Genetic predisposition (Down syndrome, osteogenesis imperfecta), rheumatoid arthritis

Clinical: Presents as acute spinal cord injury (neck pain, loss of motor function, loss of bowel/bladder function)

Diagnosis: Cervical XR

Management: Surgery

Musculoskeletal: Upper Ext

	General	Clinical	Management
Shoulder			
Shoulder Impingement Syndrome	- Compression of rotator cuff tendons/subacromial bursa between head of humerus and acromion, causing pain	- Shoulder pain with **overhead activity**, localized to **lateral deltoid** - Exam: Tenderness over rotator cuff muscles, with pain upon abduction/external rotation Special tests for impingement: - **Neer**: Passive flexion of straight, internally rotated arm - **Hawkin**: 90° Shoulder/elbow flexion → quick internal rotation	Dx: Clinical. Ultrasound can support. Tx: - Rest, Ice, NSAIDs, PT - Referral to orthopedics for failed conservative therapy for greater than 3 months for impingement/6 months for tendinopathy
Rotator Cuff Tendinopathy	- Inflammation of rotator cuff tendons - Can be caused by chronic shoulder impingement or repetitive overhead activity in sport or work		
Rotator Cuff Tear	- Risk: Acute traumatic injury or chronic degeneration with eventual rupture	- **Shoulder pain, weakness**, especially with overhead activity - Exam: Extreme weakness with external rotation - Positive **empty can test** (supraspinatus)	Dx: US or **MRI** Tx: Surgery for acute tears, conservative treatment for chronic (PT/steroid injections)
Adhesive Capsulitis	- "**Frozen Shoulder**" (chronic inflammation and fibrosis of joint capsule) - Risk: Either idiopathic or associated with prior shoulder injury	- Painful, stiff shoulder joint - **Extreme limitation** of active/passive **ROM**	Dx: Clinical Tx: Mobility exercises. Steroid injection/physical therapy if not improving.
Labral Tear	- SLAP tear most common (injury to superior portion of glenoid labrum) - Risk: Labor or athletics involving high intensity overhead activity	- **Anterior shoulder pain**, "clicking" in shoulder, decline in shoulder strength - Can occur with acute traumatic event - **O'Brien's active compression test**, crank test, anterior glide test	Dx: MRI or MR arthroscopy Tx: Conservative preferred, but surgery in some athletes
Ant. Shoulder Dislocation	- Most common type of dislocation - Occurs with traumatic blow to abducted/externally rotated arm	- Extreme pain/discomfort, with refusal of any movement - **Shoulder abducted/externally rotated** - Often complicated by fractures or axillary nerve damage	Dx: Clinical, confirmed with XR Tx: **Manual reduction**, followed by shoulder immobilization
Post. Shoulder Dislocation	- Occurs with severe blow to anterior shoulder or extreme muscle contractions (classically **seizure** or **lightening strike**)	- Extreme pain/discomfort - Shoulder adducted/internally rotated - Prominent posterior shoulder (grossly) - Often associated with fractures, labrum/rotator cuff injuries	Dx: Clinical, with XR confirmation ("light bulb sign") Tx: **Manual reduction**
AC Joint Sprain	- Caused by trauma to adducted shoulder (direct blow/fall)	- **Tenderness over the AC joint** - Positive crossover test (pain with cross-body arm adduction)	Dx: XR (shows widened AC joint, possible ant/post shift of clavicle) Tx: Minor → rest/ice/Compression, severe → surgical
Biceps Tendinopathy	- Repetitive stress to the proximal long head of biceps, resulting in tendon injury/inflammation - Associated with other mechanical shoulder issues (e.g., impingement)	- Anterior shoulder pain, worse with pulling/lifting activities	Dx: Clinical Tx: Analgesia (NSAIDs, local steroid injections), physical therapy
Biceps Tendon Rupture	- Most commonly anterior biceps tendon rupture - Occurs with clear traumatic event/associated "pop"	- Acute, severe, anterior shoulder pain, edema, and ecchymosis - **Gross deformity of biceps**	Dx: US (alt. MRI) Tx: Conservative in some, surgical repair in athletes/workers that require strength

Musculoskeletal: Upper Ext

	General	Clinical	Management
Elbow			
Medial Epicondylitis	- **"Golfer's Elbow"** - Risk: Repetitive, forceful flexion movements of elbow	- Localized pain of **medial elbow** and proximal wrist flexor muscles - Pain with passive forearm extension (with elbow extended)	Dx: Clinical Tx: Counter force bracing, NSAIDs, PT, activity modification
Lateral Epicondylitis	- **"Tennis Elbow"** - Risk: Repetitive, forceful extension movements of elbow	- Localized pain of **lateral elbow** and proximal wrist extensor muscles - Pain with passive forearm flexion (with elbow extended)	
Radial Head Subluxation	- **"Nursemaid's Elbow"** (kids) - Axial traction on forearm with arm extension, resulting in a torn or displaced **annular ligament of the radiohumeral joint**	- Arm held in **extension and pronation** - Should have no signs of fracture, such as focal bone tenderness/deformity/swelling (if they do, XR to rule out fracture)	Dx: Clinical Tx: **Manual reduction** (hyperpronation of arm)
Ulnar Collateral Ligament Injury	- Occurs in long term, competitive baseball players (can occur with acute injury or accumulated chronic trauma)	- Medial elbow tenderness, worse with the motion of throwing	Dx: MRI Tx: **Tommy John surgery** (UCL tendon repair)
Olecranon Bursitis	- Inflammation of bursa posterior to ulna - Becomes inflamed from trauma, chronic injury/overuse, or arthritis	- Swollen, tender, inflamed areas on the back of the elbow	Dx: Clinical Tx: NSAIDs, joint protection, fluid aspiration (fluid has high chance of recurring)
Hand (Nerve Issues)			
Carpal Tunnel Syndrome	- Increased pressure in the carpal tunnel, causing abnormal functioning of the **median nerve** - Risk: Obesity, diabetes, pregnancy, RA, connective tissue disease, chronic/repetitive movements of the wrist	- Painful paresthesias in median nerve distribution (**first 3.5 digits**) - Symptoms often occur at night - Provoked by movements of the wrist - Severe, chronic disease can lead to weakness or atrophy of thenar eminence - Exam: **Phalen**[A] and **Tinel** test, or manual carpal compression (causes symptoms)	Dx: Clinical - Nerve conduction studies and electromyography can support Tx: - Mild-moderate → splinting, glucocorticoid injections - Severe → surgical (cut the transverse carpal ligament)
Ulnar Neuropathy	- Compression can occur either at the elbow or the wrist (**Guyon canal**)	- Paresthesias/pain in ulnar nerve distribution (**4th/5th digits**) - Symptoms worse with elbow flexion or compression of the wrist - Chronic disease can cause weakness/atrophy	Dx: Clinical, with confirmation by nerve conduction studies Tx: Conservative (splinting, activity modification). Surgery (for severe or refractory cases).

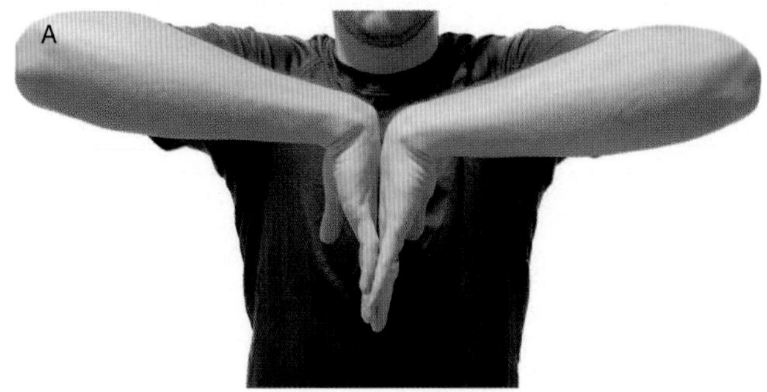

Musculoskeletal: Upper Ext

	General	Clinical	Management
Hand			
Felon	- Infection of the pulp of the finger tip	- Painful, red, swollen **distal phalanx**	- Surgical drainage
Paronychia	- Infection of the nail fold	- Painful, red, swollen **nail fold**	- Warm soaks, oral antibiotics if severe
Gamekeeper Thumb	- Also known as Skier thumb - Ulnar collateral ligament injury, from forced hyperextension/abduction of the MCP joint	- Pain/swelling on **ulnar side of MCP joint** at base of thumb - Laxity of MCP joint - XR to rule out associated fractures	- Splinting, ice, rest - Bony injury → surgery
Jersey Finger	- Injury to flexor digitorum profundus tendon at insertion in phalanx - Due to hyperextension of DIP joint	- Pain and swelling at DIP joint - **Inability to flex DIP joint**	- Surgical correction
Mallet Finger	- Injury to extensor tendon at insertion into DIP	- Pain and swelling at dorsal surface of DIP - **Inability to extend DIP joint**	- Splinting, consider surgical intervention
Trigger Finger	- Flexor tendon catching in stenotic A1 pulley over the MCP joint	- **Painless catching of the finger** during flexion/extension of the finger	- Activity modification/splinting - Glucocorticoid injection
De Quervain Tenosynovitis	- Thickening of abductor pollicis longus and extensor pollicis brevis tendons at the styloid of the radius - Risk: Repetitive movements (e.g., **mother carrying baby**)	- Radial sided wrist pain, worse with movement - Medial wrist edema/tenderness over the radial styloid (worse with stretching of the thumb, called Finkelstein test)	Dx: Clinical Tx: Splinting, NSAIDs. Steroid injection if severe/persistent.
Dupuytren Contracture	- Benign fibrous proliferative growth of palmar fascia - Risk: EtOH, northern Europeans, older age, men	- Stiff **nodule over the palmar aspect** of the hand, +/− tenderness - Decreased ROM of the fingers	Dx: Clinical Tx: Conservative (hand padding, intralesional steroids). Surgery if severe/persistent.

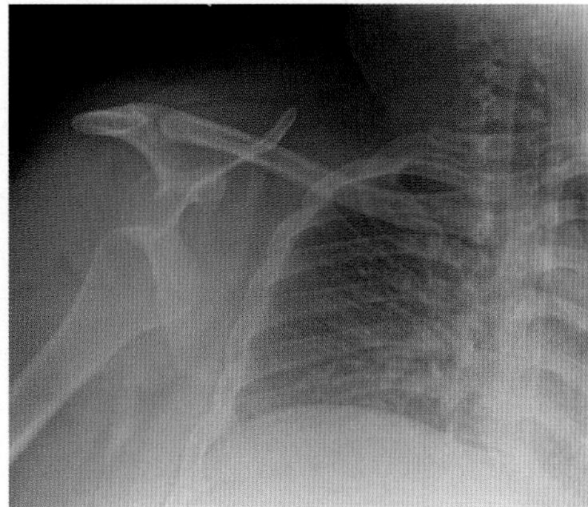

Shoulder dislocation

Musculoskeletal: Lower Ext

	General	Clinical	Management
Hip			
Trochanteric Bursitis	- Now called greater trochanteric pain syndrome	- **Lateral hip pain** with tenderness upon palpation	Dx: Clinical Tx: NSAIDs. Self-limited.
Osteoarthritis	- Degenerative hip disease	- **Groin pain**, worse with activity, improves with rest - Limited ROM, with pain elicited by movement (especially internal rotation)	Dx: Clinical. XR (not always needed, shows degenerative changes) Tx: NSAIDs, steroid injections, surgical hip replacement
Knee			
IT- Band Syndrome	- Overuse injury of lateral knee - Seen with athletes, runners, cyclists	- **Pain over lateral femoral epicondyle** where IT band inserts - Insidious onset, occurring only during activity, becoming more persistent	Dx: Clinical Tx: NSAIDs, PT
Pes Anserine Bursitis	- Pain at site of insertion of **conjoined tendon** (sartorius, gracilis, semitendinosus), associated with obesity/OA	- **Tenderness over upper/medial tibia**	Dx: Clinical. XR (to look for OA) Tx: NSAIDs, PT, weight loss
Prepatellar Bursitis	- Inflamed patellar bursa - Risk: Trauma, infection, or arthritis	- Focal swelling, erythema, and tenderness anterior to the patella/patella tendon	Dx: Aspiration (r/o infection) Tx: NSAIDs, activity modification, and bracing
Patellofemoral Pain	- Common cause of knee pain, especially in young adults	- **Pain located behind patella, worse with weight bearing** - (+) Patellofemoral compression test	Dx: Clinical Tx: PT (strength training for quads/hip muscles)
Baker Cyst	- Fluid buildup in semimembranosus/ gastroc bursa - Risk: Knee trauma, arthritis	- **Bulge behind knee**, that may cause posterior knee pain/stiffness - Can dissect into calf (presents like DVT) - **Rupture**: Calf pain, warmth, erythema	Dx: Clinical (US if unsure) Tx: Treat underlying knee disease, steroid injection
Knee (Ligament injuries)			
ACL Tear	- Noncontact injury, commonly with change of direction, with planting of leg and accidental lateral bending (valgus stress) on the knee - **"Unhappy Triad"**: ACL/MCL/Medial meniscus injuries	- **"Pop" in knee, instability, and pain** - Effusion/swelling quickly after injury - Lachman test (30° of flexion) has highest sens/spec. Anterior drawer classically used.	Dx: MRI Tx: - Can treat conservatively (but ↑ risk of OA, ligamentous injury) - Surgery (for athletes, or multi-ligament tears)
PCL Tear	- Posterior force directed at flexed knee, seen with MVC or sports (but rare)	- Can present with pain, swelling, instability (highly variable, because often have multiple other associated injuries) - Posterior drawer test (+)	Dx: MRI Tx: RICE, physical therapy/rehab
Meniscus Tear	- Can occur from acute, twisting trauma to the knee, or due to chronic degenerative process if older	- Pain along the medial or lateral aspect of the knee, worse with twisting movements - **Popping/catching or instability** (knee "giving out") - **McMurray's test** (+)	Dx: MRI Tx: Can be treated conservatively or surgically corrected (if bad symptoms or athlete)
MCL Injury	- Injured by valgus stress to knee - Ranges from minor injury (grade I) to complete tear (grade III)	- **Tenderness over MCL, pain, instability** - Increased joint space opening upon valgus stress test	Dx: MRI Tx: RICE, physical therapy/rehab
LCL Injury	- Rare, often occur with other knee injuries - Due to blow to the medial part of knee	- **Tenderness over LCL, pain, instability** - Increased joint space opening upon varus stress test	Dx: MRI Tx: RICE, physical therapy/rehab

Musculoskeletal: Lower Ext

	General	Clinical	Management
Shin/Ankle			
Medial Tibial Stress Syndrome	- **"Shin Splints"** - Risk: Excessive physical activity (running)	- **Pain along the medial tibia** (**diffuse**, vs point tenderness of stress fracture) - Worse with activity	Dx: Clinical Tx: Activity reduction, ice
Ankle Sprain	- Most commonly injury to **ATFL**, from inversion injury (medial sided deltoid ligaments rarely damaged) - Classifications: Grade 1: Stretching/microscopic tear Grade 2: Incomplete tear Grade 3: Complete tear	- **Swelling, ecchymosis, tenderness over lateral ankle** - History of traumatic mechanism consistent with sprain	Dx: Clinical. XR if meets Ottawa. Ottawa ankle rules (for XR) - Focal bony tenderness over distal 6 cm of either malleolus - Unable to weight bear Tx: RICE, physical therapy
Achilles Tendinopathy/ Rupture	- Tendinopathy is from chronic overuse - Rupture occurs acutely, with explosive movement	- Pain or stiffness in area 2-5 cm superior to the calcaneus - Worse with activity, improves with rest - **Rupture**: Acute pain, swelling, complete loss of plantar flexion	Dx: Clinical Tx: Physical therapy, stretching for tendinopathy. Surgery for ruptures.
Foot			
Plantar Fasciitis	- Pain caused by the plantar fascia, possibly due to the development of bone spurs - Risk: Obesity, excessive standing, flat feet	- **Pain in heel, worse with walking** - Point tenderness over the heel on exam	Dx: Clinical Tx: Activity modification, shoe inserts, stretching, short course of NSAIDs
Morton Neuroma	- Benign interdigital growth from chronic nerve entrapment	- Numbness/burning pain between **3rd/4th distal metatarsal** - Clicking sensation when palpating this space	Dx: US Tx: Orthotics or other pressure unloading devices

Musculoskeletal: Neurovascular

Brachial Plexus Lesions

Roots	Clinical Manifestation
Upper trunk (C5-C6) **Erb Palsy**	- Often occurs during infant delivery (lateral traction on neck) or due to trauma in adults - Presents as **adduction/internal rotation of the arm** (supra/infraspinatus, deltoid weakness) - Tx: PT/observation for recovery, with surgery if no improvement
Lower trunk (C8-T1) **Klumpke Palsy**	- Risk: Traumatic birth, trying to catch something while falling - Paralysis of intrinsic hand muscles, resulting in **claw like grasp**, +/– Horner syndrome
Entire plexus (C5-T1)	- Complete arm paralysis

Thoracic Outlet Syndrome

General: Collection of syndromes from neurovascular compression in thoracic outlet (area between first rib/behind clavicle). Can have different presentations depending on nerve, arterial, or venous involvement.

Risk: Rib/muscle abnormalities (trauma, congenital, repetitive movements)

Clinical:

- **Neuro**: UE pain, weakness, paresthesias. Muscle atrophy (if chronic).
- **Arterial**: Presents with thromboembolism to extremity (pain, pallor, cool)
- **Venous**: UE venous thrombosis, swelling, cyanosis

Diagnosis: CT/MRI, US, or electrodiagnostic testing (depending on subtype)

Management:

- Nerve: Conservative (PT). If refractory → Thoracic decompression.
- Arterial: Embolectomy, thoracic decompression, anticoagulation
- Venous: Thrombolysis, thoracic decompression, anticoagulation

Specific Nerve Lesions

Nerve	Clinical Manifestation
Upper Extremity	
Axillary	- **Sensory loss over lateral shoulder** - Risk: Shoulder trauma (dislocation, humeral head fracture)
Radial	- **Wrist drop**, weakness of wrist/finger extensors, sensory loss over back of hand - Risk: Compression of nerve in spinal groove ("Saturday night palsy"), or injury with midshaft humeral fracture
Long thoracic	- **Winged scapula** (ask to press arms against wall) - Risk: Trauma, or iatrogenic (breast surgery)
Lower Extremity	
Lateral femoral cutaneous	- **Meralgia paresthetica** (paresthesias/pain radiating down lateral thigh) - Risk: Compression (under inguinal ligament)
Superior gluteal	- **Trendelenburg gait** (pelvis tilts on downward on the side contralateral to the lesion) - Risk: Iatrogenic (surgery or injection in upper medial gluteus)
Common peroneal	- **Foot drop, steppage gait**, sensory loss over dorsum of foot/lateral shin - Risk: Compression at point nerve wraps around fibula (at knee), most commonly from prolonged immobilization/pressure or casting
Posterior tibial	- **Tarsal tunnel syndrome** (compression of nerve at ankle as it passes under tarsal ligament) - Presents as paresthesias/sensory loss over the plantar surface of foot/toes - Risk: Trauma (fracture/dislocation), arthritis

Rheumatology Pharm

	Mechanism	Indication	Side Effects/Management
Anti-inflammatory			
Acetaminophen	- COX inhibitor of CNS (mostly inactivated peripherally)	- Analgesia - Antipyretic	- Hepatotoxic (at high doses)
NSAID Ibuprofen Naproxen Indomethacin Ketorolac Diclofenac Meloxicam	- Reversibly inhibit COX1/COX2	- Analgesia - Antipyretic - Anti-inflammatory	- Gastritis/PUD (resulting in GI bleeds) - Renal: Interstitial nephritis, ischemia, prerenal AKI (vasoconstriction of afferent arteriole) - Increased risk of cardiovascular events
Celecoxib	- Reversibly inhibits COX2, spares COX1 (platelet effects)	- Analgesia, anti-inflammatory	- Increased risk of cardiovascular events
Colchicine	- Inhibit microtubule polymerization (↓ neutrophil chemotaxis and degranulation)	- Anti-inflammatory (gout, familial mediterranean fever)	- GI issues (**diarrhea**, nausea, vomiting) - Agranulocytosis
Hypouricemic			
Allopurinol	- Inhibits xanthine oxidase	- Gout - Tumor lysis syndrome	- Hypersensitivity reactions (SJS/TEN) - Myelosuppression, hepatitis
Febuxostat	- Inhibits xanthine oxidase		- Increased death/MI (compared to allopurinol)
Probenecid	- Inhibits tubular resorption of uric acid in PCT		- Inhibition of renal tubular anion channels (reduces excretion of many drugs) - Uric acid nephrolithiasis
Pegloticase Rasburicase	- Recombinant uricase that catalyzes uric acid to water soluble product	- Tumor lysis syndrome	- Methemoglobinemia (if G6PDH deficiency)
Bones			
Bisphosphonate Alendronate Ibandronate Risedronate Zoledronate (IV)	- Pyrophosphate analog that inhibits osteoclastic activity, induce apoptosis	- Osteoporosis - Hypercalcemia - Paget of bone - Metastatic bone disease	- **Esophagitis** (drink with water, stay upright 30 minutes, empty stomach) - **Jaw osteonecrosis** (in those with high doses, most commonly cancer patients) - ↑ risk for atypical femur fractures - Bone/joint pain
Teriparatide	- Recombinant PTH analog given subcutaneously	- Osteoporosis	- Transient hypercalcemia
Abaloparatide	- PTHrP analog	- Osteoporosis	
Calcitonin	- Antagonizes parathyroid hormone effects (inhibits osteoclastic bone resorption) - Administered intranasally	- Hypercalcemia - Osteoporosis (second-line agent)	- Hypocalcemia - Rhinitis
Denosumab	- RANK-L antagonist	- Hypercalcemia (malignancy) - Osteoporosis - Prevention of skeletal events metastasis or myeloma	- ↑ Infection risk - Jaw osteonecrosis - ↑ risk for atypical femur fractures - Bone/joint pain
Romosozumab	- Anti-sclerostin antibody	- Osteoporosis	

Rheumatology Pharm

	Mechanism	Indication	Side Effects/Management
DMARD (Disease-Modifying Anti-Rheumatic Drugs)			
Methotrexate	- Folic acid analog, inhibiting dihydrofolate reductase, ↓ DNA production	- Rheumatoid arthritis - Autoimmune conditions	- Myelosuppression (reversible with use of leucovorin) - Hepatotoxicity - Stomatitis - Pneumonitis/fibrosis
Leflunomide	- Inhibits pyrimidine synthesis		- Hepatotoxicity - Teratogen
Hydroxychloroquine	- Immunosuppression via impaired neutrophil chemotaxis and complement activity		- Retinal toxicity
Sulfasalazine	- Unclear MOA, but known immunosuppressive effects		- Hypersensitivity (sulfa drug) - Megaloblastic anemia/↓ folate absorption - Hemolytic anemia (G6PDH deficiency)
Biologic Anti-Rheumatic Agents			
Adalimumab Certolizumab Etanercept Infliximab	- TNF inhibitors	- Rheumatoid arthritis - Severe psoriasis - IBD	- Opportunistic infections (including reactivation of TB, fungal infections)
Anakinra	- IL-1 receptor antagonist	- Rheumatoid arthritis	- ↑ infection risk - Neutropenia
Tocilizumab	- IL-6 receptor antagonist	- Rheumatoid arthritis - Juvenile idiopathic arthritis - Temporal arteritis	- ↑ infection risk (including increased URIs)
Abatacept	- T-cell costimulation modulator	- Rheumatoid arthritis	- ↑ infection risk

Dermatology Basics

Physical Exam/Terms

Morphology	Features	Example
Macule	- Flat lesion < 1 cm in diameter	- Freckle
Patch	- Flat lesion > 1 cm in diameter	- Cafe-au-lait spot
Papule	- Elevated lesion < 1 cm in diameter	- Acne
Plaque	- Flat, elevated lesion > 1 cm in diameter	- Psoriasis
Vesicle	- Fluid containing lesion < 1 cm	- Chickenpox
Bullae	- Fluid containing lesion > 1 cm	- Bullous pemphigoid
Nodule	- Solid, round, raised dermal lesion	- Erythema nodosum
Pustule	- Vesicle containing purulent fluid	- Folliculitis
Wheal	- Transient, edematous papule or plaque	- Urticaria
Petechiae	- Flat, nonblanching red spot < 3 mm	- Thrombocytopenia
Purpura	- Flat, nonblanching red spot 3-10 mm	- Thrombocytopenia
Ecchymosis	- Flat, nonblanching red spot > 10 mm	- Bruise
Scale	- Flaking off of skin	- Eczema
Crust (serum)	- Dry exudate	- Impetigo
Lichenification	- Thickening of skin	- Lichen simplex chronicus
Erosion	- Partial loss of epidermis	- Minor skin trauma
Ulceration	- Full thickness loss of epidermis	- Pressure ulcer
Hyperkeratosis	- Increased thickness of stratum corneum	- Callus
Parakeratosis	- Hyperkeratosis + retained nuclei in corneum	- Psoriasis
Acanthosis	- Epidermal hyperplasia	- Acanthosis nigricans
Acantholysis	- Loss of adhesion of epithelial cells	- Pemphigus vulgaris

Topical Steroids

Group	Class	Drugs (selected options)
Mild	Classes 6 and 7	- Hydrocortisone acetate 1% (OTC)
Intermediate	Classes 4 and 5	- Triamcinolone acetonide 0.1%
Potent	Classes 2 and 3	- Fluocinonide 0.05%
Super Potent	Class 1	- Clobetasol propionate 0.05% - Betamethasone dipropionate (augmented) 0.05%

General Rules:

- Steroids prescribed for 14-day course once or twice daily
- High-potency steroids are avoided on face and intertriginous areas
- Adverse effects: Cutaneous atrophy, telangiectasias, and striae with overuse

Pigmented Skin Disorders

	Clinical Presentation	Diagnosis/Management
Hyperpigmented Lesions		
Freckle (Ephelides)	- Hyperpigmented macule from enlarged melanosomes - Seen in fair-skinned children, worse with sun exposure	- Benign - Often fade with time
Lentigo	- Hyperpigmented macule from ↑ melanocyte activity - Can be simple (idiopathic, seen in kids) or **solar** ("liver spots," associated with sun exposure)	- Benign
Cafe-au-lait Spot[A]	- Hyperpigmented macule from ↑ melanogenesis - Congenital or acquired at young age - Associated with McCune-Albright, NF1	- Benign
Melasma	- Acquired hyperpigmentation of sun-exposed skin of face - Associated with pregnancy	- Sunscreen - Hydroquinone/steroid cream
Hypopigmented Lesions		
Albinism	- Group of AR-inherited disorders (often tyrosinase enzyme) of abnormal melanin biosynthesis - Presents with **lack of pigmentation** of skin, hair, and eyes - Abnormal vision	- Skin sun protection - Eye care
Vitiligo	- Acquired disorder of hypopigmentation from loss of melanocytes - Asymptomatic **depigmented patches throughout the body** - Associated with hypothyroidism, IBD, alopecia, psoriasis	- UVB light - Topical or systemic steroids
Tinea Versicolor[B]	- Common fungal skin infection seen in young adults - Caused by ***Malassezia*** - Often seen in hot/humid climates - Well demarcated hyper or hypopigmented lesions of trunk and extremities	Dx: KOH prep of skin scraping (hyphae and yeast balls) Tx: Topical azoles, selenium sulfide, or zinc pyrithione * Lesions take months to resolve
Idiopathic Guttate Hypomelanosis	- Common acquired hypopigmentation disorder of older adults - Presents with diffuse **small, round white macules** - Asymptomatic other than cosmetic change	- Benign, but generally progressive - No clear treatment

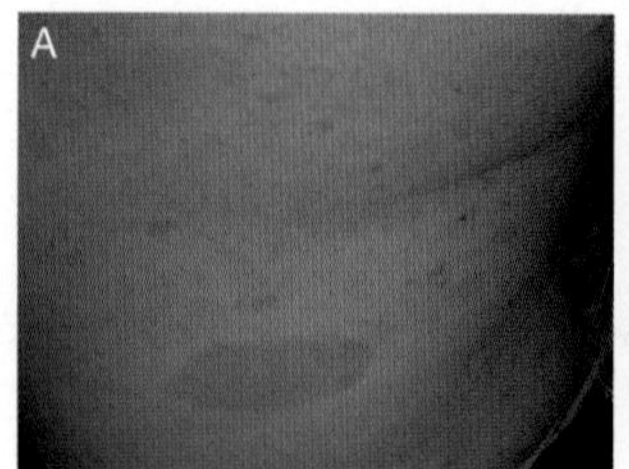

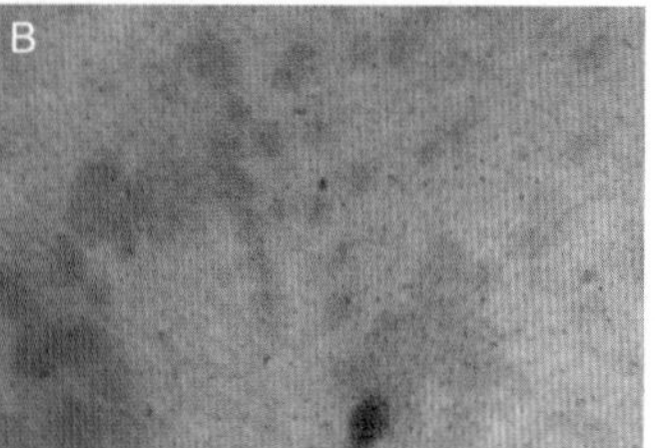

Benign Skin Disorders

	Clinical Presentation	Diagnosis/Management
Pityriasis		
Pityriasis rosea	- Exanthematous skin condition believed due to HSV-7 - Presents with **herald patch**[A] (single, large oval-shaped pink lesion), followed days later by smaller lesions on the trunk and proximal extremities (**"Christmas tree"** pattern) - Itching common	- Self-limited (resolves in 6-8 weeks) - Topical steroids for itching
Pityriasis alba	- Dermatitis (often post inflammatory) with decreased melanocyte activity - Presents with asymptomatic, fine scaled patches of hypopigmentation on the trunk, face, proximal extremities	- Self-limited - Topical steroids
Dry Skin/Scaling Disorders		
Xerosis (Dry skin)	- Common condition of **dry skin**, seen in winter months (with cold and low humidity) - Presents with scaling rash, pruritus, and fissures	- Topical emollients
Ichthyosis	- Chronic inherited skin disorder (most commonly of filaggrin gene) - Presents in **childhood as rough, scaly dry skin**	- Topical emollients *If severe: keratolytics (coal tar, salicylic acid) or topical retinoids
Cysts		
Milium	- Keratin cysts that arise from **clogged eccrine sweat ducts** - Present as 1-2 mm white papules (often on face)	- Benign - Excision if bothersome
Epidermoid Cyst **("Sebaceous Cyst")**	- Benign **keratin producing squamous epithelium nodule** - Dome-shaped freely mobile nodule, with central punctum - Can produce cheesy white discharge - Can become irritated and infected	- Often resolve spontaneously - Can be excised (cosmetic) or I&D (if infected)
Pilar Cyst	- Arise from hair follicle - Firm **subcutaneous nodules** on the **scalp**	- Excision if bothersome
Nodules		
Dermatofibroma	- Idiopathic, benign nodule from fibroblast proliferation - Firm, **hyperpigmented nodule, +/– central buttonhole**	- No treatment indicated - Excision if bothersome
Erythema Nodosum	- Delayed-type hypersensitivity resulting in **panniculitis** (inflammation of all dermal layers) - Associated with **sarcoidosis**, IBD, TB, strep, Behcet, coccidiomycosis - **Painful, erythematous, tender nodule** on the legs	- Self-limited (resolves over weeks)
Acrochordon (Skin Tag)	- Benign outgrowth of normal skin - Presents as nodule on stalk	- Excision if bothersome

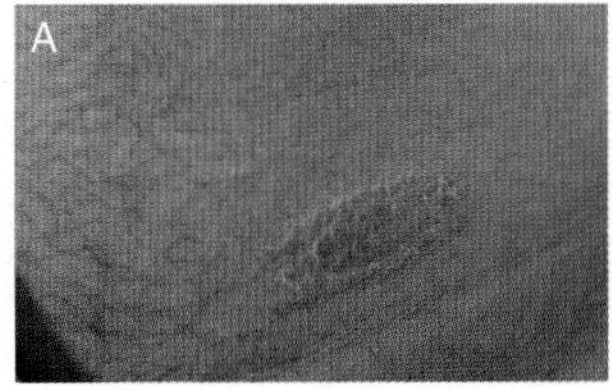

Benign Skin Disorders

	Clinical Presentation	Diagnosis/Management
Common Skin Lesions		
Seborrheic Keratosis[A]	- Common benign epidermal lesion caused proliferation of immature keratinocyte - Round, hyperpigmented, warty lesions with **stuck-on appearance** (can be pink or brown) - Generally asymptomatic, but can get irritated, itch, or bleed - **Leser-Trelat sign**: Appearance of multiple SKs, associated with underlying malignancy	- No treatment required - Cryo or excision if cosmetic concern
Actinic Keratosis	- Proliferation of atypical epidermal keratinocytes - Associated with **excessive sun exposure** - **Premalignant** (SCC) - Scaly, erythematous papules in area of chronic sun exposure	- Surgical excision or cryotherapy - Topical 5-FU for multiple lesions
Acanthosis Nigricans	- Epidermal hyperplasia causing symmetric, **velvety hyperpigmented thickening of skin** - Associated with insulin resistance (obesity, diabetes, PCOS) and occult malignancy	- Workup and treat underlying cause
Lipoma	- Benign proliferation of mature adipocytes (most common benign soft-tissue neoplasms) - Presents with **mobile subcutaneous nodule**	- Treatment not indicated - Excise if bothersome

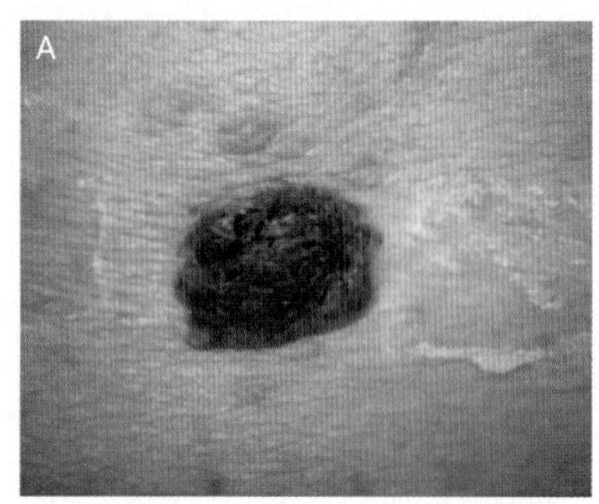

Inflammatory Skin Disorders

Acne Vulgaris

General: Acne is a common inflammatory disorder of the pilosebaceous unit. Pathogenesis involves follicular hyperkeratinization (obstructs sebaceous follicles), sebum production, *Propionibacterium acnes* proliferating in follicle, and inflammation.

Risk: Young adults, hyperandrogenism

Clinical: Lesions most common on **face, neck, chest, back**

- Open comedones (blackheads)
- Closed comedones (whiteheads)
- Inflammatory papules, pustules, or nodules
- Can lead to postinflammatory hyperpigmentation and scarring

Diagnosis: Clinical. Workup for hyperandrogenism if clinical signs.

Management:

Subtype	Description	Intervention
Comedonal	- Closed or open comedones	- Topical retinoids (tretinoin, adapalene) - Salicylic or azelaic acid
Inflammatory	- Inflamed, red papules/pustules	- Topical antimicrobial (Benzoyl peroxide, clindamycin) - Topical retinoids Refractory disease: - Oral antibiotics - Hormonal therapy (OCPs, spironolactone) - Isotretinoin (teratogen, need two negative pregnancy tests and two forms of contraception to use)
Nodular	- Large, cystic appearing nodules	

Rosacea

General: Chronic condition with unknown pathophysiology that classically causes facial redness in middle-aged individuals

Clinical:

- **Erythematous skin over the cheeks**[A] with flushing, telangiectasias
- Phymatous changes (thick skin, rhinophyma, bulbous appearance of nose)
- Papules, pustules
- Burning, stinging sensations, edema, and dryness
- Ocular involvement (in about half of patients)
    - Conjunctival injection, lid telangiectasias, scleritis

Diagnosis: Clinical

Management:

- Behavioral modification (sun protection, avoid triggers like alcohol/sunlight)
- Facial erythema: Topical brimonidine or laser therapy
- Papules/pustules: Topical antibiotics (metronidazole) or PO tetracycline if severe

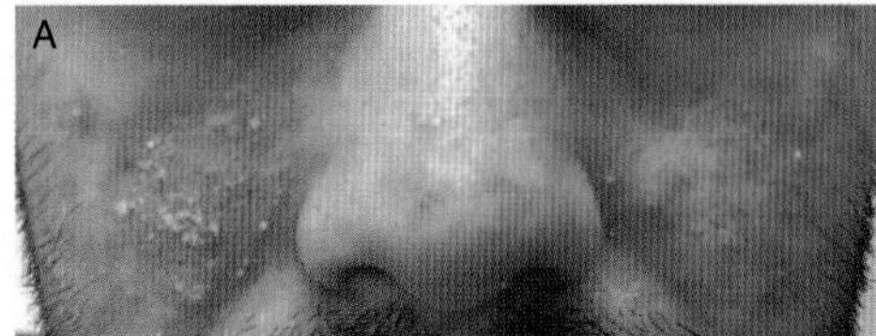

Inflammatory Skin Disorders

	Clinical Presentation	Diagnosis/Management
Seborrheic Dermatitis	- Chronic, relapsing dermatitis in areas with sebaceous glands - Possibly associated with *Malassezia* Clinical - Mild: **Scaly, flaky scalp rash** (dandruff) - Severe: Yellowish, oily, thick flakes at hairline, ears, skin folds - **"Cradle Cap"** in infants	- Mild: Ketoconazole (zinc pyrithione/ selenium sulfide) shampoo - Severe: Ketoconazole shampoo + topical high potency corticosteroid - Infants: Emollients
Allergic Dermatitis (Eczema)	- Common childhood pruritic inflammatory skin disease - Risk: Personal/family history of **atopy**, low humidity - Clinical: Presents as **pruritic, scaly dry erythematous rash** - Extensor surface at young age, flexor surfaces when older - Lichenified plaques at older ages	- Topical **corticosteroids, emollients.** Topical calcineurin inhibitor if severe. - Complications: Cellulitis, eczema herpeticum (vesicular eruption over eczema, treat with acyclovir)
Allergic Contact Dermatitis	- Type IV hypersensitivity reaction against allergen (poison ivy, oak, iodine, rubber, nickel, other metal) - Acute: **Erythematous papules and vesicles with oozing** - Severe pruritus - Chronic: Skin thickening, excoriations	- Identify/avoid allergen - Topical corticosteroids - Oral corticosteroids if > 20% of body surface OR need rapid improvement
Irritant Contact Dermatitis	- Local inflammatory skin response to chemical/physical agent - Agents include detergents, acids, alkalis, metal, wood - Skin **erythema, edema, vesicle formation** - Most commonly on hands	- Topical corticosteroid, emollient - Avoid irritant exposure
Lichen Planus	- Chronic inflammatory mucocutaneous disorder - Associated with hepatitis C - Skin lesions: **Pruritic, polygonal, purple, papules/plaques** - **White, lace-like pattern** (Wickham striae) - Can also involve scalp (alopecia), oral mucosa (ulcers or Wickham striae), genitals	- High potency topical steroids - Systemic steroids or phototherapy if extensive

Psoriasis

General: Chronic inflammatory skin disease causing plaques, from epidermal hyperproliferation and immune dysregulation

Clinical:

- **Well-demarcated, erythematous plaques with silver scale**[A]
    - Auspitz sign: Pinpoint bleeding after removing scale
- Most common on extensor surface of knee/elbow, scalp, gluteal cleft
- Certain subtypes can result in pustules, nail involvement, or "reverse" psoriasis (involvement of intertriginous areas rather than extensors)

Diagnosis: Clinical. Biopsy (if uncertain) reveals epidermal hyperplasia, parakeratosis, neutrophils in the stratum corneum.

Management:

Mild-moderate	- Topical steroids, emollients - Alternative: Topical vitamin D (calcipotriene), topical retinoids, tar
Moderate-severe	- UV light therapy PLUS topical therapy (as above) - Systemic therapy (refractory cases): Methotrexate, cyclosporine, biologics (anti-TNFα, IL-17, IL-23)

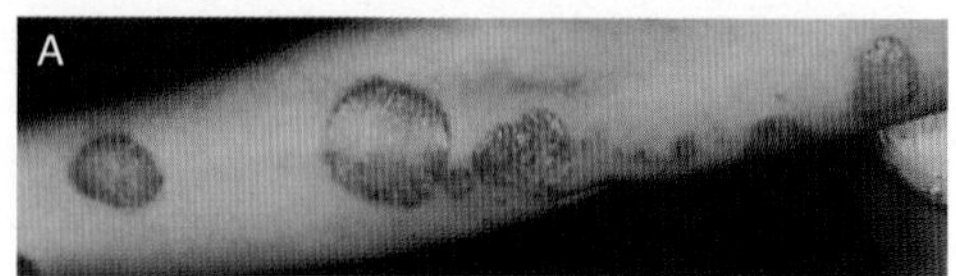

Inflammatory Skin Disorders

Drug Eruptions

General: Adverse reactions to drugs can cause a diverse set of dermatologic eruptions. Differential includes:

- Drug-induced exanthems
- DRESS
- Erythema multiforme or SJS/TEN
- Erythroderma
- Urticaria/angioedema/anaphylaxis
- Cutaneous small vessel vasculitis/serum sickness
- Photosensitivity

Condition	Clinical Features	Management
Drug-Induced Exanthem	- **Morbilliform or maculopapular drug eruption**[A] - Most common adverse drug reaction - Presents within 3-14 days of med use with diffuse maculopapular rash, predominantly on trunk/proximal extremities	- Withdraw offending drug - Antihistamines and topical corticosteroids for symptoms
Serum Sickness	- Immune complex formation due to antibody formation against nonhuman protein (type III hypersensitivity) - Common causes include monoclonal/chimeric antibodies (Rituximab, anti-thymocyte globulin) - Serum sickness "like" reactions seen with a variety of drugs (penicillins, TMP-SMX, cefaclor) - Presents with fever, rash, and polyarthritis within 1-2 weeks of drug exposure	- Withdraw offending agent - Supportive care - Systemic steroids if severe
DRESS (Drug reaction with eosinophilia and systemic symptoms)	- T-cell mediated hypersensitivity to certain drugs (most commonly sulfa drugs, antiepileptics, and allopurinol) <u>Clinical</u>: (2-8 weeks after med) - Constitutional: **Fever**, lymphadenopathy - Skin: **Morbilliform skin eruption** - Heme: **Eosinophilia**, atypical lymphocytosis - Liver: **Drug-induced liver injury** - Lung: Pneumonitis - Renal: Interstitial nephritis	- Withdraw offending drug - Topical steroids (for skin) - Systemic steroids (for lung/kidney involvement)

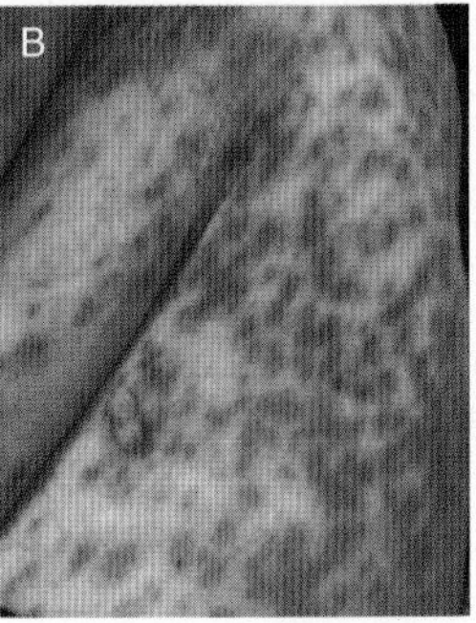

Inflammatory Skin Disorders

Erythema Multiforme

General: Immune-mediated disorder (type IV hypersensitivity) against an infectious or drug antigen that results in cutaneous/ mucosal lesions

Etiology:

- **HSV** (most common cause)
- Other infections: *Mycoplasma*, HIV, VZV, EBV
- Drugs: NSAIDs, sulfa drugs, antiepileptics, antibiotics

Clinical:

- Cutaneous: **Erythematous papules, vesicles, target lesions**[A]
  - Target lesions have dusky center, red inflammatory zone, ring of edema, and an erythematous halo
  - Generally starts on extremities with centripetal spread
- Mucosal lesions common

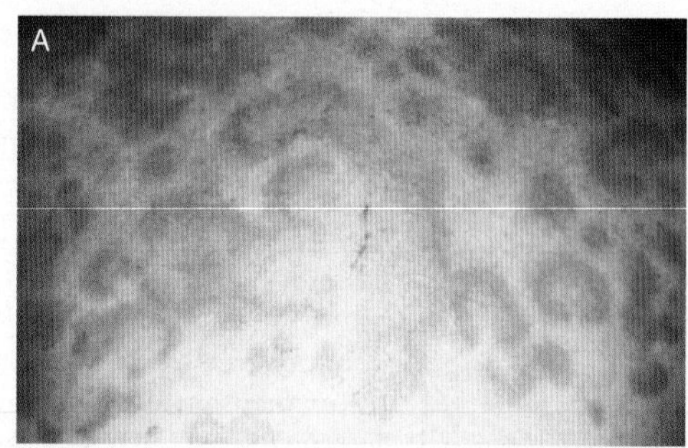

Diagnosis: Clinical. Biopsy if unsure.

Management:

- Self-limited (resolves in ~ 2 weeks)
- Supportive care (topical corticosteroids, antihistamines)

Stevens-Johnson Syndrome/Toxic Epidermal Necrolysis

General: Mucocutaneous reaction with extensive necrosis and epidermal sloughing

- SJS: < 10% of body surface involved
- SJS/TEN Overlap: 10-30% of body surface involved
- TEN: > 30% of body surface involved

Etiology:

- Drugs: Allopurinol, sulfa drugs, NSAIDs, sulfasalazine, lamotrigine, anticonvulsants
- *Mycoplasma* infection

* Risk is increased in those with malignancy or HIV

Clinical: Generally within 1 month of exposure

- **Influenza-like prodrome** (high fever, myalgias, malaise) 3 days prior to rash
- Cutaneous lesions: **Erythematous macules and vesicles**
  - Very painful skin to touch
- Skin sloughing (within days of onset)
- Mucosal erosions
- Ocular: Conjunctivitis, bullae, corneal ulceration, uveitis all possible
- Urogenital ulcers

Diagnosis: Clinical. Biopsy (if diagnosis uncertain).

Management:

- Withdraw offending agent
- Supportive care at burn center (wound care, fluids, treat pain, infection prevention)
- Adjunctive cyclosporine or corticosteroids

Inflammatory Skin Disorders

Allergic Skin Reactions

Condition	Clinical Features	Management
Urticaria	- **Edematous, fleeting wheals that cause intense pruritus** Caused by: - IgE response to antigen (latex, food, insect bite, drugs) - Direct mast cell activation (IV contrast, certain drugs [opiates]) - Certain viral or bacterial infections - NSAIDs	- Antihistamines - Oral glucocorticoids if severe
Angioedema	- **Edematous swelling of lips, tongue, throat, larynx** - Can also affect GI tract (nausea, emesis, abdominal pain) - Life-threatening if airway compromised Subtypes: - **Mast-Cell Mediated** (allergic reaction) - **Bradykinin Mediated** (ACEi)	- Protect airway - Antihistamines (mild cases) - Glucocorticoids - Epinephrine (severe) - If Bradykinin mediated: C1 inhibitor concentrate, icatibant, or FFP

Erythroderma (Exfoliative Dermatitis)

General: Diffuse erythema and scaling of ≥ 90% of body surface area, caused by a variety of underlying conditions (Note: Erythroderma is not a diagnosis, but rather a clinical sign/manifestation of condition)

Etiology:

- Exacerbation of dermatologic condition (psoriasis or atopic dermatitis)
- Hypersensitivity drug reaction (Penicillins, sulfa, etc.)
- Cutaneous T-cell lymphoma (mycosis fungoides)

Clinical:

- **Diffuse, uniformly red, warm skin on > 90% of body**
- Severe pain or itching
- Systemic symptoms (fever, chills, malaise) may be present
- Loss of fluids/electrolytes, ↑ perfusion of skin (may result in heart failure)

Diagnosis: Clinical

Management:

- Discontinue any potentially offending medications
- Supportive (fluids/electrolytes, support hemodynamics, monitor temp)
- Topical steroids/antihistamines for skin symptoms

Blistering Skin Disorders

Bullous Pemphigoid/Pemphigus Vulgaris

	Bullous Pemphigoid	Pemphigus Vulgaris
Gen	- Subepithelial bullous disorder of older adults - Autoantibody against basement membrane hemidesmosome protein (BP180/BP230, also known as BPAg)	- Intraepithelial bullous disorder with characteristic acantholysis - Autoantibody against intracellular keratinocyte adhesion molecules (desmoglein)
Clin	- **Large (> 1 cm) tense bullae** (Nikolsky sign [-])[A] - Trunks/extremities most commonly impacted - Preceded by prodrome of itchy, erythematous plaques (similar to eczematous dermatitis)	- **Flaccid blisters, which easily rupture**, leading to painful erosions (Nikolsky sign [+]) - Mucosal involvement (most common is oral mucosa, which leave painful ulcers)
Dx	- Biopsy (direct immunofluorescence showing **linear** basement membrane Ig deposition) - Serology (ELISA for anti-BM Ig)	- Biopsy (direct immunofluorescence showing **reticular** intercellular Ig deposition) - Serology (for anti-desmoglein Ig)
Tx	- Acute: High-potency topical steroids (systemic if cannot do topical) - Chronic: Often requires steroid-sparing agent (MTX, mycophenolate, azathioprine, dapsone, tetracycline)	- Acute: Systemic corticosteroids +/– Rituximab - Chronic: Immunosuppression (azathioprine or mycophenolate)

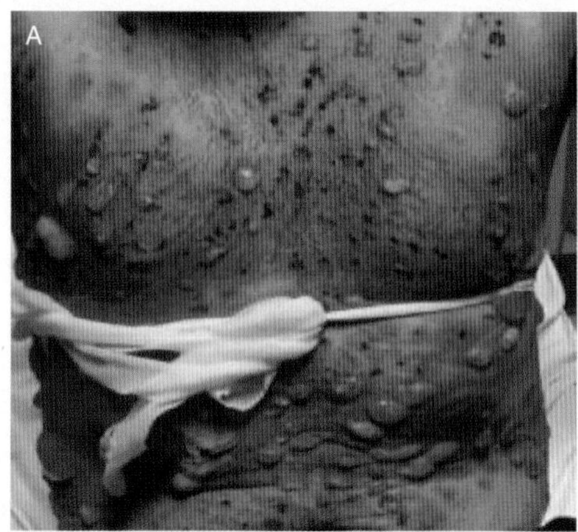

Dermatitis Herpetiformis

General: Autoimmune cutaneous eruption associated with Celiac (gluten sensitivity)

Clinical:

- **Pruritic skin eruption of papules and vesicles**
- Excoriations and erosions from itching
- Extremities, buttocks, back, scalp involvement

Diagnosis: Biopsy (direct immunofluorescence showing **IgA in the papillary dermis**)

- Celiac serology often positive. Universally all patients carry HLA DQ2/DQ8.

Management: Gluten-free diet, dapsone

Sun-Related Skin Disorders

Sunburn

General: Inflammatory skin reaction to exposure to excessive ultraviolet radiation. Repeated episodes increase risk for **skin cancer**. Also leads to:

- **Photoaging**: ↑ wrinkles and skin discoloration
- **Senile purpura**: Ecchymotic lesions on sun-damaged skin in older adults

Etiology:

- Natural sunlight
- Tanning beds or phototherapy

Clinical:

- Painful, erythematous skin within 24 hours of sun exposure
- Edema, blisters, and eventual skin sloughing all common

Management:

- Mild/moderate: Cool compress, NSAIDs, aloe vera or calamine
- Severe: Hospitalization for fluids and analgesia

Prevention:

- Wear protective clothing, avoid sun at peak hours
- Apply sunscreen (SPF ≥ 30) 30 minutes before going outside (reapply every 2 hours)

Photosensitivity/Photoallergic Reactions

Type	Features
Polymorphous Light Eruption	- Common rash (also known as sun-poisoning) that occurs with UV light exposure - Presents with **pruritic papular rash** in sun-exposed area within days of sun exposure
Phototoxicity	- Drug reaction, in which drug absorbs UV light in skin, and gives off energy, damaging surrounding tissue - Causes include tetracyclines, sulfa drugs, NSAIDs - Presents similarly to sunburn, but reaction occurs more quickly and with greater severity than expected with typical sunburn
Photoallergic	- Delayed hypersensitivity with reaction to drug metabolites produced after sun exposure - Causes include topical agents (sunscreens, fragrances), other systemic drugs - Presents with **itchy, eczematous eruptions**

Other causes of sun-related skin reactions:

- Solar urticaria (hives with sun exposure)
- Porphyria
- Autoimmune (SLE/drug-induced lupus/dermatomyositis)

Infectious Skin Disorders

	Clinical Presentation	Diagnosis/Management
Viral Skin Infections		
Warts	HPV 1-4. Subtypes: - **Common wart (verruca vulgaris)** - Flat wart (verruca plana) - Plantar wart (verruca plantaris) - Present as **flesh colored hyperkeratotic lesion**, can cause pain/discomfort	- Salicylic acid or cryotherapy
Molluscum Contagiosum	- **Poxvirus.** Transmitted skin to skin (highly contagious). - Can grow rapidly/large in immunosuppressed patients - Small papules (2–5 mm) with central umbilication, sparing palm/sole	- Cryotherapy, curettage, or podophyllin
Herpes Zoster (Shingles)	- Reactivation of VZV (must have had VZV previously) - Severe pain (neuritis) and **vesicular rash in a dermatomal distribution**[A] Complications: - Post-herpetic neuralgia (lingering neuropathic pain) - VZV ophthalmicus or oticus	- Acyclovir or valacyclovir (if within 72 hours of symptoms or new lesions still appearing) - Only contagious to those without VZV in past or immunocompromised - Recurrent disease much more common in immunocompromised
Fungal Skin Infections		
Candidal Intertrigo	- Burning **red plaques in the skin folds** with surrounding satellite macules - Inframammary fold, gluteal cleft, inguinal creases, under abdominal pannus	Dx: Clinical. KOH prep/fungal culture can confirm. Tx: Topical azoles or nystatin
Dermatophyte (tinea) infections - Caused by *Trichophyton, Microsporum*, and *Epidermophyton* - Diagnosis is generally clinical, but confirmation with KOH prep is recommended		
Tinea corporis [Ringworm]	- Risk: Skin-to-skin contact, infected animals, humidity - Presents as scaly, erythematous annular plaque, central clearing, pruritus	- Topical azoles or terbinafine
Tinea capitis	- Scaly scalp patches with alopecia, pruritus - Wood's lamp fluoresces if microsporum	- Oral griseofulvin or terbinafine
Tinea unguium Onychomycosis	- Fungal nail infection, with thickened, discolored nails, subungual debris, and separation of nail plate from bed	- Oral terbinafine (alt: Azoles)
Tinea pedis [Athlete foot]	- Interdigital, moccasin, and vesiculobullous subtypes - Redness, scaling between toes and on the foot	- Topical azoles or terbinafine
Tinea cruris [Jock itch]	- Erythematous plaques in medial thigh, perineal areas	- Topical azoles or terbinafine

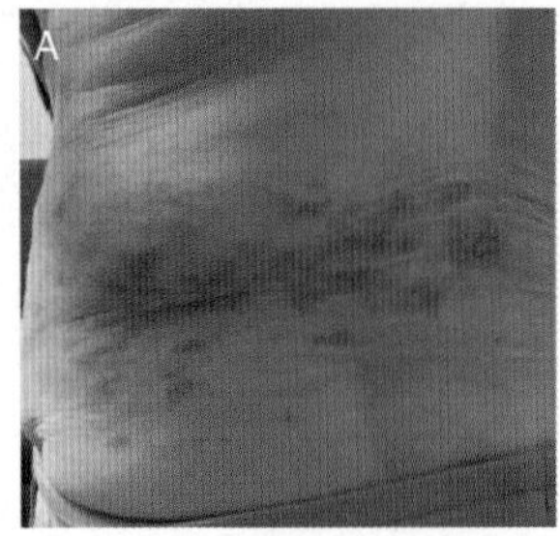

Infectious Skin Disorders

	Clinical Presentation	Diagnosis/Management
Parasitic Skin Infections		
Scabies	- *Sarcoptes scabiei* mite infection - Spreads via person-to-person contact - Mites tunnel into epidermis, lay eggs, and deposit feces, causing type IV hypersensitivity skin reaction - **Pruritic erythematous rash with burrows, excoriations** - Most commonly on wrists/hands	Dx: Clinical. Scabies microscopic prep to confirm. Tx: Topical 5% permethrin or oral ivermectin
Pediculosis Capitis[A] (Head lice)	- Common scalp infection in children - Can be asymptomatic or cause pruritus and excoriations	Dx: Visualize nits/adult lice Tx: Topical permethrin (alt: Malathion, benzyl alcohol, topical ivermectin) * No need to hold out of school, but examine household contacts
Pediculosis Pubis (Crabs)	- Sexually transmitted pubic lice infection - Presents as pubic itching	Dx: Visualize nits/adult lice Tx: Topical permethrin
Cutaneous Larva Migrans	- Hookworm (*Ancylostoma*) infection, often acquired from walking barefoot on soil/sand - Erythematous migrating cutaneous tracks	Dx: Clinical appearance Tx: Oral albendazole or ivermectin
Bed Bugs[B]	- Bugs that infest human dwellings - Presents with pruritic papules noticed upon waking	Dx: Detect bedbugs in sleeping area Tx: Professional pest eradication
Bacterial Skin Infections		
Impetigo	- Highly contagious, superficial skin infection from *Staph/Strep*, common in kids - Can be primary or secondary to minor skin trauma - **Painful pustules, "honey" crusting** - Bullae (in bullous impetigo) - Punched out ulcers (ecthyma)	- Limited: Topical antibiotics (mupirocin) - Extensive: Dicloxacillin or cephalexin
Erysipelas	- Infection of superficial dermis/lymphatics - Most common organism: *Streptococcus pyogenes* - Presents as acute onset **well-demarcated raised erythematous rash**, with systemic symptoms (fever/chill)	- *Strep* coverage (oral amoxicillin or cephalexin. IV cefazolin or ceftriaxone)
Cellulitis	- Infection of deep dermis and subcutaneous fat - Most common: *Strep*, MSSA, MRSA - Presents with **progressive skin erythema, edema**, which is poorly demarcated - Nonpurulent (more commonly *Strep*) or purulent (*Staph*)	- Nonpurulent: Cefazolin/cephalexin - Purulent: - TMP-SMX, clindamycin, doxycycline - IV vancomycin
Abscess	- Collection of pus within the dermis or subcutaneous space - Most common: MSSA/MRSA - **Fluctuant, painful erythematous nodule**, +/− exudate	- I&D +/− antibiotics (same as purulent cellulitis above)

*Note: For all skin infections, IV antibiotics are used for severe infections and those with systemic features. Oral antibiotics are appropriate for mild disease. Risk factors for MRSA dictate coverage (prior MRSA infection, purulent infection, infection resistant to empiric therapy).

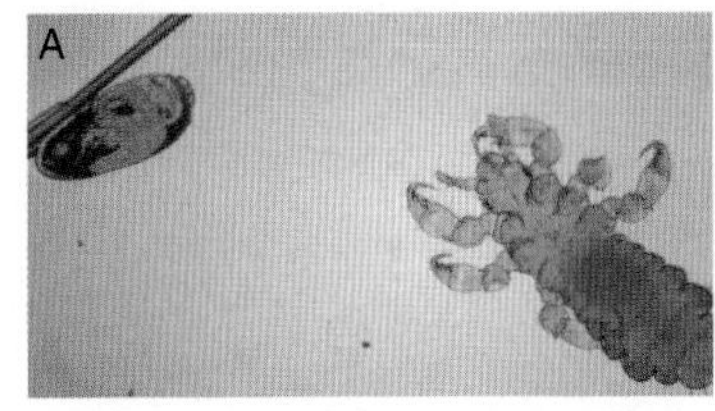

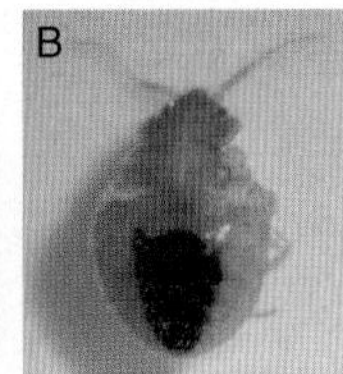

Infectious Skin Disorders

Necrotizing Soft Tissue Infections

General: Includes necrotizing cellulitis, fasciitis, myositis. Subtypes:
- Necrotizing fasciitis type I: Polymicrobial
- Necrotizing fasciitis type II: Monomicrobial (group A *Streptococcus*)
- Necrotizing myositis: Group A *Streptococcus,* other beta-hemolytic *Streptococci*
- Necrotizing cellulitis: *Clostridium perfringens* or polymicrobial

Risk: Traumatic wounds, immunosuppression, obesity, diabetes mellitus

Clinical:
- **Rapidly progressive soft tissue erythema and edema, with extreme pain**
    - Crepitus may be present (~50%)
    - Tissue bullae and necrosis
- Systemic symptoms (fever, chills, etc.)

Diagnosis: Primarily clinical: Rapidly progressive infection, **systemic signs, +/− crepitus**
- CT (can reveal **gas in soft tissue**, which is highly specific)

Management:
- Surgical exploration/debridement PLUS
- Broad spectrum antibiotics: Vancomycin + carbapenem or beta-lactam/lactamase inhibitor + clindamycin (inhibits toxin production)

Staph Scalded Skin Syndrome/Toxic Shock Syndrome

	Staph **Scalded Skin Syndrome**	**Toxic Shock Syndrome**
Gen	- *Staph* produced exfoliative toxin, which cleaves desmoglein-1 in the stratum granulosum - Seen commonly in infants or immunocompromised	- *Staph* or *Strep* produced TSST-1 "superantigen," causing massive T-cell response - Seen with tampon use, postpartum infections, and ENT surgery/sinusitis
Clin	- 24-48 hours of fever/skin tenderness followed by **generalized erythematous rash with bullae formation and sloughing**[A] - Nikolsky sign (+)	- **Fever (> 102°F), hypotension, rash** - Diffuse macular erythematous rash, skin desquamation <u>Organ involvement</u>: - Renal (AKI) - GI (emesis/diarrhea) - Liver (↑ AST/ALT) - Heme (thrombocytopenia) - MSK (myalgias, ↑ CK)
Dx	- Clinical - Culture all possible sources of infection (bullae are sterile)	- Clinical
Tx	- Supportive (fluids, skin care) - Antibiotics (cover *Staph*, e.g., nafcillin, vancomycin)	- Supportive (hemodynamic support) - Source control - Antibiotics (vancomycin + clindamycin)

Infectious Skin Disorders

Erythrasma

General: Superficial skin infection caused by *Corynebacterium minutissimum*. Seen frequently in those with diabetes, obesity.

Clinical:

- Interdigital: Scaly rash between toes
- Intertriginous: Dark erythematous to **brown scaly plaques found in groin, inframammary region, or axillae**

Diagnosis: Clinical, plus Wood lamp (coral red fluorescence)

Management: Topical clindamycin or erythromycin. Oral antibiotics if widespread.

Hidradenitis Suppurativa

General: Chronic suppurative/inflammatory soft tissue process from follicular occlusion of the folliculopilosebaceous unit

Risk: Associated with diabetes, obesity, insulin resistance

Clinical:

- **Severely painful/inflamed nodules**[A]
    - Most common in **axilla, inguinal, inframammary, perineal areas**
- Possible opening with purulent discharge
- Can be complicated by rope-like scarring, abscess or draining sinus tract formation, open comedones

Diagnosis: Clinical

Management:

- Behavioral (quit smoking, lose weight, avoid skin trauma)
- Pain control (NSAIDs)
- <u>Antibiotics</u>:
    - Topical clindamycin for mild disease
    - Oral doxycycline or clindamycin/rifampin for severe disease
- <u>Surgery</u>:
    - Intralesional steroids or surgical unroofing (to ↓ inflammation in acute, symptomatic lesions)
    - Wide excision of lesions (for chronic, refractory cases)

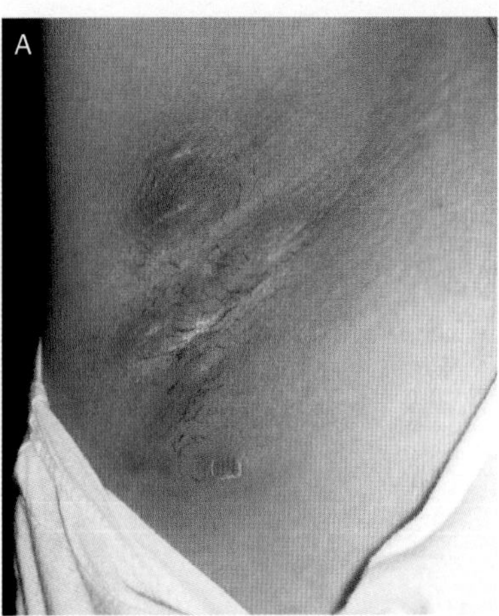

Soft Tissue Ulcers

Chronic Ulcers

Subtype	Clinical Features
Pressure	- Tissue damage from **unrelieved pressure between soft tissue and bony prominence** - Risk: Hospitalized patients, immobility Stage I: - Intact skin, but nonblanchable erythema Stage II: - Shallow ulcer with disrupted dermis Stage III: - Full thickness skin loss, possible visualization of subcutaneous fat Stage IV[A]: - Full thickness skin loss with involvement of bone, joint, or tendon Unstageable: - Full thickness tissue loss, with slough/eschar in ulcer - Management: Wound care, pain control, proper nutrition. Reposition patient at least every 2 hours.
Venous	- Ulcers that occur secondary to **chronic venous insufficiency** - Present as single or multiple shallow, exudative ulcers, most commonly over medial/lateral malleoli - Management: Compression stockings, elevate legs, diuretics
Arterial	- Ischemia from arterial obstruction, secondary to **PAD or other arterial obstruction** - Sharply demarcated ulcer at site furthest from vascular supply - Signs of arterial insufficiency (hairless legs, shiny skin, absent pulses) - Diagnosis: ABI/Doppler - Management: Revascularization
Diabetic	- Ulcers that occur due **diabetic neuropathy** (chronic trauma, abnormal vascular tone) - Most common near bony prominences (e.g., plantar surface of foot), appear punched out with irregular borders - Management: Mechanical offloading, wound care, debridement
Marjolin	- **Ulcerating squamous cell carcinoma** that occurs over an area of a chronic wound - Diagnosis: Biopsy - Management: Wide resection

Pressure ulcer stages:

Stage	FIndings
I	- Intact skin, but nonblanchable erythema
II	- Shallow ulcer with disrupted dermis
III	- Full thickness skin loss, possible visualization of subcutaneous fat
IV[A]	- Full thickness skin loss with involvement of bone, joint, or tendon
Unstageable	- Full thickness tissue loss, with slough/eschar in ulcer

Other Ulcers

Ecthyma Gangrenosum	- Occurs in immunocompromised patients with bacteremia (most commonly *Pseudomonas*) - Due to vascular bacterial invasion causing ischemic necrosis - Punched-out ulcer with crust, surrounded by violaceous margins
Pyoderma Gangrenosum	- Inflammatory ulcer from abnormal neutrophil function - Risk: Autoimmune disease (IBD, inflammatory arthritis), malignancy - Acute, progressive, painful, purulent ulcer with irregular violaceous border[B]

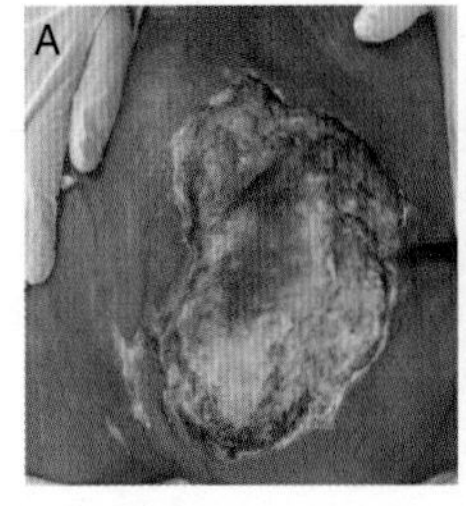

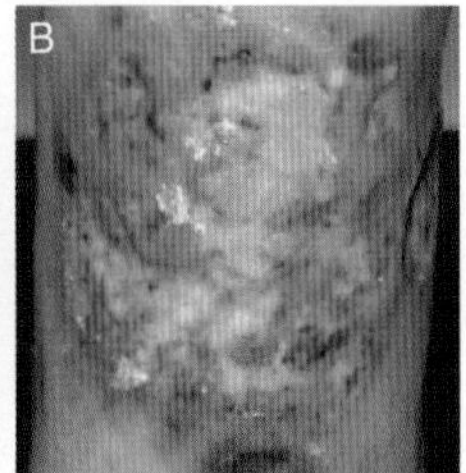

Hair Disorders

Hair Loss

Condition	Features
Androgenic Alopecia	- Selective loss of hair from the scalp due to genetic and hormonal factors (↑ DHT) - Temporal, anterior, and vertex areas of the scalp most often affected
Chemotherapy Alopecia	- Diffuse scalp hair loss from destruction of proliferating cells in the hair shaft
Alopecia areata	- Chronic autoimmune condition of relapsing episodes of hair loss - Smooth, discrete circular areas of hair loss[A] - Tx: Topical/intralesional steroids
Other	- Trichotillomania - Tinea capitis

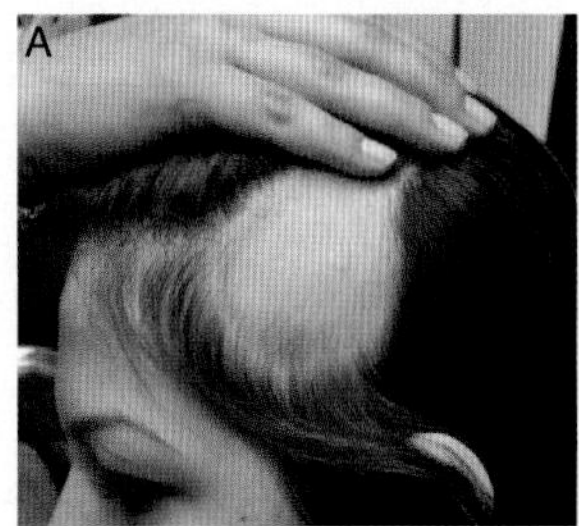

Folliculitis

General: Inflammation of the hair follicle, from infectious (bacterial/viral/fungal) or noninfectious cause

Etiology: Most commonly *Staph, Pseudomonas, Malassezia*

Clinical: Erythematous, follicular papules/pustules

Diagnosis: Clinical

Management: Topical antibiotics (clindamycin/mupirocin) or systemic antibiotics if severe

Specific Subtypes:

Hot-tub folliculitis	- *Pseudomonas* folliculitis from dirty hot tub
Tinea barbae	- "**Barber itch**." Folliculitis of beard hair in adult men. - *Trichophyton rubrum* most common culprit
Pseudofolliculitis barbae	- Noninfectious folliculitis from shaving, with beard hair growth back into follicle
Keratosis pilaris	- Common disorder of follicular keratinization - Papules on the back of extensor surface

Vascular Skin Tumors

	Clinical Presentation	Diagnosis/Management
Bacillary Angiomatosis	- Complication of *Bartonella* infection in HIV (CD4 < 100) - Presents as **friable red/purple nodule or papule**	- Doxycycline
Kaposi Sarcoma[A]	- Abnormal vascular proliferation from HHV-8 infection - Commonly associated with HIV/AIDS - **Dark red or purple skin nodules or plaques** - Can involve mouth/GI mucous membranes	Dx: Biopsy (vascular proliferation with lymphocytes) Tx: Can observe if asymptomatic. Symptomatic lesions can require local excision or chemotherapy.
Cherry Hemangioma	- Mature, adult hemangioma - Benign, unlikely to regress significantly	- Only excise if bothersome
Glomus Tumor	- Arises from the thermoregulatory glomus body - Painful red-blue tumor under fingernails	- Surgical excision
Pyogenic Granuloma[B]	- Lobulated capillary hemangioma occurring with pregnancy or trauma - **Rapidly growing, friable nodule** - Risk for ulceration/bleeding	- Surgical excision
Infantile Hemangioma[C]	- Common childhood hemangioma - Erythematous nodules that rapidly grow for a few months after birth, then regress over time	- Monitor lesions - If disfigurement or symptomatic: Propranolol or laser/surgical excision

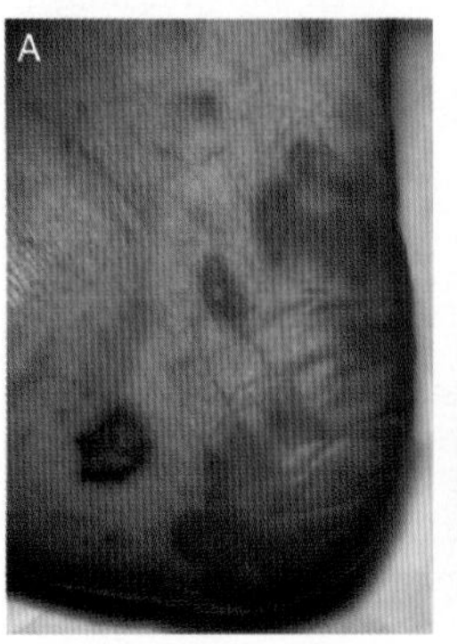

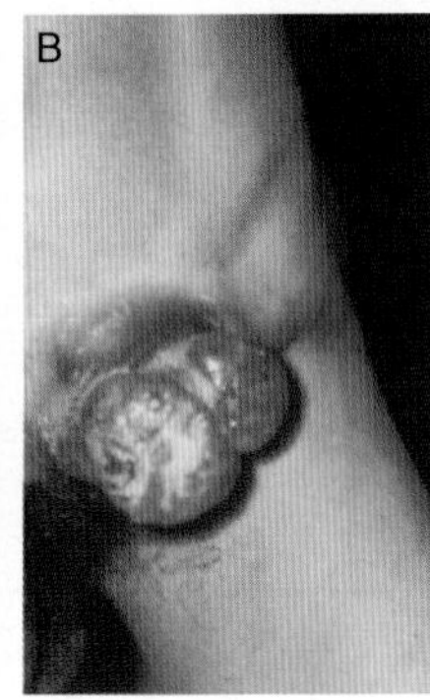

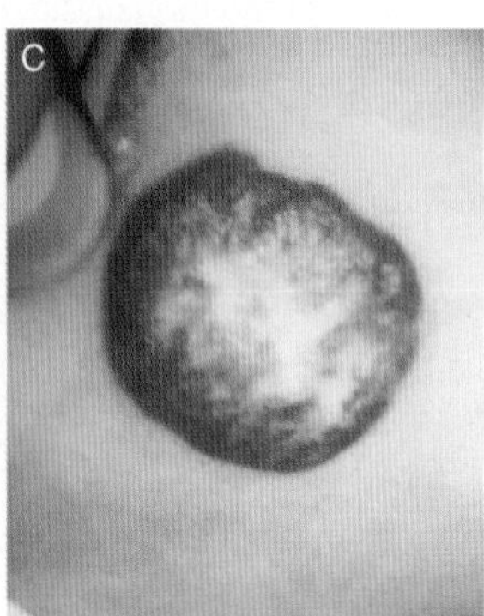

Dermatologic Malignancies

Basal Cell Carcinoma

General: Neoplastic proliferation of basal layer of the epidermis. Can be locally destructive, but have low metastatic potential.

Risk: UV light, fair skin

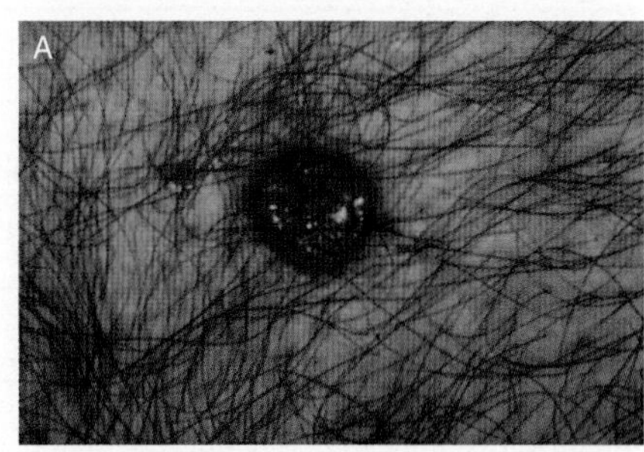

Clinical:

- Nodular[A]: **Pearly, waxy lesion, peripheral telangiectasia** (most often in head/neck area)
  - Frequent ulceration, bleeds
- Superficial: Scaly plaques

Diagnosis: Biopsy (shave, punch or excisional). Nests of atypical basal epithelium.

Management: Excision (Surgical, electrodesiccation and curettage [ED&C], MOHS)

- 5 mm margins
- MOHS for small (< 6 mm) head/neck lesions
- Topical therapy (imiquimod or 5-FU) if not surgical candidate

Squamous Cell Carcinoma

General: Neoplastic proliferation of squamous cells in the skin. Higher potential than BCC for local recurrence or metastases.

- Keratoacanthoma: Well-differentiated SCC that grows rapidly over weeks and then resolves

Risk: UV light, chronic wounds/inflammation/scars

- Actinic keratoses are precursor lesions

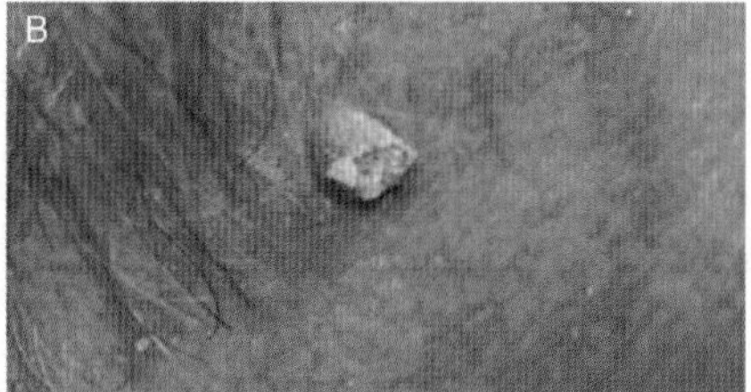

Clinical: **Erythematous plaques or nodules**[B]

- Scaling, crusting, ulceration, or increased pigment all possible

Diagnosis: Biopsy (shave, punch, or excisional)

Management: Excision (surgical, electrodesiccation, and curettage [ED&C], MOHS)

- 5-10 mm margins

Dermatologic Malignancies

Melanocytic Nevi

General: Benign proliferation of melanocytes. Associated with UV light/fair skin.

Junctional	- Dark, macular lesions. Common in children. - From basal epidermis
Compound	- Darkly pigmented papules - From basal epidermis/upper dermis interface
Intradermal	- Skin colored to tan papules. Common in adults. - From dermis
Atypical (Dysplastic)	- Still benign, but have some high risk features consistent with melanoma - ↑ risk for development of melanoma

Clinical: Varied appearance, but in general: < 6 mm, round/oval shape, regular border, even hyperpigmentation, homogenous surface

Diagnosis: Clinical. Biopsy if unsure.

Management: Observation. Excisional biopsy should be considered for lesions with atypical/concerning features OR changing over time.

Melanoma

General: Malignant melanocytic neoplasm, with characteristic radial growth phase (lateral within epidermis) followed by nodular growth (deep into dermis)

Superficial Spreading	- Long radial growth phase. Good prognosis. - Generally a macule or very thin plaque
Lentigo Maligna	- Found on elderly chronically sun damaged skin - Proliferation of melanocytes along dermal/epidermal junction - Present as tan or brown macules, with slowly progressive growth
Acral Lentiginous	- Palmar, plantar, subungual location - More common if dark skinned
Nodular	- Vertical growth phase melanomas. Poor prognosis. - Appear as darkly pigmented nodules

Risk: Sun/UV light exposure, fair skin, history of nevi, family history, xeroderma pigmentosum

Clinical: **ABCDE** (asymmetry, border irregularity, color variation, diameter [> 6 mm], elevation)
- **"Ugly Duckling Sign"** (looks suspicious[A] or different than other lesions)

Diagnosis: Clinical/dermoscopic features. Excisional biopsy (with 1-3 mm margin) for definitive diagnosis.

Management: Surgical Excision

Breslow Depth	Margins	Other surgical considerations: ≥ 0.8 mm deep: Lymphatic mapping/sentinel LN biopsy
In situ	0.5 cm	
≤ 1 mm	1 cm	
> 1 mm	1-2 cm	

Metastatic disease:
- Resection if only a few sites involved/surgery is feasible
- Systemic therapy: Immunotherapy first-line
    - Pembrolizumab and nivolumab (anti PD-1)
    - Ipilimumab (anti CTLA-4)

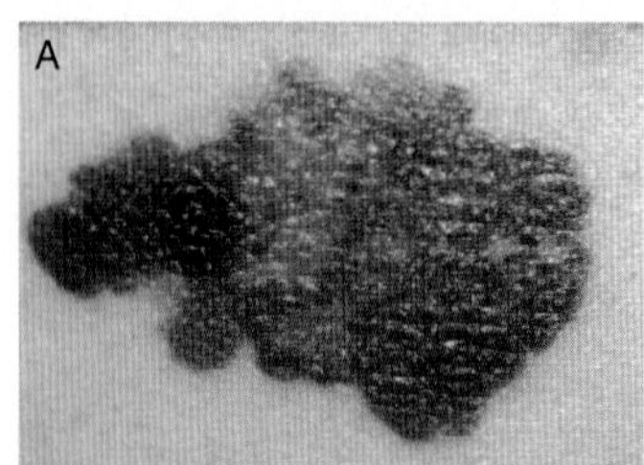

Gram-Positive Bacteria

	Clinical Presentation	Management/Antimicrobial Coverage
Staphylococcus		
Staphylococcus aureus	- Skin and soft tissue infections - Endocarditis - Septic arthritis/osteomyelitis - Pneumonia (especially post influenza) - Toxin-mediated (toxic shock, scalded skin, food poisoning)	Tx: - MSSA: Nafcillin/Oxacillin, beta-lactam/lactamase inh., cephalosporins - MRSA: Vancomycin (alt: Linezolid, daptomycin) for IV. TMP-SMX, clindamycin, doxycycline for PO.
Staphylococcus epidermidis	- Normal skin flora (often if cultured is a skin contaminant) - Can infect catheters, orthopedic prosthesis	See *Staph aureus*, risk for methicillin resistance
Staphylococcus saprophyticus	- Cause of female UTI	
Streptococcus		
Streptococcus pyogenes	- Pyogenic: Pharyngitis, cellulitis, impetigo - Immunologic: Rheumatic heart disease/glomerulonephritis - Toxigenic: Toxic shock, scarlet fever	Tx: Susceptible to most beta-lactams (including penicillin, cephalosporins)
Streptococcus agalactiae	- Infant pneumonia, meningitis, sepsis	
Streptococcus pneumoniae	- Meningitis, otitis media, pneumonia, sinusitis	Tx: Susceptible to most beta-lactams
Streptococcus viridans	- *S. sanguinis* → endocarditis - *S. mutans, S. mitis* → dental caries	
Enterococcus	- UTI, GI infections (diverticulitis, cholecystitis), subacute endocarditis	Tx: Ampicillin, vancomycin, carbapenems, others *Not susceptible to cephalosporins
Streptococcus bovis	- Subacute endocarditis (associated with colorectal cancer)	
Bacillus		
Bacillus anthracis	- Cutaneous: Painless ulcers with black eschar - Inhalation: Inhale spores → fever, pulmonary hemorrhage, mediastinitis, shock, meningitis	- Systemic: Broad antibiotics, anthrax antitoxin, supportive care
Bacillus cereus	- Food poisoning ("reheated rice syndrome"): Emesis, diarrhea	- Self-limited
Clostridium		
C. difficile	- Diarrhea [See: GI]	
C. perfringens	- Necrotizing cellulitis ("gas gangrene") - Food poisoning (spores ingested, can cause late onset GI symptoms)	
C. botulinum	**Botulism** - Produces toxin that inhibits presynaptic Ach release - Causes: - Infant botulism (ingested spores, classically raw honey) - Foodborne (ingestion of preformed toxin in food) - Wound infection (rare) - Presents with descending flaccid paralysis/bilateral cranial palsy. Prodrome of abdominal pain, nausea, emesis, dry mouth, diplopia.	- Infants (< 1 y/o): Human-derived botulism Ig - Others (> 1 y/o): Equine-derived botulism antitoxin
C. tetani	**Tetanus** - Produces exotoxin, blocks inhibitory neurotransmitter release at spinal cord - Source: Wound infections (adult), umbilical stump (infants) - Clinical: Severe, generalized muscle contraction. Trismus, risus sardonicus, opisthotonos. - Infants present with hypertonicity and failure to thrive	Active tetanus: Supportive care, tetanus Ig, Metronidazole, and benzodiazepines (for spasms) Prophylaxis (Vax=Td or TDap)

Vax	Minor/Clean Wound	Dirty/Severe Wound
≥ 3 dose	Vax (if last dose > 10 y)	Vax (if last vax > 5 y)
< 3 dose	Vax	Vax + Tet Ig

Gram-Positive Bacteria

	Clinical Presentation	Management/Antimicrobial Coverage
Corynebacterium diphtheriae	- Causes **diphtheria** (rarely seen in United States due to vaccines) - Presents with pharyngitis, characteristic gray-white pseudomembranes - Toxin can disseminate and cause myocarditis, CNS damage, and renal injury	Tx: - Antibiotics: Penicillin or erythromycin - Diphtheria antitoxin
Listeria monocytogenes	- Generally infects infants, elderly, or immunosuppressed Presents as: - Healthy: Self-limited, minor gastroenteritis - Immunosuppressed: Sepsis, invasive gastroenteritis - Pregnancy: Amnionitis, sepsis, abortion - Infants: Meningitis, granulomatosis infantiseptica (diffuse pyogenic granulomas)	Tx: Ampicillin or penicillin G
Nocardia	- Infection occurs almost exclusively in immunocompromised Presents as: - Pneumonia (similar to TB) - CNS disease (brain abscess) - Cutaneous (skin infection, lymphangitis)	Tx: TMP-SMX
Actinomyces[A]	- Bacteria that can cause cervicofacial invasion from dental infection or oromaxillofacial trauma. Pelvic actinomycosis from IUD. - Presents with mass, which progresses slowly into abscesses, draining sinus tracts (yellow sulfur granules), fistulae, and tissue fibrosis	Tx: Penicillin (or ampicillin/erythromycin)

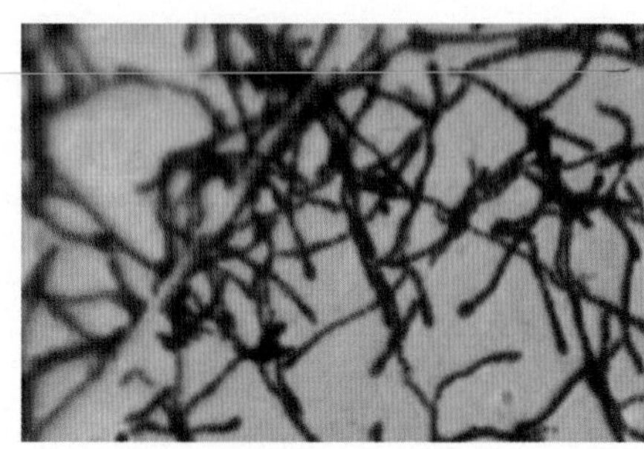

Gram-Negative Bacteria

	Clinical Presentation	Management/Antimicrobial Coverage
Neisseria meningitidis	- Cause of meningitis/meningococcemia [See: Neurology]	Tx: Penicillin or ceftriaxone *PPX (close contacts): Rifampin, ciprofloxacin, or ceftriaxone
Neisseria gonorrhoeae	- Cause of gonorrhea urethritis/cervicitis, PID, septic arthritis, and neonatal conjunctivitis [See: STI]	Tx: Ceftriaxone/azithromycin
Respiratory Gram Negatives		
Bordetella pertussis	**Pertussis** (whooping cough) - Presents with: - Catarrhal: 1-2 weeks of flu like prodrome (cough/rhinitis) - Paroxysmal: 2-6 weeks. Severe cough with inspiratory whoop, post-tussive emesis. - Convalescent stage: Eventual resolution of symptoms	Dx: Culture, PCR, serology Tx: Macrolides. Update Tdap. *Post-exposure ppx: Macrolide for close contacts
Legionella pneumophila	- Bacteria that thrives in and is transmitted from water - Pontiac fever: Mild flu-like syndrome of headache, fever, muscle aches that occurs with inhalation of *Legionella* endotoxin. Self-limited, no workup required. - **Legionnaires disease**: Atypical pneumonia, gastrointestinal symptoms, fever/myalgias, hyponatremia	Dx: Urine antigen and respiratory culture Tx: Azithromycin or levofloxacin
Haemophilus influenzae	- Nontypable: Respiratory infection (otitis, PNA, sinusitis) - Encapsulated (type B): Can cause meningitis, septic arthritis, pneumonia, and epiglottitis	Tx: Amoxicillin-clavulanate or cephalosporin
Enteric Gram Negatives (Enterobacteriaceae)		
Enterobacter *Citrobacter* *Serratia*	- Part of normal intestinal microbiota - Can cause biliary/GU infections	
Salmonella spp	- Source: Infected poultry, milk, eggs, or pets (turtles) - Gastroenteritis (diarrhea, emesis, abdominal pain, fever) *Hard to differentiate clinically from other causes of gastroenteritis	Dx: Stool culture Tx: Supportive care. Antibiotics (fluoroquinolone) if high risk or severe.
Salmonella typhi	**Typhoid**: - Obtained from ingesting contaminated food/water - Presents as abdominal pain, fever, hepatosplenomegaly - Bradycardia, pulse-temperature dissociation, and "rose-spots" (salmon colored macules)	Dx: Blood/stool culture Tx: Ceftriaxone or ciprofloxacin PPX: Typhoid vax (either live oral or IM) for travelers to endemic areas
Shigella	- Common cause of bacterial diarrhea, transmitted person to person or through food - Presents with abdominal cramps, fever, and bloody diarrhea	Dx: Stool culture Tx: Fluoroquinolone or macrolide
Campylobacter jejuni	- Common cause of acute enteritis (abdominal pain, diarrhea, sometimes bloody). Risk for GBS or reactive arthritis.	Tx: Supportive care +/− antibiotics (fluoroquinolone or macrolide)
Yersinia enterocolitica	- Common cause of acute diarrhea illness (fever, abdominal pain, diarrhea). Can be confused with appendicitis.	Tx: Supportive care
Escherichia coli		
ETEC	- Causes watery diarrhea in children or travelers	- Self-limited - Fluoroquinolone or macrolide if severe
STEC	- Invasive, bloody diarrhea in children - HUS (produces Shiga-like toxin)	- Supportive care
EPEC	- Cause of watery diarrhea in children in developing countries	- Supportive care
EIEC	- Presents similar to *Shigella* with watery/bloody diarrhea	- Supportive care

Gram-Negative Bacteria

	Clinical Presentation	Management/Antimicrobial Coverage
Klebsiella	- Pneumonia (nosocomial, rarely community-acquired) - GU infection, bacteremia, intraabdominal infection	Tx: Cephalosporins, fluoroquinolone (Note: Some strains are MDR due to ESBL)
Proteus	- GU infection, struvite stones	Tx: Ampicillin, TMP-SMX
Helicobacter pylori	- **Peptic ulcer disease** [See: GI]	
Vibrio cholera	**Cholera** - Acute secretory watery diarrhea ("rice water" diarrhea) - Caused by cholera toxin - See in many third-world countries	Tx: Aggressive fluids, antibiotics (fluoroquinolone, macrolide, or tetracycline)
Vibrio vulnificus	- Lives in marine environments. Can be ingested (oysters) or due to wound infection. - Associated with ↑ Iron (e.g., hemochromatosis) - Can present with rapidly progressive cellulitis (necrotizing infection, bullous rash) and sepsis	Tx: - Tetracycline + ceftriaxone - High mortality rate
Nosocomial		
Pseudomonas	- Feared, aggressive, water-loving nosocomial pathogen - Can cause sepsis, PNA, UTI, osteomyelitis (puncture wounds), otitis externa, skin infections (hot tub folliculitis, ecthyma gangrenosum, skin infections in burn victims)	Tx: Carbapenem, aminoglycoside, cefepime, fluoroquinolone, piperacillin-tazobactam
Burkholderia cepacia	- Opportunistic organism that can cause PNA in patients with underlying lung disease (CF) or immunocompromised	Tx: TMP/SMX, fluoroquinolone, cephalosporins
Acinetobacter baumannii	- Hospital-acquired infections (commonly PNA/bacteremia)	Tx: Often multidrug-resistant; carbapenem, polymyxin, cefepime
Zoonotic		
Yersinia pestis	**Bubonic plague** - Transmitted by fleas, with rat reservoir. - Presents as fever, chills, malaise, myalgias - Swollen/painful lymph nodes ("bubo") - Eventual disseminated infection (sepsis, pneumonia)	Dx: Culture/serology Tx: Aminoglycoside, tetracycline, fluoroquinolone
Francisella tularensis	**Tularemia** - Zoonotic infection from animal contact or tick - Nonspecific febrile illness (fever, malaise, myalgias) - Ulceroglandular: Ulcerative lesion at site of inoculation, with regional lymphadenopathy	Dx: Serology Tx: Aminoglycoside, tetracycline, fluoroquinolone
Brucella	**Brucellosis** - Zoonotic infection from contact with infected animal tissue/fluids (cow, sheep) or food products such as unpasteurized milk and cheese - Presents as insidious onset of fever, malaise, night sweats, myalgias, arthralgias - Sacroiliitis, spondylitis, endocarditis, meningitis/encephalitis	Dx: Culture/serology Tx: Doxycycline/rifampin
Pasteurella multocida	- Soft tissue infection after cat/dog bite, scratch, or lick - Rapid (within 24 hours) onset of inflammation	Tx: Amoxicillin-clavulanate
Anaerobes		
Bacteroides fragilis	- Normal organism of the GI tract - Can be implicated in GI/GU/pulmonary abscesses, as well as dental infections and skin/soft tissue infections	Tx: Metronidazole, clindamycin, or beta-lactam/lactamase inhibitors
Gardnerella	- Cause of **bacterial vaginosis** [See: GYN]	Tx: Metronidazole

Atypical Bacteria

	Clinical Presentation	Management/Antimicrobial Coverage
Chlamydia		
Chlamydia trachomatis	- Intracellular parasite - Serotype A-C: Trachoma - Serotype D-K: Urethritis, cervicitis, PID, neonatal conjunctivitis/PNA	
Chlamydophila psittaci	- **Psittacosis:** Atypical pneumonia - Obtained from inhalation of particles of bird feces	Tx: Doxycycline/macrolide
Chlamydophila pneumoniae	- Atypical pneumonia	Tx: Doxycycline/macrolide
Rickettsia		
Rickettsia rickettsii	**Rocky Mountain spotted fever** - Transmitted by dermacentor tick - Occurs in eastern US - Presents initially with fever, chills, headache, myalgias, arthralgias. Eventual development of rash (starts at wrists[A] and ankles, spreads inward [centrifugal]) - Thrombocytopenia, hyponatremia, transaminitis	Dx: Serology or clinical diagnosis Tx: Doxycycline (alt: Chloramphenicol)
Rickettsia prowazekii	**Epidemic typhus** - Rare, found in rural Africa/Asia/South America - Transmitted by louse/flea - Acute onset fever, malaise, severe headache, followed later by maculopapular rash and CNS symptoms (confusion, lethargy) - Brill-Zinsser disease: Mild recrudescence of symptoms	Tx: Doxycycline (alt: Chloramphenicol)
Rickettsia typhi	**Endemic (murine) typhus** - Transmitted by flea - Presents as acute, nonspecific flu-like illness, rash	
Spirochetes		
Treponema pallidum	- [See: STD]	
Borrelia burgdorferi	**Lyme disease** (ixodes tick vector, mouse reservoir) - Found in northeastern US - Stage 1: Erythema migrans, flu-like symptoms, arthralgias - Stage 2 (early disseminated): Carditis, AV block, facial nerve palsy, migratory myalgias/arthritis - Stage 3 (late disseminated): Encephalopathy, inflammatory arthritis	Dx: ELISA, followed by confirmatory western blot Tx: Doxycycline (alt: Amoxicillin) - Ceftriaxone if CNS/cardiac involvement PPX: - If tick bite < 36 hours: Remove tick, no ppx - If tick bite > 36 hours: Remove tick, Doxycycline
Leptospira	**Leptospirosis** - Tropical infection (in US → Hawaii) - Animal reservoir, excrete in urine, possibly into water/soil - Nonspecific illness (fever, severe myalgias, and headache) - Conjunctival suffusion - Weil disease: Occurs in ~ 5% of cases. Progressive multi-system illness. Jaundice, renal failure, pulmonary hemorrhage	Dx: PCR, serology Tx: Doxycycline or azithromycin

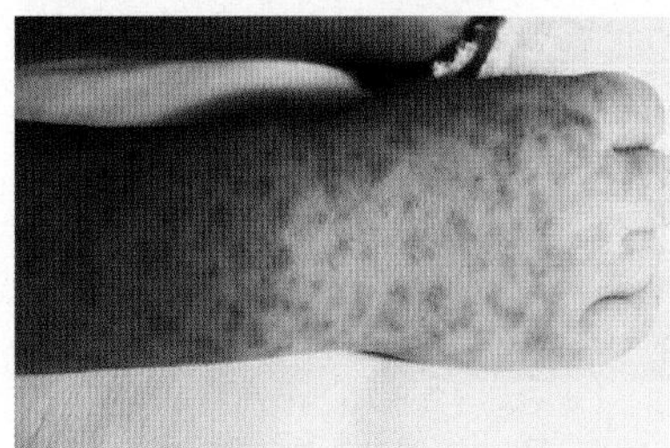

Atypical Bacteria

	Clinical Presentation	Management/Antimicrobial Coverage
***Mycobacterium* (non-TB)**		
Mycobacterium leprae	**Leprosy** - Transmitted by respiratory droplets from infected humans, rarely armadillos. - **Lepromatous:** Diffuse hypopigmented, anesthetic skin lesions. Can have nodules, papules, plaques. Palpable nerves with neuropathy. Skin thickening[A] ("lion facies") possible. - **Tuberculoid:** Few hypoesthetic, erythematous macules	Dx: Skin biopsy (with acid fast stain) Tx: Rifampin + dapsone. In lepromatous; add clofazimine.
Mycobacterium marinum	- Cause of skin/soft tissue infection in those exposed to fresh/salt water	Tx: Clarithromycin + ethambutol/rifampin
Mycobacterium kansasii	- Presents as lung disease similar to tuberculosis	
Mycobacterium avium complex	- Pulmonary disease in those with COPD, bronchiectasis - Disseminated infection in immunocompromised patients [See: HIV]	
Mycoplasma	- **Atypical pneumonia**. Young people/close proximity at risk. - Presents as: Pharyngitis, headache, malaise - Dry cough (diffuse interstitial infiltrate on CXR) - Possible cold-agglutinin (IgM)	Tx: Macrolides, respiratory fluoroquinolone
Ehrlichia chaffeensis	- Human **monocytic** ehrlichiosis (Vector: Lone-star tick) - Common in southern US - Presents as: Flu-like illness (fever, headache, myalgias) - Leukopenia, thrombocytopenia, ↑ ALT/AST	Dx: Serology (ELISA/IFA) or PCR Tx: Doxycycline
Anaplasma phagocytophilum	- Human **granulocytic** anaplasmosis (Vector: Ixodes tick) - Presents as: Flu-like illness (fever, headache, myalgias) - Leukopenia, thrombocytopenia, ↑ ALT/AST	
Coxiella burnetii	- **Q-Fever**: Zoonotic infection, most commonly exposure to spores in farm animal bodily fluids - Presents as: High grade fever, fatigue, headaches, myalgias - Possible mild pneumonia, hepatitis. Rarely endocarditis.	Dx: Serology Tx: Doxycycline
Bartonella henselae	- **Cat Scratch Disease** (due to cat scratch or bite) - Presents with papule/nodule at site of inoculation, followed by erythematous painful lymphadenopathy, +/– fever	Dx: Clinical. Confirm with serology. Tx: Azithromycin

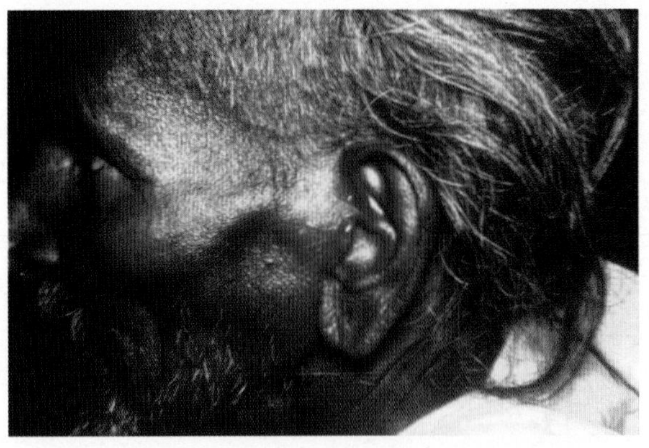

Fungal Infections

	Clinical Presentation	Management/Antimicrobial Coverage
Cutaneous	- Note: *Tinea* infections (dermatophytes, *Malassezia*) covered in dermatology	
Sporothrix schenckii	- Dimorphic fungi found in decaying plant matter - Presents with papule at site of inoculation, with ascending lymphangitis (lesions along lymphatic chain), ulceration	Dx: Culture Tx: Itraconazole
Systemic		
Histoplasmosis	- Found in soil contaminated with bird/bat droppings (caves) - Midwestern/central US (Ohio and Mississippi River valley) Clinical: (Note: Most are asymptomatic/clear organism) - Systemic symptoms (fevers, malaise, weight loss) - Pulmonary (patchy/nodular infiltrates, with hilar LA) - Other: Arthralgias, skin nodules. Rarely disseminates. - Lab: Pancytopenia, ↑ AST/ALT, LDH	Dx: Culture, serology, and urine/serum antigen. Biopsy can show granulomas/yeast forms. Tx: - Mild: Itraconazole - Severe: Amphotericin B, followed by itraconazole
Blastomycosis	- Inhalation of conidia. Occurs in similar area to Histoplasma, but extends into upper-midwest US/great lakes. Clinical: (Can disseminate even if immunocompetent) - Pulm: Acute/chronic pneumonia (most common) - Derm: Verrucous lesions, violaceous nodules, skin ulcers - MSK: Osteomyelitis, osteolytic bone lesions	Dx: Visualization or culture (sputum, tissue, purulent material). Urine/serum antigen. Tx: - Mild: Itraconazole - Severe: Amphotericin B, followed by itraconazole
Coccidioidomycosis	- Southwestern US (dust → inhale spores) Clinical: **Valley Fever** - Pneumonia (chest pain, cough) - Systemic symptoms (fever, night sweats, weight loss) - Arthralgias, erythema nodosum	Dx: Serology (IgM), culture Tx: - Mild: Itraconazole - Severe: Amphotericin B, followed by itraconazole
Opportunistic		
Candida	- Oral thrush, esophagitis, vaginitis, intertrigo, endocarditis - Can disseminate in immunocompromised patients	
Allergic bronchopulmonary Aspergillosis	- Hypersensitivity in asthma/CF patient to *Aspergillus* colonization, can lead to chronic inflammation/bronchiectasis - Presents as asthma with recurrent exacerbations, occasional coughing up of brown mucus plugs	Dx: *Aspergillus* IgE/skin testing Tx: Acute flare: Corticosteroids + voriconazole
Chronic pulmonary aspergillosis	- Risk: History of lung disease/damage (e.g., cavitary TB) - Presents with subacute onset weight loss, productive cough, hemoptysis, dyspnea, fever/night sweats	Dx: Imaging shows cavitary upper lobe lesions, possible fungus ball. (+) *Aspergillus* IgG. Tx: Surgically resect aspergilloma. Voriconazole.
Invasive aspergillosis	- Pulmonary tissue infection with vascular invasion - Risk: Immunocompromised (HIV/immunosuppressant use) - Presents with fever, chest pain, dyspnea, hemoptysis - Imaging: Pulmonary nodules/infiltrates, + halo sign	Dx: Sputum stain/culture, biomarkers (beta-D-glucan, galactomannan). Tissue biopsy if uncertain. Tx: Voriconazole (+ caspofungin if severe)
Cryptococcus	- Round yeast with thick capsule. Associated with pigeons. - Inhalation of fungus into lungs → Hematogenous spread may involve the brain and meninges - Clinical: Meningoencephalitis [See: HIV], pneumonia	Dx: CSF Ag (latex agglutination or ELISA) Tx: Amphotericin B + flucytosine (2 weeks), then fluconazole (for 1 year)
Mucormycosis	- Risk: Diabetes (ketoacidosis), steroid use, neutropenia - Presents as rapid, acute sinusitis, with necrotic invasion of surrounding structures (sinuses, palate, turbinates, skin) - Black necrotic eschar on skin and mucosa - CNS: Frontal lobe abscess, cavernous sinus thrombosis	Dx: Tissue biopsy (histopathologic analysis) Tx: Surgical debridement, amphotericin B

Protozoal Infections

	Clinical Presentation	Management/Antimicrobial Coverage
Giardia lamblia	- Source: Fresh water, foodborne. Fecal-oral spread. - Risks: Camping, traveling. IgA deficiency. - Presents with **bloating, flatulence, steatorrhea**	Dx: Stool antigen/PCR or stool microscopy (O&P) Tx: Metronidazole/tinidazole +/– nitazoxanide
Entamoeba histolytica	- Source: Contaminated water, food (especially in developing countries) Presents as: - Mild diarrhea or **severe bloody diarrhea/colitis** - Liver abscess [See: GI]	Dx: Stool microscopy (O&P)/antigen testing Tx: - Metronidazole/tinidazole - Paromomycin (for intraluminal cysts)
Cryptosporidium	- Source: Contaminated water, food. Fecal-oral spread. Presents as: - Asymptomatic or minor diarrhea in immunocompetent - **Severe, chronic diarrhea in immunocompromised**	Dx: Stool microscopy (and/or stool PCR) Tx: Nitazoxanide (for those with > 2 weeks of symptoms)
Trichomonas vaginalis	- Vaginitis [See: GYN]	
Naegleria fowleri	- Source: Freshwater lakes/ponds - Acute, **rapidly fatal meningoencephalitis**	Tx: Amphotericin B + steroids
Acanthamoeba	- Chronic meningoencephalitis - **Corneal eye infection (dirty contacts)**	
Toxoplasma gondii	- Commonly found in cats (felines) - Transmitted by oocysts (in stool), cysts in infected meat, vertical transmission (mother to fetus) - Oocysts invade intestines → Disseminates - **Immunocompetent**: Asymptomatic or mononucleosis-like illness - **Congenital**: TORCH infection - **Immunocompromised (HIV/AIDS)**: Encephalitis, ring-enhancing lesions on head imaging	Dx: - Toxo serology (IgM in active disease) - If HIV: Classic imaging, Toxo IgG + Tx: Sulfadiazine + pyrimethamine (+ leucovorin) (TMP-SMX is alternative)
Trypanosoma brucei	- Transmitted by tsetse fly - Human African trypanosomiasis ("**sleeping sickness**") - Subtypes: Gambiense → slow, chronic, rhodesiense → Rapid - Early: Painful bite site (with possible chancre), flu-like symptoms (intermittent headache, fevers, malaise, arthralgia) - Late: CNS disease (meningoencephalitis, somnolence)	Dx: Blood smear (identify trypomastigotes) Tx: Pentamidine/suramin (early blood infection) and melarsoprol (late CNS disease)
Trypanosoma cruzi	- Seen in South America. Transmitted by reduviid bug. **<u>Chagas disease</u>** - Acute: Romana sign (periorbital swelling), nonspecific systemic symptoms (fever, lymphadenopathy) - Chronic: Dilated cardiomyopathy, achalasia, progressive colonic dilatation	Dx: - Acute: Blood smear (trypomastigote) or PCR - Chronic: Serology (IgG) Tx: Benznidazole and nifurtimox
Leishmania donovani	- Seen in South Asia, East Africa. Transmitted by sandfly. **Visceral** (Kala-azar or old world) Subtype: - Spiking fevers, hepatosplenomegaly, pancytopenia **Cutaneous** Subtype: - Nonhealing, crusty, nonpainful skin ulcer	Dx: Histopathology (needle aspiration/tissue biopsy) Tx: - Visceral: Amphotericin B - Cutaneous: Paromomycin

Protozoal Infections

Malaria

General: *Plasmodium* infection, transmitted by bite of anopheles mosquito. Protozoal infection of red blood cells and liver.

Subtype	Features
P. falciparum	- Most common. sub-Saharan Africa, Haiti, Dominican - Banana-shaped gametocytes[A] - Severe symptoms, irregular fever pattern
P. vivax/ovale	- Next most common, Western Pacific and Americas - 48-hour fever cycle - Dormant form (hypnozoite) in liver can cause recurring infection
P. malariae	- Rarer form, mostly found in sub-Saharan Africa - 72-hour fever cycle

Clinical:

- **Paroxysmal fevers** (timing depends on underlying organism)
- Hemolytic anemia, jaundice
- Splenomegaly
- Systemic symptoms (fatigue, malaise, arthralgias, headache)
- Can be complicated by hypoglycemia, acidosis, renal failure, ARDS or CNS disease (seizure/coma)

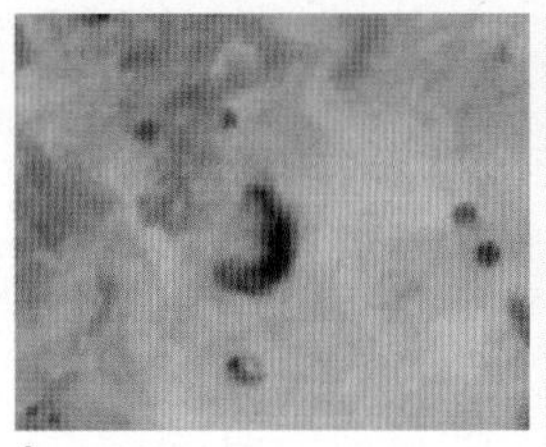
A

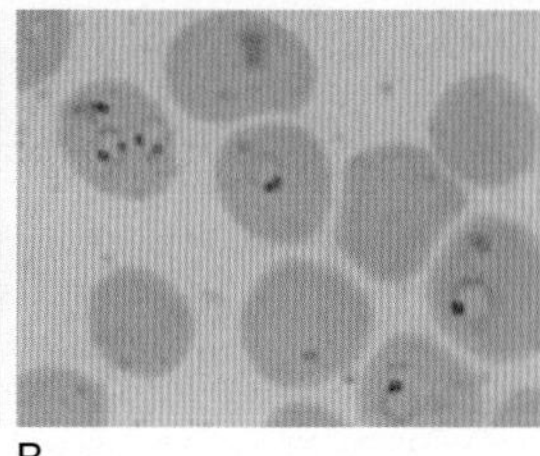
B

Diagnosis:

- Microscopy[B] (**thin/thick preps**) is gold standard
- Rapid antigen testing in resource poor areas

Management:

Subtype	Treatment
P. falciparum	- Artemisinin combination therapy (artemether/artesunate regimen)
P. vivax/ovale *P. malariae* *P. knowlesi*	- Chloroquine sensitive area: Chloroquine or artemisinin combination therapy (artemether/artesunate regimen) - Chloroquine resistant area: Artemisinin combination therapy (artemether/artesunate regimen) - Alternative: Atovaquone-proguanil, quinine + doxycycline, mefloquine - Primaquine for anti-relapse

Prophylaxis:

- Start 2 weeks before leaving and continue 4 weeks once back
- Chemoprophylaxis based on region of travel
- Regimen options: Doxycycline, atovaquone/proguanil, or mefloquine
- Mosquito protection (sprays, netting)

Babesia

General: Spread by *Ixodes scapularis* (also lyme/anaplasma) in northeastern US

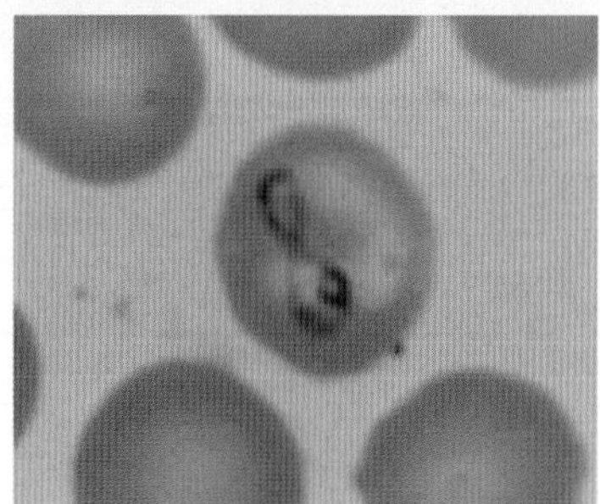

Clinical:

- Nonspecific flu-like illness (malaise, myalgias, fever, night sweats, headache)
- Hemolytic anemia, transaminitis, thrombocytopenia
- Severe disease in asplenic patients

Diagnosis: Blood smear (intraerythrocytic rings[C], "maltese cross") or blood PCR

Management: Atovaquone + Azithromycin

Helminth Infections

	Clinical Presentation	Management/Antimicrobial Coverage
Nematode (roundworms)		
Enterobius vermicularis (**pinworm**)	- Cycle: Fecal-oral (adult worms → lay eggs in perianal area → Itch and reintroduce via mouth) - Clinical: Asymptomatic OR anal pruritus	Dx: "Tape test" (look for perianal eggs) Tx: Albendazole or pyrantel pamoate
Trichuris (**whipworm**)	- Cycle: Ingest eggs, hatch larva in colon, mature to adults - Clinical: Can cause diarrhea (+/– mucus or blood), and rectal prolapse if heavy worm burden	Dx: Stool microscopy (for ova/parasite) Tx: Albendazole
Ascaris lumbricoides (**roundworm**)	- Cycle: Ingest eggs → Hatch in GI, larva migrate to lungs → cough up, swallow adult worms into GI - Clinical: - Early infection: Mild pulmonary symptoms (cough) - Late infection: GI symptoms (diarrhea, emesis, abdominal pain), with possible bowel obstruction or malnutrition	Dx: Stool microscopy (for ova/parasite) Tx: Albendazole
Ancylostoma duodenale and Necator americanus (**hookworm**)	- Cycle: Larvae in soil penetrate skin → migrate to lungs → Cough/swallow → GI → mature to adult worms - Clinical: - Cutaneous larva migrans [See: Derm] - Chronic GI symptoms, blood loss (anemia), malnutrition	Dx: Stool microscopy (for ova/parasite) Tx: Albendazole
Strongyloides stercoralis	- Cycle: Larvae in soil penetrate skin → migrate to lungs → cough/swallow → GI → mature to adult worms - Chronic asymptomatic infection may persist for many years - Immunocompromised: Hyperinfection (dissemination of larvae to lungs, liver, heart, CNS)	Dx: Stool microscopy (for ova/parasite) Note: Often need serologic testing because larva burden low Tx: Ivermectin
Trichinella spiralis	- Cycle: Fecal-oral (undercooked meat [pork or wild meat]) - Ingest cyst → Larvae released, mature in intestine → Release larva that migrate and encyst in skeletal muscle - Clinical: - Early GI symptoms (abdominal pain/diarrhea), followed by muscle stage (myositis/ ↑ CK), fever, periorbital edema, eosinophilia - Myocarditis, meningoencephalitis, pulmonary invasion	Dx: Serology. Biopsy is definitive but often unnecessary. Tx: Albendazole
Toxocara canis	- Cycle: Ingestion of eggs from soil/stool, with larvae hatching in GI, and systemic invasion - Most common in children, exposed in sandbox/playgrounds (which are contaminated with feces from puppies/kittens) - **Visceral larva migrans**: Pneumonitis, hepatitis with possible heart/CNS/muscle invasion - **Ocular larva migrans**: Unilateral ocular worm invasion	Dx: Serology Tx: Albendazole
Onchocerca volvulus	- Blackfly transmission (larva deposition in skin) - Clinical: Onchocerciasis, also known as "**river blindness**" - Ocular (keratitis/uveitis/chorioretinitis) - Dermatologic (skin nodules/papules/plaques)	Dx: Skin-snip biopsy. Slit-lamp exam. Tx: Ivermectin
Wuchereria bancrofti	- Mosquito transmission (larva deposition, lymphatic invasion) - Clinical: Acutely causes lymphangitis, with chronic disease causing lymphedema ("**Elephantiasis**")	Dx: Antigen tests, blood smears Tx: Diethylcarbamazine
Loa loa	- Transmission: Deer/horse fly transmission - Clinical: Swelling in skin, conjunctivitis (from worm invasion)	Dx: Visualization in eye Tx: Diethylcarbamazine

Helminth Infections

	Clinical Presentation	Management/Antimicrobial Coverage
Cestodes (tapeworms)		
Taenia solium	- Cycle: Ingest eggs, which hatch larvae that invade. Eggs often come from feces of asymptomatic tapeworm carrier. Note: Humans become carrier via ingestion of raw pork (contains cysticerci that hatch intestinal tapeworms) Clinical: **Cysticercosis** (cysts throughout body, especially CNS) - Intraparenchymal: Seizures, headache, focal deficits - Intraventricular: Hydrocephalus, ↑ ICP	Dx: - CT/MRI (depending on stage, calcified/edematous/enhancing brain lesions) - Serology Tx: Albendazole + praziquantel + glucocorticoids
Diphyllobothrium latum	- Fish tapeworm (transmitted from raw freshwater fish) - Nonspecific GI symptoms, vitamin B12 deficiency	Dx: Stool microscopy (for ova/parasite) Tx: Praziquantel
Echinococcus granulosus	- Ingestion of eggs in feces/soil (dogs are definitive hosts) - Clinical: Liver cysts [See: GI], lung cysts	Dx: Imaging (CT/US) and serology Tx: Albendazole +/− percutaneous intervention
Trematodes (flukes)		

Schistosoma[A]	- Cycle: Snail host, cercariae (released into water) penetrate human skin, migrate to liver where they mature
	
	Clinical:
	- <u>Acute</u>: "Swimmer's itch" (itchy rash at penetration site) and katayama fever (fever, urticaria, angioedema, eosinophilia occurring within 2 months of initial infection)
	- <u>Chronic</u>:
	  - Chronic abdominal pain, diarrhea
	  - Liver fibrosis (portal hypertension)
	  - Bladder polyps, obstruction, renal failure
		Dx: Stool/urine microscopy (for ova/parasite)
		
		Tx: Praziquantel

Clonorchis sinensis (Chinese Liver Fluke)	- Chronic infection can cause hepatobiliary disease (obstructive jaundice, pancreatitis, cholangitis, liver abscess)	Dx: Stool microscopy (ova/parasite) Tx: Praziquantel

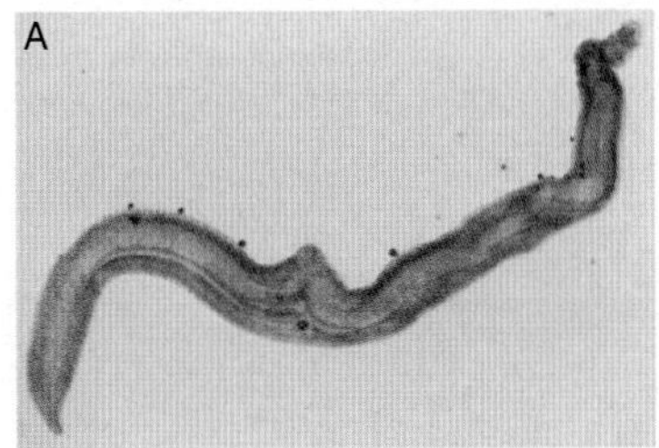

DNA Viruses

	Clinical Presentation	Management/Antimicrobial Coverage
Parvovirus B19	- Small virus, respiratory spread, infects RBC precursors Clinical: - In utero: Hydrops fetalis - Kids: **Erythema infectiosum** (fifth disease): - Low grade fever, "slapped cheek" descending rash - Adults: Flu-like illness, with **polyarthralgias** (resembles RA) - Sickle/thalassemia: Aplastic crisis	Dx: B19 Serology (IgM) or PCR test Tx: Self-limited, supportive

Human papilloma virus (HPV)	- Types 1-4: Verruca vulgaris (common wart)
	- Types 6, 11:
	  - Anogenital warts (condyloma acuminata)
	  - Laryngeal papillomatosis (respiratory tract tumors)
	- Types 16, 18, 31, 33: Anogenital cancers
	
	HPV makes E6 (inhibits P53) and E7 (inhibits Rb)	

BK polyomavirus	- Renal transplant: **Tubulointerstitial nephritis**	
JC polyomavirus	- **Progressive multifocal leukoencephalopathy** [See: HIV]	
Adenovirus	- Common, seen in individuals in close proximity (military) Clinical: - URTIs (otitis, pharyngitis, tonsillitis, pneumonia) - Epidemic conjunctivitis (pink eye) - Diarrheal illness (infants/children) - Hemorrhagic cystitis	
Pox virus	- **Smallpox** - **Molluscum contagiosum**[A]	

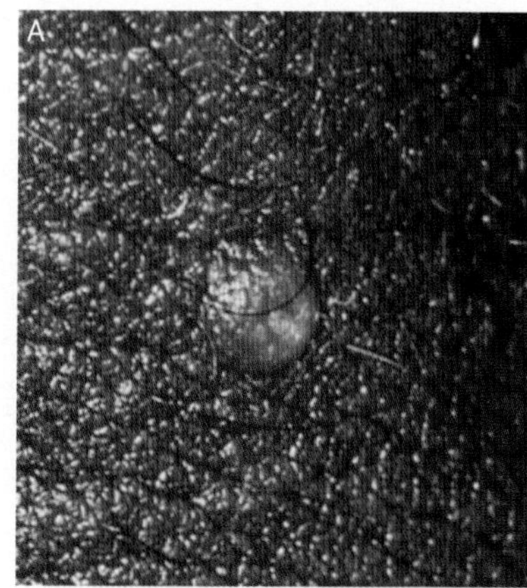

DNA Viruses (Herpes)

	Clinical Presentation	Management/Antimicrobial Coverage

HSV-1	- **Primary herpes** (gingivostomatitis/pharyngitis):
	  - Oral mucosal vesicular lesions (+/– ulceration)
	- **Recurrent** (herpes labialis):
	  - Reactivation from sensory ganglion, with vesicle on lip
	
	Other clinical manifestations:
	- Genital herpes
	- Encephalitis
	- Herpetic whitlow
	- Eczema herpeticum
	- Keratitis
		Dx: Viral culture or PCR
		
		Tx: Acyclovir, famciclovir, or valacyclovir

HSV-2	- **Genital herpes** [See: STD] - Neonatal herpes [See: OB]	
Varicella-Zoster	**Varicella (chicken pox)** - Primary VZV infection - Prodrome of fever, malaise, pharyngitis - Followed by generalized vesicular rash (red base with fluid-filled vesicle on top) - Contagious 48 hours before rash starts until skin lesions have fully crusted - Complications: Bacterial superinfection (most commonly Strep), pneumonia, encephalitis/cerebellar ataxia **Zoster (shingles)** [See: Derm] - Reactivation of VZV in sensory ganglia	Dx: Clinical Tx: - Supportive care (antihistamines, NSAIDs) - Acyclovir if > 12 y/o or immunocompromised PPX: Varicella vaccine
Epstein-Barr	**Mononucleosis** - Fever, pharyngitis, fatigue - Hepatosplenomegaly, posterior cervical lymphadenopathy - Generalized maculopapular rash (seen more commonly after amoxicillin administration) - Atypical lymphocytosis, elevated LFTs - Complications: GBS, meningoencephalitis, cranial nerve palsy - EBV associated with B-Cell lymphoma (Hodgkin), Burkitt lymphoma, nasopharyngeal carcinoma	Dx: Heterophile antibody test. Serology if unclear. Tx: Supportive *No athletics (3 weeks), no contact sports (4 weeks)
Cytomegalovirus	- Most individuals have been exposed Clinical: - Asymptomatic (if immunocompetent) - CMV Mononucleosis (mono like syndrome, but without positive heterophile antibody test) - Immunocompromised: Reactivation disease [See: HIV] - Pneumonitis, retinitis, esophagitis, colitis - Congenital infection [See: OB]	Dx: Serology/PCR (only required if presentation is heterophile negative mono OR immunocompromised) Tx: Severe infections treated with ganciclovir, cidofovir, or foscarnet
HHV 6/7	**Roseola** - High fevers for several days (seizures possible) - Followed by centrifugal maculopapular rash	Dx: Clinical Tx: Self-limited (NSAIDs for fever control)
HHV 8	**Kaposi sarcoma** [See: Derm]	

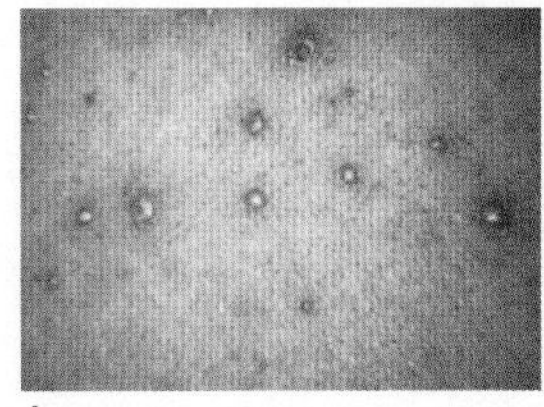
A

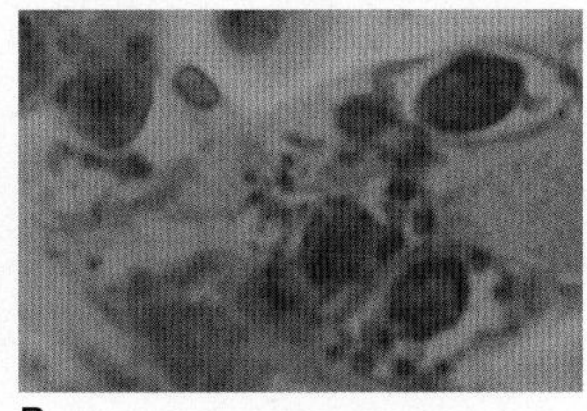
B

RNA Viruses

	Clinical Presentation	Management/Antimicrobial Coverage
Enteroviruses (Note: Most are cleared asymptomatically or cause minor febrile illness. The following are rare syndromes associated with these viruses. Young children and immunocompromised patients are most at risk.)		
Entero	- Meningoencephalitis, pneumonia, bronchiolitis	Dx: Clinical - If organism needs to be identified: RT-PCR Tx: Self-limited/supportive care
Echo	- Meningoencephalitis	
Coxsackie A	**Hand-Foot-Mouth** - Common infection in kids - Fever, oral vesicles on the buccal mucosa/tongue, and small painful lesions on the hands/feet **Herpangina** - Fever, odynophagia, vesicular lesions on tonsils/soft palate	
Coxsackie B	- Meningoencephalitis - Myocarditis, pericarditis, or pleurodynia (fever + sharp pleuritic chest pain)	
Polio	- Most clear virus asymptomatically/minor febrile illness - **Poliomyelitis**: - Only occurs in small fraction of those with viremia - Viral meningitis (fever, headache, neck stiffness) - Destruction of anterior horn motor neurons - Asymmetric flaccid proximal muscle weakness	Dx: Stool/CSF viral culture, PCR Tx: Supportive PPX: Salk (IM) or sabin (oral) vaccine
Rhinovirus	- Common cold (URTI)	
Norovirus	- Common cause of viral gastroenteritis	Dx: Clinical diagnosis. If definitive identification needed (i.e., for public health), ELISA/PCR available. Tx: Supportive Note: Rotavirus can be fatal in young infants.
Rotavirus		
Toga Viruses		
Alphavirus	- Mosquito vector. **Eastern/western equine encephalitis.**	
Chikungunya	- Aedes mosquito transmission. Endemic in Western Africa, but seen elsewhere (Central/South America, Caribbean). **Chikungunya fever**: - High fever with severe, bilateral, symmetric polyarthralgia - Headache, myalgias, maculopapular rash - Labs: ↑ AST/ALT, thrombocytopenia, leukopenia	Dx: RT-PCR or serology Tx: Supportive (fluid, NSAID pain control) *Some patients may develop chronic arthritis, requiring methotrexate or glucocorticoids
Rubivirus	**Rubella** ("German Measles") - Fever, lymphadenopathy (cervical/postauricular), arthralgias - Maculopapular rash (starts on face and spreads caudally) - Severe congenital infection	Dx: Not needed, unless concern over congenital infection (serology) Tx: Supportive
Flavi Viruses (all are mosquito-transmitted)		
Yellow fever	**Yellow fever** (mosquito-borne hemorrhagic fever) - Initial flu-like symptoms, followed by ~48-hour remission - Followed by hepatic/renal failure, hemorrhage, shock	Dx: Serology or rtPCR Tx: Supportive care. High mortality rate. PPX: Vaccination available
Dengue	**Dengue fever** ("Breakbone") - High fever, severe myalgias/arthralgias, retroorbital headache - Hepatomegaly/↑ LFTs, maculopapular rash - Hemorrhage (skin/mucosal bleeding) - Can lead to vascular leakage (shock, organ failure)	Dx: Clinical. Serology can confirm. Tx: Supportive care (Note: Acetaminophen okay, but no NSAIDs due to bleeding risk)
Zika	- Causes mild flu symptoms, polyarthralgias, rash - Associated with **fetal microcephaly**, fetal loss	Dx: Serology or rtPCR Tx: Supportive
West Nile Japanese St. Louis	- Often asymptomatic, but can cause febrile flu-like symptoms, and CNS involvement (**meningoencephalitis**)	Dx: CSF serology/PCR (for CNS disease) Tx: Supportive

RNA Viruses

	Clinical Presentation	Management/Antimicrobial Coverage
Coronavirus	- Common cause of URTIs - SARS/MERS (flu-like symptoms, followed by period of respiratory failure) - Covid-19	Dx: PCR
Influenza (orthomyxo)	- Respiratory spread, cause of the common flu - Antigenic shift (epidemics) and antigenic drift (endemics)	Tx: Oseltamivir [See: Pulm]
Ebola (filo)	**Ebola virus disease** - Initial fever, emesis, severe diarrhea (volume depletion) - Maculopapular rash, hemorrhage - Shock, multiorgan system failure (kidney/liver)	Dx: PCR Tx: Supportive care, proper precautions (isolation + contact/droplet)
Rabies (rhabdo)	- Transmitted via infected animal bite (bats/racoons/skunks in US, dogs in developing countries) Clinical: - ~1-2 months after bite, presents with prodrome (flu-like symptoms, with possible pain/paresthesias at bite site) - CNS symptoms follow: Encephalitis (hyperactivity, pharyngeal spasms, hypersalivation, hydrophobia), ascending flaccid paralysis - Coma, respiratory failure, and eventual death	Dx: Often clinical, but molecular tests available if confirmation needed Tx: Poor prognosis (experimental regimens) PPX: Rabies Vax/IVIG [See: EM] for full algorithm
Paramyxo		
Parainfluenza	- Adults: URTI/pneumonia - Children: **Croup** [See: Pulm]	
RSV	- URTI/pneumonia - Children: **Bronchiolitis** [See: Pulm]	
Metapneumovirus	- URTI/pneumonia	
Mumps	**Mumps** - Highly infectious; respiratory/fomite spread - Decreased incidence due to vaccine - Clinical: - Fever, malaise, myalgias, followed by **parotid swelling** - Complications: Orchitis/oophoritis, meningoencephalitis	Dx: Clinical (serology/rtPCR if uncertain) Tx: Supportive care PPX: MMR vaccine
Measles ("**Rubeola**")	**Measles** - Highly contagious (respiratory/airborne spread) Clinical: - Prodrome: Fever, malaise, cough, conjunctivitis, coryza, Koplik spots (white lesions on the buccal mucosa) - Exanthem: Erythematous/brown maculopapular rash, starting at head and spreading down to body, and out (spares palms/soles) Complications: - Otitis media or PNA - Encephalitis - Encephalomyelitis - Subacute sclerosing panencephalitis	Dx: Serology or rtPCR Tx: Supportive care + vitamin A PPX: MMR vaccine
Retrovirus	- HIV [See: HIV] - HTLV-I/II: Associated with T-cell leukemia/lymphoma - HTLV-I-associated myelopathy (tropical spastic paraparesis) - Progressive muscle weakness, spasticity, hyperreflexia	Dx: ELISA serology, followed by western blot Tx: - [See: Onc] for T-cell leukemia/lymphoma - Spastic paraparesis treated supportively +/– steroids

HIV/AIDS

Overview of Human Immunodeficiency Virus

General:

- **HIV**: Retrovirus that infects immune cells (T-cells, macrophages) → progressive immunodeficiency
- **AIDS**: Acquired immunodeficiency syndrome, defined as:
  CD4 cell count < 200 OR AIDS-defining condition

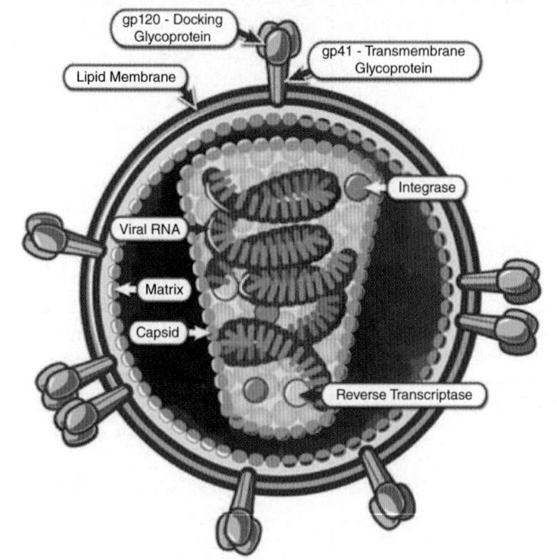

Pathophysiology:

- Envelope Proteins: gp41 (enters host cells) and gp120 (docking)
- p17 (matrix protein), p21 (capsid protein)
- **Reverse polymerase** (makes DNA from RNA), integrase (integrate HIV DNA into host cell DNA), proteases
- Virus initially infects macrophages (binding CCR5), with eventual spread to CD4 T-cells

Transmission:

- Transmission: Sexual, infected blood, or vertical at birth
  - Needlestick injury/shared needle: 20-60/10,000 exposures
  - Vaginal sex: 4-8/ 10,000 exposures
  - Anal sex (receptive): ~100/10,000 exposures
  - Vertical: ~30% (no meds). With medications, risk is < 2%.
- Increased risk if higher viral load, concurrent STIs, lack of circumcision

Clinical:

Stage	Clinical Features
Acute HIV	- ~2-4 weeks after exposure - Presents with **fever, lymphadenopathy, sore throat**, headache, myalgias. Painful mucocutaneous ulcers. - Macular rash, gastrointestinal symptoms (diarrhea) also possible *Viral load elevated, but antibody normal (no seroconversion yet)
Chronic HIV	- Asymptomatic for some period of years (~8-10 years). May have persistent generalized lymphadenopathy. - Symptomatic ("pre-AIDS"): Occurs in some patients, but not all. Prior to AIDS level disease, patient may develop increased frequency of constitutional symptoms, infections (dermatologic, fungal). - Progressive decline in CD4 count
AIDS	- CD4 cell count < 200 OR - AIDS-defining condition (most common listed below):

PCP pneumonia	Candidiasis (esophageal)	Cryptococcus
Chronic HSV	CMV (systemic or ocular)	Kaposi sarcoma
Toxoplasmosis	Prog. multifocal leukoencephalopathy	HIV wasting
MAI or TB infection	Lymphoma (brain/Burkitt)	Invasive cervical cancer
Chronic cryptosporidium	Disseminated histo/coccidio-mycosis	HIV encephalopathy

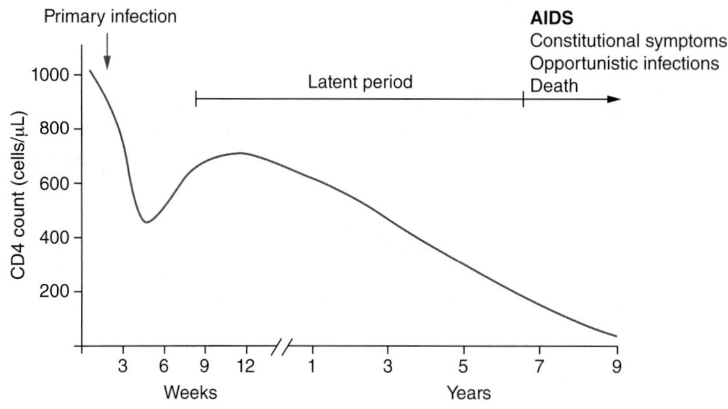

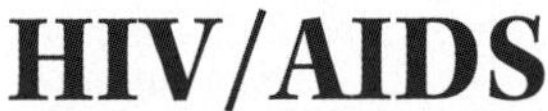

HIV/AIDS

Diagnosis of HIV

<u>Routine screening/diagnosis</u>

- **4th-generation immunoassay**
    - Detects HIV p24 antigen and HIV antibodies
- HIV-1/2 differentiation immunoassay
    - Now preferred confirmatory test (over western blot)

<u>Screening indications</u>

- One time screening between ages 13 and 75
- **Annual screening**: MSM (men who have sex with men), IV drug use, sex workers, sex with high-risk partner
- Others: Routine prenatal screening, new STI, exposure to body fluids/blood

<u>Acute HIV</u> (testing given concern for symptoms consistent with acute HIV)

- 4th-generation immunoassay PLUS
- **HIV viral load** (RNA): Should be $\uparrow\uparrow$ in acute HIV

Management of HIV

<u>Antiretroviral therapy (ART)</u>

- General considerations
    - All with HIV should be treated with antivirals, regardless of CD4 count
    - Once initiated, ART is continued indefinitely

- Regimens
    - Treatment naive: **2 NRTIs + integrase inhibitor**
        - Emtricitabine + tenofovir + dolutegravir
        - Emtricitabine + tenofovir + bictegravir
        - Abacavir + lamivudine + dolutegravir
    - Drugs modified over time based on viral resistance profile

<u>Pre-exposure prophylaxis</u>

- Indications: HIV-uninfected patients at high risk to acquire HIV
- Regimen: **Emtricitabine + tenofovir**, for as long as patient is determined to be at risk

<u>Post-exposure prophylaxis</u>

- Indications:
    - Needlestick or body fluid exposure in known HIV patient
        - Includes blood, semen, vaginal fluid
        - Does not include urine, saliva, sweat
        - Exposure to nonintact skin or mucous membrane
    - Recent sexual exposure to known HIV carrier
    - High risk sexual activity
        - Condomless sex in high HIV prevalence area, condomless MSM, sex work
    - Recent IV drug use with needle sharing
- Regimens (similar to treatment naive above)
    - Emtricitabine + tenofovir + integrase Inhibitor
- Management:
    - 28 days of therapy
    - Test patient with 4th-generation assay at start of PEP, 6 weeks, 4 months

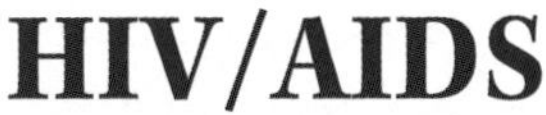

HIV Drugs

Drug	Mechanism	Side Effects/Management
NRTIs		
Abacavir Didanosine Emtricitabine Lamivudine Stavudine Tenofovir Zidovudine	- Competitive inhibitor of viral reverse transcriptase (incorporated into DNA, causing strand termination)	- Mitochondrial toxicity (neuropathy, pancreatitis) - Lactic acidosis - Myopathy - Pancreatitis - Lipoatrophy (especially zidovudine/stavudine) - Hepatotoxicity - Renal insufficiency (tenofovir) <u>Abacavir hypersensitivity</u> - Associated with HLA-B*5701 - Fever, rash, GI problems, malaise
NNRTIs		
Efavirenz Etravirine Nevirapine Rilpivirine	- Binds reverse transcriptase at site outside active site, causing conformational change that ↓ enzymatic activity	- Efavirenz: Teratogenic, vivid dreams, other CNS symptoms (confusion), psychiatric changes (irritability, anxiety) - Mild hepatotoxicity across class
Integrase Inhibitor		
Bictegravir Dolutegravir Elvitegravir Raltegravir	- Inhibits enzyme that aids in viral DNA incorporation into host DNA	- Generally well tolerated - Levels boosted by CYP 3A4 inhibitors
Protease Inhibitor (PI)		
Atazanavir Darunavir Indinavir Lopinavir	- Prevent viral maturation by inhibiting cleavage of key polyproteins to their active components	- Insulin resistance/hyperglycemia - Hyperlipidemia, lipodystrophy - Hepatotoxicity * Generally used with boosting agents
Fusion Inhibitor		
Maraviroc	- CCR5 entry inhibitor	- Both infrequently used, unless many other drugs failed
Enfuvirtide	- gp41 blocker	
Boosting Agents		
Cobicistat Ritonavir	- Cyp 3A4 inhibitors, boosting the levels of protease inhibitors and elvitegravir - Note: Ritonavir is a PI that has some antiviral efficacy, but is primarily used in low doses as booster	- Cobicistat: Mild renal insufficiency - Ritonavir: See PI class side effects

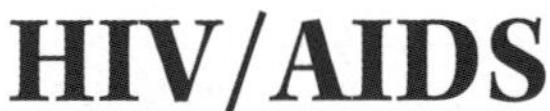

HIV/AIDS

Overview of HIV Complication Prophylaxis

Infection	Indication	Regimen
Tuberculosis	- Screen all HIV patients with IFN-γ or PPD	- Treat latent TB if present
Pneumocystis	- CD4 $\leq$ 200	- TMP-SMX - Alt: Atovaquone, dapsone, or aerosolized pentamidine
Toxoplasma	- CD4 $\leq$ 100 and - Positive toxo IgG serology	- TMP-SMX - Alt: Dapsone + pyrimethamine
MAC	- CD4 $\leq$ 50 and no ART - Not indicated if on ART	- Azithromycin
Coccidiomycosis	- CD4 $\leq$ 250 AND in Arizona/California	- Fluconazole
Histoplasmosis	- CD4 $\leq$ 150 AND in highly endemic area (usually not needed in US)	- Itraconazole

Vaccinations in HIV

Vaccination	Indications
Live vaccines (MMR/Varicella)	- Contraindicated if CD4 $\leq$ 200 - MMR/varicella vaccines if CD4 > 200 and patient has not previously received
Influenza, TDAP, HPV	- All have same indications as normal adult
Pneumonia	- PCV20 alone or PCV15 followed by PPSV23 $\geq$ 8 weeks later
Hepatitis A	- If chronic liver disease or high risk (MSM, IV drug use)
Hepatitis B	- If not immune
Meningitis (ACWY)	- All HIV infected, regardless of age

Mucocutaneous/Cutaneous HIV Complications

Disorder	Clinical Features
Oral thrush	- Oropharyngeal candidiasis: Most common HIV opportunistic infection. Seen with CD4 < 200. - Presents with white plaques on the buccal mucosa, palate, tongue - Tx: Topical nystatin or clotrimazole. Oral azoles if severe.
Oral hairy leukoplakia	- EBV-mediated disorder of tongue epithelium - White plaques on the side of tongue - Cannot be scraped off (differentiates from *Candida*) - Tx: Often no treatment required. Antivirals (acyclovir) effective.
Bacillary angiomatosis	- Bartonella infection, seen with CD4 < 100 - *B. Henselae* → Cats. *B. Quintana* → lice exposure (homeless). - Presents with vascular cutaneous lesions (with varied appearance). Often red-purple nodules/papules. - Systemic symptoms (fevers/chills/malaise) - Dx: Biopsy - Tx: Doxycycline/erythromycin. ART.
Kaposi sarcoma	[See: Derm] - Tx: ART therapy usually leads to resolution (without requiring systemic chemotherapy)

HIV/AIDS

Pneumocystis Pneumonia

General: Pulmonary opportunistic fungal infection with pneumocystis jirovecii. Occurs almost exclusively in immunocompromised patients (HIV, chronic steroid use). Caused by inhalation of yeast, resulting in pulmonary infection.

Clinical:

- **Indolent onset fever, dry cough, dyspnea, hypoxemia**
    - Note: Usually slower onset in HIV, but acute fulminant respiratory failure in others
- ↑ LDH levels
- XR: **Bilateral diffuse infiltrates**

Diagnosis:

- Definitive: Organism identification in sputum or bronchoalveolar lavage
- Often treated based purely on clinical presentation

Management:

- TMP-SMX
- Alt: Pentamidine (IV), atovaquone (oral), clindamycin + primaquine, trimethoprim + dapsone
- Corticosteroids if $PaO_2 < 70$ or Aa gradient > 35

Prophylaxis: (TMP-SMX)

- HIV with CD4 < 200
- Others: Immunosuppressant use (high-dose steroids, cyclophosphamide, etc.), stem cell/solid organ transplant

Gastrointestinal Infections

Esophagitis Clinical: Presents with **dysphagia/odynophagia** Diagnosis: Clinical, with confirmation via upper endoscopy in some cases Management: Treat empirically with fluconazole - If no improvement: Upper endoscopy indicated - Acyclovir for HSV, ganciclovir for CMV	
Candidal	- White plaques, with likely oral thrush
HSV	- Round, herpetic ulcerations/vesicles
CMV	- Linear ulcerations
Diarrhea	
Cryptosporidium *Isospora* *Microsporidium*	- Parasitic gastrointestinal pathogens, CD4 < 200 - Clinical: Low-grade fever, abdominal pain, weight loss, chronic watery diarrhea - Dx: Stool O&P - Tx: Nitazoxanide (cryptosporidium), TMP-SMX (isospora), albendazole (*microsporidium*)
Mycobacterium avium complex	- CD4 count < 50, generally not on ART - Clinical: Fever, weight loss, night sweats, chronic diarrhea, abdominal pain, diffuse lymphadenopathy - **Watery diarrhea** is significant component of disseminated infection - Dx: Blood culture or tissue biopsy - Tx: Clarithromycin + ethambutol
Cytomegalovirus	- Reactivation of latent CMV infection, CD4 < 50 - Clinical: - Systemic symptoms (fever/weight loss/malaise) - **Abdominal pain/diarrhea** (can be watery +/− blood), esophagitis - **Retinitis** - Dx: Clinical symptoms + endoscopy w/ biopsy (both macroscopic and microscopic features of CMV) - Tx: Ganciclovir or valganciclovir

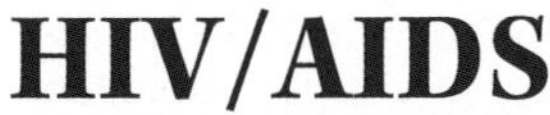

HIV/AIDS

HIV Nephropathy

General: Characterized by collapsing form of focal segmental glomerulosclerosis

Clinical: Proteinuria/nephrotic syndrome, with progressive renal insufficiency

Diagnosis: Renal biopsy (collapsing, focal areas of glomerulosclerosis, with dilated tubules and interstitial inflammation)

Management: ART. ACEi/ARB.

Neurologic HIV Complications

Disorder	Clinical Features
Primary CNS Lymphoma	- Extranodal **non-Hodgkin lymphoma** originating from CNS - Associated with **EBV** - Clinical: Confusion, memory loss, focal neurologic deficits (e.g., hemiparesis), aphasia, seizures - MRI w/ contrast: Contrast-enhancing lesion (solitary most common) - Dx: Brain biopsy - Tx: Chemotherapy (methotrexate-based), ART
Toxoplasmosis	- Common if CD4 count < 100 and not receiving PPX - Clinical: Presents with fever, headache, CNS symptoms (focal deficits, confusion, mental status change) - +/− Extracerebral manifestations (pneumonitis/chorioretinitis) - MRI: **Multiple ring-enhancing CNS lesions** - Dx: Clinical presentation + MRI + positive toxo IgG - Tx: Sulfadiazine + pyrimethamine
Progressive Multifocal Leukoencephal-opathy	- Due to reactivation of **JC Virus** - Demyelinating disease seen with HIV, leukemia/lymphoma treatment, natalizumab - Clinical: Indolent and progressive mental status changes, ataxia, focal neurologic deficits, seizures - MRI: Multiple, asymmetric, nonenhancing, hypodense white matter lesions (no surrounding edema) - Dx: LP (**CSF JC virus PCR**) - Tx: ART, but poor prognosis
Cryptococcus	- Common cause of meningoencephalitis in HIV patients - Seen if CD4 count < 100 OR no ART therapy - Clinical: Systemic symptoms (fever/malaise) with headache, neck stiffness, photophobia - Dx: CSF (culture/Ag test/India Ink stain with encapsulated yeast) - Tx: Amphotericin B + flucytosine induction, followed by prolonged fluconazole course
HIV Dementia	- HIV-associated neurocognitive disorders. Occurs in advanced AIDS. - Clinical: Difficulty with attention, memory, concentration, and informational processing - Dx: Diagnosis of exclusion - Tx: ART

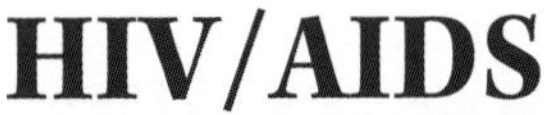

HIV/AIDS

Other HIV Complications

Disorder	Clinical Features
IRIS	- Immune reconstitution inflammatory syndrome - Worsening of a preexisting infectious processes with initiation of ART - Clinical: Presents within 1-2 months of starting ART with exacerbations of opportunistic HIV infection - Management: Treat opportunistic infection, continue ART *Generally can initiate ART within 2 weeks of treatment of opportunistic infection. Delay > 2 weeks for cryptococcal and tuberculosis meningitis.
HIV Wasting	- Rapid weight loss and tissue wasting with severe AIDS - Tx: Improves dramatically with ART

HIV-Associated Lipodystrophy Syndrome	- Multifaceted syndrome that can involve pure fat atrophy OR accumulation of fat
	- **Fat atrophy**: Preferential loss of subcutaneous fat, versus fat/muscle seen with HIV wasting
	  - Most commonly associated with NRTI (stavudine, zidovudine)
	- **Fat accumulation**: Truncal fat accumulation (like Cushing)
	  - Not associated with any specific drug regimen
	
	- Both atrophy/accumulation can be associated with **insulin resistance, hyperlipidemia**

Disseminated Fungal Infection	- Disseminated candida - Histoplasmosis, blastomycosis, coccidioidomycosis

Sexually Transmitted Infection

Chlamydia

General: Sexually transmitted gram-negative intracellular bacterium, most common bacterial STI in the US

Risk: Sexual behavior (new partner, multiple partners), inconsistent condom use, history of STI, men who have sex with men

Clinical: Variety of potential presentations
- Asymptomatic (common, especially in men)
- <u>Men</u>
    - **Urethritis** (mucoid urethral discharge/dysuria)
    - Prostatitis, epididymitis (rare)
- <u>Women</u>
    - **Cervicitis**
    - Pelvic inflammatory disease

Diagnosis: NAAT (vaginal swab or urine)
- Can also obtain NAAT from other sites, such as anal/pharyngeal
- Note: Organism does not gram stain well

Management: Azithromycin (single dose 1000 mg) or doxycycline
Note: This is for simple urethritis or cervicitis. If advanced pathology (PID, epididymitis) is present, further antibiotics are indicated.

Gonorrhea

General: *Neisseria gonorrhoeae* infection, gram-negative diplococci, second most common cause of bacterial STI in the US

Risk: [See: Chlamydia]

Clinical:
- Asymptomatic (Often in both men/females)
- Extragenital: **Proctitis, pharyngitis**, disseminated disease
- Men
    - **Urethritis** (mucoid urethral discharge/dysuria)
    - Epididymitis
- Women
    - **Cervicitis** (usually with urethritis)
    - Pelvic inflammatory disease

Diagnosis: NAAT (vaginal swab or urine)
- Can also obtain NAAT from other sites, such as anal/pharyngeal
- Gram stain: Gram-negative diplococci, PMNs

Management: Ceftriaxone + azithromycin or doxycycline

Sexually Transmitted Infection

Syphilis

General: Infection from the spirochete *Treponema pallidum*. Transmitted via sexual contact and vertically during pregnancy.
- Considered contagious during primary, secondary, and early latent disease

Clinical:

Primary (Weeks)	- **Chancre**: Papule, which ulcerates. Ulcer is nonexudative and painless. - Regional lymphadenopathy - Heals in a few weeks without therapy
Secondary (Months)	Weeks to months after chancre, presents with: - Constitutional symptoms (fever/malaise/other flu symptoms) - **Diffuse lymphadenopathy** (epitrochlear nodes are classic) - Arthritis, hepatitis, glomerulonephritis - **Rash**: Maculopapular/pustular, involving trunk, limbs, palms/soles[A] - White/gray plaques on mucous membranes/genitals (condyloma lata) - Alopecia A B
Latent	- Serologic evidence of syphilis without symptoms
Tertiary (Years)	- Widely variable number of years after primary infection - Gummas (ulcers or granulomatous nodules) that occur on skin and bone - Cardiovascular: Aortitis, aortic aneurysm <u>CNS</u>: - Early neurosyphilis: Meningitis (headache, neck stiffness, confusion), increased risk for stroke, panuveitis - Late neurosyphilis: - **General paresis**: Progressive dementia - **Tabes dorsalis**: Posterior column degeneration, with sensory ataxia, sharp pains - **Pupillary dysfunction**: Argyll-Robertson pupil, does not contract with light, but does with accommodation

Diagnosis: Screen with treponemal test, followed by nontreponemal test to confirm active infection

Treponemal (FTA-ABS, TP-EIA)	- Persistently positive after infection - More specific than nontreponemal
Nontreponemal (RPR/VDRL)	- Increases with active disease, decreases after treatment - Frequent false positives, and false negative early in disease - False positive with: SLE, certain drugs/viral infections - Lumbar puncture (CSF-VDRL) to diagnose neurosyphilis

FTA-ABS or TP EIA	+	+	−
RPR or VDRL	+	−	N/A
	Syphilis infection	Early/latent infection or treated infection	Very early infection or negative

Management:
- IM penicillin G (for primary, secondary, tertiary, and latent disease)
  - Alt: Doxycycline (best if penicillin allergy)
- IV penicillin G +/− probenecid for neurosyphilis
- Trend RPR or VDRL titer to determine response
- Jarisch-Herxheimer: Worsening symptoms for ~24 hours after treatment

Sexually Transmitted Infection

Genital Herpes

General: Genital herpes is most commonly caused by HSV-2, but HSV-1 also possible

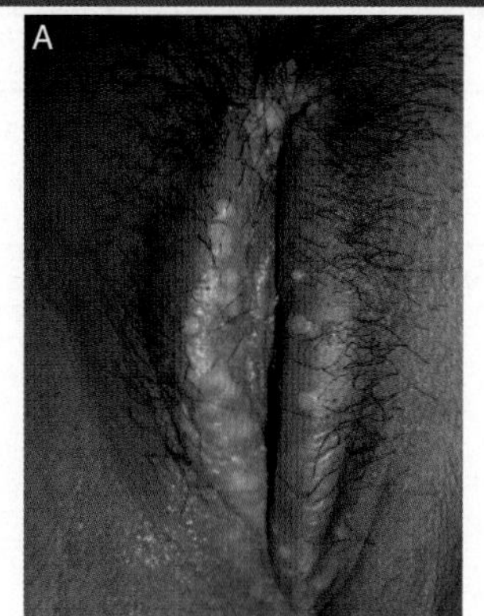

Clinical:
- **Primary**: Variable, but can have painful genital ulcers and systemic symptoms
- **Recurrent**: Episodes of genital ulcers[A] (less severe than initial episode)
    - Multiple vesicles on erythematous base is classic

Diagnosis:
- PCR/culture (sample from unroofed lesion)
- Serology if no active lesions (IgM)

Management:
- Primary infection: Acyclovir, famciclovir or valacyclovir
- Recurrent disease:
    - Chronic acyclovir suppression if ≥ 6 episodes per year
    - Episodic antiviral therapy if < 6 episodes per year
- Note: No therapy requiring if episodes infrequent/not bothersome

Ulcerative Lesions DDx

Painful Ulcers	Painless Ulcers
Herpes	***Syphilis*** (Chancre)

Chancroid
- *Haemophilus ducreyi.* Rare in US.
- Deep, painful exudative ulcer
- Dx: Clinical (no good tests)
- Tx: Azithromycin or ceftriaxone
	Lymphogranuloma venereum
	- Due to chlamydia infection (L1-L3 serotypes)
	- Small shallow ulcer clusters, followed by:
	  - Severe, painful inguinal LA (buboes)
	  - Anorectal disease (proctocolitis, anal mass)
	  - Eventual fibrosis and strictures if untreated
	- Dx: NAAT
	- Tx: Doxycycline/azithromycin

	Granuloma Inguinale (donovanosis) - Due to *Klebsiella* granulomatis - Rare in US, more common in tropics - Nodules, which ulcerate, forming extensive ulcers with granulation tissue base - Tx: Azithromycin

Other STI

Disorder	Features
Pubic lice (crabs)	- *Phthirus pubis.* Transmitted sexually or via clothing/towel. - Presents with pruritus, diagnosed when bug visualized - Tx: Topical permethrin
Anogenital warts (*Condylomata acuminata*)	- HPV 6, 11 infection. Transmitted sexually. - Variable appearance (nodular or plaque-like lesions that are white, erythematous, or skin-colored) - Tx: Imiquimod, podophyllotoxin, cryotherapy, trichloroacetic acid, surgical (Note: May resolve on own, but takes months.)

Infection Prophylaxis

Hospital Infection Prophylaxis		
Precaution	**Features**	**Indications**
Standard	- Hand hygiene - Proper gloves/gown/eye protection when exposed to body fluids	- All patients
Isolation		
Contact	- Gown/gloves	- MRSA, VRE - Multidrug-resistant gram negative - Viral (HSV, norovirus, VZV, RSV, parainfluenza) - *C. Diff* - Scabies
Droplet	- Mask	- Virus: Influenza, adeno, parvo, rubella, mumps - Bacteria: Meningococcus, HiB, pertussis, diphtheria
Airborne	- Airborne isolation room (negative pressure, proper air filtering) - N95 mask or respirator	- Tuberculosis - Measles, varicella - SARS, ebola

Post-Exposure Prophylaxis	
Organism	**Regimen/Indications**
N. meningitidis	- PPX for all close contacts (ideally within 24 hours) - Regimen: ciprofloxacin, ceftriaxone, rifampin
HiB	- PPX for household contacts of invasive type B infection that have not completed HiB vaccine OR are immunocompromised - Regimen: Rifampin
Pertussis	- Household/close contacts should receive PPX - Regimen: Macrolide
Hepatitis B	- Nonimmune patient exposed to HepB or HepB unknown - Exposure: Percutaneous or mucosal exposure to body fluids - HBIG plus HepB Vax
Varicella	Post exposure to Varicella: - VZV vaccination: For healthy VZV-nonimmune children/adults - Varicella Ig: For pregnant women, infants, and immunocompromised (not vaccine candidates)
Influenza	- Antivirals for close exposure to flu, in the following situations: - Pregnancy, high-risk for complications, nursing home outbreaks

Antimicrobials

	Mechanism	Indication	Side Effects/Management
Penicillin Beta-Lactams			
Penicillin G (IM) Penicillin V (PO)	- Blocks peptidoglycan synthesis in cell wall (blocks transpeptidases)	- Covers basic gram positives, spirochetes, meningococcus - Syphilis, actinomycosis - Sickle-cell, rheumatic fever prophylaxis	- Hypersensitivity reactions (anaphylaxis, drug rash) - Coombs (+) hemolytic anemia - Acute interstitial nephritis (AIN)
Amoxicillin (PO) Ampicillin (IV)	- Same as Penicillin, but with β-lactamase resistance	- Gram-positive and some gram-negative coverage - Listeria	
Dicloxacillin Nafcillin Oxacillin		- MSSA coverage	
Piperacillin Ticarcillin	- Used with Tazobactam (β-lactamase inhibitor)	- Broad-spectrum - *Pseudomonas* coverage	
Cephalosporins			
1st Generation Cefazolin Cefalexin	- Blocks peptidoglycan synthesis in cell wall (blocks transpeptidases) - β-lactamase resistance	- Basic gram-positive, limited negative coverage - MSSA	- Hypersensitivity reactions (some penicillin cross-reactivity [< 10%], can be used in patients with low risk PCN allergies) - Disulfiram-like reaction with EtOH (rare) - Hypoprothrombinemia (↑ bleeding risk)
2nd Generation Cefaclor Cefoxitin Cefuroxime		- Basic gram-positive, extended gram-negative coverage	
3rd Generation Ceftriaxone Ceftazidime Cefotaxime Cefdinir		- Extended gram-negative coverage - Ceftazidime: *Pseudomonas*	
4th Generation Cefepime		- Extended gram-negative coverage, plus *Pseudomonas*	
5th Generation Ceftaroline Ceftolozane		- Ceftaroline: MRSA coverage - Ceftolozane: *Pseudomonas*	
Carbapenems			
Imipenem Meropenem Ertapenem	- Blocks peptidoglycan synthesis in cell wall (blocks transpeptidases)	- Broad gram-positive, negative, and anaerobic coverage (including *Pseudomonas*)	- Seizures (imipenem) - Hypersensitivity reactions (minimal cross-reactivity with penicillin [< 1%])
Monobactams			
Aztreonam	- Blocks peptidoglycan synthesis in cell wall (blocks transpeptidases)	- Gram-negative coverage (including *Pseudomonas*)	
Vancomycin	- Binds Dala/Dala precursors and inhibits bacterial cell wall growth	- Gram-positive coverage, including MRSA	- Nephrotoxicity/ototoxic (rare) - Vancomycin infusion reaction (diffuse flushing with infusion, correct with antihistamines/slow infusion)
Aminoglycosides			
Gentamicin Neomycin Amikacin Tobramycin	- Inhibits 30s ribosome - Bactericidal	- Gram-negative infections (including *Pseudomonas*)	- Nephrotoxicity - Ototoxicity - Neuromuscular blockade (avoid in myasthenia gravis)
Tetracyclines			
Doxycycline Minocycline Tetracycline	- Inhibits 30s ribosome - Bacteriostatic	- Broad coverage, including atypicals, zoonotic, and tick-borne pathogens	- GI upset, pill esophagitis - Photosensitivity - Teratogen: Discolored teeth, inhibits bone growth

Antimicrobials

	Mechanism	Indication	Side Effects/Management
Macrolide			
Azithromycin Clarithromycin Erythromycin	- Inhibits 50s ribosome - Bacteriostatic	- Basic gram-positive and gram-negative coverage - Atypical pneumonia	- ↑ GI motility - Arrhythmia (QT prolongation) - Cholestasis - CYP 450 inhibition
Fluoroquinolones			
Ciprofloxacin Levofloxacin Moxifloxacin	- Inhibits topoisomerase II (DNA gyrase) - Bactericidal	- Gram-negative coverage, with some *Pseudomonas* activity - Levo/moxi: Respiratory infection coverage	- Tendinopathy (risk if older or if using steroids) - Cartilage damage in kids - Neurologic (insomnia, confusion, psychosis) - QT prolongation
Sulfonamides			
Sulfamethoxazole Sulfisoxazole Sulfadiazine	- Inhibit dihydropteroate synthase (part of DNA synthesis pathway)	- Gram-positive and negative coverage (including MRSA) - PCP treatment/PPX - Toxoplasmosis - Dapsone: Leprosy	- Hemolysis (G6PD deficiency) - Pancytopenia (including megaloblastic anemia) - Nephrotoxicity (including interstitial nephritis) - Hyperkalemia (from ENAC channel inhibition) - Sulfa hypersensitivity reactions
Dapsone			
Trimethoprim	- Inhibits bacterial dihydrofolate reductase		
Misc.			
Linezolid	- Inhibits 50s ribosome	- Gram-positive coverage (including MRSA, VRE)	- Myelosuppression - Peripheral and optic neuropathy - Serotonin syndrome (has MAOI activity)
Clindamycin	- Inhibits 50s ribosome	- Gram-positive and anaerobic coverage	- High risk of *C. Diff* infection
Daptomycin	- Lipopeptide that disrupts cell membrane of Gram (+) bacteria	- Gram-positive coverage (including MRSA)	- Myopathy/rhabdomyolysis - Inactivated by pulmonary surfactant (don't use for PNA)
Metronidazole	- Forms free radical toxin that damages DNA	- Anaerobes - *H. pylori, Gardnerella* - Some parasites (*Giardia, Entamoeba, Trichomonas*)	- Metallic taste - Disulfiram-like reaction
Nitrofurantoin	- Inhibits ribosome complex formation	- Used primarily for gram-negative UTIs	- Rare interstitial pneumonitis and hepatotoxicity
Anti-tuberculosis			
Rifampin Rifabutin	- Inhibit RNA polymerase	- TB, leprosy, meningococcal ppx	- Minor hepatotoxicity - Turns body fluids red - CYP450 inducer
Isoniazid	- ↓ mycolic acid synthesis	- TB	- Hepatotoxicity (usually minor transaminitis, but severe hepatitis possible) - Drug-induced SLE - B6 deficiency (peripheral neuropathy, sideroblastic anemia)
Pyrazinamide	- Unknown mechanism	- TB	- Hepatotoxicity - ↑ uric acid (gout flares)
Ethambutol	- Blocks arabinosyltransferase (mycobacterial cell wall synthesis)	- TB, MAI	- Optic neuropathy (red-green color blindness)

Antimicrobials

Multidrug-Resistant Organisms

Organism	General	Management
MRSA	- Methicillin-resistant *Staph Aureus*	- Oral Agents: Doxycycline, clindamycin, TMP-SMX - IV Agents: Vancomycin, daptomycin, linezolid
Pseudomonas	- Intrinsically resistant to numerous antibiotics - Can acquire resistance to other agents (i.e., acquire ESBL)	- Piperacillin-tazobactam - Ceftazidime, cefepime - Aztreonam - Ciprofloxacin - Carbapenems, aminoglycosides
Enterococcus	- Strains tested for sensitivity to ampicillin, vancomycin	- Ampicillin-sensitive: Ampicillin - Ampicillin-resistant: Vancomycin - VRE (vanc-resistant): Linezolid, daptomycin
ESBL gram negatives	- Extended-spectrum beta-lactamases - Inactivates most beta-lactams, cephalosporins - Carried most commonly in *Klebsiella, E. Coli*	- Carbapenems

CRE	- Carbapenem-resistant enterobacteriaceae
	- Provides resistance to all beta-lactams
	- Found in some *E. Coli, Enterobacter, Klebsiella*
		- Fosfomycin (uncomplicated UTI)
		- Severe infections:
		  - Ceftazidime-avibactam
		  - Meropenem-vaborbactam
		  - Imipenem-cilastatin-relebactam

Antifungals

	Mechanism	Indication	Side Effects/Management
Amphotericin B	- Binds ergosterol, creating pores in cell membrane - Delivered in liposomes to decrease host toxicity	- Severe fungal infections	- "Shake and Bake": Fevers, chills with infusion - Phlebitis - Nephrotoxicity - Electrolyte abnormalities (hypomag/hypokalemia)
Nystatin	- Same as amphotericin - Delivered topically	- Thrush, intertrigo, diaper rash	
Azoles Fluconazole Itraconazole Voriconazole Posaconazole Isavuconazole	- Inhibits ergosterol synthesis	- Cover basic fungal infections - Itraconazole: Endemic fungi - Voriconazole: *Aspergillus*	- Inhibits CYP 450 - Hepatotoxicity - Voriconazole: Vision changes, hallucinations, photosensitivity reaction - Ketoconazole: Hepatotoxicity (rarely used)
Echinocandins Caspofungin Micafungin	- Inhibit the synthesis of β-glucan in fungal cell wall	- *Candida* systemic infections - *Aspergillus*	- Flushing (with IV formulations)
Terbinafine	- Inhibits squalene epoxidase (part of ergosterol synthesis)	- Topical dermatophytes, including onychomycosis	- GI disturbances (including abnormal taste) - Hepatotoxicity
Griseofulvin	- Disrupts microtubules, inhibiting fungal cell mitosis	- Topical dermatophytes	- CYP 450 inducer - Teratogen

	Yeast (Candida, Crypto)	Endemic Fungi (Histo/blasto/coccidio)	Molds (Aspergillus)	Molds (Mucor)
Amphotericin				
Fluconazole				
Itraconazole				
Voriconazole				
Micafungin				

Antimicrobials

	Mechanism	Indication	Side Effects/Management
Antivirals			
Oseltamivir Zanamivir	- Inhibit neuraminidase (prevent release of progeny virus)	- Influenza	- Nausea/vomiting
Acyclovir Famciclovir Valacyclovir	- Guanosine analog, inhibit viral DNA prolongation	- Herpes viruses (including HSV, VZV)	- Obstructive crystalline nephropathy (when given IV, administered with fluids)
Ganciclovir Valganciclovir	- Guanosine analog, inhibits viral DNA kinase in CMV	- CMV	- Myelosuppression (leading to cytopenias) - Nephrotoxicity
Foscarnet	- Viral DNA/RNA polymerase inhibitor	- CMV/HSV (second-line agent)	- Nephrotoxicity - Electrolyte issues (hypocalcemia, hypokalemia)
Cidofovir	- Viral DNA polymerase inhibitor	- CMV retinitis - HSV (acyclovir-resistant)	- Nephrotoxicity
Anti-helminth/louse			
Albendazole	- Inhibits microtubule assembly	- Variety of parasitic worm infections	- Hepatotoxicity
Pyrantel pamoate	- Neuromuscular blockade		
Diethylcarbam-azine	- Inhibitor of arachidonic acid metabolism	- Filariasis, loiasis	
Ivermectin	- Increases parasitic cell membrane permeability	- Parasitic worm infections - Lice, scabies	- Neurotoxicity
Praziquantel	- Increases parasitic cell membrane permeability	- Parasitic worm infections (especially *Schistosoma*)	- GI disturbances
Permethrin	- Na channel blocker	- Anti-louse	- Skin irritation (at site of application)

Neurologic Exam

Mental Status	- Attention (repeat back series of numbers)
	- Memory (remember 3 words after 5 minutes of distraction)
	- Language
	  - Repetition: Repeat complex phrases (no ifs, ands, or buts)
	  - Naming: Name objects
	  - Comprehension: Follow simple one-step commands
	  - Read/write
	- Visuospatial: Copy diamond or cube
	- Calculations: Serial sevens

Cranial Nerves	- CN II (Optic): Pupillary reaction, visual acuity (Snellen), visual fields, fundoscopy - CN III, IV, VI: Extraocular movements - CN V: Facial sensory, muscles of mastication - CN VII: Facial movement - CN IX: Uvula deviation, gag reflex - CN XI: "Shrugging" motor strength - CN XII: Tongue movements
Motor	- Muscle bulk/appearance - Strength testing (0/5 is no movement, 3/5 can overcome gravity, 5/5 is full strength)
Sensory	- Spinothalamics: Sharp/dull testing, temperature - Posterior column: Vibration testing (tuning fork), proprioception
Reflexes	- Achilles (S1/S2) - Patellar (L3/L4) - Biceps (C5/C6) - Triceps (C7/C8) - Babinski response (upper motor neuron sign) - Grading: 2+ normal (1+ hyporeflexia, 3+ hyperreflexia, 4+ clonus)
Coordination	- Finger-to-nose, heel-to-shin - Rapid alternating movements
Gait	- Romberg (stand in place with eyes closed) - Walk (check balance, speed, use of arms/legs) - Heel/toe walk (test of balance)

Stroke

Transient Ischemic Attack

General: Episode of transient neurologic dysfunction secondary to transient CNS ischemia that does not result in infarction

Etiology:

- **Embolic**: Embolic thrombus, either artery-to-artery or from heart (e.g., AF or LV thrombus)
- **Low Flow**: From arterial stenosis (atherosclerosis)
- **Lacunar**: Thrombosis over lipohyalinosis of small penetrating arteries

Clinical: **Focal neurologic deficit**, that spontaneously **resolves within 24 hours**

- Often resolves quickly (low-flow in minutes, embolic in hours)

Diagnosis: MRI (preferred) or CT

- Source localization: Duplex US (or CTA/MRA), cardiac monitoring, TTE

Management: ASA +/– Clopidogrel (dual-antiplatelet [DAPT] used in short-term for high-risk TIAs)

- Secondary prevention (weight loss, smoking cessation, statin)
- Outpatient evaluation for stroke source (see above)

Stroke Risk: Overall risk ~8% at 30 days and 10% at 90 days. High risk for stroke if MRI shows area of focal ischemia.

Ischemic Cerebrovascular Accident (CVA)

General: Inadequate brain oxygenation, leading to infarction of the brain parenchyma

Subtype	Etiology/Risk	Clinical Features
Thrombotic	- Atherosclerosis (**hypertension**, HLD, DM, smoking) - Small vessel lipohyalinosis (lacunar infarcts)	- **Local thrombotic obstruction of artery** - Fluctuating severity of symptoms initially, with periods of improvement
Embolic	- Atrial fibrillation - Carotid disease (artery-to-artery) - Endocarditis/valve disease - Septal defects (PFO/ASD)	- **Thrombus derived from outside CNS** - Can have multiple infarcts in different vascular territories - Sudden onset of focal deficits - Maximal severity early on
Hypoperfusion	- Shock	- Global, nonspecific deficits

Diagnosis:

- **Noncontrast CT** (rule-out hemorrhage, occasionally see signs of ischemia)
    - Needed quickly to help determine tPA candidacy
- MRI (used later to help identify extent of ischemia and stroke subtype)
- Source localization: Duplex US (or CTA/MRA), cardiac monitoring, TTE

Management:

Thrombolytic (IV alteplase)	- Given for clear ischemia with measurable deficits - Must be given within **3-4.5 hours** of symptoms - Exclusion criteria: Active bleeding, hx of intracranial lesion or stroke, stroke/head trauma within 3 months, recent intracranial surgery, BP > 185/110, plt < 100 K, INR > 1.7, PTT > 40s - Relative exclusion: Minor or improving neurologic deficits, recent major surgery/trauma/MI/GI bleed
BP control	- ≤ 185/110 if tPA used, ≤ 220/120 if not - Labetalol, nicardipine, and clevidipine
Antiplatelets	- Aspirin (within 48 hours of stroke) *If tPA used, do not start ASA for at least 24 hours
Statin	- For all

Note: Mechanical thrombectomy utilized with increased frequency for proximal large artery obstruction

Secondary Prevention:

- Lifestyle modification (HTN, DM control, smoking cessation)
- Antiplatelet (aspirin, clopidogrel, or aspirin-dipyridamole)
- Statin

Carotid Artery Disease

Carotid Artery Disease

General: Atherosclerotic stenosis of the carotid artery. Plaques develop just inside the internal carotid at the bifurcation. Considered "symptomatic" if the patient has stroke symptoms (i.e., stroke, TIA, amaurosis fugax) in the previous 6 months. Events occur due to thrombus formation, which either causes low flow state or embolizes.

Clinical:

- **Stroke** (anterior circulation TIA/stroke features [MCA, ACA, retinal])
- Amaurosis fugax
- Hollenhorst plaques in retina. Rare, but specific.
- Carotid bruit

Diagnosis: Imaging (the following modalities have similar efficacies)

- Carotid duplex US
- MRA
- CTA

Management:

Symptomatic	Intervention
100% stenosis	- Medical management
70-99% stenosis	- Carotid endarterectomy (ideally performed between 3-14 days after stroke symptoms) - Carotid artery stenting (if high risk for surgery or lesion is not surgically accessible)
50-69% stenosis	- Carotid endarterectomy (if reasonable life expectancy)
$<$ 50% stenosis	- Medical management
Asymptomatic	**Intervention**
$\geq$ 70% stenosis	- Intensive medical therapy (statin, antiplatelet, BP control, etc.) - +/− Carotid revascularization (if low surgical risk/long life expectancy)
$<$ 70% stenosis	- Intensive medical therapy (statin, antiplatelet, BP control, etc.)

Subclavian Steal

General: Flow reversal in vertebral artery ipsilateral to significant stenosis of subclavian artery

Clinical: Exercise-induced arm ischemia and/or vertebrobasilar ischemia

- BP on affected side $>$ 15 mmHg less than normal arm, pulse differential

Diagnosis: Clinical (pulse exam, BP) plus duplex US scan

Management: Bypass surgery or stenting

Stroke

Stroke Syndromes	
Subtype	**Clinical Features**
Cortical	
Anterior Cerebral	- Impacts medial cortex - Contralateral motor/sensory deficit, with **lower extremity predominance** - Behavioral changes (abulia, dyspraxia, emotional change)
Middle Cerebral	- Impacts frontal, parietal, and temporal lobes - Most commonly embolic from carotid artery disease - Contralateral motor/sensory deficit, with **upper extremity and face predominance** - Aphasia (dominant) or neglect (nondominant) - Eye deviation toward side of infarction (frontal eye fields) - Homonymous hemianopsia
Posterior Cerebral	- Impacts occipital lobe, medial temporal lobe or thalamus - Most commonly from atherosclerosis of vertebral or basilar arteries - **Contralateral hemianopia with macular sparing** - Possible sensory symptoms (from lateral thalamic infarct)
Brainstem	
Anterior Spinal	**Medial medullary syndrome** - Contralateral upper/lower limb paralysis - Ipsilateral hypoglossal (tongue deviates toward lesion) - Loss of proprioception (medial lemniscus)
Posterior Inferior Cerebellar (PICA)	**Wallenberg syndrome** (lateral medullary) - Dysphagia/Hoarseness - ↓ Pain/temp from ipsilateral face/contralateral body - Ipsilateral Horner syndrome - Vertigo, nystagmus, ataxia, dysmetria
Anterior Inferior Cerebellar (AICA)	**Lateral pontine syndrome** - Ipsilateral facial paralysis (facial nucleus) - ↓ Pain/temp from ipsilateral face/contralateral body - ↓ Decreased lacrimation/salivation/taste from anterior tongue - Vertigo, nystagmus, ataxia, dysmetria
Basilar	- Medial pons, possible **"Locked-in syndrome"** - Corticospinal: Unilateral or bilateral paresis - Bulbar: Unilateral or bilateral face weakness, dysarthria, dysphagia, limited jaw movement - Oculomotor: Horizontal gaze palsy, internuclear ophthalmoplegia
Lacunar	
Pure Motor	- Internal capsule (posterior limb) - Unilateral paralysis of face, arm, leg without sensory loss
Pure Sensory	- Thalamus (VPL/VPM) - Unilateral sensory deficit of face, arm, leg without motor loss
Ataxic Hemiparesis	- Internal capsule, basis pontis, or corona radiata - Unilateral weakness and limb ataxia
Dysarthria-Clumsy Hand	- Genu of internal capsule, basal pons - Unilateral face weakness, dysarthria, with hand weakness/clumsiness

Stroke

Intracerebral Hemorrhage

General: Parenchymal brain bleeds, second most common stroke (after ischemic)

Etiology:

- Hypertensive vasculopathy (penetrating vessels develop pseudoaneurysms which rupture)
- Cerebral amyloid angiopathy
- Vascular malformations
- Conversion from ischemic stroke

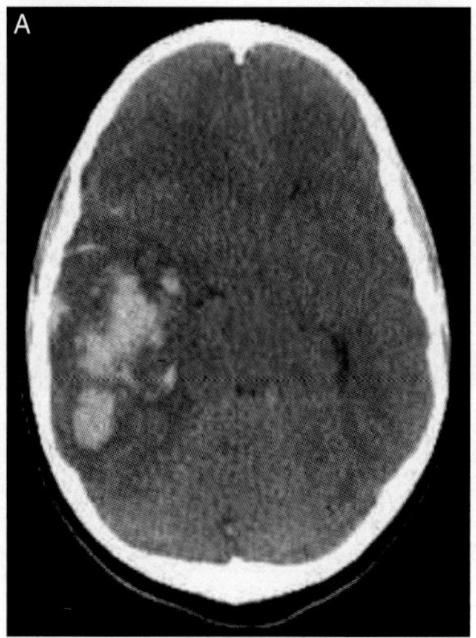

Clinical:

- Acute, progressive focal neurologic deficit (depending on location)
- Signs of increased ICP if large (headache, drowsiness, emesis, seizures)

Diagnosis:

- **Noncontrast CT**[A] (reveals bleed/hematoma)
- MRI (can aid in determining underlying cause)

Management:

- ICU level supportive care
- Stop antiplatelets/anticoagulants (and use reversal agents if available)
- BP control (target MAP of 110, or 160/90): Nicardipine, labetalol, enalapril
- ICP control: Elevate head of bed, use sedation (propofol)
    - If concern over ICP, can use invasive monitoring
    - Mannitol/hypertonic saline, hyperventilation, CSF drainage

Subarachnoid Hemorrhage

General: Bleeding into the subarachnoid space (between arachnoid/pia)

Etiology:

- **Ruptured saccular (berry) aneurysms**
- Other causes: Vascular malformations, arterial dissection, trauma

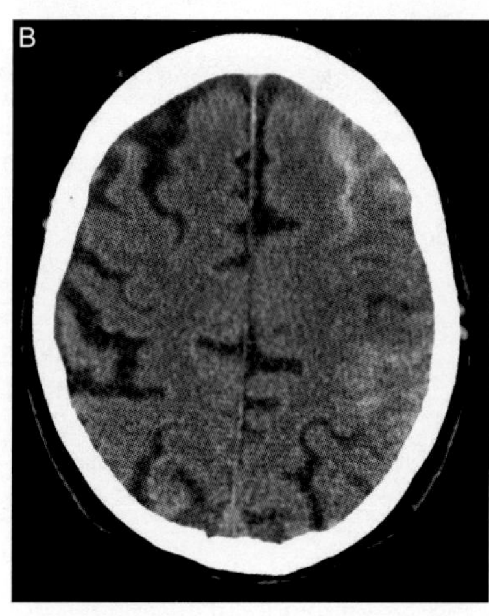

Clinical: Universally causes **sudden, severe headache**

- Fever, nuchal rigidity, loss of consciousness all possible

Diagnosis:

- **Noncontrast CT**[B]
- LP (if CT negative, but suspicion high; xanthochromia is classic)
- CTA/MRA to identify aneurysms

Management:

- Supportive ICU level care
- BP (< 160 systolic): Nicardipine, labetalol, or enalapril
- Nimodipine (improves outcomes)
- Aneurysm: Surgical clipping or endovascular coil (↓ risk of rebleed)
- Seizure PPX (if seizure is part of presentation or high risk bleed)

Complications:

- Rebleeding (surgical intervention helps prevent)
- Vasospasm (no well-validated intervention, but hyperdynamic therapy is used)
- Hydrocephalus (consider shunt placement)
- Hyponatremia (SIADH)

Stroke

Unruptured Cerebral Aneurysm

General: Also called saccular ("berry") aneurysms. ↑ Risk for rupture and SAH.
- Most common sites: (1) Anterior communicating, (2) posterior communicating, (3) MCA

Risk: Polycystic kidney disease, Ehlers-Danlos, Marfan, hypertension, smoking

Clinical: Generally asymptomatic unless ruptured. Large aneurysms can cause headache, visual loss, or cranial nerve deficits.
- Anterior communicating: Compression causes bitemporal hemianopia
- Posterior communicating: Compression causes ipsilateral CN III palsy

Diagnosis: CTA or MRA

Management: Small aneurysms observed/monitored, and large symptomatic aneurysms intervened upon endovascularly

Venous Sinus Thrombosis

General: Thrombosis of cerebral veins or dural sinuses, leading to backup of blood, with eventual CNS dysfunction

Etiology: Prothrombotic states (genetic thrombophilia, OCP, pregnancy, malignancy, surgery)

Clinical: Highly variable presentation, usually gradual onset over days
- **Headache**
- Other signs of increased ICP (**vomiting, papilledema, and visual problems**)
- Focal neurologic deficits in some
- Seizures

Diagnosis: **CT or MR venography** + Brain MRI

Management: Anticoagulation (LMWH or IV heparin)
- Long-term warfarin or DOAC

Cavernous Sinus Thrombosis

General: Thrombosis of the cavernous sinus, which multiple cranial nerves run through (CN III, IV, V1, V2, VI)
- Associated with infection (septic thrombosis), following facial infection. *Staph aureus* most common.

Clinical:
- Early signs: Headache, orbital pain, proptosis
- Lateral gaze palsy (CN VI)
- CN III (oculomotor) deficits (mydriasis, eyelid drooping, diplopia)
- Changes in sensation in the V1/V2 dermatomes

Diagnosis: CT or MRI with contrast

Management:
- Heparin
- Antibiotics (if infection)
- Surgical drainage in severe cases

Subdural/Epidural Bleeds

Subdural Hematoma

General: Bleed into potential space between dura and the arachnoid membranes, due to rupture of bridging veins

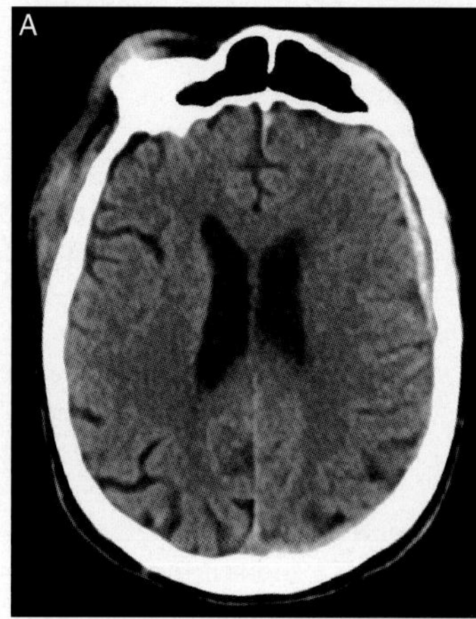

Etiology:

- Trauma (MVA, assault, falls in elderly)
    - ↑ Risk: Elderly (cortical atrophy), TBI, EtOH, anticoagulation

Clinical:

- Acute: Increased ICP (headache, emesis), anisocoria, CN palsies, coma
- Chronic: Progressive headaches, neurologic impairment, somnolence

Diagnosis:

- **Contrast CT**[A] (crescentic hyperdense lesion, possible midline shift)
- MRI (higher sensitivity)

Management: Acute Subdural

Operative	- Indicated if signs of herniation/severely ↑ ICP, clot thickness ≥ 10 mm or midline shift ≥ 5 mm - Surgical craniotomy (or alternative decompressive method)
Nonoperative	- Serial CT scans - ICP management (head elevation, hyperventilation, and mannitol)

Chronic subdural: Surgery if clinically severe/progressive neurologic decline, clot thickness ≥ 10 mm or midline shift ≥ 5 mm

Epidural Hematoma

General: Bleeding into potential space between dura/skull, most commonly from sphenoid damage/rupture of middle meningeal artery

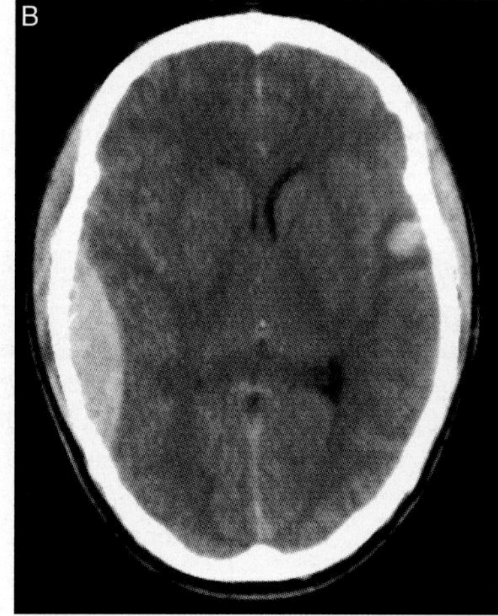

Etiology: Trauma (often fracture of temporal bone)

Clinical:

- Altered consciousness, confusion, drowsiness
- Headache, vomiting, seizures
- Possible loss of consciousness, followed by "**lucid interval**" (transient recovery), subsequent deterioration

Diagnosis: Noncontrast CT[B] (biconvex hyperdense lesion)

Management: Urgent/emergent surgical hematoma evacuation

Intracranial Hypertension

Overview of ICP

General: Intracranial pressure is normally ≤ 15 mmHg, intracranial hypertension defined as **≥ 20 mmHg**
- Cerebral perfusion pressure: CPP = MAP – ICP

Etiology:
- Cerebral edema
- Intracranial mass lesion or bleed (tumor, hematoma, hemorrhage)
- Hydrocephalus (increased CSF production/decreased CSF absorption)
- Idiopathic intracranial hypertension

Clinical:
- Headache, papilledema, CN VI palsy
- **Cushing triad**: Bradycardia, respiratory depression, and hypertension
- Herniation syndromes (see below)

Management:
- ICP monitoring (intraventricular/intraparenchymal)
- Interventions
    - Head elevation, hyperventilation, mannitol
    - Sedation (propofol), which reduces brain metabolic demand
    - BP control (maintain CPP > 60 mmHg), fever control

Idiopathic Intracranial Hypertension

General: Elevated pressure in the subarachnoid, due to poor arachnoid reabsorption

Risk: Women of childbearing age, obesity, retinoids, tetracycline

Clinical: Headaches, worse in mornings, associated with nausea, **tinnitus (pulsatile)**
- Transient visual obscurations, papilledema, **CN VI (abducens) palsy**

Diagnosis: MRI (rule out causes of ↑ ICP). LP (elevated CSF pressure).

Management: Acetazolamide (alt: Topiramate). LP/steroids can help acutely.
- If visual loss (despite therapy): Optic nerve sheath fenestration or CSF shunt

Herniation

Syndrome	Clinical Manifestations
Transtentorial (uncal)[A]	- Midbrain compression - Mydriasis and down/out gaze (compression of CN III) - Contralateral homonymous hemianopia (compression of PCA) - Hemiparesis - Eventual central herniation/death
Transtentorial (central)[B]	- Thalamus and temporal lobe herniation through tentorium cerebelli - Causes somnolence, loss of consciousness, posturing. Often fatal.
Subfalcine[C]	- Cingulate gyrus under falx cerebri → ACA infarction
Tonsillar[D]	- Cerebellar tonsils herniate downward through the foramen magnum, compressing medulla - Respiratory depression and cardiac instability/death

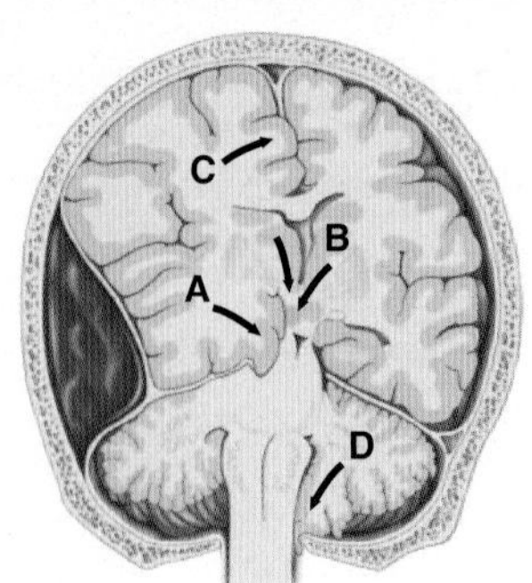

Traumatic Brain Injury

Overview of Traumatic Brain Injury (TBI)

General: TBI is a heterogenous term that includes brain trauma of a variety of mechanisms and varying severity. Often occurs from direct trauma, rapid acceleration/deceleration, or penetrating injury. Includes:

- Concussion
- Brain contusions
- Diffuse axonal injury (due to shearing mechanism)
    - Especially poor prognosis (present with coma/increased ICP)
    - Imaging shows blurring of gray/white junction
- Hemorrhages (subdural, epidural, intracranial)

Subtypes:

GCS 13-15	Mild TBI (concussion). See below.
GCS 9-12	Moderate TBI
GCS < 9	Severe TBI

Mild TBI (Concussion)

General: Mild brain injury from blunt force or acceleration/deceleration injury

Clinical:

- No focal neurologic deficits
- Headaches, dizziness, or imbalance
- Possible loss of consciousness at time of event
- Confusion and amnesia (for events just before and after trauma)

Diagnosis:

- Clinical (see above)
    - Can use clinical scoring tool like SAC or SCAT5
- CT head in select patients

Adult CT Indications (Canadian CT head rules)	Child CT Indications (2-18 y/o)
- GCS < 15 two hours after injury - Focal neuro deficits - Skull fracture - Seizure - Anticoagulant use - Age > 65 y/o - ≥ 2 episodes of vomiting - Severe mechanism of injury - Retrograde amnesia to event > 30 minutes	- GCS < 15 - Focal neuro deficits - Skull fracture - Prolonged loss of consciousness - Seizure Can observe OR CT the following: - Headache, vomiting, severe mechanism, loss of consciousness

Management:

- 24 hours of monitoring (for worsening symptoms)
    - CT for worsening symptoms
- Graduated return to play for sports (do not return until asymptomatic, off medication for symptoms)
- Cognitive rest (e.g., from work) until symptoms resolve

Traumatic Brain Injury

Carotid/Vertebral Artery Dissection

General: Separation of arterial wall layers, leading to creation of false lumen and compromised blood flow

Etiology:
- Trauma: Sports, sex, yoga, chiropractic manipulations
- Connective tissue disorder: Marfans, Ehlers-Danlos, fibromuscular dysplasia

Clinical:
- **Unilateral neck pain or headache**
- TIA/CVA symptoms
    - Carotid: Anterior circulation stroke symptoms (MCA, ACA)
    - Vertebral: Posterior circulation stroke symptoms (brainstem, cerebellar)
- Horner syndrome
- Audible bruit

Diagnosis: MRA/CTA

Management:
- Aspirin or anticoagulation
- tPA (used if ischemic stroke symptoms and meets criteria)
- Endovascular stenting

Skull Fractures

Subtype	Clinical	Management
Linear	- Simple, linear fracture through full thickness of calvarium - Generally not clinically significant	Dx: CT Tx: No intervention required if patient has no underlying brain injury/ bleed
Depressed	- Segment of skull driven below the plane of adjacent skull - Associated with TBI - Risk for infection, bleeding, seizures - Can have "step off" on physical exam	Dx: CT Tx: Tdap, antibiotic prophylaxis, +/− surgical repair
Basilar	- Fracture of bone forming base of skull (sphenoid, occipital, cribriform plate, petrous temporal) - High risk for bleeds and dural tears (causing CSF leaks) Clinical: - **Battle sign**: Bleed behind ear/mastoid - Periorbital ecchymosis[A] ("raccoon eye") - Clear/blood tinged rhinorrhea or otorrhea (concern for CSF leak) - Hemotympanum	Dx: CT - CSF Leak: "Halo-sign" or beta-2 transferrin level Tx: Surgery (for bleeds)

Hypokinetic Movement Disorders

	General/Clinical	Management

Parkinson	- Loss of dopamine containing neurons in the substantia nigra in the midbrain, causing reduced excitatory input to the motor cortex
	- Risk: ↑ Age, family history. Smoking is protective.
	
	Clinical: (Cardinal 4 symptoms numbered)
	(1) **Bradykinesia** (slow movements)
	(2) **Tremor** (pill-rolling rest tremor, improves with movement)
	(3) **Rigidity** (increased resistance to passive movement)
	(4) **Postural instability** (impaired postural reflex, manifested as imbalance)
	
	- Masked facial expression, hypophonia
	- Gait: Shuffling, short-steps, "freezing"
	- Neuropsychiatric or cognitive dysfunction
	- Neurogenic orthostatic hypotension
		Dx: Clinical diagnosis (bradykinesia + tremor or rigidity, without any evidence of an alternative diagnosis)
		
		Tx:
		- **Levodopa-carbidopa** (first-line)
		
		- Dopamine agonists (ropinirole, pramipexole)
		  - Adjunctive agents in advanced disease
		- MAO-B inhibitors (selegiline, rasagiline)
		  - Adjunctive agent
		- COMT inhibitors (tolcapone, entacapone)
		  - Adjunctive agent in advanced disease
		
		- Anticholinergics (trihexyphenidyl, benztropine)
		  - Treats tremor, used in early disease
		- Amantadine
		  - Mild effects, useful in early disease
		
		- Surgical: Deep brain stimulation

Parkinson Plus		
Multiple Systems Atrophy	- Overarching term for multiple diseases (olivopontocerebellar atrophy, Shy-Drager, and striatonigral degeneration), which all have Parkinsonian features plus other symptoms Clinical: - **Parkinsonian features** (bradykinesia, rigidity, tremor) - **Dysautonomia** (orthostasis, erectile dysfunction) - **Cerebellar dysfunction** (ataxia)	Dx: Clinical. - Some improve on levodopa/carbidopa but a lack of improvement would indicate MSA over Parkinson. Tx: Levodopa (see if response). Otherwise care is purely supportive, no other effective treatments.
Progressive Supranuclear Palsy	- Tau-positive neurodegenerative disease, resulting in rapidly progressive Parkinsonism Clinical: - Parkinsonian features (postural instability causing falls) - Supranuclear ophthalmoplegia (vertical gaze palsy) - Others: Cognitive issues, dysarthria, dysphagia	Dx: Clinical. MRI findings can be supportive (midbrain atrophy, "Hummingbird" sign). Tx: Supportive. No effective therapies. Poor response to levodopa.
Corticobasal Degeneration	- Progressive tau-positive neurodegenerative disease Clinical: - Initially presents with focal akinesia, dystonia, myoclonus, or apraxia - Progressive cognitive issues/behavioral changes - Can progress to diffuse Parkinsonian features - CT/MRI shows asymmetric frontal cortical atrophy	Dx: Clinical. Poor response to levodopa. Tx: No effective therapies
Other "Parkinson plus" (covered elsewhere) - Lewy body dementia - Pick disease		

Hyperkinetic Movement Disorders

	General/Clinical	Management
Tremors		
Resting Tremor	- Usually due to Parkinson disease - "Pill-rolling" tremor, disappears with movement (4-6 hz freq)	Tx: [See: Parkinson]
Physiologic Tremor	- Normal low-amplitude, high-frequency (10-12 hz) - Normally subclinical, but apparent with ↑ sympathetic activity	
Essential Tremor	- AD, familial tremor - Action tremor, most commonly of hands/forearms (6-12 hz)	Tx: Propranolol (alt: Primidone, moderate EtOH)
Intention Tremor	- Associated with neurologic disease (stroke, multiple sclerosis) - Tremor occurs with goal-directed movements, worsening as hand gets close to target	
Functional Tremor	- Psychogenic tremor with varying presentation (frequency and characteristics), but disappears with distraction	
Myoclonus	- Brief, shock-like, involuntary movements - **Physiologic** (jerks associated with sleep) - **Essential** (idiopathic, can be acquired or hereditary) - **Epilepsy** (associated with seizures)	Tx: Antiepileptics (levetiracetam or valproate) or benzodiazepines
Fasciculations	- Small, local, involuntary muscle contraction - Appears as flicker under skin - Can be sign of motor neuron disease (ALS), but often benign	
Tardive Dyskinesia	- Writhing movements of the mouth, face and limbs - Secondary to chronic antipsychotic medication use	Tx: Discontinue antipsychotic med, but often irreversible

Chorea

General: Movement disorder characterized by involuntary quick, random, and irregular movements

Chorea	- Involuntary, brief, unpredictable contractions. Most commonly affect distal limbs, but also face and trunk.
Athetosis	- Slow, writhing, "snake-like" movements
Ballism	- Large amplitude (flinging/kicking) movements of proximal arms/legs - Hemiballism (unilateral) most common, due to lesions involving the subthalamic nucleus

Etiology:

- Hereditary (Huntington, other rare syndromes)
- Secondary (infections, autoimmune disease, drugs)
- Sydenham chorea with rheumatic heart disease

Huntington Chorea

General: Progressive neurodegenerative disorder. AD CAG nucleotide repeat in the huntingtin gene on chromosome 4. Causes loss of GABA-producing neurons in the striatum.

Clinical: Gradual and progressive onset of symptoms between 30-50 y/o

- Chorea, progressive motor function decline
- Psychiatric: Irritability, depression, or psychotic symptoms, progressive cognitive decline
- MRI: Can show caudal atrophy (in late-stage disease)

Diagnosis: Clinical/family history, confirmatory **genetic testing**

Management: Supportive, multidisciplinary care

- Chorea: Tetrabenazine, reserpine (alt: Antipsychotics)
- Behavioral symptoms (psychosis): Atypical antipsychotics

Hyperkinetic Movement Disorders

Dystonia

General: Sustained, prolonged muscle contractions, causing repetitive abnormal, stereotypical movements

Adult Onset Focal Dystonia:

Cervical	- Spasmodic torticollis: Horizontal turning of neck with lateral tilt
Blepharospasm	- Involuntary blinking and involuntary eye closure
Spasmodic Dysphonia	- Laryngeal muscle involvement, resulting in voice breaks that interrupt normal speech
Oromandibular/ Lingual	- Involuntary jaw clenching, chewing, opening - Tongue protrusion
Task-Specific	- Writer's cramp - Musician's dystonia

Management:

- If related to antipsychotic medication: Benztropine
- Trial of levodopa (see if responsive)
- Botulinum toxin injection

Stiff Person Syndrome

General: Progressive, full body stiffness. Associated with anti-GAD antibodies in CSF (decreases available GABA, resulting in uninhibited muscle contraction).

Clinical:

- Progressive **axial muscle spasms, stiffness, and rigidity**
- Spasmodic episodes, impaired ambulation

Diagnosis: Clinical, plus EMG (continuous motor activity, improves with diazepam)

Management: **Benzodiazepines** or baclofen

Restless Leg Syndrome

General: Idiopathic disorder characterized by uncomfortable urge to move legs

Etiology: Idiopathic, but associated with low central iron stores (↓ ferritin)

Clinical:

- Uncomfortable urge to move legs during periods of inactivity (e.g., at night)
- Felt in lower legs, varied sensation (restless, cramping, electric)
- Transient relief with movement

Diagnosis: Clinical (but work up for low iron with ferritin levels)

Management:

- Iron replacement (for low or borderline low ferritin)
- Nonpharmacologic therapy (massage, heat, exercise)
- Avoid exacerbating agents (anti dopaminergic agents, antihistamines)
- Pharm: **Pramipexole, ropinirole** (alt: Gabapentin/pregabalin)

Cerebellar/Gait Disorders

Clinical Manifestations of Cerebellar Dysfunction

General: Cerebellum functions to modulate movement, especially aiding with coordination and balance

Lesion	Abnormality
Lateral Cerebellum	- Ipsilateral limb dysmetria (test with finger/nose, heel/shin) - Intention tremor - Ipsilateral dysdiadochokinesia (test with rapid alternating movements)
Medial Cerebellum	- Truncal ataxia ("wide-based" cerebellar gait)
Flocculonodular	- Vertigo - Nystagmus

Abnormal Gaits

Subtype	Clinical Features	Etiologies
Hemiplegic	- Drags affected leg in semicircle (circumduction)	- Stroke
Neuropathic	- "Steppage gait." Patient with foot drop lifts leg high to avoid tripping over it.	- Motor neuropathy (e.g., L5 nerve disease OR motor neuron disease like ALS)
Myopathic	- Hip drop on contralateral side due to weak ipsilateral gluteal muscles - "Trendelenburg sign"	- Myopathy (muscular dystrophy)
Cerebellar	- Staggering, wide-based gait with ataxia	- Cerebellar disease (e.g., stroke) - EtOH intoxication
Parkinsonian	- Stooped, head forward posture - Walks with shuffling, short steps - Decreased arm swing	- Parkinson - Movement disorders
Sensory	- Lack of proprioception, so slams foot to help localize/feel	- Peripheral sensory neuropathy, dorsal column degeneration
Vestibular	- Unsteady, falling over - Complain of associated features such as vertigo	- Any cause of vertigo
Frontal	- Gait apraxia, difficulty starting to walk - Freezing, "magnetic" gait - En bloc turns. Falls backwards.	- Dementia - Normal pressure hydrocephalus

Cerebellar/Gait Disorders

	General/Clinical	Management
Genetic		
Spinocerebellar Ataxia	- Wide variety of genetic mutations responsible. Mutations can be inherited (most commonly AD) or sporadic. - Clinical: Cerebellar ataxia, with other symptoms depending on specific mutation	Tx: No effective therapies

Friedreich Ataxia	- AR GAA-trinucleotide expansion (frataxin gene). Most common inherited spinocerebellar ataxia.
	
	<u>Clinical</u>:
	- Cerebellar atrophy (limb and gait ataxia)
	- Degeneration of multiple spinal cord tracts
	  - **Spinocerebellar**: Ataxia, dysarthria
	  - **Dorsal column**: Loss of sensation/proprioception
	  - **Corticospinal**: UMN weakness
	- Hypertrophic cardiomyopathy
	- Other: Diabetes mellitus, kyphoscoliosis, hammer toes
		Dx: Clinical. Confirm with genetic testing.
		
		Tx: No specific disease altering therapy. Supportive, multidisciplinary care.

Toxin Mediated		
EtOH Cerebellar Degeneration	- Degeneration of cerebellar vermis from chronic alcohol use - Clinical: Poorly coordinated, wide-based gait	Dx: Clinical Tx: EtOH cessation, nutritional supplementation
Inflammatory Cerebellar Disease		
Acute Cerebellar Ataxia (Post infectious Cerebellitis)	- Occurs weeks after certain viral/bacterial infections or rarely post vaccination. Seen in young children. - Autoimmune white matter demyelination of the cerebellum - Clinical: Acute, rapid onset of gait disturbance, ataxia	Dx: Clinical Tx: Self-limited. Most fully recover.

Central Demyelinating Disease

Multiple Sclerosis

General: CNS inflammatory demyelinating disease, believed to be due to autoreactive lymphocytes. Typical clinical courses below:
- **Relapsing-Remitting**: Episodes followed by partial/complete recovery
- **Secondary Progressive**: Initial relapse-remit, then progressive disease
- **Primary Progressive**: Progressive worsening (temporary improvements possible, but overall worsens)

Risk: Female, aged 20-40, ↑ distance from equator, ↓ vitamin D

Clinical:
- **White matter CNS lesions, separated by space and time**
  - Optic neuritis (blurry vision, painful eye movements)
  - Internuclear ophthalmoplegia (nystagmus of abducting eye contralateral to lesion)
  - Transverse myelitis (spinal cord lesions causing sensory or motor deficits)
  - CNS white matter lesions
  - Cerebellar disease (ataxia, intention tremor, dysarthria)
- Bladder incontinence
  - Urge incontinence initially (from detrusor overactivity)
  - Eventually can develop overflow incontinence
- Autonomic dysfunction (erectile dysfunction , constipation)
- Fatigue, depression, neuropathic pain, cognitive decline
- Classic signs:
  - Uhthoff: Symptoms worse with heat (axons conduct worse)
  - Lhermitte: Electric sensation with neck flexion
  - Charcot triad: Scanning speech, intention tremor, nystagmus

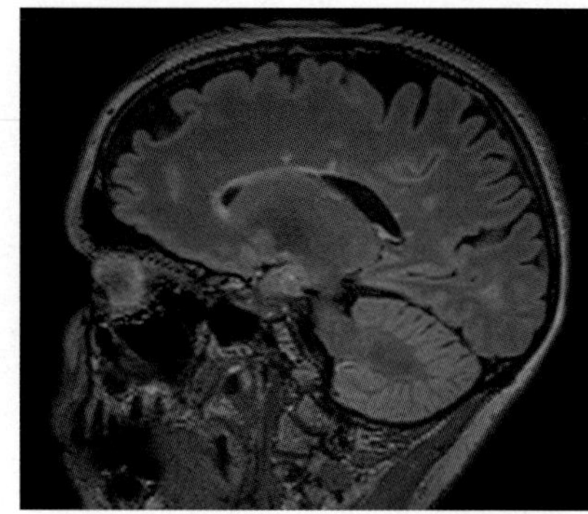

Diagnosis: Combination of **clinical symptoms and MRI lesions**
- MRI: New and old white matter lesions in multiple typical CNS areas
  - New lesions enhance with contrast
  - Dawson fingers[A] from corpus callosum (classic sign)
- Other supportive tests:
  - LP (CSF shows oligoclonal IgG bands). Used if above is equivocal.
  - Visual evoked potentials: Latency of P100 peak

Management:

Acute exacerbation	- High-dose IV methylprednisolone
Chronic Management	
Relapse-remit	Disease-modifying therapy: - Glatiramer, IFN-β (both safe, less efficacious) - Fingolimod, dimethyl fumarate, teriflunomide (intermediate effectiveness) - Natalizumab, ocrelizumab, alemtuzumab (more side effects, but more effective) - Vitamin D for all
Primary progressive	- Ocrelizumab
Secondary progressive	- Ocrelizumab, rituximab

Central Demyelinating Disease

Acute Disseminated Encephalomyelitis (ADEM)

General: Postinfectious, autoimmune central demyelinating disorder. More common in kids than adults.

Etiology: Post infection or vaccination

Clinical:

- Multiple focal neurologic deficits (can present with motor, sensory, or cranial nerve defects)
- Encephalopathy

Diagnosis:

- MRI: Multifocal, asymmetric, white matter lesions
- LP: Increased protein, lymphocytosis

Management: IV methylprednisolone +/− IVIG

Neuromyelitis Optica

General: Inflammatory CNS disorder, due to autoantibodies against aquaporin-4

Clinical:

- Acute episodes of optic neuritis PLUS
  - Transverse myelitis
  - Brainstem syndromes (area postrema; intractable hiccups, emesis)

Diagnosis: MRI plus AQP-4 antibody test

Management:

- Acute: IV methylprednisolone
- Chronic: Azathioprine, rituximab, or others

Progressive Multifocal Leukoencephalopathy

General: Inflammatory central demyelinating disorder due to reactivation of JC virus of CNS oligodendrocytes → white matter demyelination

Risk:

- HIV
- Natalizumab
- Hematologic malignancies (leukemia/lymphoma)

Clinical: Progressive, subacute focal neurologic deficits

- Encephalopathy, motor dysfunction, sensory issues, ataxia

Diagnosis:

- MRI: Multifocal, asymmetric white matter lesions
- LP: CSF shows JC virus IgG
- Brain biopsy (definitive, but rarely used due to side effects)

Management: Supportive. No effective therapy.

- Treat underlying disorder (e.g., start ART)

Peripheral Demyelinating Disease

Guillain Barre/AIDP

General: Acute immune-mediated peripheral neuropathy, believed due to molecular mimicry, causing immune-mediated damage to peripheral nerves. Variants include:

- Acute inflammatory demyelinating polyneuropathy (AIDP)
  - Most common, with typical presentation (see clinical)
- Acute motor axonal neuropathy (like typical AIDP, but no sensory symptom)
- Acute motor and sensory axonal neuropathy (more sensory involvement)
- Miller Fisher syndrome (ophthalmoplegia, ataxia, areflexia)

Etiology: Associated with infections (***Campylobacter jejuni***, EBV, CMV, HIV), rarely post immunization

Clinical:

- Rapidly **ascending extremity weakness**/paralysis/loss of DTR
  - Time to maximum weakness < 4 weeks
- Can involve respiratory, facial, and bulbar muscles
- **Autonomic dysfunction** (arrhythmias, tachycardia, postural hypotension)
- Paresthesias

Diagnosis: Clinical diagnosis, supported by following labs

- LP: CSF analysis shows ↑ protein, but normal cell count ("**Albuminocytologic dissociation**")

Management:

- Supportive care (hemodynamic monitoring, respiratory support)
  - Monitor FVC and negative inspiratory force
- Plasma exchange or IVIG
- Corticosteroids not effective

Chronic Inflammatory Demyelinating Polyneuropathy (CIDP)

General: Acquired disorder of chronic demyelination of the peripheral nervous system. Progresses over at least 8 week time course.

Clinical:

- Progressive or relapsing/remitting peripheral neuropathy
  - Motor usually more pronounced than sensory deficits
  - Hyporeflexia or areflexia

Diagnosis: Clinical, plus the following diagnostic evidence

- Electrodiagnostic (↓ conduction velocities, supporting demyelination)
- Nerve biopsy
- LP: CSF analysis shows ↑ protein, but normal cell count

Management: IVIG, plasma exchange, or glucocorticoids

Spinal Cord Lesions

Spinal Cord Syndromes

Syndrome	Clinical Findings
Brown Sequard (Hemisection)	- Ipsilateral hemiparesis - Ipsilateral dorsal column signs (vibration/proprioception) - Contralateral loss of pain and temp (from spinothalamic which crosses two levels above the level of the loss of sensation)
Central Cord	- Loss of pain/temperature at the level of the lesion - Weakness (more pronounced in upper extremities compared to lower extremities)
Ventral Cord	- Loss pain/temperature, motor weakness
Dorsal Cord	- Loss of proprioception, vibration, fine touch
Transection	- Loss of all sensation and motor function - Bladder dysfunction

Spinal Cord Disorders

Disorder	Clinical Findings
Syringomyelia	- Fluid-filled dilation of the spinal cord - Most commonly in cervical or thoracic spine (C8-T1) - Associated with Chiari I malformation, but also infection, tumor, inflammation, or trauma - Causes central cord syndrome (**"cape-like" loss of pain/temp**)
Subacute Combined Degeneration	- Associated with B12 deficiency - Leads to degeneration of posterior column and corticospinal tracts - Presents with problems walking, + Romberg, spastic paresis in legs, hyperreflexia
Transverse Myelitis	- Associated with MS, and other autoimmune conditions - White matter lesion, usually 1-2 segments, in thoracic cord
Spinal Cord Infarctions	- Most commonly anterior spinal infarct - Causes ventral cord syndrome ("spinal shock," flaccid paralysis below lesion)
Compressive Lesions	- Epidural abscess or hematoma - Neoplasms - Cervical spondylotic myelopathy
Tabes Dorsalis	- Advanced neurosyphilis (now rare with antibiotics) - Posterior column disease (sensory ataxia and sharp pains) - Argyll-Robertson pupils (do not respond to light, but do contract with accommodation)

Neuromuscular Disease

Amyotrophic Lateral Sclerosis

General: Motor neuron degeneration, with **combined lower and upper motor neuron degeneration**

Etiology: Sporadic (90%): Increased risk with ↑ age, family history, and smoking
- Hereditary (10%): Many genes. SOD 1 (superoxide dismutase type 1) is common subtype.

Clinical: **Asymmetric limb weakness**, with other UMN and LMN signs, and progressive cognitive impairment
- Upper motor signs: Muscle weakness, spasticity, hyperreflexia
- Lower motor signs: Muscle weakness, fasciculations, atrophy
- Bulbar (dysphagia, dysarthria) symptoms also possible
- Progressive worsening of disease, with prognosis of ~3-5 years on average

Diagnosis: Clinical diagnosis (combination of UMN/LMN signs, without evidence of an alternative cause, plus the following)
- EMG: Reveals evidence of acute/chronic denervation
- MRI: Typically normal

Management: Riluzole (improved survival), edaravone (slows neurodegeneration), sodium phenylbutyrate-taurursodiol
- Symptom control: (PEG tube for dysphagia, PPV for respiratory compromise, antispasmodics, mucolytics)

Spinal Muscular Atrophy

General: Inherited degeneration of the anterior horn cells that results in muscular atrophy. Presents in kids. Due to AR SMA gene mutation.

Clinical: Diffuse symmetric proximal muscle weakness (UE > LE). Flaccid, unable to sit upright, "Frog-leg" posture.
- Weak cry, difficulty sucking/swallowing, hyporeflexia/areflexia

Diagnosis: Genetic testing

Management: Supportive care (respiratory, nutritional)
- Nusinersen (intrathecal injection of antisense DNA that increases SMN gene expression)

Muscular Dystrophy

	General/Clinical	Management
Muscular Dystrophy		
Duchenne (DMD)	- X-linked dystrophin mutation (frameshift mutation) Clinical: (onset < 5 y/o) - **Proximal muscle weakness** (with ↑ CK, aldolase) - Starts with **lower extremity** (i.e., hip-girdle), then progresses - Cardiomyopathy - Scoliosis, bone fractures - Calf pseudohypertrophy, Gowers sign	Dx: Genetic testing confirms. Muscle biopsy (with dystrophin stain) used in equivocal cases. Tx: - Prednisone for motor function - Multidisciplinary supportive care (physical therapy, nutritional, monitoring of cardiac/respiratory function) - DMD: Poor prognosis (most die in 10-20s from respiratory failure, cardiomyopathy) - BMD: Improved prognosis vs DMD
Becker (BMD)	- X-linked dystrophin mutation (nonframeshift mutation) Clinical: - Similar presentation to DMD, but later onset (i.e., 10-15 y/o) - **Milder disease course**	
Myotonic	- AD inheritance of DMPK gene CTG trinucleotide repeat Clinical: (Presents in late teens/young adults) - Muscle weakness (skeletal and respiratory muscle) - Myotonia, cataracts, arrhythmias, balding, hypogonadism	Dx: Genetic testing Tx: No disease-modifying therapies available. Supportive care only.
Limb-Girdle	- Group of AR or AD muscular dystrophy - Clinical: Weakness in the pelvic and/or shoulder girdle	Dx: Genetic testing. Biopsy if uncertain. Tx: Multidisciplinary supportive care
Facioscapulo-humeral	- AD (but frequently sporadic) mutation in DUX4 gene - Clinical: Onset as young adult. Asymmetric muscle weakness of face, scapula, upper arms, lower abdomen.	Dx: Genetic testing (alt: Muscle biopsy, EMG) Tx: Multidisciplinary supportive care

Neuromuscular Disease

Myasthenia Gravis

General: Autoimmune dysfunction of neuromuscular junction, due to autoantibody formation against acetylcholine receptor

Clinical:

- Skeletal muscle weakness (**muscles weaken with use**)
  - Initially transient symptoms, eventually more frequent/severe
  - Preserved reflexes/sensory function
- Ocular symptoms (most common initial): **Ptosis, diplopia**
- Bulbar symptoms: Fatigue with chewing, dysphagia, and dysarthria
- Thymoma (seen ~15% of MG cases, rule out with CT chest)
- Myasthenic crisis: Respiratory distress due to respiratory muscle fatigue
  - Exacerbated by certain drugs (hydroxychloroquine, fluoroquinolone, aminoglycoside, beta-blockers)

Diagnosis:

- Lab: AChR-Ab (alt: MuSK) autoantibodies (confirms diagnosis if symptomatic, but can have seronegative disease)
- Electrophysiologic tests:
  - Repetitive nerve stimulation (progressive decline in compound muscle action potential)
- Bedside ice-pack test OR edrophonium (tensilon) infusion test. Both should improve muscle strength.

Management:

Myasthenia Crisis	- Plasmapheresis/exchange and IVIG, plus glucocorticoids - Monitor vital capacity and maximum inspiratory pressure (if low, may require invasive ventilation)
Chronic	- Acetylcholinesterase inhibitors (pyridostigmine) first line - Most require chronic immunotherapy (glucocorticoids, azathioprine, mycophenolate, cyclosporine) - Thymectomy: Indicated in those with thymoma, all patients < 60 y/o with MG

Lambert-Eaton Syndrome

General: Neuromuscular junction disorder due to autoantibody against presynaptic voltage-gated Ca channels

Etiology: Most commonly associated with small-cell lung cancer

Clinical:

- **Progressive, symmetric proximal muscle weakness** (improves with activity)
- Autonomic dysfunction (erectile dysfunction, dry mouth) and decreased reflexes

Diagnosis: VGCC antibody titers

- ↑ compound motor action potentials (CMAPs) with repeated stimulation

Management: 3,4-diaminopyridine (alt: Guanidine +/− Pyridostigmine)

- IVIG/prednisone if refractory

Ventricular Pathology

	General/Clinical	Management

Hydrocephalus	- Excessive CSF in the ventricles with dilatation and ↑ ICP
	
	Causes:
	- Noncommunicating: **Blockage of flow**
	  - Aqueductal stenosis
	  - Chiari malformation
	  - Dandy-Walker malformation
	
	- Communicating: **CSF not being absorbed from arachnoid**
	  - Scarring from meningitis, intraventricular hemorrhage
	
	Clinical:
	- ↑ ICP (headache, vomiting, papilledema, etc.)
	- Irritability, behavioral changes, altered mental status
	- In children: Increased head-circumference
		Dx: CT/MRI (ventriculomegaly)
		
		Tx: Surgical correction in symptomatic patients (CSF shunt or endoscopic third ventriculostomy)

Normal-Pressure Hydrocephalus	- Enlarged ventricles but normal opening pressure on LP - Due to impaired CSF absorption Clinical: ("**Wet, wobbly, wacky**") - Cognitive impairment - Gait ataxia (slow, wide-based gait) - Urinary incontinence	Dx: - MRI or CT (ventriculomegaly[A] out of proportion with sulcal/cortical atrophy) - Lumbar puncture (check pressure, improvement of symptoms after tap) Tx: Ventricular shunting
Hydrocephalus Ex-vacuo	- Cortical atrophy with enlarged ventricles (see in older people or those with dementia), in proportion to increased size of sulci	

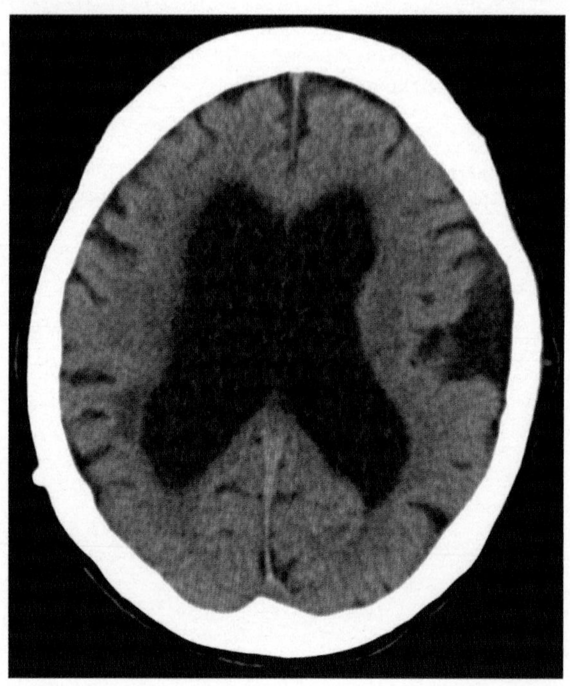

Dementia

Neurocognitive Disorder

Center disorder	Findings/Criteria
Normal Aging	- Slight decreases in fluid intelligence (processing new information, problem solving, working memory) - Word finding difficulties (expressive aphasia) - Sleep changes (advanced sleep-wake cycle) - No loss of function
Mild Neurocognitive Disorder	- Deficit in at least one cognitive domain that cannot be attributed to normal aging - Usually impaired memory - Unlike dementia, function is primarily intact
Major Neurocognitive Disorder (Dementia)	- Significant decline in ≥ 1 cognitive domains (executive, learning/memory, language, attention, motor, social) - Requires assistance in IADLs or ADLs - Not caused by delirium or medical condition - MMSE (mini-mental state exam) is generally < 24/30

IADL/ADL

IADL	ADL
- Higher-level activities to remain independent - Often can receive aid from outside to remain independent	- Basic self-care activities that must be performed to stay self-sufficient
- Shopping, cooking, finances, med management, telephone use	- Bathing, dressing, feeding, toileting, continence, transferring

Dementia Causes

	General/Clinical	Diagnosis/Management
Alzheimer Disease (AD)	- Most common cause of dementia. Almost always presents > 65 y/o. - Early onset (< 60): Rare. Can be idiopathic or associated with genes mutations in Presenilin 1, 2, or APP (amyloid precursor protein) - Involves β-amyloid plaques and tau neurofibrillary tangles - Risk: ↑ age, females, family history of dementia, APOE4 allele <u>Clinical</u>: - Generally starts with **memory impairment** - Progressive to other domains (executive, language, and visuospatial) - Neuropsychiatric/behavioral, motor symptoms late in disease	Dx: Clinical. MRI can show cortical/hippocampal atrophy Tx: - Cholinesterase inhibitor (donepezil, galantamine, and rivastigmine) - Memantine in severe disease
Vascular	- Due to large/small artery strokes and chronic vascular injury <u>Clinical</u>: (Often presents in **stepwise fashion**) - Executive dysfunction (memory mostly preserved, vs AD) - Focal cortical deficits (aphasia, neglect, etc.) - Focal subcortical deficits (motor, gait, etc.)	Dx: Clinical. MRI can show focal white matter lesions, with cortical and or subcortical infarcts Tx: Treat underlying vascular disease
Lewy Body	- Seen > 65 y/o. Path shows cortical Lewy-body formation. <u>Clinical</u>: - Dementia (progressive cognitive decline) - **Parkinsonism** develops at least **1 year after cognitive symptoms** - Visual hallucinations, REM sleep-behavior disorder	Dx: Clinical. MRI can show cortical atrophy (w/o significant hippocampal disease) Tx: Cholinesterase inhibitors, low-dose anti-psychotics, levodopa (for parkinsonism)
Frontotemporal "Pick Disease"	- Cause of early onset dementia (50s-60s y/o) - Pathophys: Involves tau, TDP-43 <u>Clinical</u>: - Behavioral subtype: Disinhibition, loss of sympathy, increased apathy, compulsive behaviors, hyperorality - Aphasia subtype: Progressive language issues, with cognition intact	Dx: Clinical. MRI can show unilateral or bilateral frontal and temporal atrophy Tx: No disease-modifying therapy

Prion Disease

General: Neurodegenerative disease due to prions, which are abnormally conformed proteins. Once exposed, the abnormal protein induces conformational change in the host's normal PrP, which then forms a chain reaction, aggregates, and causes cell death.

Etiology: Most commonly spontaneous mutation, but can also be acquired or familial

Management: No effective therapies. Universally fatal.

Subtype	Features
Creutzfeldt-Jakob	- Pathophys: Spongiform change and accumulation of abnormal PrP Clinical - Rapidly progressive cognitive deterioration - Behavioral changes (depression, apathy, mood changes) - Myoclonus (startle) - Extrapyramidal signs (ataxia, nystagmus) or corticospinal (motor dysfunction) Diagnosis - MRI: Abnormal signal in putamen/caudate - EEG: Periodic, **triphasic sharp "spike" wave complexes** - CSF: 14-3-3 protein, **RT-QuIC** - Brain biopsy (definitive but rarely performed)
Bovine Spongiform Encephalopathy	- "Mad Cow Disease." Variant of Creutzfeldt-Jakob caused by ingestion of infected meat products.
Kuru	- Neurodegenerative prion disease seen in Papua New Guinea groups that practice cannibalism
Fatal Familial Insomnia	- Neurodegenerative disease from inherited or acquired PrP mutation - Presents with progressive mental status change, behavioral change, and insomnia

Altered Mental Status

Encephalopathy Overview

General: Clinical syndrome of change in cognitive and psychological functioning. Due to an underlying medical condition. Commonly develops in **acutely hospitalized patients**.

- Terms: Altered mental status, delirium, encephalopathy used interchangeably
- Sundowning: Variant of delirium, behavioral change in evening

Etiology: "MIST"

Metabolic	- Electrolyte disturbances (hyponatremia, hypernatremia, hypercalcemia) - Hypo/hyperglycemia - Uremia - Hypoxemia/hypercapnia - Endocrine issues (hypo/hyperthyroidism, adrenal insufficiency) - Nutritional deficiencies (including vitamin B1, B12 deficiency)
Infection	- Any, including UTI, pneumonia, bacteremia
Structural (CNS)	- Brain bleeds (SDH, SAH, intracranial hemorrhage) - Mass lesions - Seizures - Encephalitis, meningitis
Toxin	- Drugs (opiates, benzodiazepines, alcohol) - Substance withdrawal (e.g., alcohol withdrawal)

Clinical:

- Acute deterioration in mental status (over hours-to-days)
- Fluctuating level of awareness, orientation
- Loss of concentration
- Visual hallucinations
- Subtypes:
    - Hyperactive: Agitation, mood lability, uncooperative
    - Hypoactive: Decreased psychomotor activity (drowsy/lethargic), slow to respond

Diagnosis: Clinical diagnosis

- Workup and evaluate for the above causes (electrolytes, glucose, urinalysis/culture, tox screen, etc.)

Management:

- Treat underlying cause
- Protocols to prevent delirium
    - **Orientation protocols** (clocks, dates visible, etc.)
    - Avoid polypharmacy (especially benzos)
    - Avoid physical restraints (use one-to-one sitter if necessary)
    - Frequent reorientation from familiar persons
    - Nonpharmacologic sleep aids
- Severe agitation or psychosis: Haloperidol or atypical antipsychotic

Altered Mental Status

Coma

General: A state of unarousable unresponsiveness

Etiology: Variety of causes, including trauma, metabolic, drug/toxins, and CNS lesions

Glasgow Coma Scale:

	Eye	Motor	Verbal
1	Does not open eyes	None	No verbal
2	Opens to pain	Decerebrate posture	Incomprehensible
3	Opens to voice	Decorticate posture	Inappropriate words
4	Opens spontaneously	Withdraws from pain	Confused
5		Localizes pain	Appropriate, oriented
6		Moves with command	

Persistent Vegetative State

General: State of wakefulness without awareness (of environment, stimuli). No response to visual, auditory, painful stimuli. Preserved reflexes/autonomic function.

Etiology: Severe anoxic brain injury

Brain Death

General: Irreversible loss of cortical and brainstem function. Legally equivalent to cardiopulmonary death in US.

Diagnosis: Algorithm below

- If the patient does not meet the criteria, ancillary tests (CTA/MRA, EEG, evoked potentials) may be performed

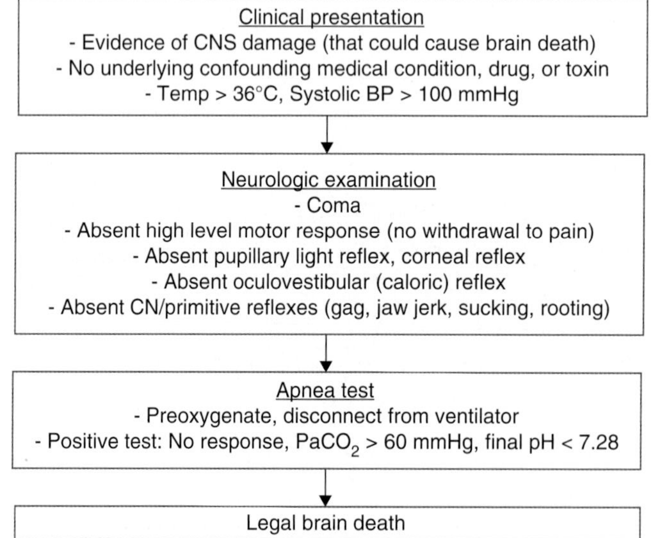

Headache

	General/Clinical	Diagnosis/Management
Tension	- Most common headache subtype - Precipitants: Mental tension and stress Clinical: - Generalized, **bilateral aching headache** of mild-to-moderate pain - Often with tender muscles (e.g., posterior neck muscles) - Normal neurologic examination, lacks photophobia or aura - Can occur infrequently or be chronic (i.e., >15 days per month)	Dx: Clinical Tx: NSAIDs (ibuprofen, naproxen) first-line therapy. Caffeine can be added. PPX: TCA (amitriptyline) only drug with established prophylactic evidence
Migraine	- Pathophys: Cortical spreading depression with trigeminal activation - Risk: Female, family history - Triggers: Fasting, stress, menstruation, weather change, EtOH/wine Clinical: Episodic. passing through multiple phases - Prodrome: Depression, irritability, neck stiffness, tiredness - Aura: Visual (flashing lights), sensory (paresthesias), or auditory - Headache: **Pulsating, unilateral, throbbing pain** - Nausea, vomiting, and photophobia are common	Dx: Clinical. Neuroimaging not necessary unless atypical presentation/want to rule out other pathology. Tx: - Abortive: High-dose NSAIDs or triptans - In ED: IV metoclopramide, diphenhydramine, NSAID PPX: - General measures (good sleep/diet, regular exercise) - Pharm (see below)
Cluster	- Rare. Seen primarily in men. Thought to be due to overactivation of trigeminal/hypothalamic pathway. Clinical: **Excruciating, unilateral headache behind eye** - Autonomic phenomena (rhinorrhea, congestion, ptosis, miosis, lacrimation, facial flushing, conjunctival injection) - Episodes are short (~15 minutes to 2 hours), and can occur multiple times per day, usually daily over a period of weeks with complete remission between "cluster" periods	Dx: Clinical. Head imaging to rule out other dangerous causes of headache. Tx: Inhaled O_2. Sumatriptan. PPX: Verapamil

Migraine PPX

General: Indicated in anyone that has impaired quality of life from migraines. All have equal efficacy, so pick based on possible treatment of comorbid conditions.

Agent	Comorbid Conditions Treated
Beta-blocker (propranolol, timolol)	- HTN, other heart diseases
Amitriptyline and venlafaxine	- Depression, mood disorder, insomnia (amitriptyline)
Valproate and topiramate	- Epilepsy
Verapamil	- Hypertension, arrhythmia rate-control
CGRP antagonists (erenumab, fremanezumab, rimegepant)	

Differential Diagnosis for Headaches

"VOMIT"

- Vascular (subarachnoid hemorrhage, subdural hematoma, epidural hematoma, ICH, temporal arteritis)
- Other (malignant hypertension, pseudotumor cerebri, post lumbar puncture)
- Meds (nitrates, chronic analgesic abuse)
- Infection (meningitis, encephalitis, cerebral abscess, sinusitis)
- Tumor

Red Flag Symptoms: Sudden onset, "worst ever," new onset without previous episode, increasing in severity and frequency over time, worse after lying down, mental status change, focal neurologic deficits, trauma, fever, stiff neck

Other Causes of Headache:

Medicine rebound	- Due to excessive (> 3x per week) amounts of acute symptomatic medication use for chronic headaches - Tx: Abruptly stop medication
Paroxysmal hemicrania	- Presents as 5-30-minute unilateral excruciating headaches in trigeminal distribution - Episodes happen multiple times a day, occurring a couple of times per year with remission between - Tx: Indomethacin usually effective
Low pressure	- Occurs post lumbar puncture or epidural anesthesia. Orthostatic headache (better laying down, worse sitting up). - Tx: NSAIDs +/– epidural blood patch

Vertigo

	General/Clinical	Management

Vertigo
(OVERVIEW)
	- Sensation of spinning and dizziness
	- Caused by abnormalities of the vestibular system
	
	- **Peripheral**: Vestibular canal/CN VIII problem
	  - BPV, vestibular neuritis, Meniere
	- **Central**: Cerebellum or brainstem lesion
	  - Vertebrobasilar stroke, cerebellar stroke, tumor
		Dx: HINTS Exam (can help differentiate central from peripheral vertigo):
		- **H**ead **i**mpulse
		- **N**ystagmus
		- **T**est of **s**kew
		
		Tx: Acute episodes can be treated with antihistamines, antiemetics, and benzodiazepines

Differential Diagnosis		
Benign Paroxysmal Positional Vertigo	- Canalithiasis (calcium debris) in semicircular canal - Clinical: Recurrent episodes of vertigo (< 1 min), often triggered by head movements	Dx: Dix-Hallpike maneuver (causes nystagmus) Tx: Particle repositioning (Epley) maneuver
Vestibular Neuritis (Labyrinthitis)	- Acute viral or postinflammatory CN VIII disorder <u>Clinical</u>: - Acute, single, episode of vertigo - Persistent and lasts for several days - Possibly associated with or following viral symptoms	Dx: Clinical Tx: Antiemetics, antihistamines (like meclizine)

Meniere	- Due to increased endolymph/pressure
	
	<u>Clinical</u>:
	- Episodic vertigo (often episodes last > 0.5 hour)
	- Hearing loss
	- Tinnitus/ear fullness
		Dx: Clinical
		
		Tx:
		- Acute: Antihistamine (meclizine) or anticholinergic (scopolamine)
		- Chronic:
		  - Diet/lifestyle (limit salt intake, caffeine, EtOH)
		  - Diuretics (HCTZ)
		  - Surgery (endolymphatic sac surgery)

Migraine	- Migraine symptoms (headache, aura) PLUS vertigo during episodes	Dx: Clinical Tx: Treat as migraine
Stroke	- Stroke in brainstem (vestibular nuclei) or cerebellum	

Seizures

Overview of Seizures

General: Episode of abnormal activity caused by excessive, synchronous electrical activity in the cerebral cortex

Etiology:

Infants (< 6 M)	- CNS disease (hypoxic-ischemic encephalopathy, CNS hemorrhage/infection) - Metabolic (hypoglycemia, hypocalcemia) - Rarely neonatal onset epilepsy syndrome
Children	- Febrile (usually 6 months to 5 y/o) - Epilepsy (variety of genetic and idiopathic subtypes)
Adults	- Stroke (ischemic/hemorrhagic, subarachnoid hemorrhage), subdural hematoma, anoxic brain injury - Infection (abscess, meningitis, encephalitis) - Brain mass or vascular malformation - Alcohol withdrawal - Drug intoxication - Metabolic disturbances (HypoNa, HyperNa, HypoCa, hypoglycemia) - Epilepsy (usually presents in childhood, but rare subtypes can present later in adulthood)

Clinical:

- **Abnormal motor activity, sensory changes,** and/or **autonomic activity** (sweating, piloerection, pupillary change)
    - Tonic: ↑ tone
    - Atonic: Loss of tone, can drop if standing
    - Myoclonic: Muscle jerks
- First sign can be vocalization (cry): Pharyngeal muscles tighten
- Can maintain awareness (simple) or be without awareness (complex)
- Transient perioral cyanosis (most commonly in children)
- Tongue biting, incontinence, and self-injury are all classic signs
- **Postictal state**: Confusion or disorientation after seizure
- **Todd's paralysis**: Persistent muscle weakness following a seizure, resolves over hours
- **Status epilepticus:** > 5 minutes of continuous seizure activity or cluster of seizures without normal recovery

Diagnosis: Clinical diagnosis. MRI and EEG for further evaluation if cause unknown.

Management of Seizure

Active Seizure	- Most are self-limited (~ 2 minutes) - First aid: Protect bystanders, loosen tight clothing, nothing in mouth, place on side to avoid aspiration - Actively seizing: Can give benzo (e.g., IV lorazepam, IM midazolam)
Status Epilepticus	- ABCs (airway, breathing, and circulation) - IV lorazepam or diazepam - Fosphenytoin (or phenytoin, valproate, levetiracetam) - Refractory: IV midazolam, propofol, or pentobarbital

Chronic Prevention	- Antiepileptic indicated if recurrent, unprovoked seizures
	- Drug choice is complex, without clear evidence of superiority of any specific drug
	
	- **Broad spectrum agents** (for both generalized and focal):
	  - Levetiracetam, lamotrigine, topiramate, valproate
	- **Narrow spectrum agents** (for focal seizures):
	  - Carbamazepine, oxcarbazepine, phenytoin
	  - Ethosuximide (used for absence)
	- Refractory cases: Epilepsy surgery, vagus nerve stimulation, ketogenic diet
	
	- Period of seizure free (6-12 months) required before resuming driving

Seizures

Seizure Subtypes

	General/Clinical	Management
Focal Seizures	- Originates from one hemisphere Clinical: - Motor features: **Movements/jerks in one part of body** - Sensory features: Paresthesias, auditory/visual symptoms	
Generalized Seizures **(Previously Grand-mal)**	- Originates focally, but spreads and involves both hemispheres Clinical: - Motor features: **Diffuse movements/jerks throughout body** - Sensory, autonomic features also possible	
Absence Seizures	- Common type of seizure in children - Presents with episodes of "**spacing out**", < 20 seconds - Can recur multiple times per day - Automatisms (eyelid flickers, tongue smacking), tone intact	Dx: EEG (3 Hz spike and wave pattern), provoked by hyperventilation Tx: Ethosuximide (alt: Valproate)
Febrile Seizures	- 6 months to 5 y/o - Occur with **viral or bacterial infection** - **Generalized tonic-clonic activity** most common - Must not have prior history of epilepsy Note: Children with febrile seizures are at risk for recurrent febrile seizures and have small ↑ risk for epilepsy	Dx: Clinical diagnosis. MRI, EEG, LP only required if atypical features (suspicion for meningitis, other serious pathology) Tx: IV Lorazepam if seizing for > 5 min - If back to baseline after, can reassure and send home. No evidence for antipyretics or antiepileptic.

Psychogenic Nonepileptic Seizures	- Clinically present like epileptic seizures, but no focal CNS changes are found on workup
	- Subtle features can hint that episode is not true seizure
	  - Movements more variable, changing in type and magnitude
	  - More writhing, thrashing
		Dx: EEG (no abnormal EEG activity during seizure)
		
		Tx: Patient/family education. Psychotherapy (CBT) and treat underlying psych disorders.

Epilepsy Syndromes

Temporal Lobe Epilepsy	- Most common focal epilepsy syndrome - Caused by mesial temporal sclerosis - Focal seizures with impairment of consciousness
Childhood Absence Epilepsy	- Syndrome of chronic, recurring absence seizures - Occurs in kids ~5-10 y/o - Usually remits by puberty
Juvenile Myoclonic Epilepsy	- Often history of absence seizures (~ 5 y/o), followed by myoclonic seizures later (~15 years) - Full tonic-clonic seizures - Hallmark: Myoclonic jerks on awakening
Benign Rolandic Epilepsy	- Most common form of childhood epilepsy - Occurs between 6 and 10 years old, often remitting after a few years - Focal seizures are characteristic, often starting in face and spreading to other body areas
Lennox-Gastaut	- Presents in children between 3 and 5 y/o - Multiple seizure subtypes (tonic, atonic, myotonic, and atypical absence seizures) - Impaired development, intellectual disability

Neuropathy/Neuropathic Pain

Overview

	Features	Etiology
Neuropathy		
Mononeuropathy	- Peripheral insult to one nerve, most commonly due to compression	- Carpal tunnel, cubital tunnel - Meralgia paresthetica
Mononeuritis multiplex	- Multiple, single nerve abnormalities	- Vasculitis (e.g., Polyarteritis Nodosa)
Polyneuropathy	- Diffuse peripheral nerve disease	- Diabetes mellitus, B12 deficiency - GBS - Toxins (e.g., EtOH, chemotherapy)
Radiculopathy	- Compression of nerve root, causing weakness, sensory loss, and/or pain	- Disc herniation - Osteoarthritis, spinal stenosis
Myelopathy	- Spinal cord dysfunction, most commonly from compression	- Trauma, spinal stenosis, mass

Management: Treat underlying condition
- Pharm (for neuropathic pain): Gabapentin/Pregabalin, TCA (amitriptyline), topical capsaicin or lidocaine

Complex Regional Pain Syndrome

General: Previously named reflex sympathetic dystrophy. Disorder of extremities with localized pain that is disproportionate to any trauma or underlying pathology. Pathophysiology unknown (thought due to neurogenic inflammation and abnormal CNS pain pathway).

Clinical: Limb pain, sensory/motor impairments, autonomic symptoms, atrophy
- Examples: Burning skin, muscle spasms, vasospasm, skin/nail changes, edema

Management: Patient education, PT/OT
- Pharm: NSAIDs, amitriptyline, gabapentin
- PPX: Vitamin C (after distal limb surgery/fracture)

Neuropathic Syndromes

	General/Clinical	Management
Trigeminal Neuralgia	- Caused by: - Compression of CN V nerve root (e.g., by artery, vein, tumor) - Herpes-Zoster or demyelination (e.g., multiple sclerosis) - Sudden, quick, severe, unilateral, episodes of shock-like pain in the distribution of CN V	Tx: Carbamazepine (alt: Oxcarbazepine)
Facial Nerve Palsy	- Paralysis of facial muscles due to CN VII lesion - **Bell palsy** (idiopathic facial palsy) - Nonidiopathic causes: Lyme disease, otitis media - Isolated, acute-onset, unilateral facial paralysis - Involves both lower (cheek) and upper (forehead) muscles - Associated with decreased lacrimation, hyperacusis, loss of taste/sensation on the anterior ⅔ tongue	Tx: Self-limited (resolves within weeks to months). **Prednisone**. Antivirals if severe.
Ramsay Hunt (Herpes-Zoster Oticus)	- Reactivation of VZV in multiple cranial nerves - Triad of unilateral facial paralysis, vesicles in ear, and ear pain	Tx: VZV antivirals (acyclovir, valacyclovir)
Post Herpetic Neuralgia	- Pain left in distribution of VZV reactivation (shingles)	Tx: Gabapentin, pregabalin, TCA, or topical capsaicin
Drug-Induced Neuropathy	- Common agents: Vincristine/vinblastine, cisplatin, paclitaxel - Clinical: Sensory neuropathy (stocking-glove distribution), rare motor involvement	

CNS Infections

Meningitis

General: Inflammatory disease of the leptomeninges. Infectious agent spreads via hematogenous spread, contiguous spread (sinusitis, otitis media, trauma, surgery), or retrograde transport up nerves.

Etiology	Organism
Bacterial Meningitis	
Neonates	- Group B *Streptococci*, gram-negatives (*E. Coli*), *Listeria*
Children	- *Neisseria meningitidis, S. pneumoniae, H. influenzae*
Adults	- *S. pneumoniae, N. meningitidis, H. influenza. Listeria* in elderly.
Immunocomp	- *Listeria*, gram-negative (*E. Coli*), *S. pneumoniae*
Trauma/Surg	- MRSA, coagulase-negative *Staph*, gram-negatives
Aseptic	- Enterovirus (coxsackie, echo), HIV, HSV, mumps, VZV. Syphilis, lyme.
Other	- Tuberculosis, fungal (*Cryptococcus, Coccidioides*)

Clinical: **Fever, nuchal rigidity, headache**

- Lethargy, but intact sensorium (vs encephalitis). Seizure, focal deficits (occur in some).
- Maculopapular rash (with meningococcus)
- **Kernig sign**: Inability to extend knees with patient supine and hips flexed
- **Brudzinski sign**: Leg flexion elicited by passive flexion of neck

Diagnosis: **Lumbar puncture** (CSF findings are diagnostic)

Subtype	WBC	Diff	Protein	Gluc	Gram Stain
Normal	< 5	--	15-60	50-75 (66% serum)	--
Bacterial	> 1000	> 80% PMN	↑↑	↓	(+)
Viral (aseptic)	5-500	> 50% Lymph	↑	↔	--
Fungal	20-2000	> 50% Lymph	↑	↔	--
TB	20-2000	> 80% Lymph	↑	↓	(+) in some

CT (needed before LP?)

- Previously universally performed to rule out ↑ ICP in fear of herniation
- Usually not required. Only indicated if: History of mass lesion or stroke, new onset of seizure, papilledema, focal neurologic deficit, abnormal consciousness, or immunocompromised (e.g., HIV)

Management:

- Empiric antibiotic therapy: Start immediately after LP is performed. Adjust per culture/sensitivity.
- Steroids: Indicated in some (see below), has been shown to reduce complications in certain groups

Type	Group	Antibiotic/Drug Regimen
Bacterial	Neonate (< 1 month)	- Ampicillin + gentamicin or cefotaxime
	Children (> 1 month)	- Vancomycin + ceftriaxone (or cefotaxime) - Dexamethasone (for HiB, controversial w/ *S. Pneumo*)
	Adults	- Vancomycin + ceftriaxone (or cefotaxime) - Add ampicillin if > 50 y/o - Dexamethasone (if pneumococcus, started empirically in most cases)
	Immunocomp	- Vancomycin + ampicillin + cefepime or meropenem
	Trauma, surgery, nosocomial	- Vancomycin + cefepime or meropenem
Aseptic		- Observe, consider acyclovir if HSV suspected

Complications: Hearing loss (evaluate all children after for hearing loss), seizures, intellectual disability, hydrocephalus

CNS Infections

Encephalitis

General: Diffuse inflammation of the brain parenchyma. Differentiated from meningitis by abnormalities in brain function (e.g., altered mental status).

Etiology	Specific Findings
HSV-1	- Red cells in CSF - Temporal lesions/hemorrhage - Occurs any time of year (versus the below arboviruses)
West Nile	- Associated with ascending flaccid paralysis - Peaks in late summer/early fall in the US
Mumps	- Associated with parotitis, lack of vaccine status
Powassan	- Tick-borne virus (*Ixodes*), occurs in Northeastern US
Others	- St. Louis encephalitis virus - Eastern/Western equine encephalitis virus - California encephalitis virus - Rabies

Clinical:

- **Altered mental status** (confused, agitated, or unresponsive)
- Seizures
- Focal deficits (cranial palsies, motor/sensory deficit)
- Meningismus and headache (in those with meningoencephalitis)

Diagnosis: LP (CSF cell count/glucose/protein, PCR for HSV, serology for West Nile)

- WBC < 250 (usually lymphocyte predominance)
- Protein mildly increased, glucose normal

Management: Supportive care. Empiric acyclovir (for possible HSV).

Brain Abscess

General: Focal collection of pus within the brain parenchyma. Usually due to contiguous spread (sinusitis, otitis, mastoiditis) or hematogenous spread (bacteremia).

Etiology:

- *Strep viridans*, other *Strep*
- *Staph aureus*, other *Staph*
- Gram negatives, anaerobes

Clinical:

- Headache, fever
- Focal neurologic deficits (cranial nerve defects, hemiparesis), papilledema

Diagnosis:

- MRI (or CT): Ring-enhancing brain lesion
- CT-guided aspiration

Management:

- Aspiration or surgical drainage
- Empiric antibiotics (vancomycin + ceftriaxone + metronidazole)
- Glucocorticoids

CNS Malignancies

Brain Malignancy

Etiology:

- Primary (see next page) -- 30% of cases
- Secondary (metastasis) -- 70% of cases

Clinical:

- May be asymptomatic
- **Seizures and focal neurologic deficits**
- ↑ ICP (headache, vomiting, papilledema)
    - Headache (early morning, worse bending over/with valsalva)

Diagnosis: **MRI with contrast** (best for visualization compared to CT)

Paraneoplastic Syndromes of CNS

Disorder	Features
Paraneoplastic Encephalomyelitis	- Autoantibody formation against CNS antigens. Can cause encephalitis, myelitis, or both. - Common antigens include Hu (SCLC), Ma-2 (testicular), and CMPR-5 (SCLC, thymoma) - Clinical: Neuropsychiatric issues (impaired cognition, psychosis, memory loss, etc)
Anti-NMDA Receptor Encephalitis	- Subtype of paraneoplastic/autoimmune encephalitis - Often associated with teratomas, but can also be idiopathic autoimmune condition - Clinical: Psychiatric disturbance, memory deficits, seizures, dyskinesias, autonomic instability - Dx: CSF finding of anti-NMDA IgG - Tx: Corticosteroids, IVIG, tumor resection
Opsoclonus-Myoclonus Ataxia Syndrome	- "Dancing eyes, dancing feet" - Occurs most commonly with neuroblastoma (in children) and SCLC (adults) - Clinical: Ataxia, myoclonus, opsoclonus (multi directional rapid eye movements)
Paraneoplastic Cerebellar Degeneration	- Associated with SCLC, Hodgkin lymphoma, breast cancer - Antibodies against Hu, Yo, Tr antigens in Purkinje cells - Clinical: Gait instability, dizziness, nausea, vomiting

Brain Metastasis

General: Most common primary cancer site lung, breast, kidney, melanoma

Clinical:

- Focal deficits, cognitive dysfunction, and headache all possible
- Must work up for brain mets in any cancer patient presenting with new neurologic symptoms

Diagnosis: MRI (one or more lesions, most commonly occur at **gray-white junction**[A])

Management:

- Single lesion: Surgical removal, stereotactic radiosurgery
- Multifocal lesions: Whole brain radiation therapy
- Glucocorticoids (↓ edema/ICP)

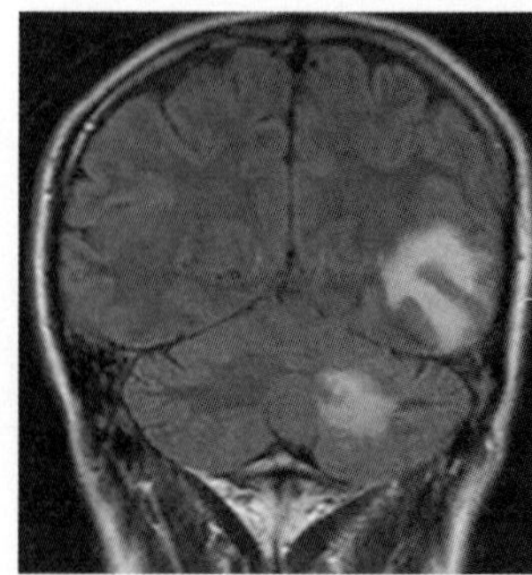

CNS Malignancies

	General/Clinical	Management
Adult Tumors (Usually supratentorial)		
Glioblastoma Multiforme	- Most common primary brain tumor in adults - High grade glioma, with poor prognosis - Rapidly progressive neurologic symptoms	Dx: MRI: Butterfly appearance, central necrosis Tx: Surgical resection. Neoadjuvant radiation therapy and Temozolomide.
Meningioma	- Derived from meninges and located along dura - Risk: Radiation, NF2 - Often asymptomatic, but can cause focal findings where compression occurs	Dx: MRI: Extra-axial, dural based mass Tx: Surgical resection or observation
Vestibular Schwannoma	- Also known as acoustic neuroma - Schwann cell tumors derived from CN VIII - Presents with loss of hearing, tinnitus, and vertigo - Can compress cranial nerves (CN V, VII)	Dx: MRI: Tumor at cerebellopontine angle Tx: Surgical resection or radiation therapy
Oligodendroglioma	- Rare, slow growing glioma - Associated with IDH mutation, deletion of 1p/19q - Slow growing, progressive symptoms over years - Most common symptom is seizure	Dx: MRI: Most commonly frontal cortex Tx: Surgical resection, radiation, chemo
Pediatric Tumors (usually infratentorial)		
Pilocytic Astrocytoma	- Well-differentiated, low grade, glioma - Posterior fossa tumor, cystic +/− solid components - Presents with cerebellar dysfunction (ataxia)	Dx: MRI. Confirm with histology. Tx: Surgical resection (often achieves cure)
Medulloblastoma	- Highly malignant primary brain tumor - Can metastasize inferiorly to spinal leptomeninges - Cerebellar dysfunction (truncal ataxia) - Can compress fourth ventricle (hydrocephalus, ↑ ICP)	Dx: MRI (midline, enhancing cerebellar mass, often causing obstructive hydrocephalus) Tx: Surgical resection + chemoradiation
Ependymoma	- Glial tumor of ependymal lining of ventricles - Can cause hydrocephalus	Tx: Surgical resection + radiation
Craniopharyngioma	- Childhood supratentorial tumor, also seen in adults - Derived from ectodermal remnant of Rathke pouch - Headache, visual issues (bitemporal hemianopsia), endocrine (hyperprolactinemia, diabetes insipidus, or panhypopituitarism)	Dx: MRI (calcified, solid or cystic masses in the suprasellar area) Tx: Surgical resection + radiation
Pinealoma	- Germ cell tumor arising from pineal gland - Presents with ↑ ICP and hydrocephalus - **Parinaud syndrome**: Vertical gaze palsy, eyelid retraction, diplopia, pupils do not react to light - Can produce β-hCG (causing precocious puberty)	Tx: Radiation therapy
Brain Stem Glioma	- Can be low grade (focal brainstem glioma) or high-grade (diffuse intrinsic pontine glioma, which has poor prognosis)	Tx: Surgical resection + chemoradiation

Hearing Loss

Etiology of Hearing Loss

	Conductive	Sensorineural
Path	- Caused by lesions in the outer or middle ear, which interfere with mechanical conduction	- Due to lesions in the cochlea or CN VIII (inner ear)
Clin	- Worse with low frequency	- Worse with high frequency OR intensity - Poor sound discrimination - Possible tinnitus
Cause	<u>External Ear</u> - External otitis - Cerumen - Exostoses (bony outgrowths in auditory canal) <u>Middle Ear</u> - Otitis media - Cholesteatoma - Otosclerosis - Tympanic membrane perforation	<u>Inner Ear</u> - Hereditary/congenital hearing loss - Presbycusis - Noise-induced hearing loss - Ototoxic drugs - Meniere - Acoustic neuroma - Multiple sclerosis - CVA - Complication of CNS infection (meningitis, neurosyphilis) - Sudden sensorineural hearing loss

Evaluation of Hearing Loss

(1) Clinical evaluation
- Whispered voice test, or tone-emitting otoscopes
- External auditory canal exam (rule out cerumen, external otitis, etc.)
- Rinne/Weber Test (differentiates conductive vs sensorineural hearing loss)

	Rinne	Weber
Normal	Air > Bone	Equal both ears
Conductive	Bone > Air in affected ear	Lateralized to affected ear
Sensorineural	Air > Bone	Lateralized to unaffected ear
Mixed	Bone > Air in affected ear	Lateralized to unaffected ear

(2) Audiologic testing (for all that do not have obvious cause of hearing loss)
(3) MRI (or CT) for asymmetric disease

Hearing Loss

	General/Clinical	Management
Conductive		
Cerumen Impaction	- Accumulation and obstruction of ear wax - Due to cerumen overproduction or tortuous/narrow ear canal	Tx: Mineral oil or hydrogen peroxide, irrigation, mechanical removal
Cholesteatoma	- Growth of desquamated squamous epithelium debris in the middle ear - Can be primary (from negative pressure retraction pocket) or secondary (perforation from trauma or chronic inflammation) - Present with hearing loss and ear drainage - Pearly mass behind tympanic membrane[A]	Dx: Clinical. MRI/CT can aid in ruling out cranial involvement. Tx: Surgical (tympanomastoidectomy)
Otosclerosis	- Bony overgrowth of the stapes, resulting in mechanical failure of sound conduction in the inner ear	Tx: Hearing aids or surgical correction (stapedectomy plus prosthesis)
Sensorineural		
Presbycusis	- Age-related hearing loss - Caused by generalized damage to cochlea or inner ear - Presents with gradual, progressive symmetric hearing loss, difficulty with high pitches and voice discrimination	Tx: Hearing aids
Noise-Induced	- Chronic exposure to sounds > 85 dB	
Ototoxicity	- Aminoglycosides and Cisplatin most common - Aspirin, Quinine, Chloroquine, loop diuretics	
Sudden Sensorineural Hearing Loss	- Acute, unilateral, hearing loss, due to idiopathic, autoimmune, or viral etiology	Dx: MRI. Audiology used to rule out other disorders. Tx: Steroids. Generally regain hearing in a week.

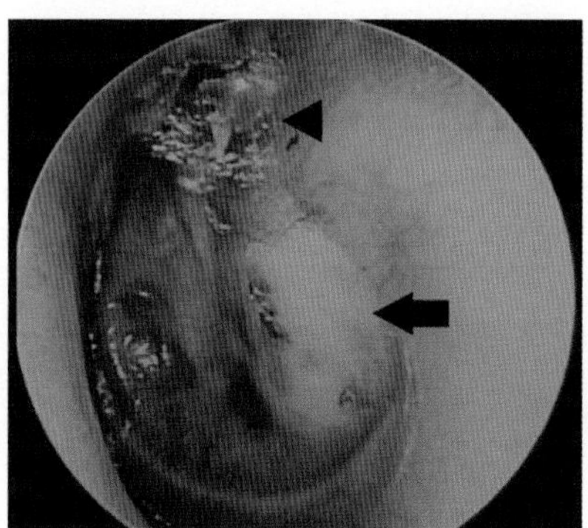

Ophthalmology

	General/Clinical	Management
Eyelid Pathology		
Hordeolum (stye)	- Small abscess of the eyelid (most commonly *Staph aureus*) - Presents as small, painful, erythematous swelling, either externally at eyelid margin, or internally on conjunctiva	Dx: Clinical Tx: Self-limited. Warm compress. I&D if persistent.
Chalazion	- Chronic granulomatous infection of meibomian gland - Presents as painless, localized eyelid nodule - Occurs on inner eyelid - Less painful, red, and angry compared to stye	Dx: Clinical Tx: Self-limited. Persistent lesions: I&D or steroid injection.
Xanthelasma	- Cholesterol-filled yellow plaques associated with hypercholesterolemia	Dx: Cholesterol panel Tx: Intervention not required
Dacryocystitis	- Infection of lacrimal sac from nasolacrimal duct obstruction - Pain, erythema, swelling over the medial canthus	Dx: Clinical Tx: Oral antibiotics
Blepharitis	- Inflammation of the eyelids occurring near eyelid margin - Present with erythematous, swollen, itchy eyelids - Associated symptoms include blurry vision, excessive tearing, gritty sensation, flaking/scaling	Dx: Clinical Tx: Eyelid massage, warm compress, and washing. Topical antibiotics for severe or refractory cases.
Conjunctival Disorders		
Conjunctivitis		
Bacterial	- *Staph aureus*, pneumococcus, *H. influenzae*, most common - Erythema, thick mucoid discharge - Eye often stuck shut in morning - **Most often unilateral**	- Erythromycin ointment or trimethoprim/polymyxin drops
Viral	- Can occur as part of viral syndrome (e.g., URI like **Adenovirus**) - Erythema, mucoid/serous discharge, burning/gritty sensation - **Most often bilateral**[A]	- Self-limited. Artificial tears, antihistamines.
Allergic	- Bilateral erythema, watery discharge, and itching - History of atopy (atopic dermatitis, asthma)	- Avoid allergens, rubbing eyes - Acute: Topical antihistamine/vasoconstrictor (naphazoline/pheniramine) - Chronic: Antihistamine/mast cell stabilizer (olopatadine, azelastine)
Trachoma	- Most common infectious cause of blindness in the world - Infection with *Chlamydia trachomatis* - Active trachoma causes **mild conjunctival inflammation** - Repeated episodes can lead to **cicatricial disease**[B] - Chronic eyelid inflammation and scarring turns lids inwards (entropion), ingrown eyelashes (trichiasis), and blindness	Dx: Clinical. Culture/PCR for chlamydia if unsure. Tx: Antibiotics (azithromycin, tetracycline). Surgery for trichiasis.
Subconjunctival Hemorrhage	- Can be idiopathic or occur with trauma/eye contact - Presents as focal collection of blood between conjunctiva and sclera	Tx: Self-limited (resolves in a few weeks)
Dry Eye	- Also referred to as **keratoconjunctivitis sicca** - Decreased tear production or excessive tear evaporation - Presents with chronic dry eye, irritation, burning	Tx: Artificial tears

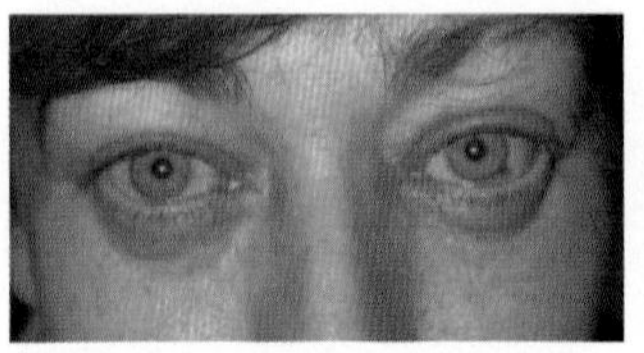

A

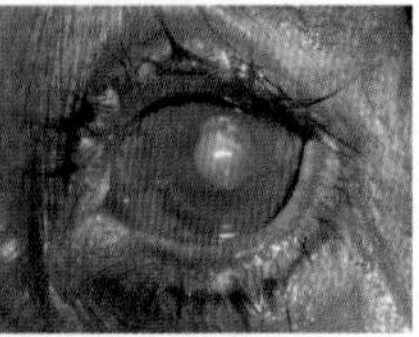

B

Ophthalmology

	General/Clinical	Management
Sclera Disorders		
Scleritis	- Acute inflammation of the sclera. Potentially blinding. - Often associated with RA or vasculitis (GPA) - Presents with ocular redness, severe pain (worse with eye movements), eye watering, possible visual impairment	Dx: Clinical/slit-lamp examination Tx: NSAIDs. Prednisone + rituximab for severe cases.
Episcleritis	- Inflammation of the episclera. Benign and self-limited. - Usually idiopathic, can be associated with rheumatologic condition - Presents with focal erythema/injection, vasodilation of the episcleral vessels, possible irritation, **but no visual loss**	Tx: Self-limited
Lens Disorders		
Cataracts (adult)	- **Opacification of the lens** (present in 50% over 75 y/o) - Risk: ↑ Age, smoking, EtOH, light exposure, diabetes, steroids - Decreased visual acuity (especially in the dark, with glare around bright lights) - Myopic shift: ↑ refractive power of the lens → nearsightedness	Dx: Clinical (slit-lamp exam) Tx: Surgical extraction/artificial lens replacement
Presbyopia	- **Loss of accommodating power of lens**, occurring with ↑ age - Presents with difficulty reading close, fine print	Tx: Reading glasses
Refractive Errors	- Myopia (nearsightedness) - Hyperopia (farsightedness) - Astigmatism (abnormal corneal shape)	Dx: Snellen chart (worse than 20/25) Tx: Glasses, contact lenses, or refractive surgery (Lasik)
Corneal Disorders		
Corneal Abrasion	- Corneal insult from direct trauma, foreign bodies, contact lens - Presents with severe eye pain - Foreign body sensation in eye, irritation - Photophobia, refusal to open eye	Dx: Fluorescein examination Tx: Usually improve within 2-3 days. Topical antibiotic prophylaxis (erythromycin). Oral or topical NSAIDs for analgesia.
Keratitis	- **Inflammation of the cornea**, with bacterial, viral, fungal causes - Risk: Contact lens use, immunosuppression, trauma - Presents with corneal infiltrate +/− mucopurulent discharge - Red eye, photophobia, foreign body sensation	Dx: Penlight exam (infiltrate appears like small white spot, stains (+) with fluorescein) Tx: See specific etiology below
Bacterial Keratitis	- *Staph aureus, Pseudomonas* most common	Tx: Topical antibiotics
Viral Keratitis	- Most commonly HSV - Corneal lesion is dendritic, forming from initial vesicular lesions	Tx: Oral or topical antivirals
Amebic Keratitis	- *Acanthamoeba* infection - Associated with poor contact lens hygiene - Can rapidly lead to vision loss if not treated	Tx: Topical antiparasitic agents (polyhexamethylene biguanide, hexamidine)
Misc. Eye Disorders		
Globe Rupture	- Can be caused by blunt trauma or penetrating trauma - Presents with eye deformity and volume loss - Eccentric pupil, pupillary defects, decreased visual acuity	Dx: Clinical. CT is used to better characterize. Tx: Prophylactic antibiotics, tetanus. Avoid increasing eye pressure. Primary surgical closure is definitive.
Optic Neuritis	- Acute inflammatory demyelination of optic nerve - Associated with MS, NMO - Presents with monocular vision loss - Possible color desaturation, afferent pupillary defect - Possible optic nerve inflammation or atrophy on exam	Dx: MRI Tx: High-dose steroids

Ophthalmology

Glaucoma (Chronic)

General: Increased IOP leading to damage to optic neuropathy and irreversible vision loss (peripheral vision, followed by central)

	Open Angle	Closed Angle
Path	- ↑ Aqueous humor production or ↓ outflow	- Narrowing of the anterior chamber angle, ↓ aqueous humor outflow
Risk	- ↑ Age, family history, Black	- Primary: ↑ Age, family history, hyperopia - Secondary: Fibrosis, inflammation, mass, or neovascularization
Clin	- Asymptomatic - Progressive peripheral visual field loss with eventual "tunnel vision," followed by central vision loss	- Can present with acute blockage (see below) OR - Chronic, asymptomatic process (like open angle) with progressive peripheral visual field loss
Dx	- Fundus examination (cupping)[A] - Tonometry: ↑ IOP (> 25 mmHg) is consistent with glaucoma, but not diagnostic - Gonioscopy (diagnostic for closed-angle, allows for visualization of angle)	
Tx	- First line therapy: Pharm and surgery equal efficacy Pharm - Prostaglandins (latanoprost), beta-blockers (Timolol) Surgery: Trabeculoplasty	- Surgery: Laser peripheral iridotomy is definitive treatment Note: Treat/remove underlying cause if secondary to another process

Drug	Class/Mechanism	Side Effects
Timolol	Beta-blocker	- Generally well-tolerated
Bimatoprost latanoprost	Prostaglandins	- Heterochromia, ↑ eyelash length - Conjunctival hyperemia
Acetazolamide	Carbonic Anhydrase Inh.	
Pilocarpine Physostigmine	Cholinomimetics	- Miosis (if chronic use)
Epinephrine Brimonidine	Alpha-agonist	- Ocular hyperemia, blurred vision, discomfort - Mydriasis

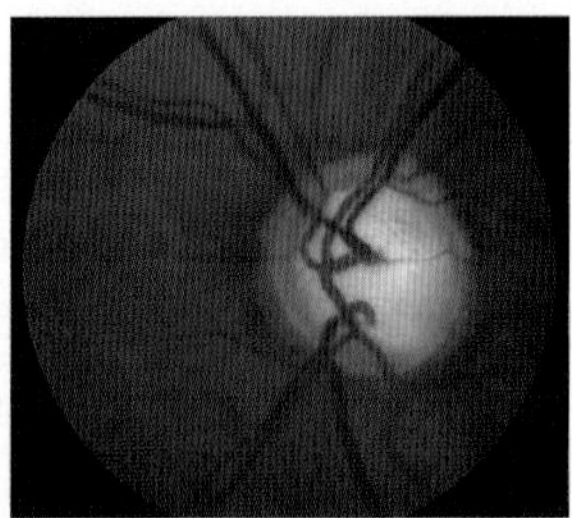

Acute Angle Closure Glaucoma

Clinical:

- Decreased visual acuity, abnormal halo around light
- Headache/severe eye pain, associated with nausea and vomiting
- Conjunctival erythema, dilated pupils

Management:

- Emergent therapy/ophtho referral
- Topical beta-blocker (timolol), alpha-agonist (brimonidine, apraclonidine), miotic agents (pilocarpine)
- Acetazolamide or mannitol
- Laser iridotomy

Ophthalmology

	General/Clinical	Management
Sudden Visual Loss		
Central Retinal Artery Occlusion[A]	- **Acute occlusion of retinal artery** - Similar etiology to CVA (atherosclerosis, embolic) - Presents with acute, painless single sided visual loss - Poor prognosis, often leads to permanent visual loss	Dx: Clinical plus fundoscopy (pale retina with cherry red spot) Tx: Ocular massage, anterior chamber paracentesis, reduce intraocular pressure
Central Retinal Vein Occlusion	- **Thrombotic occlusion of retinal veins**, with resulting ischemia - Risks: Coagulopathy, hyperviscosity, atherosclerosis - Presents with acute/subacute progressive loss of visual acuity (less sudden than arterial). Can be asymptomatic.	Dx: Fundoscopy (disc swelling, venous dilation, hemorrhages, cotton wool spots) Tx: Observation. anti-VEGF injections if macular edema, laser treatment for neovascularization.
Retinal Detachment[B]	- Separation of the neurosensory retina from the retinal pigment epithelium, leading to ischemia and vision loss - Evolves from posterior vitreous detachment or retinal tears - Risk: Eye trauma, diabetes mellitus, myopia - Presents with floaters/flashes of light, which can progress to peripheral vision loss ("curtain over visual field")	Dx: Fundoscopy (retinal breaks/abnormalities, gray elevated retina, pigmented cells in vitreous) Tx: Laser retinopexy or cryoretinopexy
Vitreous Hemorrhage	- Leakage of blood into vitreous humor of the eye - Associated with retinal tears, trauma, and child abuse - Presents with impaired vision, floaters, and light flashes	Dx: Fundoscopy (retina obscured by floating cells in vitreous) Tx: Elevated head, allow hemorrhage to settle. Treat underlying cause.
Retinal Disorders		
Diabetic Retinopathy[C]	- Associated with DM1 and DM2 Classification - **Nonproliferative**: Microaneurysms, hemorrhages, exudates, and cotton wool spots - **Proliferative**: Neovascularization (leads to vitreous hemorrhage and/or retinal detachment) - Generally asymptomatic until late stage	Dx: Fundoscopy (screen yearly) Tx: - Glycemic control (Hgb A1C < 7%), BP control - Proliferative: Photocoagulation or anti-VEGF
Hypertensive Retinopathy[D]	- Retinal changes directly associated with chronic hypertension - Arterial wall thickening, AV nicking, flame hemorrhage, exudate, cotton-wool spots, optic disc edema/papilledema	Dx: Fundoscopy Tx: Manage underlying hypertension
Macular Degeneration	- Most common cause of blindness in developed countries - Risk: ↑ Age, smoking, EtOH use, family history - Presents with central vision loss, scotomas, metamorphopsia Classification - **Dry**: Degeneration of the central retina, drusen deposition - **Wet**: Leakage of serous fluid/blood with neovascularization	Dx: Fundoscopy (areas of retinal atrophy, depigmentation, drusen). Edema, hemorrhage, and neovascularization in wet MD. Tx: - Dry: Supportive. Eye vitamins, quit smoking - Wet: anti-VEGF injections
CMV Retinitis	- Reactivation of latent CMV, full thickness inflammation of retina - Common disease in **AIDS with CD4 < 50** - Presents with loss of central vision, scotoma/floaters	Dx: Fundoscopy (fluffy retinal lesions, hemorrhage) Tx: Ganciclovir (either oral or intravitreal), ART
Retinitis Pigmentosa	- Inherited progressive retinal degeneration - Presents with night blindness, peripheral visual field loss - Ophthalmoscopy: Pigment deposits, pale optic nerve	Dx: Clinical, plus advanced retina testing

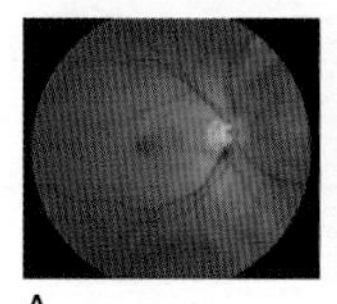
A

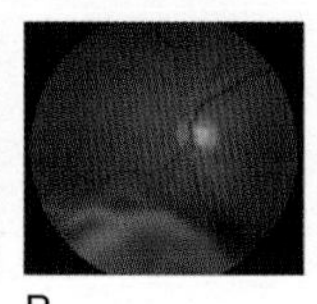
B

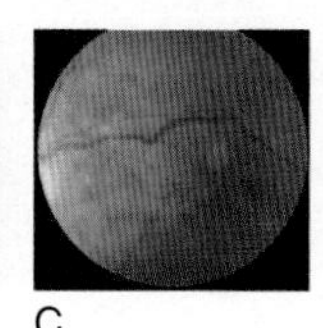
C

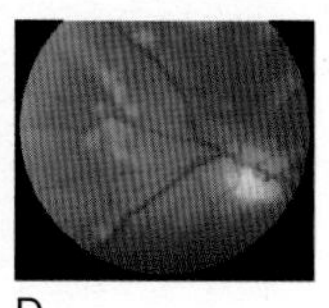
D

Ophthalmology

Uveitis

General: Intraocular inflammation

Etiology:

- Systemic inflammatory conditions (sarcoidosis, IBD, spondyloarthritis)
- Viral (HSV, VZV), parasitic (toxoplasmosis)

	Anterior	Posterior
Path	Anterior chamber inflammation, including: - Iritis - Iridocyclitis	Inflammation posterior to lens, including: - Vitritis - Pars planitis - Chorioretinitis
Clin	- Red eye, **pain**, photophobia, possible ↓ visual acuity	- Presents with ↓ visual acuity, **painless**
Dx	- Clinical (history + slit lamp) - Leukocyte/protein accumulation in anterior chamber	- Clinical (history + slit lamp) - Chorioretinal inflammation, leukocytes in vitreous humor
Tx	- Topical glucocorticoids	- Intraocular glucocorticoids

Associated Conditions:

Sympathetic Ophthalmia:

- Anterior uveitis that occurs ~ 1 year after penetrating trauma to other eye
- Believed due to systemic antigen exposure, autoimmune response

Acute Retinal Necrosis:

- Reactivation of HSV, HZV or other viruses seen in severe immunocompromised states
- Presents with prodrome of keratoconjunctivitis, then progresses to bilateral necrotizing retinitis
- Clinical diagnosis (ophthalmoscopy shows retinal/vitreal inflammation, retinal vascular arteriolitis)
- Treat with acyclovir/valacyclovir

Endophthalmitis

General: Infection within eye, including vitreous/aqueous humor

Etiology: Post surgery, penetrating eye trauma, keratitis

Clinical: Presents with eye pain, decreased visual acuity, conjunctival injection, hypopyon (WBCs in anterior chamber)

Management: Vitrectomy. Intravitreal antibiotics.

Ophthalmology

Eye Movement Disorders

Lesion	Features

CN III	- Parasympathetic (external nerve fibers):
	  - Subject to compression
	  - Causes pupillary dilation with abnormal light reflex
	
	- Motor (internal nerve fibers):
	  - Damaged from vascular disease (diabetes mellitus)
	  - Causes down/out gaze, ptosis, diplopia

CN IV	- Innervates superior oblique muscle - Presents as vertical/oblique diplopia, worse with downward gaze - Patients often head tilt toward side of lesion - Worsening misalignment (eye moves upward) with adduction of eye
CN VI	- Impaired abduction on side of lesion
Internuclear Ophthalmoplegia	- Lesion in medial longitudinal fasciculus (normally coordinates CN VI/CN III movements) - Lesions cause conjugate horizontal gaze palsy - Example (right MLF): With leftward gaze, left eye abducts with nystagmus, right eye has impaired adduction (does not move past midline)
Frontal Eye Field Lesions	- Lesions in the frontal eye field result in eyes deviated toward the side of the lesion

Pediatric Eye Disorders

	General/Clinical	Management
Cataracts	- Can be idiopathic, or associated with trauma, glucocorticoid use, or congenital infections - Presents with asymmetric red reflex, leukocoria, photophobia, decreased visual acuity	Dx: Clinical (slit-lamp exam) Tx: Surgical extraction
Dacryostenosis	- Due to **congenital nasolacrimal duct obstruction** - Presents with persistent tearing and discharge - Debris in eyelids, possible swelling in medial eye	Dx: Clinical Tx: Lacrimal sac massage, self-limited
Amblyopia ("Lazy Eye")	- Decreased visual acuity from **abnormal visual development** - Due to strabismus, refractive errors, or other structural eye issues	Dx: Routine screening < 5 y/o (fixation testing for preverbal, visual acuity if verbal) Tx: Treat underlying condition. Encourage use of lazy eye (patch/atropine drops for other eye).
Strabismus	- **Abnormal ocular alignment** - Primary (congenital) or secondary (acquired ocular/CNS disorder) - Definitions: Esotropia (nasal), exotropia (temporal), hypertropia (upward), and hypotropia (downward) - Presents with asymmetry of red or corneal light reflexes, possible head tilt, abnormal cover-uncover test - Amblyopia can develop if not treated	Tx: - Occlusion therapy (patch good eye) OR penalization therapy (cycloplegic drops in good eye) - Eyeglasses (to correct refractive errors) - Surgery if refractory
Retinopathy of Prematurity	- **Overproliferation of retinal blood vessels** - Caused by excess O_2 exposure - Seen in **premature**, low birth weight babies - Common cause of childhood blindness	Dx: Retinal examination Tx: Monitor mild disease, laser coagulation and VEGF inhibitors for severe disease
Retinoblastoma	- Most common childhood ocular malignancy - Can be heritable (germline RB1 mutation) or sporadic - Presents with leukocoria, strabismus	Dx: Retinal exam, plus ocular US/MRI Tx: Laser or cryotherapy, +/− chemotherapy

Congenital Neurologic Disease

Disorder	Features
<u>Neural tube defects</u> Risk factors: **Folate deficiency**/antagonists, **neuroleptic drugs** (valproate, carbamazepine, phenytoin)	
Spina bifida occulta	- Failure of fusion of the vertebral bodies, without herniation of spinal cord - Ranges asymptomatic to neurologic dysfunction (including weakness and autonomic symptoms) - Can have skin abnormalities (dimple, tuft of hair) overlying lesion - Tx: Surgery if any neurologic dysfunction
Meningocele	- Meninges (but no neural tissue) herniate through bony defect. Rare. - Usually asymptomatic - Tx: Surgically repair, with good prognosis
Meningomyelocele	- Meninges and neural tissue herniate through bony defect - Almost always has **Chiari II malformation** - Associated with severe neurologic deficits (paralysis below the level of lesion, bladder dysfunction) - ↑ AFP on prenatal screening, confirmed with US - Tx: Surgically repair (emergently)
Anencephaly	- Malformation of anterior neural tube, resulting in abnormal forebrain, open calvarium - ↑ AFP on prenatal screening, confirmed with US - Not compatible with life
Holoprosencephaly	- Failure of separation of the left and right hemispheres - Often associated with other midline defects, such as cleft lip, midface cleft and cyclopia - Severe defects not compatible with life
Encephalocele	- Skull/dural defect, with herniation of meninges +/− brain - Tx: Surgical repair
Posterior Fossa Malformations	
Chiari I	- Ectopic, downwardly displaced cerebellar tonsils[A] through foramen magnum - Associated with syringomyelia - Manifests with headaches, cerebellar dysfunction (ataxia, especially with cough/valsalva) - Symptoms start in adolescence/adulthood
Chiari II	- Downward displacement of the cerebellar tonsils and vermis - Associated with myelomeningocele - Causes hydrocephalus and hind brain dysfunction (paralysis below the level of the lesion)
Dandy-Walker	- Agenesis of cerebellar vermis with cystic enlargement[B] of fourth ventricle - Associated with noncommunicating hydrocephalus, spina bifida

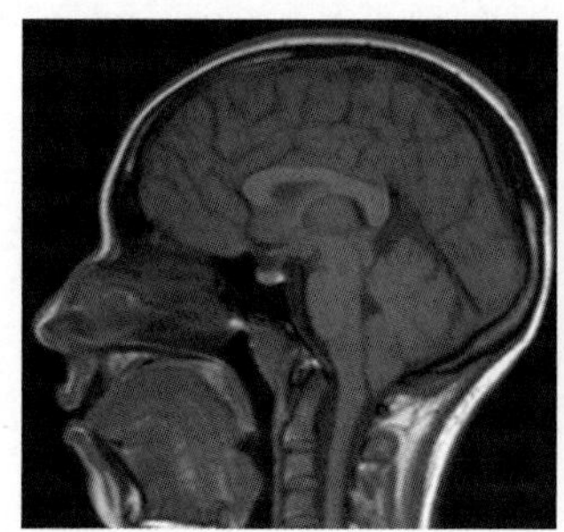
A

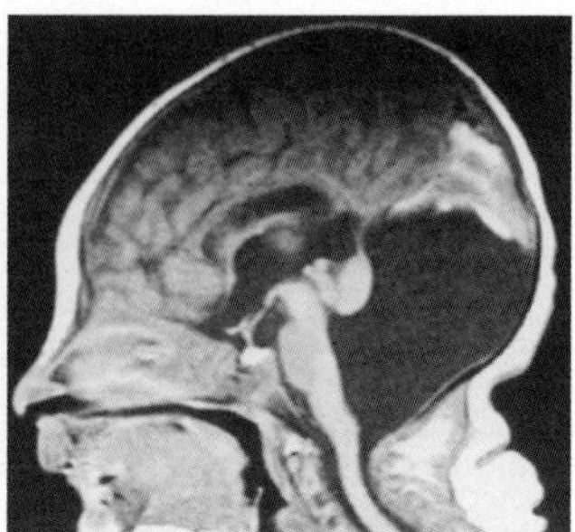
B

Congenital Neurologic Disease

	General	Clinical	Management
Neurofibromatosis (von Recklinghausen)	- AD NF1 mutation on chromosome 17	- Café-au-lait macules - Axillary freckling - Lisch nodules (iris hamartomas) - Neurofibromas - Other: Optic glioma, long bone dysplasia, pheochromocytoma	Dx: Clinical + genetic testing Tx: Careful medical supervision with treatment of complications
Neurofibromatosis 2	- AD NF2 mutation on chromosome 22 (Merlin tumor suppressor gene)	- Bilateral acoustic schwannomas - Tumors (meningiomas, spinal tumors) - Neuropathy, cataracts, skin lesions	
Tuberous Sclerosis	- AD TSC1/2 gene mutations, most often sporadic	- Derm: - Ash-leaf spots (hypopigmented patches) - Shagreen patches (thick orange peel skin) - Angiofibromas - CNS: - Glioneuronal hamartomas ("Tubers") - Subependymal nodules - Epilepsy, intellectual disability - CV: Cardiac rhabdomyoma - Renal: Angiomyolipoma	Dx: Clinical + genetic testing Tx: Antiepileptics, screening brain MRI
Sturge-Weber	- Sporadic mosaic mutations in GNAQ gene	- Port wine stain (facial capillary malformation) - Ipsilateral leptomeningeal cavernous angioma - Glaucoma, heterochromia of iris, vascular malformations in the eye - Epilepsy, intellectual disability	Dx: Clinical, plus MRI with contrast to determine extent of CNS disease Tx: Medically manage complications

Cerebral Palsy

General: Abnormal fetal CNS development, resulting in permanent motor dysfunction

Risk: Prematurity, low birth weight, multiple gestation, IUGR, intrauterine infection, perinatal hypoxic-ischemic injury

Clinical:

Subtype	Risk	Clinical Features
Spastic diplegia	- Preterm - PVL	- Lower extremities usually affected - Spasticity, UMN signs, muscle contractures
Spastic hemiplegia	- Neonate stroke - Congenital CNS maldevelopment	- Unilateral arm/leg involvement - Spasticity, UMN signs, muscle contractures
Spastic quadriplegia	- SGA/preterm - Variety of global brain abnormalities	- Entire body - Spasticity, UMN signs, muscle contractures
Dyskinesia (athetoid)	- Kernicterus - Hypoxic-ischemic	- Hypotonia, reduced purposeful movements - Development of involuntary movements - Choreiform, athetoid, and dystonic movements all possible
Ataxic	- Cerebellar hypoplasia	- Hypotonia, poor coordination, ataxia

Comorbidities: Intellectual disability, epilepsy, behavioral issues, visual/hearing defects, orthopedic (hip subluxation, scoliosis)

Diagnosis: Clinical (combination of symptoms, plus characteristic MRI findings)

Management:

- Physical/occupational/speech therapy
- Spasticity: Botulinum toxin, antispasmodics (baclofen), surgical (selective dorsal rhizotomy)
- Preventative: Magnesium (in moms at risk of premature birth)

Neuro Pharm

	Mechanism	Indication	Side Effects/Management
GABA Targeting Antiepileptics			
Barbiturates Phenobarbital Pentobarbital Thiopental	- GABA potentiator (↑ duration of action)	- Seizures (acute, status) - Anesthesia - Alcohol withdrawal	- Respiratory/CNS depression (especially with EtOH) - CYP 450 Induction
Benzodiazepine Diazepam Lorazepam Midazolam Chlordiazepoxide Alprazolam	- GABA potentiator (↑ frequency of opening)	- Seizures (acute, status) - Alcohol withdrawal - Anxiety - Spasticity - Insomnia	- Respiratory/CNS depression - Tolerance over time (limits usefulness chronically) - Dependence/withdrawal - Overdose can be reversed with **flumazenil**
Tiagabine	- ↑ GABA concentration and activity	- Narrow-spectrum antiepileptic	
Vigabatrin			- Vision loss
Ca^{2+} Channel Blocking Antiepileptics			
Ethosuximide	- Blocks T-type Ca^{2+} channels	- Absence seizure	- GI Upset - Drowsiness
Na^{+} Channel Blocking Antiepileptics			
Phenytoin Fosphenytoin	- Blocks Na^{+} channels	- Status epilepticus - Narrow-spectrum antiepileptic	- Gingival hypertrophy, ↑ body hair - SJS (HLA-B*1502, most commonly Asian) - Confusion, blurry vision, ataxia (long term) - ↓ Folate/megaloblastic anemia - Teratogen/fetal hydantoin syndrome - CYP450 induction - ↓ Vitamin D/osteopenia
Carbamazepine Eslicarbazepine Oxcarbazepine	- Blocks Na^{+} channels	- Narrow-spectrum antiepileptic	- Sedation - Hyponatremia/SIADH - Myelosuppression - SJS (HLA-B*1502, most commonly Asian) - CYP450 induction
Lacosamide	- Blocks Na^{+} channels	- Narrow-spectrum antiepileptic	- Well-tolerated
Lamotrigine	- Blocks Na^{+} channels	- Broad-spectrum antiepileptic	- SJS
Topiramate	- Blocks Na^{+} channels, ↑ GABA activity, blocks NMDA receptors	- Broad-spectrum antiepileptic - Headache prophylaxis	- Weight loss - Mental dulling, sedation - Inhibits carbonic anhydrase (metabolic acidosis, nephrolithiasis)
Valproate	- Blocks Na^{+} channels, ↑ GABA concentration	- Broad-spectrum antiepileptic - Mood stabilizer (Bipolar)	- Nausea/vomiting - Hepatotoxicity - Weight gain - Thrombocytopenia, tremor - Teratogen
Misc. Antiepileptic Drugs			
Gabapentin	- GABA analog, but acts mainly inhibiting Ca^{2+} channels	- Narrow-spectrum antiepileptic - Neuropathic pain - Used off label for EtOH use disorder, fibromyalgia, hot flashes	- Sedation - Dizziness, ataxia - Toxicity with renal failure
Levetiracetam	- Unclear mechanism	- Broad-spectrum antiepileptic	- Well-tolerated (possible somnolence)

Neuro Pharm

	Mechanism	Indication	Side Effects/Management
Parkinson Drugs			
Levodopa-carbidopa	- L-Dopa crosses BBB, converted to dopamine in CNS - Carbidopa inhibits peripheral breakdown of L-Dopa	- Parkinson disease	- Headache, nausea, sleepiness, dizziness - **Dopaminergic stimulation**: Confusion, psychosis, hallucinations, orthostatic hypotension - "**Wearing-Off Effect**": Motor fluctuations, dyskinesias that develop years after beginning levodopa
Pramipexole Raniperole	- Dopamine agonist	- Parkinson disease (early disease) - Restless leg syndrome	- Similar dopaminergic stimulation effects as levodopa
Entacapone Tolcapone	- COMT inhibitors (prevents peripheral L-Dopa breakdown)	- Parkinson disease (L-dopa adjunct only, no effect on own)	
Selegiline	- MAO-B inhibitors (prevents dopamine breakdown)	- Parkinson disease (only modest efficacy)	- Similar dopaminergic stimulation effects as levodopa - Rare risk for serotonin syndrome
Amantadine	- ↑ synaptic dopamine availability	- Parkinson disease (mainly used early in mild disease)	- Livedo reticularis - Lower extremity edema
Benztropine Trihexyphenidyl	- Anticholinergic agents	- Parkinson disease (mainly tremor)	- Anticholinergic side effects (confusion, dry mouth, urinary retention, blurry vision)
ALS Drugs			
Riluzole	- ↓ glutamate-induced excitotoxicity	- ALS	
Edaravone	- Free-radical scavenger	- ALS	
Huntington Drugs			
Tetrabenazine	- VMAT2 inhibitor (blocks dopamine packaging into vesicles)	- Huntington (for chorea)	- Akathisia, parkinsonism
Dementia Drugs			
Memantine	- NMDA antagonist	- Dementia	
Donepezil Galantamine Rivastigmine	- Acetylcholinesterase inhibitor		- Nausea, vomiting, diarrhea
Multiple Sclerosis Drugs (selected)			
Glatiramer	- Peptides similar to myelin basic protein	- Multiple sclerosis	- Local injection site reactions
Interferon beta	- Anti-inflammatory cytokine		- Flu-like symptoms
Dimethyl fumarate	- Unknown		- Flushing, GI symptoms
Fingolimod	- Sphingosine analogue that modulates the S1PR		- Macular edema - Bradycardia, heart block
Misc. Neurologic Agents			
Rizatriptan Sumatriptan	- 5-HT1B/1D agonist	- Migraine abortant	- Coronary vasospasm and myocardial ischemia - Paresthesias
Baclofen	- GABA-B agonist at spinal cord	- Muscle relaxant	- Drowsiness, dizziness - Withdrawal syndrome (similar to benzo/alcohol)
Zolpidem Zaleplon Eszopiclone	- Acts on BZ1 subtype GABA receptor	- Insomnia	- Headaches - ↓ cognitive functioning (possibly lasting into next day) - Tolerance/dependence over time (less risk compared to benzos)

Adult Preventative Care

	Male	Female
Screening (Note: The following are for average risk adults unless noted. For high-risk conditions, refer to specific sections for screening intervals)		
HTN	- Optimal screening not known, but typically performed every visit	
HLD	- 1x screen between 17 and 21 y/o - Lipid screens once > 35 y/o (> 25 for high risk)	- 1x screen between 17 and 21 y/o - Lipid screens once > 45 y/o (> 35 for high risk)
Diabetes	- Screen those with HTN, HLD, or 35-70 y/o and BMI > 25	
Osteoporosis	- DEXA screen in clinical signs of low bone density, fracture history, or fracture risk factors	- DEXA scan all > 65 y/o, < 65 with risk factors (i.e., elevated FRAX) - q5 years if T-score > −1
Colon Ca	- 45-75 y/o - Methodology and risk determines interval [See: GI]	
Prostate Ca	- PSA screening (> 50 y/o) is an individual decision (discuss pros/cons with patient)	
Lung Ca	- Annual low dose CT scan - Indications: 50-80 y/o, 20 pack-year history, and either current smoker or quit within last 15 years	
Breast Ca		- Mammography, starting at age 40-50 (societies vary on age), with q1-2 yr repeat testing
Cervical Ca		- 21-29 y/o: Pap smear (q3 yr) - > 30 y/o: Pap smear (q3 yr) OR Pap + HPV (q5 yr) - Stop at 65 y/o if adequate negative prior screening
STD	- Chlamydia/gonorrhea (all sexually active females < 25 y/o, and all male and females > 25 with risk factors) - HIV: One time between 13 and 75 y/o. Annual screening if high risk.	
Hep B	- Screening reserved for high risk individuals (risks include IV drug use, high risk sexual activity, MSM, inmates, history of liver disease, close contact of Hep B patient, individuals born in endemic areas)	
Hep C	- One time screen for those between 18 and 79 y/o	
Abd Aortic Aneurysm	- 1x between 65 and 75 y/o in smokers OR first-degree family history of AAA	
Other Preventative Care		
Aspirin (daily low dose)	- Highly controversial, but overall evidence lacking for use of aspirin for primary prevention of cardiovascular events given elevated bleeding risk - Should be considered in those with significantly elevated cardiovascular risk	

Adult Preventative Care

Vaccine	19–26 years	27–49 years	50–64 years	≥65 years
Influenza inactivated (IIV4) or **Influenza recombinant** (RIV4)	1 dose annually			
or	or			
Influenza live, attenuated (LAIV4)	1 dose annually			
Tetanus, diphtheria, pertussis (Tdap or Td)	1 dose Tdap each pregnancy; 1 dose Td/Tdap for wound management (see notes)			
	1 dose Tdap, then Td or Tdap booster every 10 years			
Measles, mumps, rubella (MMR)	1 or 2 doses depending on indication (if born in 1957 or later)			
Varicella (VAR)	2 doses (if born in 1980 or later)	2 doses		
Zoster recombinant (RZV)	2 doses for immunocompromising conditions (see notes)		2 doses	
Human papillomavirus (HPV)	2 or 3 doses depending on age at initial vaccination or condition	27 through 45 years		
Pneumococcal (PCV15, PCV20, PPSV23)	1 dose PCV15 followed by PPSV23 OR 1 dose PCV20 (see notes)			1 dose PCV15 followed by PPSV23 OR 1 dose PCV20
Hepatitis A (HepA)	2 or 3 doses depending on vaccine			
Hepatitis B (HepB)	2, 3, or 4 doses depending on vaccine or condition			
Meningococcal A, C, W, Y (MenACWY)	1 or 2 doses depending on indication, see notes for booster recommendations			
Meningococcal B (MenB)	2 or 3 doses depending on vaccine and indication, see notes for booster recommendations			
	19 through 23 years			
***Haemophilus influenzae* type b** (Hib)	1 or 3 doses depending on indication			

Recommended vaccination for adults who meet age requirement, lack documentation of vaccination, or lack evidence of past infection; Recommended vaccination for adults with an additional risk factor or another indication; Recommended vaccination based on shared clinical decision-making; No recommendation/Not applicable

Vaccine	General Indications	Special Considerations
Influenza	- All patients, yearly	
Tdap/Td	- Booster q10 years (at least 1x should be Tdap)	
Varicella	- All (without documented evidence of immunity)	- Contraindicated if pregnant or immunodeficiency
Zoster	- All > 50 y/o - Note: Historically, only live vax (ZVL) was available, but now new recombinant vax (RZV) is preferred	- ZVL (contraindicated for pregnant women and adults with severe immunodeficiency)
HPV	- Recommended all < 26 y/o	- Approved up until 45 y/o
PCV15 **PCV20** **PPSV23**	<u>≥ 65 y/o</u>: PCV20 OR PCV15 1x followed by PPSV23 (1 year after PCV 15) <u>19-64 y/o</u>: - Vaccinate (as above) those at risk for for pneumococcal infection (immunocompromised, smoking, COPD, asplenia, chronic heart disease, CKD, etc.)	
MenACWY	- 11-18 y/o	- Used outside age range for those at increased risk, including: travel to endemic area, military, microbiologist working with meningococcus, asplenia, complement deficiency, eculizumab use, or recent epidemic in area of living
Men-B	- 16-23 y/o	
Hep A	Patients that want protection (personal preference)	- High risk individuals (travel to endemic area, MSM, IV drug use, chronic liver disease, etc.)
Hep B	All adults 19-59 y/o, and those at high risk > 59 y/o	- High risk individuals (travel to endemic area, MSM, IV drug use, chronic liver disease, etc.)

<u>True contraindications</u>: Previous anaphylactic reaction, anaphylaxis to egg (for egg prepared live vaccines, like MMR, yellow fever), immunocompromised/ pregnant (no live vaccine), household of immunocompromised (no oral polio)
<u>False contraindications</u>: Mild illness, convalescent phase of an illness, recent exposure to communicable disease, breastfeeding, current antibiotic use

Smoking/Obesity

Smoking

General: Smoking is the leading preventable cause of mortality. Increases risk for:
- Cardiovascular disease (#1 reversible risk factor)
    - Atherosclerosis (CAD, stroke)
- COPD
- Malignancy (lung, esophageal, pancreatic, genitourinary)
- Peptic ulcer disease
- Osteoporosis

Clinical: Withdrawal can cause increased appetite/weight gain, irritability, anxiety, or depression

Smoking Cessation: Behavioral intervention + pharm is first line

Drug	Mechanism	Side Effects/Contraindications
Varenicline	- Partial agonist of $\alpha4\beta2$ (of nicotinic Ach receptor)	- Nausea - Sleep disturbance (insomnia, atypical dreams) *No issue with increased suicidality
Nicotine replacement	- Long acting patch + short-acting gum/lozenge/inhaler	- Irritation at site of drug - Headache, nausea possible
Bupropion	- ↑ NE and D release	- Increases seizure risk - Headache, dry mouth, insomnia

Hospitalized patients: Nicotine replacement (usually patch + short-term breakthrough)

Obesity

Increases Risk For: Type II DM, metabolic syndrome, CAD, HTN, HLD, OSA

Evaluation: BMI should be calculated at each visit
- Waist circumference: ≥ 40" in men and ≥ 35" in women → ↑ Cardiometabolic risk
- Should screen for obesity related comorbid conditions

Class	BMI Range
Underweight	< 18.5 kg/m²
Normal weight	≥ 18.5 to 24.9 kg/m²
Overweight	≥ 25.0 to 29.9 kg/m²
Obese	≥ 30 kg/m²
Severely obese	≥ 40 kg/m²

Management:
- Behavior modification and counseling (first line): Diet (most important) and exercise
- Pharmacotherapy (if BMI > 30 and failed behavior modification)
- Bariatric surgery: Indicated if BMI > 40 or > 35 + comorbidity

Drug	Mechanism	Side Effects
Orlistat	- Inhibits fat absorption through lipase inhibition	- GI (flatulence, cramps, steatorrhea)
Liraglutide Semaglutide	- GLP-1 analog, often used in diabetics	- Nausea, vomiting - ↑ risk pancreatitis
Lorcaserin	- Serotonin 2C-R agonist	
Phentermine-Topiramate	- Stimulant (↑ NE)	- Dry mouth, constipation - Avoid in those with cardiovascular disease
Bupropion-Naltrexone	- ↑ NE/D (unclear how naltrexone modulates)	- Avoid in those with cardiovascular disease

Geriatrics

Normal Aging

System	Normal Findings
CNS	- Minor forgetfulness, word finding difficulty, and memory loss - Functional loss not normal - Decreased brain weight, enlarged ventricles/sulci - Impaired vision (presbyopia) and hearing
Pulmonary	- ↓ Alveolar surface area (increased dead space) - Decreased lung compliance
Renal	- ↓ Creatinine clearance
GI	- ↑ Reflux - Constipation
Endocrine	- Erectile dysfunction and dyspareunia
Heme	- ↓ Bone marrow reserves (increased risk for cytopenias) - ↑ Risk for clotting
MSK	- Decreased muscle, increased fat - Increased fracture risk
Sleep	- ↓ REM latency and total REM - Decreased total sleep - Advanced sleep cycle - Increased frequency of nocturnal awakenings

Vitamins/Minerals

Fat-Soluble Vitamins

	Overdose	Deficiency
A	- Caused by excessive supplements or dietary source (liver of wild animals, like bear) - Acute: Nausea/vomiting, vertigo, blurry vision - Chronic: Alopecia, dry skin, hepatotoxicity, arthralgias, pseudotumor - Severe teratogen	- Xerophthalmia (dry conjunctiva, keratomalacia, Bitot spots [areas of corneal keratinization]) - Night blindness (nyctalopia) - Abnormal bone development - Hyperkeratosis
D	- Due to inappropriate use of vitamin D supplement - Symptoms are that of hypercalcemia (confusion, polyuria, polydipsia, nausea, vomiting, weakness)	- Rickets (children) - Osteomalacia (adults)
E	- Possible increased bleeding risk	- Hemolytic anemia - Acanthocytosis - Neuromuscular (spinocerebellar tract demyelination, manifesting as ataxia, weakness)
K	- Not known	- Increased bleeding risk (presents as easy bruising, mucosal bleeding, melena, hematuria)

Water Soluble Vitamins

Vitamin	Deficiency Syndrome
B1 (Thiamine)	***Risk:*** Alcohol use disorder, eating disorders, bariatric surgery ***Clinical:*** - **Beriberi**: Rare. Wet (high output heart failure). Dry (peripheral neuropathy). - **Wernicke-Korsakoff** - Wernicke: Triad of confusion, ophthalmoplegia, and ataxia - Korsakoff: Irreversible memory loss
B2 (Riboflavin)	***Risk:*** Rare ***Clinical:*** Stomatitis, glossitis, cheilosis, corneal vascularization
B3 (Niacin)	***Risk:*** Developing countries (corn dependent), carcinoid tumors, isoniazid toxicity, Hartnup syndrome ***Clinical:*** **Pellagra** - Dermatitis (blistering rash in sun-exposed skin)[A] - Diarrhea - Dementia (altered mental status, depression, poor concentration)
B6 (Pyridoxine)	***Risk:*** Isoniazid (inactivates B6) ***Clinical:*** Stomatitis, glossitis, cheilosis, CNS (confusion, depression), **peripheral neuropathy**, anemia Note: Can cause toxicity with massive intake (neuropathy)
B7 (Biotin)	***Risk:*** Rare. Occurs with large consumption of raw egg whites. ***Clinical:*** Dermatitis, alopecia, conjunctivitis, altered mental status
B9 (Folate) B12	[See: Heme/Onc]
C	- **Scurvy**: Hemorrhages/hemarthrosis/skin petechiae (bone and gums) - Gingivitis, poor wound healing, periosteal hemorrhage, corkscrew hairs

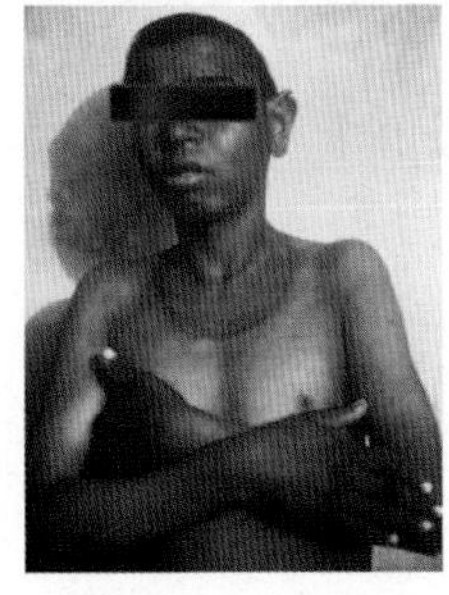

Vitamins/Minerals

Minerals	
Mineral	**Deficiency**
Chromium	- Decreased sensitivity to insulin (diabetic patients)
Copper	- Brittle hair - Skin depigmentation - Osteoporosis - Sideroblastic anemia - Peripheral neuropathy
Selenium	- Cardiomyopathy - Muscle dysfunction
Zinc	- Impaired growth (children) - Alopecia - Impaired wound healing - Rash (pustules in perioral/perianal region) - Dysgeusia, anosmia - Hypogonadism *Can be caused by acrodermatitis enteropathica (AR genetic disorder, causing ↓ zinc GI absorption)

Malnutrition	
Marasmus	- Complete energy (protein + nonprotein) deficient state - Very thin, from loss of protein/body fat
Kwashiorkor	- Pure protein-deficient state (seen in parts of world where people live off starches) - Generalized edema, abdominal distension[A], skin hypo/hyperpigmentation, and thin/sparse hair

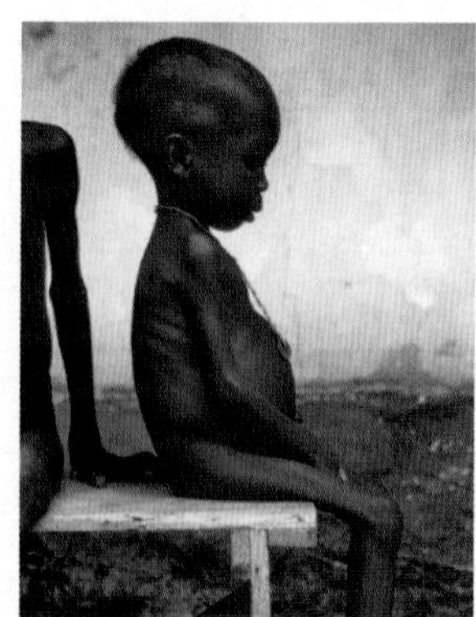

Toxicology

	General	Clinical	Management
Carbon Monoxide	- Binds hemoglobin, left-shifting oxyhemoglobin curve - Risk: Smoke, fuel-burning devices with poor ventilation, poorly functioning furnace	- Mild: Headache, nausea, dizziness, malaise - Severe: Altered mental status, seizure, coma, cardiac ischemia Dx: ABG with co-oximetry (> 15% carboxyhgb)	- 100% O_2 - Mechanical ventilation/ hyperbaric O_2 if severe
Methemoglob-inemia	- Exposure to oxidizing substance (turns Fe^{2+} to Fe^{3+}), which has poor affinity for O_2 - Risk: Dapsone, topical anesthetics, NO, other sulfa/nitrite drugs	- **Cyanosis**, dark blood - Nonspecific symptoms (HA, dyspnea, fatigue) Dx: ABG with co-oximetry (>10% methgb)	- IV methylene blue
Cyanide	- Inhibits electron transport chain Risk: - Fires - Industrial exposure - Iatrogenic (e.g., nitroprusside)	- Flushing ("cherry red") - CV: Arrhythmia, bradycardia/hypotension - Pulm: Respiratory depression - CNS: Confusion, coma, seizure - Lactic acidosis *Bright red blood/lacks cyanosis (high oxyhemoglobin concentration)	- Supportive care - Decontamination (depending on type of exposure) - Hydroxocobalamin + sodium thiosulfate - Nitrites are alternative
Organophosphates	- Cholinesterase inhibitors → Excessive cholinergic activity - Risk: Insecticides, "nerve gas" (i.e. Sarin). Exposure can be cutaneous, ingestion, inhalation.	**DUMBELS** – Defecation, urination, miosis, bronchorrhea/bronchospasm/bradycardia, emesis, lacrimation, salivation	- Atropine, pralidoxime - Intubation, 100% O_2 *Avoid succinylcholine
Arsenic	- Binds to sulfhydryl groups, affecting cellular respiration - Risk: Pesticides, pressure-treated wood, contaminated well water	- Acute: GI (watery diarrhea, vomiting, pain), **garlic breath**, QT prolongation - Chronic: Hypo/hyperpigmentation of skin, hyperkeratosis, sensory/motor neuropathy, ↑ cancer risk (skin/bladder)	- Supportive - Decontamination - Dimercaprol chelation
Iron	- Damages via free radicals and lipid peroxidation - Risk: Ingestion of iron supplements	- GI: Pain, **hematemesis/melena** - Hypotensive shock/metabolic acidosis - Radiopaque pills on XR - After initial episode: GI obstruction, hepatic toxicity	- IV deferoxamine - Gastric lavage/bowel irrigation (if pills on xray)
Salicylate	- COX inhibitor, increases respiratory drive, interferes with metabolism - Risk: ASA overdose	- Tinnitus, vomiting, dizziness, altered mental status - **Mixed respiratory alkalosis/metabolic acidosis**	- Sodium bicarbonate - Supportive care
Ricin	- Ribosome inhibitor - Found in castor beans, potential agent of terror	- Inhalation → Respiratory distress/pulm edema - Ingestion → GI bleeding/inflammation	- Supportive care - Decontamination (skin, or GI via charcoal/lavage)
Seafood Toxins			
Tetrodotoxin	- Pufferfish - Binds Na channels	- Nausea, diarrhea, paraesthesia, paralysis	- Supportive
Ciguatoxin	- Reef fish (barracuda, snapper) - Opens Na channels	- Cholinergic poisoning symptoms (nausea, vomiting, abdominal pain, paresthesias)	- Supportive
Histamine (scombroid)	- Dark meat fish (tuna, mahi-mahi) - Bacterial histidine decarboxylase forms histamine	- Anaphylaxis-like symptoms - Burning, flushing, erythema, diarrhea	- Diphenhydramine - Epi/Albuterol for anaphylactoid symptoms

Toxicology

Acetaminophen Overdose

General: Metabolized to NAPQI by CYP system, forms toxic-free radicals, damaging DNA, proteins, and lipid membranes

Risk: Overdose usually > 150 mg/kg for kids or > 7.5 g in adults

Clinical: Acute hepatic failure (AST and ALT > 1,000, ↑ INR/PT)
- Hypovolemia, jaundice, renal failure all possible

Diagnosis: **Serum acetaminophen concentration**

Management:
- If within 4 hours: Activated charcoal
- **N-acetylcysteine** (either IV or oral protocols available). Indicated if:
  - Acetaminophen level > 10 ug/mL at any point in time
  - Above line on Rumack-Matthew Nomogram
  - Evidence of liver injury
  - High-risk liver condition

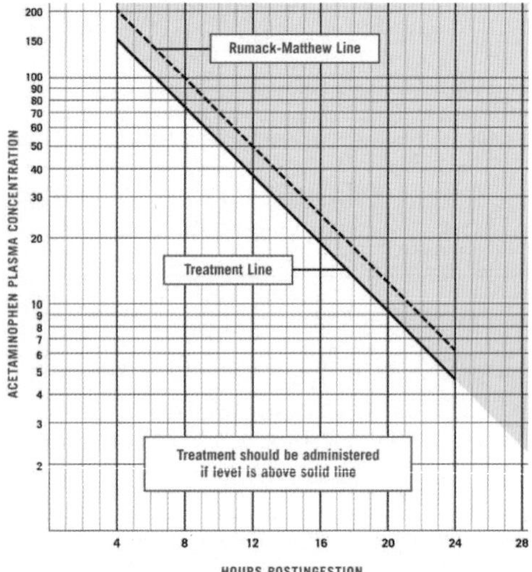

Alcohol Toxicity

Type	Source	Clinical	Management
Ethanol	- EtOH beverages	- CNS depression/inebriation	- Supportive
Isopropyl	- Rubbing alcohol - Antifreeze - Solvent	- CNS depression - Ketonemia (acetone) with normal AG	- Supportive
Methanol	- Moonshine - Solvents	- Metabolized to formic acid - CNS depression - **Visual changes** (scotoma, blurry vision) dueto retinal toxicity - AG metabolic acidosis	- Fomepizole - Sodium bicarb - Hemodialysis (if end organ damage, high alcohol levels)
Ethylene Glycol	- Antifreeze	- Renal: AKI, **oxalate nephrolithiasis** - CNS depression - AG metabolic acidosis	

*Note: All the above present with elevated osmolar gap, but only methanol and ethylene glycol cause significant elevation in the anion gap.

Ingestions

Caustic Esophageal Injury

General: Ingestion of alkali or acidic material, causing mucosal damage
- **Alkali** (e.g., ammonia, NaOH): Liquefactive necrosis, more damage to esophagus, buffered by stomach
- **Acid**: Coagulation necrosis. Causing pain immediately in oropharynx, often limiting ingestion. Causes more gastric damage.

Clinical: Can cause oropharyngeal, chest, or abdominal pain. Dysphagia, odynophagia, vomiting.

Diagnosis: Upper GI endoscopy within 24 hours to determine extent of injury
- Contraindicated if signs of hemodynamic instability/surgical complication

Management:
- Supportive care
- Contraindicated: Emetics, NG tubes, neutralizing agents, NG lavage/charcoal
- Surgery if complicated by peritonitis, mediastinitis, etc.

Complications: Strictures, perforation, ↑ cancer risk

Foreign Body Ingestion

General: Objects most commonly become stuck in esophagus/stomach. Often asymptomatic, unless complete obstruction (causes dysphagia, impaired swallowing of secretions, etc.).

Object	Features	Management
Coins[A]	- Most often in stomach and pass without problem	- Most pass spontaneously - Remove if in esophagus > 24 h
Flat Battery	- Can conduct electricity across esophagus, causing necrosis	- Urgent removal (if in esophagus)
Sharps/Bones	- High perforation risk	- Urgent removal
Magnets	- Multiple magnets can attract across bowel layers, causing necrosis, obstruction	- Urgent removal (if multiple)
Food Impaction	- Often in adults with esophageal strictures	- Emergent removal if complete obstruction (otherwise within 24 h)

Diagnosis: Multiple view plain XR

Management: Flexible endoscope is preferred method for removal. In general, if not a high risk object, can observe for 24 hours for spontaneous passage into lower GI tract, then follow with serial radiographs
- Note: Any signs of obstruction or complications is indication for removal
- If any object is stuck in esophagus for > 24 hours, removal is indicated
- Once object passes beyond proximal duodenum, follow with serial radiographs and monitor for any complications

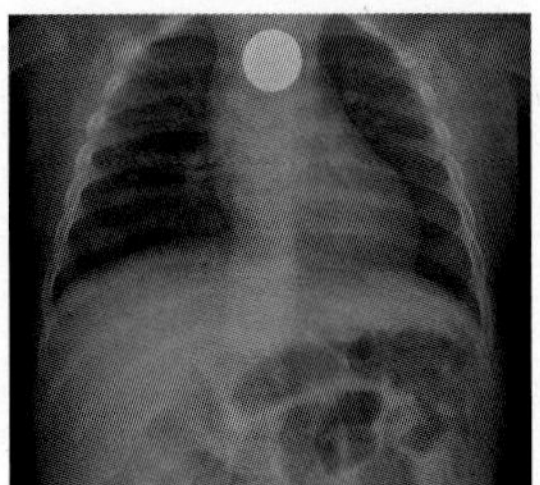

Environmental Injury

Heat Injury

General: Group of disorders caused by the failure of thermoregulation, most commonly in extreme heat/humidity

Risk: Exercise during hot/humid weather, dehydration, poor physical fitness

Disorder	Features	Management
Heat Cramp	- Exercise-induced muscle cramps	- Cool, rehydrate
Heat Syncope	- Syncope associated with physical activity in high temperature areas	- Cool, rehydrate
Heat Exhaustion	- Inadequate cardiac output secondary to heat, which results in inability to continue exercising - Temperature usually > 101°F - No neurologic dysfunction or end organ damage	- Remove from play, remove excess clothing - Cool patient (cold water or evaporative therapy) - Rehydration
Heat Injury	- Temp > 104°F with end-organ damage (but no CNS dysfunction) - Often complicated by DIC, ARDS, organ failure	- Remove from play, remove excess clothing - Cool patient (cold water or evaporative therapy) - Rehydration - Hospital level supportive care
Exertional Heat Stroke	- Temp > 104°F, CNS dysfunction, and end-organ damage	- Rapid cooling (ice-water immersion) - Fluid and electrolyte repletion - Supportive care for organ dysfunction
Non-exertional Heat Stroke	- Temp >> 104°F, CNS dysfunction, and end-organ damage - Seen in elderly, with chronic medical conditions that can impair thermoregulation	- Supportive (ABC's, intubation if necessary) - Rapid cooling (evaporative)

Hypothermia

General: Core temperature < 35°C

Risk: Outdoor extreme cold, water submersion, EtOH abuse, sepsis, hypothyroidism

Class	Temp (C)	Clinical Findings
Mild	32-35°	- Shivering, tachycardia, tachypnea, ataxia, dysarthria
Moderate	28-32°	- CNS depression, bradycardia, hypoventilation, loss of shivering reflex
Severe	< 28°	- Hemodynamic instability, CNS depression (coma), ventricular arrhythmias/asystole

Management:

Class	Management
Mild	- Supportive care (ABC's, intubate if necessary) - Warmed IV crystalloid - Remove wet clothing, passive external warming (e.g., blankets)
Moderate	- Above, plus: Active external warming (warm blankets, heating pads)
Severe	- Above, plus: Active internal warming if refractory to above options (warmed pleural/peritoneal fluids)

Environmental Injury

Frostbite

General: Freezing and subsequent necrosis of tissue. Frequently occurs in distal extremities, ears, nose, and other parts of the face. Other types of cold injury include:

- **Frostnip**: Completely reversible paresthesias due to cold exposure. Pale/red skin. Resolves with rewarming.
- **Pernio** (chilblains): Painful, erythematous lesions from repetitive damp cold exposure. Resolves over weeks.
- **Trench foot**: Due to consistent exposure of feet to wet/cold. Results erythematous, painful, edematous foot.

Risk: Cold wind exposure, or conductive loss through cold water/metal

Clinical:

- Coldness, paresthesias
- Superficial pallor with hard/waxy texture
- Eventual development of bullae[A], eschar formation. May lead to amputation if severe.

Diagnosis: Clinical. Bone scan (Tc-99) can help determine extent of injury/prognosis.

Management:

- External rewarming (warm water), analgesia, wound care
- tPA/Heparin if at risk for amputation (due to clotting in affected tissues)

Drowning

General: Aspiration of water, causing pulmonary edema/laryngospasm, pulmonary edema, with eventual hypoxemia

Management:

- Immediate: Rescue breaths, followed by CPR (if breaths fail)
- Airway: Often requires supplemental O_2/intubation
- Supportive care (manage hypothermia, end organ damage, etc.)

Electrical Injuries

General: Electrical current through tissues, causing various degrees of thermal injury

Etiology:

- Electrical (work related in adults, accidental in children)
- Lightning (DC current. Extremely high voltage. Severe, frequently fatal.)
- Stun guns/tasers (may cause minor superficial injury, but severe organ injury is rare)
    - No medical care necessary if < 15 seconds of stun gun discharge

Clinical: If severe, findings include

- Burns: Severity of internal burns may not be apparent on the skin
- Cardiac: Arrhythmias, asystole [DC] and ventricular fibrillation [AC]
- CNS: Altered mental status, neuropathy, autonomic failure, etc.
- Renal: Rhabdomyolysis
- MSK: Bone necrosis, dislocations, compartment syndrome

Management:

- Supportive care
- Burn management

Bites/Stings

Bug/Sting Bites

Type	Features	Management
Spider		
Black Widow	- Muscle pains/spasms - Localized diaphoresis - Abdominal pain, autonomic hyperactivity	- Wound care, tetanus, analgesia - Benzodiazepines - Antivenom if severe
Brown Recluse	- Bite site develops erythema, with possible necrosis/ulceration over next few days	- Wound care, tetanus, analgesia - Debridement if severe
Snake		
Coral	- "Red on yellow, kill a fellow" - Neurotoxin causes muscle weakness (anticholinergic) - Possible respiratory failure	- Antivenom - Atropine + neostigmine - Intubation (if necessary)
Crotalinae	- Rattlesnake, copperhead, or water moccasin - Causes local tissue damage - Can be complicated by rhabdo, coagulopathy	- Antivenom
Other		
Scorpion	- Pain, swelling at sting site - Certain species cause autonomic/neuromuscular toxicity	- Wound care, tetanus, analgesia - Antivenom for neurologic

Mammal Bites

Type	Organism
Human	- Organisms: *Staph, Strep, Eikenella*, anaerobes (*Fusobacterium,Peptostreptococcus*). Usually polymicrobial.
Cat/Dog	- *Pasteurella, Staph, Strep*, anaerobes

Diagnosis: Wound culture only if appears infected

Management: Wound care, irrigation, debridement if necessary
- Closure
  - Primary intention: If not infected, < 12 hours, not on hands/feet
  - Secondary intention: All others
- Antibiotics (amoxicillin-clavulanate, etc.)
  - Indicated if infected
  - Prophylactic: If high risk, especially cat bites
- Tetanus vaccination, rabies prophylaxis if indicated (see below)

Rabies Prophylaxis

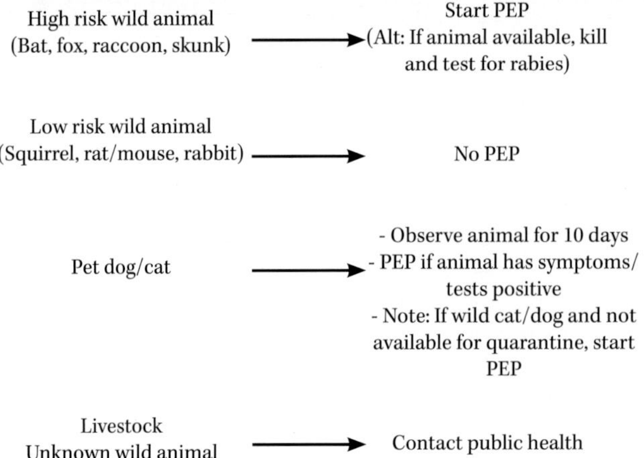

Psychiatry Basics

Mental Status Exam

General: Mental status examination is the core "physical exam" in psychiatry, with the components below

Component	Examples
Appearance	- Well-groomed, poorly-groomed. Can also note physical build, appeared age, etc.
Behavior	- Eye contact, attitude (level of cooperativity)
Speech	- Rate, rhythm, articulation
Mood	- Mood based on the patient's words (e.g., "happy")
Affect	- Observer's assessment of the patient's mood. Common descriptions include euphoric, dysphoric, neutral. - Range of emotions described flat, blunted, constricted, or full
Thought process	- Description of the patient's pattern of thoughts - Common descriptors include logical/linear, circumstantial, tangential, flight of ideas
Thought Content	- Types of thoughts the patient is having
Hallucinations	- Sensory perceptions that occur without actual stimulus - Illusions: Abnormal perception of actual stimulus
Suicidal/Homicidal Ideation	- Assessment of patients risk toward self and others - Always assess for actual plan
Cognition	- Assessment of patient's orientation, memory, concentration, consciousness, etc.
Insight	- Patient's awareness of their own problem
Judgment	- Patient's ability to approach their problems in an appropriate manner

Defense Mechanisms

Type	Features	Example
Immature		
Acting out	- Avoiding emotions by bad behavior	- Temper tantrums
Denial	- Refusing to accept unpleasant reality	- Reject new diagnosis from doctor
Projection	- Attributing feelings/emotions to another person	- Cheater accuses classmate of cheating
Regression	- Reverting to behavior of child	- Hospitalized child wets bed
Psychotic		
Displacement	- Transferring unwanted feelings to another person or object	- Mother yells at her child, because her husband yelled at her
Isolation of affect	- Separation of emotion from stressful life event	- Description of death without any emotion
Intellectualization	- Avoiding emotions through reasoning	- Focus on statistics after life-threatening diagnosis
Rationalization	- Distorting events so outcome is positive	- "Needed a change" after being fired
Reaction formation	- Actions in opposition of feelings	- Mother who despises child shows extreme love
Repression	- Withholding of memory or fact from consciousness (unconscious)	- Person does not remember episode of sexual abuse
Splitting	- Categorizing as extremes (all good or all bad)	- Person says that all the nurses here are great but all doctors are bad
Undoing	- Action or words designed to cancel some disapproved thoughts, impulses, or acts	- Think about physically hurting someone, but act nicely instead
Mature		
Altruism	- Alleviating negative feelings through charity	- Cancer survivors run charity
Humor	- Relief of anxiety with jokes or laughter	- Joking about poor test performance
Sublimation	- Transferring unwanted feelings into more appropriate activity	- Aggressive man becomes boxer
Suppression	- Intentionally withholding an idea or feeling from conscious	

Psychotic/Delusional Disorder

Disorder	Overview	DSM-5 and Clinical Features	Management
Schizophrenia	Pathophysiology: - Excess dopamine - Hypofunction of NMDA-R - MRI: Enlarged ventricles Risk factors: - Presents between 18 and 35 y/o (men earlier, poorer prognosis) - Family history - Living in urban area - **High suicide risk**	* ≥ 2 of the following, with at least 1 being #1-3 (1) **Delusions** (2) **Hallucinations** (3) **Disorganized speech** (4) Disorganized or catatonic behavior (5) Negative symptoms (flat affect, apathy, anhedonia) **Brief Psychotic** (< 1 month) - Rare. Associated with borderline personality - Triggered by extreme stressor **Schizophreniform** (1-6 months) **Schizophrenia** (> 6 months)	Antipsychotics: - Typical and atypical have equal efficacy, but atypical preferred due to side effect profile - Clozapine if refractory Psychotherapy: - Family therapy (want decreased home stress) - Behavioral/group therapy
Schizoaffective		- Meet criteria for major depressive or manic episode with concurrent psychotic symptoms - **Psychotic symptoms for ≥ 2 weeks** in the absence of mood symptoms	- Antipsychotics (atypical) - Treat mood disorder (SSRI for depression, mood stabilizer if manic)
Psychotic Disorder Due to Medical Condition	- Etiologies include dementia, Parkinson, CVA, encephalitis, and other neurologic/ endocrine abnormalities	- Hallucinations or delusions - Evidence of a nonpsychiatric cause	- Treat underlying
Substance-Induced Psychotic Disorder	- Corticosteroids, antiepileptic, anticholinergics, others - Drug use or withdrawal	- Hallucinations or delusions - Evidence of medication or substance - Not better explained by psychotic disorder	- Withdraw substance

Clinical Features of Psychosis

Positive Symptoms:
- Hallucinations, delusions, bizarre behavior, disorganized speech
- Ideas of reference (draw conclusions from every day sensory experiences)
- Respond to antipsychotics

Negative Symptoms:
- Flat or blunted affect, anhedonia, apathy, alogia (poverty of speech), and lack of interest in socialization
- Resistant to antipsychotics

Cognitive Symptoms:
- Impairments in attention, executive function, and working memory
- Neologisms (newly coined words that only have meaning to patient)
- Eye tracking defects

Phases:
- Prodromal: Decline in functioning that precedes the first psychotic episode
    - Often becomes socially withdrawn with atypical behavior
- Psychotic: Hallucinations, delusions, and disordered thoughts

Delusional Disorder

General: Presence of delusion without functional impact or other psychotic features. Often have poor insight into condition.

Subtypes of Delusions:
- **Persecutory**: Delusion of being persecuted
- **Grandiose**: Delusions of having great talent
- **Erotomanic**: Belief that other person is in love with the patient
- **Somatic**: Delusion of physical abnormality
- **Folie a deux** (Shared delusion disorder)
    - Two people share delusion (started by one, imposed on the other). Should interview separately.

DSM-5: **≥ 1 delusion for at least 1 month**
- Functionality is NOT significantly impaired, delusions not obviously bizarre
- Psychotic symptoms (i.e., hallucinations, disorganized thought) not present

Management: Establish patient rapport (patients often reject that they have condition). Antipsychotic therapy and/or CBT.

Mood Disorders

Manic Episode

DSM-5: At least three of the following **[DIG FAST]**

1. Distractibility
2. Irresponsibility (excessive involvement in activities that have potential for painful consequences)
3. Grandiosity
4. Flight of ideas
5. Agitation
6. Sleep (decreased need)
7. Talking (pressured speech)

Mania	Hypomania
≥ 7 days - **Severe** functional impairment - Possible psychotic features	**≥ 4 days** - **No marked** functional impairment - No psychotic features

Bipolar Disorder

Condition	DSM-5 Definition
Bipolar I	- Mania (at least one episode) +/– hypomania or depressive episodes
Bipolar II	- Hypomania + ≥ 1 major depressive episodes
Cyclothymic	≥ 2 years with periods of hypomania and depressive symptoms - No episodes qualify as mania or major depressive episodes

Management:

Situation	Intervention
Acute Mania	- Mild: Antipsychotic (atypical) - Severe: **Mood stabilizer (Lithium, Valproate) PLUS antipsychotic** - Refractory: Change drugs. ECT if failure to respond to > 4-5 different meds.
Acute Bipolar Depression	- Mood stabilizer (quetiapine, lurasidone, lamotrigine, lithium, valproate, or olanzapine + fluoxetine)
Chronic Bipolar	- Mood stabilizer (lithium first line, with alternatives: Valproate, quetiapine, or lamotrigine) - Refractory: Lithium or valproate PLUS antipsychotic - Patients typically require lifelong treatment
Pregnancy	- Acute mania: Typical antipsychotics. ECT also safe option. - Prenatal maintenance: Lamotrigine, atypical antipsychotics

Mood Disorders

Major Depressive Episode

***DSM-5:* 5 of the following for at least a two week period (SIG E CAPS)**

1. Depressed mood
2. Anhedonia (loss of interest in pleasurable activities)
3. Change in appetite or weight
4. Feelings of worthlessness or guilt
5. Inability to concentrate
6. Fatigue or loss of energy
7. Psychomotor agitation or retardation
8. Sleep disturbances (insomnia or hypersomnia)
9. Recurrent thoughts of death or suicide

Major Depressive Disorder

Pathophysiologic Changes:

- Decreased CSF 5-HIAA, ↑ cortisol, ↑ Total REM sleep, ↓ REM latency
- Multifactorial genetic inheritance

Condition	DSM-5 Criteria
Major depressive disorder	- **≥ 1 major depressive episode** - No mania
Persistent depressive disorder (dysthymia)	- **Depressed mood for at least 2 years** - ≥ 2 of the following (1) Hopelessness (2) Decreased appetite (3) Sleep problems (4) Low energy (5) Low concentration (6) Low self-esteem

Specifiers:

Atypical	- **Mood reactivity**, increased eating and sleeping, leaden paralysis - Hypersensitivity to interpersonal rejection
Melancholic	- Anhedonia, dysphoric affect, loss of sleep/appetite
Catatonic	- See catatonia
Psychotic	- Major depressive episodes contain hallucinations and delusions (that are not present outside the episode) - Themes tend to be consistent with mood
Anxious	- High levels of anxiety
Seasonal	- Symptoms start during one season, remit during another

Management of Depression

Inpatient Hospitalization: If high potential for self-harm/suicide

Psychotherapy: Cognitive-behavioral therapy or interpersonal psychotherapy

Pharmacotherapy: Ideal treatment is combination **psychotherapy plus pharmacotherapy**

- **SSRI** (first line)
- SNRI, atypical agents generally second line. MAOi, TCA are alternatives, but rarely used.
- Atypical antipsychotics: Adjunctive agent/treat psychotic features

Management of antidepressants:

- Must give around **4-6 weeks** to assess for efficacy of drug
- If patient still symptomatic, either increase dose or try different drug
- Phases:
  - Acute: Remission is induced (minimum 1.5-2 months in duration)
  - Continuation phase: Remission is preserved and relapse prevented (usually 5-10 months)
  - Maintenance phase: Susceptible patients are protected against relapse (many require indefinite therapy)

- Refractory (patient that fails at least two drug monotherapy trials)
  - Augment with atypical antipsychotic, lithium, or thyroid hormone
  - Electroconvulsive therapy (for severe, refractory cases)

Mood Disorders

Electroconvulsive Therapy

Procedure:

- Anesthesia given, then generalized seizure is induced via electricity across the brain
- Repeated ~6-10 times over a few weeks

Side Effects:

- **Retrograde and anterograde amnesia** (usually resolve within 6 months)
- Note: Benzodiazepines avoided (increase seizure threshold), lithium dose lowered

Indications:

- Severe, refractory depression, catatonia, or mania
- Emergent correction required (won't eat, imminent suicide risk)

Contraindications:

- No absolute contraindication
- Increased risk in those with: Recent MI or CV risk, recent stroke/aneurysm, or space occupying brain mass

Suicide

Risk Factors: [SAD PERSONS]

- Sex (male 3x more completion, but women make more attempts)
- Age (young adults or elderly)
- Depression
- Prior attempt (highest risk group)
- EtOH/Substance abuse
- Rational thought loss (psychosis)
- Social supports lacking
- Organized plan
- No significant other
- Sickness

Management:

Highest risk (ideation/intent/plan)	- Hospitalize with constant observation - Ensure safety
High risk (ideation, w/o plan)	- Close follow-up, use social supports to monitor patient - Treat underlying psychiatric conditions - Reduce access to firearms/other means of suicide

Catatonia

General: State of immobility and abnormal stuporous behavior, associated with mood disorders and schizophrenia

Clinical:

- **Immobility, stupor, mutism, echolalia, echopraxia**
- Negativism (resistant to instructions)
- Catalepsy (remains in fixed position for prolonged time)
- Posturing or waxy flexibility (resistant to movement)

Management: **Benzodiazepines** (first line), ECT for refractory cases

Grief

Typical Grief	< 6 months - Shock, numbness, distress, crying, sleep issues, decreased appetite, poor concentration, survivor guilt - Hallucinations of loved one
Prolonged Grief Disorder (Complex Grief)	> 6 months - **Loss of function** - Emotional dysregulation, preoccupation with death
Major Depression	- **Meets criteria for major depressive episode** - Signs include suicidal ideation, self-loathing, lack of breakthrough happiness

Anxiety Disorders

Panic Disorder

General: Spontaneous episodes of intense fear and other symptoms

Clinical: Panic attacks characterized by the following symptoms (minutes-to-hours)
- Dyspnea, chest pain, palpitations, diaphoresis
- Paresthesias (hyperventilation), abdominal pain/nausea
- Dizziness, derealization, depersonalization, fear of dying

DSM-5:
- **Recurrent unexpected panic attacks without trigger**
- ≥ 1 attacks followed by > 1 month of continuous worry about experiencing subsequent attacks
    - +/− behavior change to avoid potential triggers

Management:
- Acute episode: Benzodiazepine
- Chronic prevention: SSRI, CBT

Agoraphobia

General: Intense fear of **public places, where escape may be difficult**

DSM-5:
Intense fear/anxiety about > 2 situations for ≥ 6 months (due to concern of escape or inability to obtain help)
- Fear of triggering situation out of proportion to actual danger posed
- Situations often include both open spaces (e.g., bridges) and confined spaces (e.g., stores, crowds)
- Causes significant functional impairment

Management: Cognitive-behavioral therapy, SSRI

Specific Phobia/Social Anxiety Disorder

General: Irrational fear and anxiety of a specific feared object or situation
- **Specific**: Intense fear of a specific object or situation
- **Social**: Fear of scrutiny by others or of acting in an embarrassing way

DSM-5: > 6 months with the following features:
- Persistent, excessive fear elicited by a specific situation or object
- Exposure to the situation triggers an immediate fear response
- Situation or object is avoided
- Functional impairment

Management:

Specific phobia	- Cognitive-behavioral therapy
Social phobia	- Cognitive-behavioral therapy, SSRI - PRN beta-blockers for performance anxiety/public speaking

Generalized Anxiety Disorder

General: Persistent, excessive anxiety regarding many facets of daily life

DSM-5:
- **Excessive anxiety/worry about various daily events for > 6 months**
- Associated with ≥ 3 of the following:
    - Restlessness, fatigue, impaired concentration, irritability, muscle tension, insomnia

Management:
- Cognitive-behavioral therapy
- SSRI (can augment with buspirone)
- Benzos have been used, but dependence limits their utility

Anxiety Disorders

Obsessive Compulsive Disorder

General: Presence of distressful and impairing **obsessions and compulsions**
- **Obsessions**: Recurrent intrusive, anxiety producing thoughts
- **Compulsions**: Repetitive behaviors aimed to alleviate stressor
- Common patterns:
    - Contamination/cleaning
    - Doubt or harm/checking multiple times to avoid danger
    - Can be dark (e.g., obsessed over child being harmed, patient stabs self to relieve these thoughts)
- **Ego-dystonic**
- Commonly occurs with schizophrenia, bipolar disorder, eating disorders

DSM-5:
- Experiencing obsessions and or compulsions
- Time consuming (> 1 h/day) OR cause significant distress/dysfunction

Management:
- **CBT (exposure and response therapy)**
- SSRI
    - Alternative: Venlafaxine, clomipramine
    - Augment with atypical antipsychotics

Post-Traumatic Stress Disorder

General: Recurrent, negative symptoms after exposure to one or more traumatic events

DSM-5:
- Exposure to **death, threatened death, serious injury, or sexual violence**
- Plus > 1 month of the following symptoms:
    - Persistently re-experienced event (i.e., **flashbacks, nightmares**)
    - **Avoidance of trauma-related stimuli**
    - At least two symptoms of negative mood: Negative feelings of self/others/world, self-blame, anhedonia
    - At least two symptoms of arousal and reactivity: Hypervigilance, exaggerated startle, irritability/angry outbursts, impaired concentration, insomnia

Management:
- <u>Pharmacotherapy</u>:
    - SSRI or SNRI (venlafaxine)
    - Prazosin (for nightmares, sleep disruption)
    - Augmentation with atypical antipsychotics if severe
- <u>Psychotherapy</u>: CBT (containing eye movement desensitization and reprocessing)

Acute Stress Disorder:
- < 1 month of symptoms that occur within 1 month of a traumatic event
- Tx: Mobilize social supports, brief CBT, treat symptoms (insomnia/anxiety)

Adjustment Disorder

General: Behavioral or emotional symptoms develop after a stressful life event

DSM-5: **Emotional or behavioral symptoms within 3 months** in response to an **identifiable stressful life event**:
- Marked distress in excess of what would be expected after such an event
- Impairment in daily functioning
- Symptoms resolve within 6 months after stressor has ended
- Does not meet criteria for other mental disorder (including normal grief)

Management: Psychotherapy

Anxiety Disorders

Disorder	DSM-5 and Clinical Features	Management
Selective Mutism	- **Situational mutism**, often seen in children - > 1 month of consistent failure to speak in select social situations - Able to speak in other situations, and no underlying communication disorder	- CBT
Body Dysmorphic Disorder	- Preoccupation with **perceived defects or flaws in physical appearance** - Not observable/minimal defect to other observers	- CBT +/− SSRI
Excoriation Disorder	- **Recurrent skin picking** resulting in lesions - Repeated attempts to reduce skin picking - Repetitive behaviors in response to concerns	- CBT +/− SSRI
Trichotillomania	- **Recurrent episodes of pulling out hair**, resulting in hair loss - Usually involves the head or eyebrows/lashes, but can involve any hair - Not due to another medical condition (e.g., alopecia) or psych disorder	- CBT > SSRI
Hoarding Disorder	- Persistent **inability to discard possessions**, regardless of value - Accumulation of possessions that fill living areas and affect use	- CBT
Gambling Disorder	- Persistent and recurrent **problematic gambling** for at least a year - Issues seen include preoccupation with gambling, need to gamble for pleasure, jeopardizing relationships, lying about gambling	- Support group - CBT

Personality Disorders

General: Pervasive, **maladaptive personality change** that cause significant functional impairment
- Lack of insight
- Ego-syntonic
- Increased risk for other psych disorders

DSM-5:
- Enduring pattern of behavior that deviates from person's culture
- The pattern is pervasive, inflexible, and has an onset no later than adolescence or early adulthood

Cluster A ⟶ Eccentric, peculiar withdrawn [Weird]. Associated with psychotic disorders.

Cluster B ⟶ Emotional, dramatic, inconsistent [Wild]. Associated with mood disorders.

Cluster C ⟶ Avoidant, dependent, obsessive-compulsive [Wacky]. Associated with anxiety.

Management:
- Generally very difficult to treat, patients unaware that they need help
- Psychotherapy is cornerstone of care

Personality	Overview	DSM-5 and Specific Clinical Features	Management
Cluster A			
Paranoid	- Pervasive distrust and suspiciousness of others	- Distrust of others, with ≥ 4 of the following: Suspicion of exploitation or deception, preoccupation with doubts of loyalty, reluctance to confide in others, interpretation of benign remarks as threatening, persistence of grudges	- Individual psychotherapy - Antipsychotics (if psychotic)
Schizoid	- Lifelong pattern of social withdrawal - Eccentric and reclusive	- Voluntary social withdrawal and restricted emotions - ≥ 4 of the following: Chooses solitary activity, no desire for relationship, little interest in sexual activity, few friends, lack of emotion	- Generally lack insight for therapy
Schizotypal	- Eccentric behavior and peculiar thought patterns - Magical thinking (i.e., belief in superstition, telepathy, bizarre fantasies)	- Eccentric behavior, perceptual distortions, and discomfort with relationships - ≥ 5 of the following: Ideas of reference, magical thinking, illusions, suspiciousness, restricted affect, odd appearance/behavior, odd beliefs, few friends, social anxiety	- Psychotherapy - Antipsychotics (if required)
Cluster B			
Antisocial	- Exploitive of others, lacks empathy/compassion - Violates the law - Begins in childhood as conduct disorder - Must be ≥ 18 y/o	- Pattern of disregard for and violation of the rights of others + history of conduct disorder - ≥ 3 of the following: Fails to conform to social norms, deceitfulness/lies for personal gain, impulsivity, irritability/aggressiveness, lacks remorse, irresponsible, reckless	- Low utility for psychotherapy or pharmacotherapy
Borderline	- Unstable moods, behaviors, interpersonal relationships - **Splitting** is characteristic - Associated with childhood physical, emotional, sexual abuse - High rate of psychotic episodes	- Pervasive pattern of impulsivity and unstable relationship - ≥ 5 of the following: Unstable relationships, unstable self-image, unstable mood, SI/self-mutilation, anger, paranoid ideation, impulsivity (sexually/spending/substance use)	- Dialectical behavior therapy (CBT plus mindfulness skills) - Pharm: Mood stabilizers, antipsychotics, SSRI

Personality, Dissociative Disorders

Personality	Overview	DSM-5 and Specific Clinical Features	Management
Cluster B			
Histrionic	- Attention seeking behavior and emotionally labile	- ≥ 5 of the following: Provocative behavior, exaggerated emotion, easily influenced, perceives intimacy, wants to be center of attention, uses appearance for attention	- Psychotherapy
Narcissistic	- Pattern of grandiosity, need for admiration, and lack of empathy	- ≥ 5 of the following: Exaggerated sense of importance, requires admiration, entitled, takes advantage of others, lacks empathy, arrogant, envious, belief they are special	- Psychotherapy
Cluster C			
Avoidant	- Social inhibition, hypersensitivity, and feelings of inadequacy	- ≥ 4 of the following: Avoids interpersonal contact, cautious, unwilling to interact, afraid of criticism/ rejection, feels socially inept	- Psychotherapy
Dependent	- Excessive need to be taken care of that leads to submissive and clinging behavior	- ≥ 5 of the following: Feels helpless alone, seeks relationships, fear of being alone, seeks support from others, needs other to assume their responsibilities	- Psychotherapy
Obsessive-Compulsive	- Preoccupation with orderliness, control, and perfectionism - Unlike OCD, ego-syntonic	- ≥ 4 of the following: Perfectionism, excessive devotion to work, rigid/stubborn, preoccupied with detail	- Psychotherapy

Dissociative Amnesia

General: Inability to remember important autobiographical information
- Usually **post-traumatic event** or extreme stressors
- Procedural memory preserved
- Rarely generalizes to complete memory loss

DSM-5:
- Inability to recall important **autobiographical information**, usually due to traumatic or stressful event
- Often with dissociative fugue: Wandering from home

Management: Generally self-limited, psychotherapy

Depersonalization/Derealization Disorder

General: Detachment from one's self or surroundings
- **Depersonalization**: "Out of body experience"
- **Derealization**: "In dream or movie"

DSM-5:
- Recurrent experience of either depersonalization or derealization
- Reality testing remains intact during episode

Management: Psychotherapy

Dissociative Identity Disorder (Multiple Personality)

General: Presence of more than one distinct personality state
- Often occurs in victims of childhood trauma

DSM-5:
- Disruption of identity manifested as **two or more distinct personality states**
- Extensive memory lapses in autobiographical information, daily occurrences, and/or traumatic events

Management: Psychotherapy

Somatic and Factitious

Somatic Symptom Disorder

General: Perseveration over subjective symptom, which is not related to medical condition

DSM-5: > 6 months

- **≥ 1 somatic symptoms** causing distress/functional impairment
- Excessive thoughts, feelings, behaviors related to the somatic symptoms

Management:

- Regular visits with **single primary care physician**
    - Minimize unnecessary medical workups and treatments
    - Address psychological issues slowly (patients likely to resist)

Conversion Disorder

General: Neurological symptoms without underlying neurologic condition

- Onset often in adolescence or early adulthood
- Neurologic conditions include: **Weakness/paralysis, non-epileptic seizure, vision or speech problems**
- Often calm and unconcerned (la belle indifference)

DSM-5:

- ≥ 1 symptoms of altered voluntary motor or sensory function
- Incompatibility between the symptom and recognized neurological or medical conditions

Management:

- First line: Education, with self-help techniques and family education
- Second line: CBT
- Often spontaneously recover, but remission rate is high

Illness Anxiety Disorder

General: Excessive concern about having medical condition

- Previously called **hypochondriasis**

DSM-5: > 6 months of:

- **Preoccupation with having or acquiring a serious illness**
- None or minimal somatic symptoms
- High level of anxiety about health
- Performs excessive health-related behaviors

Management:

- Regularly scheduled visits (establish good relationship with PCP)
- CBT

Somatic, Factitious, Impulse

Factitious Disorder

General: Intentionally falsify medical or psych symptoms to assume the role of a sick patient. Previously called **Munchausen.**

- Risk populations:
    - Healthcare workers
    - Associated with personality disorders
- Common scenario:
    - Medical: Fever, infection, hypoglycemia, seizures
    - Psych: Hallucinations, depression

DSM-5: **Falsification of physical/psychiatric symptoms OR induction of injury or disease**

- Absence of obvious external rewards
- Done for primary (internal) gain from illness

Management:

- Collect collateral information from medical providers and family
- Collaborate with PCP and treatment team to avoid unnecessary procedure
- Patients may require confrontation

Malingering

General: Intentional reporting of physical or psychological symptoms in order for **external (secondary) gain**

- Examples: Obtain narcotics, avoid police, receive monetary reward

DSM-5: Not a medical condition

Impulse Control Disorders

Disorder	Clinical Features	Management
Intermittent Explosive Disorder	- Recurrent behavioral outbursts, characterized by verbal and/or physical aggression - Either weekly for > 3 months OR outbursts result in physical damage to people or property	- CBT + SSRI (first line)
Kleptomania	- Failure to resist urge to steal objects, despite having no personal or monetary need - Objects often discarded or returned - High rate of comorbid bulimia, and other anxiety/mood disorders	- CBT
Pyromania	- At least two episodes of deliberate fire setting - Tension before act, with gratification after watching - Excessive fascination with fires	- Often remits on own - CBT/SSRI can be used

Eating Disorders

	Overview	DSM-5 and Other Clinical Features	Management
Anorexia Nervosa	- Low body weight (BMI < 18.5 kg/m^2), with limited caloric intake and preoccupation with weight Subtypes: - **Restricting** (weight limitation from ↓ caloric intake/ excessive exercise) - **Binge-purging**	- ***DSM-5:*** Restriction of energy intake relative to requirements, leading to **low weight** - **Fear of gaining weight** or becoming fat - **Distorted body image**/concern with weight ***Complications:*** - CV: Cardiomyopathy, arrhythmia - Endocrine: Amenorrhea (↓ GNRH/LH/FSH), hypothyroidism, hypopituitary, osteoporosis - Heme: Cytopenias - Fluid/electrolyte abnormalities - Lanugo hair, alopecia	- **Nutritional rehabilitation** - **Psychotherapy** - Pharm: Not standard, but can use olanzapine - Hospitalization (indications include dehydration, hemodynamic instability, arrhythmia, very low weight/ refusal to eat) * Monitor for refeeding syndrome (hypophosphatemia)
Bulimia Nervosa	- Eating disorder characterized by **binge eating/purging** Methods of purge: - Laxative - Ipecac - Induced vomiting - Diuretics - Fasting/excessive exercise	- ***DSM-5:*** Recurrent episodes of binge eating, with compensatory **purging behaviors** (at least once per week for 3 months) - Perception of self excessively influenced by physical appearance ***Complications:*** - Parotid enlargement, dental erosions/caries - Hand calluses ("Russell sign") - Mallory-Weiss tear/acid reflux - Hypokalemia, hypochloremia, metabolic alkalosis	- CBT + SSRI (fluoxetine)
Binge Eating Disorder	- Periods of overeating without sense of control over eating	- Recurrent episodes of binge eating (at least once per week for 3 months) ≥ 3 of the following: Rapid eating, eating until too full, eating when not hungry, eating alone, feeling disgusting/gross after eating	- Psychotherapy (CBT) - If overweight: Behavioral modification for weight loss - Pharm: SSRI, topiramate

Sex/Gender Disorders

Transgender Care/Gender Dysphoria

General: Distress accompanying incongruence between patient's expressed gender and assigned gender
Common terms include;
- **Gender**: Individual's sense of feeling male, female, neither
- **Sex**: Biologic/anatomic sex
- **Transgender**: Gender identity is different from birth-designated sex
- **Transvestism**: Wearing clothes of the opposite sex

DSM-5: Gender dysphoria is defined by > 2 of the following:
- Difference between experienced gender and primary/secondary sex characteristics
- Strong desire to be other gender
- Strong desire to be treated as other gender
- Strong desire for primary/secondary sex characteristics of the other gender
- Strong belief one has typical feelings/reactions of the other gender

Management:
- Child/Adolescents: Provide education, support, and mental health referral
    - Treat comorbid psych conditions
    - Gender dysphoria that persists into onset of puberty is unlikely to subside
- Onset of puberty: **Pubertal suppression and social transition**
    - GnRH agonists are preferred
- **Gender-affirming hormones**
    - Androgens or estrogen + spironolactone
- Surgical sex reassignment
    - Indicated after 1 year of living in gender role + hormonal therapy in desired gender role

Paraphilias

General: Sexual arousal to atypical situations, fantasies, individuals, or acts. DSM recognizes the following subtypes:

Pedophilia	- Sexual interest in children (generally < 13 y/o, while individual is > 5 y/o)
Transvestic	- Sexual arousal from cross dressing
Fetishistic	- Sexual arousal from use of nonliving objects or nongenital body parts (e.g., feet)
Sexual masochism	- Arousal from being beaten, bound, humiliated, etc.
Sexual sadism	- Arousal from physical or psychological suffering of another
Exhibitionism	- Arousal from exposure of one's genitals to others
Voyeuristic	- Arousal from observing an unsuspecting individual
Frotteuristic	- Arousal rubbing against/touching nonconsenting person

DSM-5:
- > 6 months of engaging in unusual sexual activities or preoccupation with unusual sexual urges
- Occurs either with nonconsenting person and/or causes loss of functioning

Management:
- Psychotherapy, support groups

Sex/Gender Disorders

Psychologic Sexual Dysfunction

General: Sexual dysfunction include a variety of problems with sexual response

DSM-5:

- Significant clinical distress from a sexual dysfunction, which cannot be better explained by another mental or medical disorder

Disorder	**Definition** (for all: > 6 months of the following symptoms)
Men	
Premature ejaculation	Recurrent ejaculation during sex within 1 minute
Erectile dysfunction	Difficulty in getting or maintaining an erection
Delayed ejaculation	Marked delay in or absence of orgasm
Women	
Sexual interest/ arousal disorder	Absence or deficiency of sexual thoughts, desire
Female orgasmic disorder	Marked delay in or absence of orgasm

Management:

- Psychotherapy
    - Sex therapy
    - CBT
- Pharm/mechanical
    - SSRI (if premature ejaculation)
    - Hormone replacement
    - Phosphodiesterase inhibitors
    - Vacuum devices, rings, etc.

Normal Aging:

- Desire does not usually change as people age
- Men require more direct stimulation of the genitals and more time to achieve orgasm
- Women experience vaginal dryness and thinning

Sleep Disorders

Overview of Sleep Disorders

Awake (eyes open)	Beta	
Awake (eyes closed)	Alpha	
Non-REM N1	Theta	Light sleep
Non-REM N2	Spindles/K-complex	Deeper sleep
Non-REM N3	Delta	Deepest non-REM sleep
REM	Beta	

<u>Classes of sleep disorders</u>:
- Insomnia
- Sleep-related breathing disorders
- Central disorders of hypersomnolence (narcolepsy)
- Circadian rhythm sleep-wake disorders
- Parasomnias (unusual sleep-related behaviors)
- Sleep-related movement disorders

<u>Nonpharmacologic sleep advice</u>:
- Sleep hygiene (avoid caffeine/EtOH around bedtime, avoid naps, exercise regularly, relaxing activities near bedtime)
- Relaxation (progressive muscle relaxation, guided imagery, meditation)
- Stimulus control (go to sleep when you feel sleepy, try for 10 minutes max, use bed only for sleep, regular schedule, avoid naps)
- Sleep restriction

Insomnia

General: Difficulty initiating or maintaining sleep. Can be:
- Primary (idiopathic)
- Secondary (adverse med effect, symptoms of concurrent psych disorder, or related to medical disorder)

Can also be defined as:
- Acute (< 3 months): Most often related to stressor
- Chronic (> 3 months, see DSM criteria below)

DSM-5: > 3 days a week for > 3 months of:
- **Difficulty initiating or maintaining sleep, or waking up too early**
- Adequate opportunity/chance for sleep
- Functionally impairing, often causing daytime symptoms (hypersomnolence)

Management:
- Sleep Hygiene
- CBT (therapy preferred over medication)
- Pharm (for refractory cases):
  - **Sleep onset insomnia**: Melatonin, trazodone, zaleplon/zolpidem
  - **Sleep maintenance insomnia**: Orexin antagonist (suvorexant, daridorexant), eszopiclone

Sleep Disorders

	Overview	Clinical Features	Management
Obstructive Sleep Apnea	- Intermittent oropharyngeal airflow obstruction (20-30 seconds of hypoxemia, which awakens patient) Risks: - **Obesity** - Structural (tonsils, uvula) - Increased neck circumference - Family history - Alcohol	Clinical: Snoring, daytime somnolence, interruptions in breathing while sleeping Diagnosis: **Polysomnography** - > 5 episodes of apnea or hypopnea in 1 hour (in symptomatic patient) is diagnostic - > 15 episodes diagnostic if not symptomatic	- Behavioral modification (weight loss/exercise) Mild-to-moderate: - **CPAP** - Oral appliance (alternative) Severe: - CPAP is preferred - Uvulopalatopharyngoplasty - Tracheostomy (refractory)
Central Sleep Apnea	- Repetitive decrease in airflow and ventilatory effort during sleep - Primary: Idiopathic - Secondary: CHF, stroke, medical conditions, drugs, Cheyne-Stokes (periodic crescendo-decrescendo breathing pattern)	Clinical: Daytime somnolence, insomnia, signs of nocturnal hypoxia (e.g., morning headaches) Diagnosis: Polysomnography - > 5 apneic episodes per hour	- CPAP - Supplemental O_2
Obesity Hypoventilation Syndrome	- Alveolar hypoventilation secondary to **obesity (BMI > 30)**	Clinical: Hypersomnolence plus witnessed hypopnea. Presents similarly to OSA. Diagnosis: Elevated bicarbonate plus ABG (CO_2 > 45 mmHg) * Should perform polysomnography to rule out OSA	- CPAP - Tracheostomy (if refractory)

Narcolepsy

General: Inherited disorder of REM dysregulation, resulting in hypersomnolence

Clinical:

- **Daytime hypersomnolence**
- **Cataplexy** (loss of muscle tone with emotional stimulus)
- Sleep paralysis
- Hypnagogic hallucinations (going to sleep)
- Hypnopompic hallucinations (awakening)

DSM-5: Irrepressible need to sleep or daytime lapses into sleep occurring for ≥ 3 months PLUS either

(1) **Low CSF hypocretin-1 concentration** or
(2) **Cataplexy and ↓ sleep/↓ REM latency on polysomnogram**

Management:

- Education/behavioral modification (sleep hygiene, scheduled naps, avoid car accidents)
- Daytime sleepiness: Modafinil or other stimulants
- Cataplexy: Venlafaxine, fluoxetine, or sodium oxybate at night

Sleep Disorders

Circadian Sleep-Wake Disorders		
Disorder	**Description**	**Management**
Delayed	- Delayed onset of sleep, delayed wake time	- Morning bright light - Nighttime melatonin
Advanced	- Early sleep onset, early wake time	- Nighttime bright light
Non-24-H	- Circadian rhythm off 24-hour cycle - Results in wakefulness at times during night, drive for sleep during day	- Phototherapy - Melatonin
Irregular	- Failure to consolidate periods of sleep and wakefulness (e.g., 4 hours of sleep, 4 hours wake, etc.)	- Phototherapy - Melatonin
Jet Lag	- Excess daily sleep time due to poor sleep/misaligned circadian rhythm - > 2 time zones	- Self-limited - Melatonin
Shift Work	- Sleep-wake difficulties due to shifts off of the light-dark cycle	- Change schedule - Sleep hygiene/melatonin

Diagnosis:

- Sleep diaries
- Actigraphy (sensor tracking movement during sleep)

Parasomnias/Sleep Movement Disorders			
	Overview	**Clinical Features**	**Management**
Parasomnias			
Sleepwalking (Somnambulism)	- Ambulation and other acts occurring during slow wave sleep - Risks: Stress, irregular sleep, fatigue	- Sitting up, walking around, eating, and other acts during sleep - Open eyes, blank stare, glassy look - Difficulty arousing, may become agitated	- Lifestyle modification - Low-dose clonazepam
Sleep Terror	- Awakening from sleep from sudden terror, occurring during slow wave sleep	- Screaming, agitation, and fear, with event - Autonomic symptoms (flushing, sweating) - Usually little recall of event - Difficult to arouse	- Lifestyle modification - Low-dose clonazepam
Nightmare Disorder	- Dysphoric dreams occurring during REM sleep	- Repeated episodes of extended, extremely dysphoric, and well-remembered dreams - Cause significant distress/functional impairment	- Often self-limited - Lifestyle modification - Psychotherapy - Prazosin
Sleep Movement Disorder			
REM Sleep Behavior Disorder	- Dream movements that occur after the loss of REM atonia - High association with movement disorders (e.g., Parkinson)	- Dream enactment (sleep talking, yelling, walking, punching, etc.) - Generally remember dream - Dx: Polysomnography (see loss of REM atonia, dream enactment)	- Make sleep environment safe - Melatonin, clonazepam
Periodic Limb Movement Disorder	- Involuntary myoclonic limb movements occurring during sleep	> 15 periodic limb movements/h of sleep - Significant sleep disturbance or functional impairment - Dx: Polysomnography	Similar to RLS: - Pramipexole/ropinirole - Gabapentin

Child Psychiatry

Intellectual Disability

General: Severely impaired cognitive and adaptive/social functioning (replaces mental retardation)

Etiology:

- About 50% are idiopathic
- **Fragile X (most common inherited), Down (most common genetic)**
- Common comorbid conditions: Autism, ADHD, learning disorders

DSM-5:

- Significant **limitations in both adaptive and intellectual function**
- Onset during developmental period
- Deficits affect multiple domains: Conceptual, practical, and social
- IQ > 2 SD below mean

Severity	~ IQ	Description
Mild	50-70	- Can often live/function if provided some support
Moderate	35-50	- Requires high amounts of supervision
Severe	20-35	- Not independent, needs help with self-care
Profound	< 20	- Needs nursing care throughout life

Management:

- Multidisciplinary support (educational assistance, family counseling, physical/occupational/speech therapy)

Other Developmental/Learning Disorders

Diagnosis	Features
Global developmental delay	- Failure to meet expected developmental milestones in several areas (motor, social, communication)
Specific learning disorder	- Delayed development in a particular academic domain (reading, writing, arithmetic)
Language disorder	- Difficulty learning and using language - Reduced vocabulary, limited sentence structure
Fluency disorder (stuttering)	- Dysfluency and speech motor production issues
Speech-sound disorder	- Difficulty producing articulate, intelligible speech

Autism Spectrum Disorder

General: Disorder of impaired social communication/interaction and restrictive repetitive behaviors/interests

Etiology: Multifactorial. High comorbid rate with ID. Also associated with genetic disorders (Fragile X, Down, Rett).

DSM-5:

- **Problems with social interaction and communication** (lack of interest in peers, poor eye contact, impaired social interactions)
- **Restricted, repetitive patterns of behavior**, interests, and activities (peculiar interest, adherence to rituals, repetitive movements)
- Symptoms not accounted for by ID, learning disorder, deafness (rule out with audiology)

Management:

- Early intervention
- Multidisciplinary (special education, behavior therapy, speech/language/occupational therapy)

Child Psychiatry

Attention Deficit Hyperactivity Disorder

General: Characterized by inattention, hyperactivity, impulsivity. Subtypes include inattentive, hyperactive, or mixed.

DSM-5: Symptoms **> 6 months and present in at least two settings, onset before age 12**
- At least six inattentive symptoms and/or six hyperactive symptoms
- Functional impairment

Inattentive	Hyperactive
- Difficulty sustaining attention	- Difficulty remaining seated
- Does not appear to listen	- Fidgets/squirms
- Difficulty organizing	- Runs about or climbs excessively
- Loses things	- Talks excessively
- Easily distracted	- Blurts out answers
- Careless mistakes	- Interrupts others
- Struggles following instructions	- Difficulty taking turns

Management: Combination of pharmacologic plus educational/behavioral interventions
- Nonpharm: Behavior modification, educational intervention
- Pharm:
    - Stimulants: Methylphenidate, dextroamphetamine
    - Atomoxetine, alpha-2 agonists (clonidine, guanfacine)

Tic Disorders

General: Tics are repetitive, stereotyped movements or vocalizations, that are generally spontaneous and difficult to repress

Risk: Behavioral disorders, ADHD, and OCD are frequently comorbid with Tourette

Clinical:

Syndrome	DSM-5 Criteria
Persistent Chronic Motor Tic Disorder	- ≥ 1 motor tic (repetitive, stereotyped movement) - Occurs for at least 1 year
Persistent Chronic Vocal Tic Disorder	- ≥ 1 vocal tic (repetitive, stereotyped vocalization) - Occurs for at least 1 year
Tourette Syndrome	- **Multiple motor and vocal tics** - Occurs for at least 1 year

Management:
- Therapy (psychoeducation, habit reversal therapy)
- Pharm (indicated if tics are bothersome)
    - **Tetrabenazine**
    - Fluphenazine, risperidone (haloperidol/pimozide in the past)
    - Guanfacine/clonidine (especially if also have ADHD)

Disruptive Mood Dysregulation Disorder

General: New disorder to DSM-5. Described as chronic severe persistent irritability occurring in childhood and adolescence.

DSM-5: > 12 months of the following symptoms
- **Severe recurrent verbal and/or physical outbursts** (> 3x /week)
- Occur in at least 2 settings
- Persistently irritable or angry mood most of the day/nearly every day (*differentiates from intermittent explosive)
- No mania (i.e., no bipolar disorder), or underlying substance/medical issue

Management:
- Psychotherapy (CBT)
- Pharm (none have great evidence yet): Atypical antipsychotics or antidepressants

Child Psychiatry

Separation Anxiety Disorder

General: Excessive anxiety due to separation from parents

DSM-5:

- Excessive and developmentally inappropriate **fear/anxiety regarding separation from attachment figures**
- ≥ 4 weeks in children/adolescents and ≥ 6 months in adults
- ≥ 3 of the following:
  - Separation leads to extreme distress
  - Constant worry about harm
  - Reluctance to leave home
  - Reluctance to be alone
  - Reluctance to sleep alone
  - Complaints of physical symptoms when separated
  - Nightmares of separation

Management: Psychotherapy (CBT, family therapy, school therapy)

Oppositional Defiant Disorder

General: Maladaptive pattern of irritability/anger, defiance, or vindictiveness

DSM-5: At least four symptoms present for ≥ 6 months

- **Anger/Irritability**: Touchy, loses temper, easily annoyed, often angry
- **Vindictiveness**: Multiple spiteful acts in the past
- **Defiant behavior**: Breaks rules, argues with authority figures, annoys others

Management: Therapy (behavior modification), parent management training

Conduct Disorder

General: Serious disruptive behaviors, which violate the rights of other humans and animals, generally without guilt

DSM-5: Recurrent (at least 3 over the last year) **acts that violate rights of others or societal norms**. Examples below:

- Aggression to humans/animals (bullies, fights, physically harms animals/other people, rape)
- Property destruction
- Theft (steals items, breaks into home/car, lies to get goods)
- Serious rule violation (runs away from home, breaks curfew)

Management: Psychotherapy (behavior modification), parent management training

Elimination Disorder

General: Developmentally inappropriate elimination of urine or feces

- Incontinence normal at young age (feces until 4 and urine until 5 y/o)
- Can be primary (idiopathic, continence never achieved) or secondary (continence achieved, then later lost)

DSM-5:

<u>Enuresis</u>

- Recurrent urination into clothes or bed-wetting
- ≥ 5 y/o
- 2×/week for ≥ 3 consecutive months

<u>Encopresis</u>

- Recurrent defecation into inappropriate places
- ≥ 4 years old
- 1×/month for ≥ 3 consecutive months

Management: Psychoeducation (high spontaneous remission rate for both conditions)

<u>Enuresis</u>

- Bladder training (limit caffeine, nighttime fluid intake, scheduled voids), urine alarm
- Pharm if refractory (desmopressin or imipramine)

<u>Encopresis</u>

- Behavioral program (bowel retraining). If constipation, initial "clean out," followed by stool softeners/high-fiber diet

Substance Use

	Overview	Intoxication	Withdrawal
EtOH	- Activates GABA receptors	***Clinical:*** - CNS depressant, slurred speech, ataxia, stupor, coma ***Management:*** - Supportive care - Thiamine, folate - GI evacuation (only if significant EtOH intake in last hour)	***Clinical:*** - **Mild withdrawal (6-24 h)**: Anxiety, tremors, diaphoresis, palpitations, insomnia - **Seizures (24-48 h)** - **Alcoholic hallucinosis (24-48 h)**: Visual, auditory, or tactile hallucinations, but orientation is normal and vital signs stable - **Delirium tremens (48-96 hr)**: Agitation, hallucinations, hypertension, fever ***Management:*** - Benzodiazepines (CIWA scale protocol) - Normal liver → Diazepam - Liver failure → Lorazepam - Thiamine, folate, vitamins ("Banana bag")
Benzodiazepine	- Potentiate GABA channels	***Clinical:*** (Similar to EtOH) - Drowsiness, confusion, slurred speech - Incoordination, ataxia ***Management:*** - Supportive care - **Flumazenil**	***Clinical:*** - Similar to EtOH (hallucinations, tremors, anxiety, and seizures) ***Management:*** - Long-acting benzo (requires gradual tapering over months)

Alcohol Use Disorder

General: Recurrent drinking that causes functional impairment. ↑ Risk if family history (multifactorial genetic basis).

DSM-5: Recurrent drinking, resulting in failed obligations, hazardous situations, social problems, tolerance, history of withdrawal, inability to cut back, alcohol cravings

Clinical Complications:

- GI: Gastritis, hepatitis, cirrhosis, pancreatitis. ↑ risk esophageal, oropharyngeal cancers.
- Cardiac: Dilated cardiomyopathy, hypertension
- CNS: Neuropathy, cerebellar degeneration
    - **Wernicke** (thiamine deficiency)
        - Nystagmus, ataxia, ophthalmoplegia, confusion
        - Precipitated by glucose administration in those with alcohol use disorder
    - **Korsakoff**: Amnestic disorder with confabulation + apathy. Irreversible.

Management:

- Support groups (alcoholics anonymous)

<u>Pharm</u>

- **Naltrexone** (opioid receptor blocker)
    - Decreases desire/craving and "high" associated with alcohol
    - Can be initiated without complete alcohol abstinence
    - Cannot be used with severe hepatitis (mild liver disease is okay)
- **Acamprosate** (glutamate transmission modulator)
    - Should be started post-detoxification for relapse prevention
    - Can be used in patients with liver disease, but not in severe CKD

Other options: Baclofen, disulfiram, topiramate, gabapentin, SSRI, ondansetron

- Disulfiram (inhibits aldehyde dehydrogenase)
    - Causes adverse reaction to EtOH (flushing, headache, vomiting, palpitations, dyspnea)

Screening: CAGE (cut down, annoyed, guilt, eye opener), or validated tool (AUDIT, MAST)

Substance Use

	Overview	Intoxication	Withdrawal
Cocaine	- 5-HT, dopamine, epi, norepi reuptake inhibitor	***Clinical:*** - Increased energy, decreased need for sleep, euphoria, heightened self-esteem, hypertension/tachycardia, dilated pupils, fever - Paranoia/hallucinations - Rhabdomyolysis, seizures, MI, or arrhythmias ***Management:*** - Supportive care, benzodiazepines - ACS/MI: Aspirin, benzo, stenting	- Abrupt abstinence not life-threatening (symptoms usually last ~1 week) - Can experience depression, anxiety, anhedonia, cravings, and increased sleep
Amphetamines	- Block reuptake and facilitate release of dopamine and norepi	***Clinical:*** - Euphoria, dilated pupils, tachycardia, diaphoresis - Hyperthermia, dehydration, rhabdo - Can develop psychosis ***Management:*** - Supportive care, benzodiazepines	- Similar to cocaine
Marijuana	- CB receptor activator (THC is active substance in cannabis)	***Clinical:*** - Euphoria, anxiety, poor coordination - Perceptual disturbance or psychosis - Conjunctival injection, dry mouth, ↑ appetite ***Management:*** - Purely supportive - Benzodiazepines if agitation	***Clinical:*** - Only occurs after heavy/prolonged use - Irritability, anger, depressed mood, insomnia

Opioid Use Disorder

General: Misuse of opioid medications or use of illicitly obtained heroin/fentanyl

DSM-5: Problematic pattern of opioid use, causing impairment or distress, manifested by ≥ 2 of the following, within a 12-month period:

- Opioids taken longer than intended, significant cravings, social/interpersonal problems due to opioids, unsuccessful efforts to cut down, tolerance, failure to fulfill major role obligations

Clinical:

- **Intoxication**: Slurred speech, sedation, and miosis (exception: meperidine)
  - Hypothermia, seizures, respiratory depression if severe
- **Withdrawal**: Dysphoria, insomnia, lacrimation, rhinorrhea, restlessness, yawning, nausea, abdominal cramps

Management:

- **Intoxication:** ABCs, ventilation if needed, naloxone (intranasal, subQ, IV)
- **Withdrawal:**
  - Methadone, buprenorphine-naloxone, or clonidine
    - Adjunctive symptomatic meds: Ibuprofen, loperamide, ondansetron, hydroxyzine
- **Long-term OUD Therapy**:
  - **Buprenorphine-naloxone**: Partial opioid agonist, administered by transmucosal film/tab or injection
    - Can precipitate withdrawal (high affinity for opioid receptor, displaces other opioids)
  - **Methadone**: Long-acting opioid agonist, administered daily in an opioid treatment program

Complications:

- IVDU: Bloodstream infections, endocarditis, HIV, hepatitis B/C

Substance Use

Substance	Clinical Features
MDMA	- ↑ release of serotonin, inhibition of serotonin reuptake - Mild hallucinogenic properties - Clinical: Euphoria, alertness, ↑ **sociability**, ↑ **sexual desire**, bruxism - Hypertension, tachycardia, hyperthermia - Complications: **Serotonin syndrome**, hyponatremia
LSD	- Activates D, 5-HT, NE - Hallucinogenic - Clinical: Perceptual distortion (visual, auditory), depersonalization, anxiety, paranoia, psychosis

PCP
"Angel dust"
	- NMDA antagonist
	- Clinical: Agitation, depersonalization, hallucinations, impaired judgment, memory impairment, aggression
	- Nystagmus (rotary, horizontal, vertical), ataxia, dysarthria, hypertension, tachycardia, muscle rigidity
	- Overdose: Seizures, delirium, coma, death
	- Management:
	  - Monitor (dark quiet room, restraints only if necessary)
	  - Benzos/haloperidol (if needed)

Psilocybin	- 5-HT2 stimulating hallucinogenic - Found in certain mushrooms
Mescaline	- 5-HT2 stimulating hallucinogenic - Found in peyote
Inhalants	- Inhaled CNS depressant drugs - Types include toluene (solvents, paint thinners), glue, nitrous, and amyl nitrite (poppers)
Caffeine	- Adenosine receptor antagonist > 250 mg: Anxiety, insomnia, muscle twitching, rambling, diuresis > 1 g: Tinnitus, severe agitation, visual light flashes

Psychotherapy

General: Interpersonal therapy that attempts to alleviate psychological symptoms

Subtypes	Features
Cognitive-Behavioral Therapy	- Helps the patient identify and correct maladaptive beliefs - Utilizes cognitive/behavioral techniques (education, relaxation, stress management, coping skills)
Psychodynamic	- Developing insight on patient's past experiences and relationships that may affect unconscious thought patterns
Interpersonal	- Emphasizes current relationships and the connection with depressive feelings
Supportive	- Conversational therapy that focuses upon current problematic relationships and maladaptive patterns of behavior - Promotes coping skills and improved self-esteem
Dialectical	- Promotes mindfulness, emotional regulation, in addition to other CBT type techniques - Designed for **borderline personality** patients
Motivational Interviewing	- Technique utilized to encourage patients to change maladaptive behaviors

Technique	Features
Systematic Desensitization	- Relaxation techniques while being exposed to increasing doses of an anxiety-provoking stimulus
Flooding	- Confronted with an anxiety-provoking stimulus and not allowed to withdraw until they feel calm and in control
Aversion	- Negative response (e.g., shock the patient) when specific behavior occurs
Biofeedback	- Monitor physiologic data as patients try to control their physiologic state (HR/BP) - Used in patients with anxiety, chronic pain, hypertension, migraines

Psychopharmacotherapy

	Mechanism	Indication	Side Effects/Management
SSRI			
Fluoxetine Sertraline Paroxetine Citalopram Escitalopram Fluvoxamine	- Inhibitor of 5-HT reuptake at synapse	- Depression/GAD - Panic disorder - OCD (fluvoxamine) - Bulimia - PTSD - Premenstrual dysphoric disorder - Premature ejaculation	- Headache, insomnia, vivid dreams, anorexia, nausea, diarrhea (these symptoms usually subside) - Mania (if underlying bipolar) - Platelet dysfunction - Sexual dysfunction: Anorgasmia, decreased libido (does not subside, ~40% occurrence) - Lower dose, change med, or add bupropion or sildenafil - Rare/life-threatening: Seizures (rare), SIADH, serotonin syndrome - Discontinuation syndrome: Fatigue, HA, myalgias, paresthesias for rapidly stopping SSRI (except fluoxetine, which has long half-life)
SNRI			
Venlafaxine Desvenlafaxine Duloxetine Milnacipran Levomilnacipran	- Inhibitor of 5-HT and norepi reuptake	- Depression, GAD - PTSD, panic disorder, OCD - Neuropathy/fibromyalgia	- Side effects similar to SSRIs (PLUS noradrenergic symptoms like diaphoresis/dizziness) - Hypertension at higher doses
TCA			
Tertiary Amine Amitriptyline Imipramine Clomipramine Doxepin **Secondary Amine** Desipramine Nortriptyline	- Inhibitor of 5-HT and norepi reuptake - Highly anticholinergic	- Amitriptyline: Chronic pain, migraines, insomnia - Imipramine: Enuresis - Clomipramine: OCD - Doxepin: Chronic pain	- Antihistamine: Sedation, weight gain - Anti $\alpha 1$: Orthostasis, dizziness - Anticholinergic: Dry mouth, constipation, urinary retention, blurry vision - Anti-5-HT: Erectile dysfunction ***TCA Overdose*** - Presents with encephalopathy, anticholinergic symptoms, seizures, cardiac issues (QRS prolongation, heart block, risk for VTach/VFib) - Tx: $NaHCO_3$ (for > 100 ms QRS interval) - Benzo for seizures
MAO-I			
Tranylcypromine Phenelzine Isocarboxazid Selegiline	- Inhibits monoamine oxidase	- Refractory/atypical depression	Serotonin Syndrome - Must wait weeks before switching from SSRI to MAO (and from MAO to SSRI) - Can be precipitated if used with: SSRI, TCAs, St John wort, meperidine, dextromethorphan Hypertensive crisis - Precipitated by tyramine-rich foods (red wine, cheese, chicken liver, fava beans, cured meats) - HA, diaphoresis, photophobia, autonomic instability - Tx: Nifedipine or phentolamine

Psychopharmacotherapy

	Mechanism	Indication	Side Effects/Management
Atypical Antidepressants			
Bupropion	- Increased dopamine and norepinephrine	- Depression - Smoking cessation	- Tachycardia, insomnia, anxiety, headache - Decreased seizure threshold (Contraindicated: Epilepsy, eating disorder) - No sexual side effects
Mirtazapine	- α2 antagonist (increases NE/5-HT release) - 5-HT, H1 antagonist	- Depression	- Sedation - Weight gain - Dry mouth
Trazodone Nefazodone	- Inhibitor of 5-HT2, α1 adrenergic, and H1	- Insomnia	- Sedation - Dizziness, orthostatic hypotension - Priapism (Tx: Epi injection into corpus) - Nefazodone → Black box warning for liver failure
Stimulants			
Amphetamines Methylphenidate	- Increases catecholamines in synaptic cleft	- ADHD	- Decreased appetite, weight loss - Possible growth delay (reversible with stopping) - Insomnia - Irritability/mood change - BP elevation - Exacerbation of tics - Decreased seizure threshold
Atomoxetine	- Inhibits norepi synaptic uptake	- ADHD	- Less abuse potential and side effects, but less effective
Antipsychotics (first generation)			
Low Chlorpromazine Thioridazine *Mid* Perphenazine *High* Haloperidol Fluphenazine Pimozide	- D2 Receptor Blocker	- Schizophrenia - Bipolar - Antiemetic	- Anti-H → Sedation, weight gain - Anti-α → Orthostatic hypotension - Anti-M → Dry mouth, tachycardia, urine retention - QT prolongation - Increased prolactin (tuberoinfundibular) - Decreased libido, galactorrhea, gynecomastia - Extrapyramidal symptoms - Chlorpromazine → Blue gray skin deposition, photosensitivity, jaundice - Thioridazine → Pigmented retinopathy
Antipsychotics (second generation, or atypical)			
Clozapine Risperidone Quetiapine Olanzapine Ziprasidone Aripiprazole *Newest:* Paliperidone Iloperidone Lurasidone	- D2, 5-HT receptor blocker (Note: Aripiprazole is a partial D2 agonist)	- Schizophrenia - Bipolar - Borderline personality - Tic disorders	- Metabolic syndrome (monitor with weight, waist, BP, glucose, lipids) - AntiHis, antiα, anti-M (see above) - QT prolongation - Elderly: Increased risk of mortality - Clozapine: **Agranulocytosis** (must monitor WBC for 6 months weekly, next 6 months bi-weekly, then monthly). Stop if neutrophils < 1500. Can also cause seizures, myocarditis. - Quetiapine: Sedation, cataracts - Risperidone: Excreted in breast milk

Psychopharmacotherapy

Extrapyramidal Symptoms

	Features	Management
Dystonia	- Involuntary muscular contraction - Specific examples include oculogyric crisis, torticollis, opisthotonus	- Diphenhydramine - Benztropine
Bradykinesia (Parkinsonism)	- Slowed movements	- Benztropine - Amantadine
Akathisia	- Restlessness	- Reduce dose - Benzo, beta-blocker, or benztropine
Tardive Dyskinesia	- Writhing movements of mouth and tongue, choreoathetoid movements of extremities - Believed due to D2 upregulation and hypersensitivity - Often irreversible	- Discontinue medication - Clozapine (if antipsychotic needed) - Valbenazine (inhibits VMAT2)

Neuroleptic Malignant Syndrome and Serotonin Syndrome

	NMS	Serotonin Syndrome
Gen	- Occurs in those using antipsychotics - Highest risk with first generation	- Precipitated by the use of multiple serotonergic meds (MAO-I, SSRIs, SNRIs, TCAs, triptans, meperidine, dextromethorphan, St. John wort, linezolid)
Clin	- Encephalopathy - **Fever (often > 40°C)** - Muscle contractions, **rhabdomyolysis** - Autonomic instability (tachycardia, arrhythmias, tachypnea, diaphoresis) - Elevated CK, leukocytosis	- **Neuromuscular hyperactivity** (clonus, hypertonia, hyperreflexia, tremors) - **Autonomic instability** (tachycardia, arrhythmias, tachypnea, diaphoresis) - **Agitation/confusion**
Tx	- Stop neuroleptics - Supportive (fluids, cooling) - Dantrolene/bromocriptine	- Stop offending medications - Supportive care - Benzos for agitation/spasms - Cyproheptadine

	Mechanism	Indication	Side Effects/Management
Mood Stabilizers			
Lithium	- Unknown	- Bipolar disorder - Augmentation of antidepressant * Contraindicated with renal failure	- Acute side effects: Tremor (Tx: propranolol), nausea, diarrhea, ataxia, weakness - Chronic side effects: Nephrogenic DI, hypothyroidism, hyperparathyroidism, teratogen (Ebstein), benign leukocytosis Toxic levels - Precipitated by: Illness/dehydration, NSAIDs, ACE-I, thiazides, metronidazole, tetracycline - Altered mentation, tremors, convulsions, delirium - Tx: Hemodialysis if lithium level > 5 or > 2.5 with severe symptoms Management - Prior to start: ECG, chemistries (Cr/BUN), CBC, TSH, pregnancy test, urinalysis - Blood levels at 5 days, then every 2-3 days until therapeutic (after that every 6-12 months) - Monitor Cr/TSH q3-6 months
Carbamazepine Lamotrigine Valproate	[See: Neuro]		

Neonatology

Delivery Room Care (Initial)

Immediately After Birth:
- Dry infant, clear airway secretions, provide warmth. Stimulate the infant.
- Apgar score (at minutes 1 and 5. Helps to assess neonatal status, does not predict prognosis or mortality)

	Sign	0	1	2
A	Appearance	All blue	Blue extremities	All pink
P	Pulse	Absent	< 100 bpm	> 100 bpm
G	Grimace	Absence	Weak grimace	Cough/cry
A	Activity	Limp	Some flexion	Fully active
R	Respiratory	Absent	Weak cry	Good cry

- APGAR > 7: Good status. Do not require any resuscitation. Give to mom for skin-to-skin contact and early breastfeeding.

Neonatal Resuscitation

Situation	Intervention (in order of escalation of care)
HR < 100 bpm Apneic/gasping	(1) Positive pressure ventilation (intubation if prolonged/inadequate) (2) Chest compressions (if no improvement despite ventilation) (3) Epinephrine (if no response to compressions)
HR > 100 bpm Labored breathing	- Clear airway - Supplemental O_2 with pulse oximetry monitoring

Newborn Nursery

Eye Care	- Erythromycin ophthalmic ointment Note: Serves as prophylaxis for gonococcal conjunctivitis (not chlamydia)
Vitamin K	- Single IM dose - Prevents vitamin K deficiency-related bleeding
Hepatitis B Vaccine	- First vaccine within 24 hours of delivery (regardless of maternal status)
Umbilical Cord	- Sterile clamp/cutting, with "dry cord care" (keep clean/dry) - **Umbilical granuloma**[A]: Friable, pink pedunculated lesion at umbilical stump. Tx: Silver nitrate - **Omphalitis**: Infection of umbilicus/surrounding tissue. Tx: IV antibiotics
Feeding	- 8-12 feeds per day. Helps prevent hypoglycemia. Note: Up to 10% weight loss is typical in first few days after birth, but should be regained by 14 days
Screening	- O_2 saturation (to monitor for congenital heart disease) - **Genetic panel**: "Blood spot" testing, which is sent to identify a variety of inherited disorders - Hearing screening
Monitoring	- Glucose - Bilirubin
Circumcision	- Elective procedure that is controversial - Generally believed that benefits > risks, but should be shared decision with parents/doctor - Benefits: ↓ risk of penile cancer, UTI, foreskin retractile disorders. ↓ transmission of HIV/HPV. - Risks: Bleeding, infection, glans injury (extremely rare), fistula formation, excess skin removal

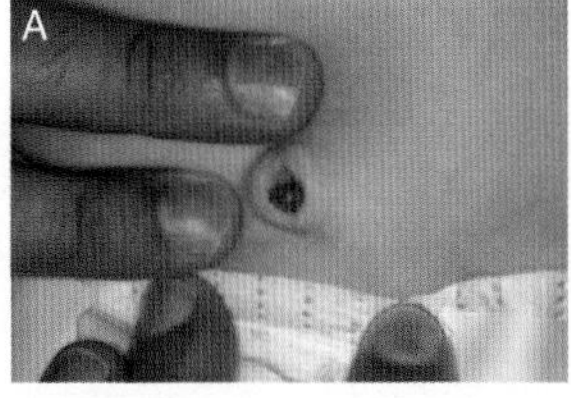

Neonatology

Breastfeeding

	Benefits	Contraindications
Infant	- Improved immunity (↓ risk of acute illnesses, such as sepsis, respiratory disease, gastroenteritis, UTI) - Improvement of GI function/maturity - Possible long-term benefits (cancer, obesity)	- Galactosemia
Maternal	- Reduced rates of breast and ovarian cancer - Maternal-infant bonding - Accelerated recovery from childbirth - Quicker return to prepartum weight - Improved child spacing (from suppression of normal cycle)	- Active herpetic breast lesions - HIV (without virologic suppression) - Current chemotherapy or radiation therapy - Use of illicit drugs or alcohol

Prematurity

General: Birth at < 37 gestational weeks. Associated with increased risk for multiple complications (see below).

- **Corrected gestational age**:
  - Chronologic age minus number of weeks born before 40 weeks
  - Useful until age of 2 y/o, when preemies should be caught up

Complications:

Immediate	Long-Term
- Hypothermia, hypoglycemia, hypotension, hypocalcemia - RDS, apnea of prematurity, bronchopulmonary dysplasia - GI (gastroesophageal reflux, NEC), hyperbilirubinemia - Intraventricular hemorrhage - Retinopathy of prematurity - ↑ infection/sepsis risk	- Overall increased mortality, morbidity (↑ hospitalizations) - Neurodevelopmental delay - Growth impairment - Impaired respiratory function

Postterm

General: Birth at > 42 gestational weeks. Associated with the below complications:

Immediate	Long-Term
- Meconium aspiration syndrome - Polycythemia - Neonatal asphyxia - Dysmaturity syndrome - Overall ↑ neonatal morbidity/mortality	- N/A

Weight

General:

- Small for gestational age [SGA] (< 10 percentile) or 2500 g
- Large for gestational age [LGA] (> 90 percentile) or 4000 g

Risk:

- SGA: IUGR, genetic abnormalities
- LGA: Diabetes mellitus (both gestational and preexisting), excessive weight gain, fetal sex (male), ↑ gestational age

Complications:

Small for Gestational Age	Large for Gestational Age
- Perinatal asphyxia - Hypothermia, hypoglycemia - Polycythemia	- Hypothermia - Birth injuries common (clavicle fracture, brachial plexus injury, facial nerve palsy, shoulder dystocia)

Neonatology

Indirect Hyperbilirubinemia

General: Almost all newborns have elevated levels of indirect bilirubin, and severely ↑ levels (> 25 mg/dL) put at risk for bilirubin-induced neurologic dysfunction (BIND)

Etiology	General	Clinical/Timing
Physiologic	- High bilirubin production, low hepatic UDPGT, low levels of bile-metabolizing intestinal flora	- Within days of birth
Hemolysis	- ABO incompatibility - Anti-Rh disease	- Within 24 hours of birth
Breast Milk Jaundice	- High β-glucuronidase in breast milk	- Starts ~3-5 days, peaks at 2 weeks - Jaundice, but normal otherwise without issues feeding
Breastfeeding Jaundice	- Failure of lactation, resulting in ↑ enterohepatic circulation	- Around 1 week - Poor feeding - Often have signs of dehydration
Others	- Crigler-Najjar - Congenital hypothyroidism - Galactosemia - Chronic disorders of hemolysis (spherocytosis) - Increased RBC load from birth trauma	

Clinical: Jaundice (yellow discoloration of conjunctiva/extremities)

Diagnosis: Serum bilirubin or transcutaneous bilirubinometer

Management:
- Phototherapy (for any with hyperbilirubinemia based on nomogram)
- Exchange transfusion (for any with signs of neurologic dysfunction)
- IVIG (for isoimmune hemolytic disease)

Direct Hyperbilirubinemia

General: Elevation of direct bilirubin is always pathologic in neonates

Etiology:
- Biliary atresia
- Choledocal cysts
- Hepatitis
- Genetic/inherited metabolic conditions

BIND/Kernicterus

Bilirubin-induced neurologic dysfunction (BIND): Acute neurologic deficits from hyperbilirubinemia
- Lethargy, hypotonia initially
- Progresses to coma, seizures, hypertonia (opisthotonos/retrocollis) if not treated

Kernicterus: Long-term sequelae of CNS bilirubin deposition
- Cerebral palsy
- Hearing loss
- Gaze defects
- Dental enamel hypoplasia/dysplasia

Neonatology

Birth Trauma

Disorder	Clinical Findings
Cephalohematoma[A]	- **Subperiosteal collection of blood**, causing head mass - Usually self-limited, resolve over next few months
Subgaleal Hemorrhage[B]	- Blood accumulation **between periosteum of the skull and the aponeurosis** - Usually due to dural venous sinus injury - High risk for massive blood loss in this space - Presents with shifting, fluctuant, skull mass, plus eventual hemodynamic instability
Caput Succedaneum[C]	- **Swelling of the scalp above the periosteum** - Presents as irregular swelling that crosses suture lines - Usually self-limited, resolves over few days
Clavicle Fracture	- **Most common fracture associated with birth** - Presents with immobility of affected arm, crepitus, edema - Dx: XR - Tx: Reassurance, NSAID analgesia, long sleeved garment, pin arm to chest
Others	- Intracranial hemorrhage (subdural, epidural, etc.) - Fracture (humeral, femur)—all rare - Nasal septal dislocation - Brachial plexus injury

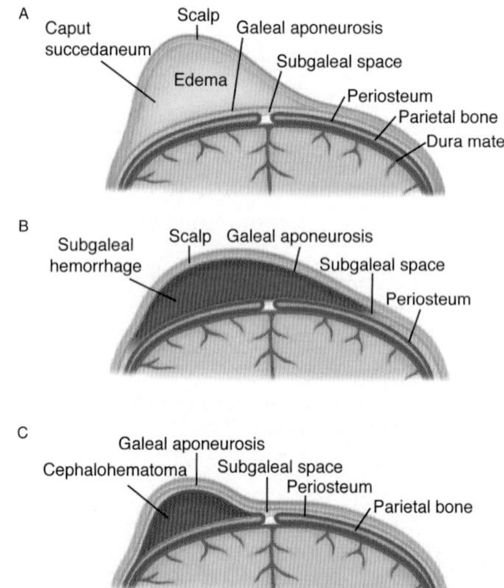

Other Neonatal Musculoskeletal Issues

Neonatal Torticollis	- Postural deformity of the neck, characterized by lateral neck flexion and neck rotation - Hypertonic sternocleidomastoid muscle - Associated with multiple gestation, breech, oligohydramnios - Risk for developing craniofacial abnormalities or plagiocephaly - Dx: Clinical - Tx: Positioning changes, physical therapy. Surgery if refractory.
Positional Plagiocephaly	- Head asymmetry from pressure on head from prolonged sleeping position - Tx: Change positioning

Neonatology

Neonatal Skin Rashes

Condition	Features	Management
Congenital Melanocytic Nevus	- Large benign moles - Low rate of malignant transformation, but monitor closely	- Monitor - Biopsy if suspicious
Congenital Dermal Melanocytosis	- "**Mongolian Spot**[A]" - Hyperpigmented, congenital blue-grey patches over low back - Benign, fades spontaneously over first few years of life	- Monitor, document well
Nevus Sebaceous	- Overgrown epidermis/hair follicles - Presents with smooth, yellow, hairless patch, oval in shape - Scalp most common location	- Monitor, usually benign
Aplasia Cutis Congenita	- Congenital lesion of abnormal skin development - Presents with erosion/ulcerative lesion - Scalp most common, but can occur anywhere	- Wound care or surgical closure
Nevus Simplex	- "**Stork Bite**[B]." Common neonatal finding. - Benign vascular proliferation found on glabella, neck, eyelid - Presents as blanchable, pink-red patches	- Fades within years
Nevus Flammeus	- "**Port wine stain**" vascular malformation - Associated with Sturge-Weber (if in V1 formation)	- Grows with child
Erythema Toxicum Neonatorum	- Scattered erythematous papules, pustules throughout the body	- No treatment - Resolves within days
Neonatal Acne	- Inflammatory papules/pustules on face	- No treatment - Resolves within days
Seborrheic Dermatitis	- Yellow, erythematous, greasy plaques - Can appear on scalp ("**cradle cap**"), face, body	- Mild: Reassurance, emollients - Severe: Ketaconazole shampoo, topical corticosteroids
Miliaria (Heat Rash)	- Blockage of sweat ducts, causing small papules on head/upper torso	- Resolves with cooling/ avoiding excess clothes
Neonatal HSV	- Clusters of vesicles on skin and mucous membranes - CNS, organ system involvement possible	- Acyclovir

Neonatal Conjunctivitis (ophthalmia neonatorum)

Type	Clinical	Management
Chemical	- Conjunctivitis from ointments used for bacterial conjunctivitis PPX - Commonly due to silver nitrate (no longer used in US)	- Self-limited - Lubricant eye drops
Gonococcal	- Within 2-5 days of birth - Severe exudates/swelling of eyelids[C], corneal edema/ulceration - Dx: Gram stain/culture	- IM ceftriaxone - Eye irrigation
Chlamydial	- Presents at 5-14 days post birth - Watery/ mucopurulent eye discharge	- PO erythromycin
HSV	- Presents at 5-14 days - Unilateral serous discharge	- Acyclovir

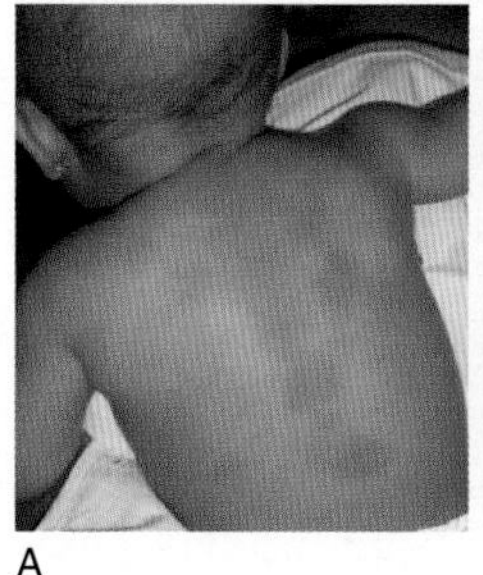
A

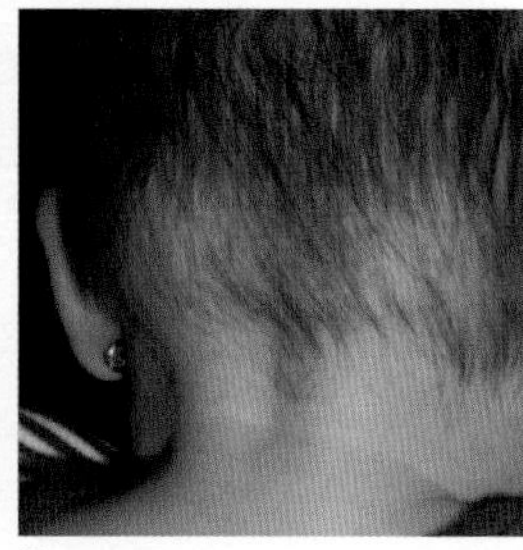
B

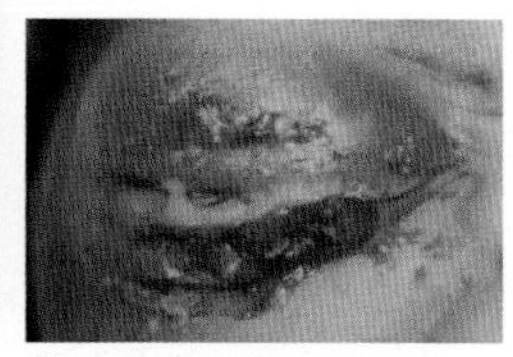
C

Neonatology

Germinal Matrix Hemorrhage/Intraventricular Hemorrhage

General: Germinal matrix hemorrhage due to vascular fragility in premature babies

Risk: **Prematurity**, low birth weight, respiratory distress/neonatal resuscitation

Clinical: Can be clinically silent, or result in **altered level of consciousness, hypotonia, seizures, coma**

Diagnosis: Cranial US

Management:
- Purely supportive (maintain proper hemodynamic status, correct fluid/electrolytes, proper nutrition)
- Monitor for complications with serial US

Complications:
- Ventricular dilation:
    - May result in ↑ ICP and further neurologic damage
    - Tx: Serial lumbar punctures or ventricular drain

Respiratory Failure

	General	Clinical	Management
Neonatal Respiratory Distress Syndrome	- Diffuse atelectasis from insufficient quantity of **surfactant** - Risk: Prematurity, C-section, maternal diabetes	- Severe respiratory distress and cyanosis - CXR (diffuse ground glass, low lung volumes) - Complications: PDA, bronchopulmonary dysplasia	- Supplemental O_2 (+ CPAP or intubation if needed) - Surfactant - PPX: [See: OBGYN]
Transient Tachypnea of Newborn	- Mild **pulmonary edema** from failed alveolar fluid clearance at birth - Risk: Prematurity, C-section, maternal diabetes	- Tachypnea starting at birth, and improving within days - CXR shows bilateral perihilar linear streaks	- Supportive - Supplemental O_2 (+ CPAP or intubation) as needed
Persistent Pulmonary Hypertension	- Right-to-left shunt from persistently **elevated pulmonary pressures** post birth - Risk: Meconium aspiration, perinatal asphyxia	- Tachypnea and cyanosis - CXR (clear lungs, possible ↓ pulmonary vasculature)	- Supportive care - 100% O_2 (helps to ↓ PVR) - If severe: inhaled NO, Sildenafil, or ECMO
Meconium Aspiration	- **Aspiration of meconium-stained amniotic fluid**	- Diagnosis of exclusion - Respiratory distress, tachypnea - Trachea may have meconium - CXR (patchy densities and areas of hyperinflation)	- Avoid suctioning, intubation immediately after birth - Supplemental O_2 - Antibiotics
Apnea of Prematurity	- **Periods of apnea** in premature neonate from immaturely developed respiratory drive or airway obstruction	- Cessation of breathing > 20 seconds OR - Shorter period of apnea that causes hypoxemia or bradycardia	- Supportive care - CPAP therapy - Methylxanthine (caffeine)

Neonatology

Hypoglycemia

General: Blood sugar < 50-60 mg/dL

Risk: Preterm infant, fetal growth restriction, maternal diabetes. Fetal macrosomia.

Clinical:

- Often asymptomatic
- Can manifest as **jitteriness**, irritability, poor tone, lethargy, poor suck/feed, seizures

Management:

- Oral feedings (if asymptomatic/not severe)
- Parenteral glucose (if symptomatic/severe)

Polycythemia

General: Hematocrit > 65%

Risk: Delayed cord clamping, twin-to-twin transfusion, maternal diabetes. Fetal macrosomia.

Clinical: Often asymptomatic

- **Plethora**
- Possible lethargy, poor feeding
- Hyperviscosity symptoms
- Associated with hypoglycemia

Management:

- IV hydration/glucose
- Partial exchange transfusion: Reserved for severe or progressive symptoms

Neonatal Sepsis

General: Systemic signs of infection plus isolation of a bacteria from blood. Most commonly due to group B *Strep* and *E. Coli.*

Risk: Chorioamnionitis, prematurity, prolonged rupture of membranes

Clinical:

- **Fever, respiratory distress, tachycardia**
- Poor feeding, lethargy, irritability
- Highly associated with low Apgar score (< 6)

Diagnosis: Blood, urine, and CSF cultures

Management: Empiric antibiotics (ampicillin and gentamicin)

Pediatric Vaccinations

Vaccine	Birth	1 mo	2 mos	4 mos	6 mos	9 mos	12 mos	15 mos	18 mos	19–23 mos	2–3 yrs	4–6 yrs	7–10 yrs	11–12 yrs	13–15 yrs	16 yrs	17–18 yrs
Hepatitis B (HepB)	1st dose	← 2nd dose →					← 3rd dose →										
Rotavirus (RV): RV1 (2-dose series), RV5 (3-dose series)			1st dose	2nd dose	See Notes												
Diphtheria, tetanus, acellular pertussis (DTaP <7 yrs)			1st dose	2nd dose	3rd dose			← 4th dose →				5th dose					
Haemophilus influenzae type b (Hib)			1st dose	2nd dose	See Notes		← 3rd or 4th dose, See Notes →										
Pneumococcal conjugate (PCV13)			1st dose	2nd dose	3rd dose		← 4th dose →										
Inactivated poliovirus (IPV <18 yrs)			1st dose	2nd dose			← 3rd dose →					4th dose					
Influenza (IIV4)							Annual vaccination 1 or 2 doses								Annual vaccination 1 dose only		
or													or				
Influenza (LAIV4)											Annual vaccination 1 or 2 doses				Annual vaccination 1 dose only		
Measles, mumps, rubella (MMR)					See Notes		← 1st dose →					2nd dose					
Varicella (VAR)							← 1st dose →					2nd dose					
Hepatitis A (HepA)					See Notes			2-dose series, See Notes									
Tetanus, diphtheria, acellular pertussis (Tdap ≥7 yrs)														1 dose			
Human papillomavirus (HPV)														See Notes			
Meningococcal (MenACWY-D ≥9 mos, MenACWY-CRM ≥2 mos, MenACWY-TT ≥2years)								See Notes						1st dose		2nd dose	
Meningococcal B (MenB-4C, MenB-FHbp)															See Notes		
Pneumococcal polysaccharide (PPSV23)														See Notes			

Types of Vaccines:

- Live, attenuated Virus (e.g., MMR, varicella)
  - Weakened viral vaccine
  - Contraindications: Immunocompromised, pregnancy
- Killed, inactivated virus (e.g., influenza, hepatitis A)
  - Completely inactivated viral vaccine
- Conjugate (e.g., HiB)
  - Bacterial polysaccharide conjugated to a protein
- Toxoid (e.g., Tdap)
  - Modified protein toxin

Contraindications/Precautions:

Contraindications (do not give vaccine in future)	**Precautions** (defer vaccines until the condition is improved)
- Anaphylaxis after prior administration - Severe immunodeficiency → No live vaccines - Pregnancy → No live vaccines - Encephalopathy within 7 days (pertussis-containing vax) - Intussusception, SCID (rota vax)	- Moderate or severe acute illness, +/− fever (defer vaccines until resolution) - MMR/VZV: IVIG within year prior to administration (may prevent proper immune response to vaccine) - DTap/Tdap: Progressive neurologic disorder (infantile spasms, epilepsy, progressive encephalopathy) → Defer until neurologic condition stabilized

Developmental Milestones

	Motor	Social	Cognitive	Communication
2 M	- Lifts head	- Social smile	- Recognizes parent	
4 M	- Holds head w/o support - Grasps toy if placed in hand	- Chuckles	- Opens mouth for bottle/breast	- Cooing
6 M	- Rolls over - Puts things in mouth	- Knows familiar people - Laughs	- Puts things in mouth - Reaches for toys	- Squealing noises
9 M	- Sits without support - Transfers objects	- Stranger anxiety - Laughs with peek-a-boo	- Separation anxiety - Object permanence	- Says "mamamama," "bababa"
12 M	- Stands/begins to walk	- Plays pat-a-cake	- Puts object in container	- Says mama and dada - Waves bye
15 M	- Few steps on own	- Shows affection - Copies others while playing	- Stacks two objects	- Follows basic command (with voice/gesture)
18 M	- Walks independently - Scribbles	- Points to something interesting	- Copies you doing chores	- > 3-word vocab
2 Y	- Runs - Kicks a ball	- Notices if others hurt/upset	- Plays with > 1 toy at same time	- 2-word combo (e.g. "more milk")
3 Y	- Uses fork - Clothes self	- Sees other children, joins to play	- Draws circle	- Basic conversation - Usually intelligible
4 Y	- Catches large ball - Serves self food/water	- Avoids danger - Likes to be a "helper"	- Names color of a few items - Draws person with > 3 parts	- ≥ 4 word sentences
5 Y	- Skips/hops	- Follows rules - Sings, dances, or acts	- Counts to 10 - Names some letters	- Tells simple story

* Based on updated 2022 CDC/AAP guidelines

Primitive Reflexes

	Description	Disappears by
Hand grasp	- Reflex grasp of object placed in palm	3M
Sucking	- When roof of mouth is touched	4M
Moro	- Abduction/extension of arms after startle	4M
Rooting	- Turn head toward side of cheek stimulus	6M
Galant	- Stroke spine, causing baby to laterally flex torso toward side of stimulus	9M
Plantar	- Dorsiflexion of foot and flexion of toes with plantar stimulation	12M

Screening

General: Based on American Academy of Pediatrics (AAP) Bright Futures screening guidelines. Selected tests include:

Test	Timing/Frequency	Details
Iron Deficiency (CBC)	- 1 y/o - Risk factors: Low birth weight, drinks lots of cows milk	
Lead	- Blood screen: 1 years, 2 years - Risk assessment: 6, 9, 12, 18, 24 months	- Screening should be adjusted to location (CDC recommendations)
Developmental Screen	- 9, 18, 30 months	- Variety of questionnaires, such as Parents Evaluation of Developmental Status
Autism Screen	- 18, 24 months	- MCT-RF
Hearing	- Start at 4 y/o	- Tone audiology, tympanometry
Vision	- Start at 3 y/o	- Test for strabismus - Test for visual acuity (as soon as child old enough to perform test)
Oral Health	- Referral to a dental home at 1 y/o	
Tuberculosis	- Risk assessment: 6, 12 months, then annually - Targeted screening if risk factors present (TST)	
Lipids	- Once 9-11 y/o - Once 17-21 y/o	
Hypertension	- Annual BP	
Drug/Alcohol	- Annually starting at 11 years	- CRAFFT screen
Depression	- Annually starting at 12 years	
Anxiety	- Screen in individuals between ages 8 and 18 y/o	
STD	- Chlamydia/gonorrhea: Annually screen sexually active females < 25 y/o - HIV: One time screen (after age 15 y/o)	

Anticipatory Guidance

General: Based on American Academy of Pediatrics (AAP) Bright Futures guidelines. Informs parents on expected growth and development, recommends safety measures.

Topic	Advice
Weight	- Infants can lose up to 10% of weight in first few days of life, but should **regain birth weight by 2 weeks** - Infants double birth weight by 4M and triple birth weight by 1Y - Infants gain ~20-30 g per day - Gain about 2 kg (4-5 lb)/yr after this
Height	- Height increases 50% by 1 year, doubles by 4 years, triples by 13 years - Height growth velocity varies, but is **~2-4 inches/year between 1 and 10 years**, progressively slowing as pubertal growth spurt approaches
Diet	- Feed infants every 2-4 hours (8-12 times/day), ~15 minnutes per breast - Supplement vitamin D if breastfeeding - Energy requirement 100 kcal/kg/day (which should be more if premature or low birth weight) - Introduce **iron-fortified cereals ~6 months** and slowly add other solid foods - Switch to whole milk (~12 months) - Encourage healthy food choices, avoiding sweets. Limit juice to < 5 oz due to risk of dental caries.
Dental	- Teeth erupt around 6 months and onwards - See dentist within 6 months of first tooth eruption - Ensure proper fluoride (usually tap water sufficient, but depends on area) - Start brushing teeth once they emerge
Bowel Movements	- Over first week, stool transitions from meconium, to yellow/seedy, and eventually more brown - 4/day during the first week, 2/day by 1 year, and 1/day by 4 years
Urine	- For first week, # of wet diapers should be about the age of child in days - **After first week, ≥ 4 wet diapers/day** - Can start toilet training around 18 months, usually successful by 3-4 y/o
Sleeping	- Initially sleep 3-4-hour stretches for 18-20 hours per day - As child gets older, they sleep less overall and for longer stretches - Many sleep through night by 6 months - 1-2 naps/day normal in years 1-4
Car Seats	**< 2 years: Rear-facing car seat (in rear)** 2-4 years: Forward facing car seat (in rear) 4-8 years: Belt-positioning booster seat (until reach 4'9" tall) < 12 years: Should ride in rear seats
Safety	Infant: - Sleep on back, hot water heater < 120°F, avoid objects that can be aspirated - Weapons and pet safety - Sunscreen 1 y/o - Childproof house 3 y/o - Helmets, street safety, stranger danger, water safety/swimming lessons

Anticipatory Guidance

Misc. Infant/Toddler Problems

Diaper Rash	- Irritant contact dermatitis from constant contact with diaper - Involves anywhere, but spares skin folds (if impacts folds, concern for *Candida*) - Tx: Topical barrier ointments (petrolatum, zinc oxide), topical steroids if severe
Breath Holding Spells	- Involuntary, harmless breath holding events - Toddler can become cyanotic or pallid (pale/limp) - Reassurance
Temper Tantrum	- Angry outbursts from fatigue or frustration - Decrease as child gets older
School Phobia	- Vague physical complaints only prior to school

Adolescents: Puberty

Puberty (Females)

- Girls start puberty between 8 and 13 y/o
  - Breast buds appear (age 10-11 years)
  - Pubic hair appears (age 10-11 years)
  - Growth spurt (age 12 years)
  - Menarche (age 12-13 years)
  - Attainment of adult height (age 15 years)

Tanner	Breast	Pubic Hair
1	Elevation of papilla	None
2	Breast bud (elevation of breast/papilla)	Sparse hair along labia
3	Further growth in breast/papilla	Darker hair grows along labia
4	Projection of breast/papilla (secondary mound)	Coarse, curly hair covering symphysis pubis
5	Normal adult contour	Adult hair extends to medial thigh

Puberty (Males)

- Boys start puberty between 10 and 15 y/o
  - Growth of testicles (age 12 years)
  - Pubic hair appears (age 12 years)
  - Growth of penis, scrotum (age 13-14 years)
  - First ejaculations (age 13-14 years)
  - Growth spurt (age 14 years)
  - Attainment of adult height (age 17 years)

Tanner	Phallus	Pubic Hair
1	Prepubertal testes	None
2	Testes start to enlarge	Sparse, long
3	Testes continue to enlarge Penis length increases	Some dark, coarse, curly hair
4	Penis length/width further increases	Dark coarse curly hair of symphysis pubis
5	Adult sized testes/penis	Dark coarse curly hair extending to medial thigh

Anticipatory Guidance

Adolescents: Guidance/Screening

Early adolescence (10-13 y/o)	- Starts to desire independence from family - Preoccupation with pubertal changes - Risk-taking behaviors
Middle adolescence (13-18 y/o)	- Conflicts with family - Preoccupation with physical appearance/presentation - Peer-group involvement, begins romantic relationships
Late adolescence (18-21 y/o)	- Development of self separate from parents - Comfortable with body image

Screening (also see the screening/vaccination charts):

Social Hx	HEADSSS (home, education, activities, drugs, sex, suicide, safety)
Drugs/EtOH	CRAFT - Have you ever ridden in a CAR driven by someone (including yourself) who was "high" or had been using alcohol or drugs? - Do you ever use alcohol or drugs to RELAX, feel better about yourself, or fit in? - Do you ever use alcohol/drugs while you are by yourself, ALONE? - Do you ever FORGET things you did while using alcohol or drugs? - Have you gotten into TROUBLE while you were using alcohol or drugs?
Confidentiality	- Important to create rapport with adolescents, and keep most discussions confidential from parents - **Includes**: Pregnancy, birth control, mental health, drugs/EtOH - **Excludes**: Abuse (sexual/physical), suicidal/homicidal ideation

Minors/Consent

General: For minors (age < 18), only parents can provide consent

- Exceptions:
    - Emergencies
    - Emancipated minors (married, military, living separately from parents)
    - Special circumstances (treatment of STIs, contraceptives, prenatal care)

Growth Disturbances

Failure to Thrive

General: Abnormal weight gain in first 2 years of life. No definitive definition, but considered when weight < 2nd percentile, weight falls more than 2 lines on growth curve, or weight gain is less than linear growth velocity.

	Organic	Non-organic
Definition	- Acute/chronic medical disorder - Have signs/symptoms associated with medical condition	- No underlying disease or disorder - Due to malnutrition for caregiver neglect, stress, or lack of parenting skills
Etiologies	- Cystic fibrosis - Congenital heart defects - Chronic vomiting (e.g., bowel obstruction or GERD) - HIV - CNS (cerebral palsy, hydrocephalus)	- Poverty - Poor feeding techniques - Inadequate breast milk or formula

Diagnosis: Clinical diagnosis based on definition provided above

Management:
- Interdisciplinary care (nutritionist, OT, speech therapy, social worker)
- Nutritional catch-up: Calculate daily energy requirement, provide enough calories to overcome this level
    - High calorie formulas for infants, high calorie additions for those eating solid foods
- Hospitalization for severe cases

Differential for Microcephaly

General: Occipitofrontal circumference < 2 SD below mean for age

Etiology:

Congenital	Acquired
- TORCH infections - Teratogen exposure (EtOH) - Trisomy 13, 18, 21	- Late pregnancy infections - Meningitis - Ischemic brain insults - Metabolic (hypothyroidism)

Clinical: Associated with small brain size
- Often occurs with intellectual disability, developmental delay, cerebral palsy

Differential for Macrocephaly

General: Occipitofrontal circumference > 2 SD above mean for age

Etiology:
- Increased brain size: Anatomic or familial megalencephaly
- Increased CSF: Hydrocephalus
- Hemorrhage, mass lesions

Clinical: Workup if single measurement > 2 SD OR cross multiple lines on the head circumference growth curve

Diagnosis: Ultrasound (for infants with open fontanelle), otherwise MRI

Management: Treat underlying condition

SIDS/Child Abuse

Sudden Infant Death Syndrome (SIDS)

General: Sudden death of infant < 1 y/o, with no clear underlying cause after thorough autopsy and evaluation. Pathophysiology unknown. **Most common cause of death between 1M and 1Y.**

Risk Factor	Prevention
- Smoking (in household) during/after pregnancy	- Smoke avoidance
- Prone/side sleep position	- Supine sleeping
- Soft sleep surface with loose bedding	- Firm surface, without extra blankets/pillows
- Bed sharing	- Avoid bed sharing
Other: - Maternal age < 20 - Prematurity - Sibling who died from SIDS	Other: - Use pacifier

Clinical: Often no signs, but can have evidence of terminal event like bloody froth in mouth, clenched fists

Child Abuse

General: Physical injury inflicted on a child by a caretaker

Risk: Single/young parents, low parental education, parental substance use

Clinical:

- Bruises (in pre mobile infant, located on butt/back, in pattern of striking object)
- Oral injuries
- Burns (if well-demarcated, appear due to immersion injury[A])
- Fractures:
    - Multiple fractures in different healing stages
    - Most commonly ribs/sternum, metaphyseal corner, bilateral long bone, skull
- Head trauma:
    - Retinal hemorrhages
    - Skull fractures
    - Bulging fontanelles
    - Encephalopathy
- Suspect if:
    - **Inconsistent stories from caregiver**
    - Story is out of proportion with injury, vague history

Diagnosis:

- Skeletal survey
- Head CT (if head trauma suspected)

Management:

- Remove from caregiver's care
- Contact appropriate authorities (must be reported to protective services -- **doctors are mandated reporters**)
- Manage patient's injuries

Colic/Pediatric Constipation

Colic

General: Crying for no clear reason, lasting for ≥ 3 hr/day and occurring on ≥ 3 days/week, in healthy infant < 3 months old

Clinical:

- Paroxysmal episodes of crying
- Compared to normal crying, colic is higher pitched, louder, and involves clenched fists and facial flushing
- Normal physical examination/developmental history

Management:

- Most often improves as child gets older
- Provide parental support
- Soothing techniques (pacifier, rocking baby, rubbing tummy)
- Feeding techniques (fix underfeeding/overfeeding, inadequate burping)

Differential:

Normal crying	- Intermittent, < 2 hr/day - Generally consolable with soothing methods

Pediatric Constipation

General: Common primary care presentation in preschool-aged children

Risk: Excess cow's milk, newly introduced solid foods, toilet training, school entry

Clinical:

- Painful, firm/small bowel movements
- Refusal to defecate, with eventual encopresis possible
- Can be complicated by anal fissure, hemorrhoid, or UTIs

Management:

- Increase fiber intake, increase water intake, minimize cow's milk to < 24 oz
- Laxatives (polyethylene glycol or lactulose)
- Suppositories/enemas if necessary

Growing Pains

General: Pain that wakes child at night, not associated with musculoskeletal disease

Clinical: Bilateral pain in thighs or calves that occurs at night, resolves in morning

Management:

- Education/reassurance
- Stretching, massage, heat, analgesics

Chromosomal Abnormalities

	General/Clinical	Management
Trisomy 13 (Patau)	- **Microphthalmia, cleft lip/palate, polydactyly** - Holoprosencephaly, severe intellectual deficits - Cardiovascular defects (ASD/VSD/PDA) - Umbilical hernia, omphalocele	Dx: Karyotype (alt: FISH) Tx: None. Most die within days to weeks after birth.
Trisomy 18 (Edwards)	- **Micrognathia, low-set ears, prominent occiput** - Clenched fists with overlapping fingers - Cardiovascular defects (VSD, PDA) - Renal (horseshoe kidney) - GI (Meckels diverticulum and malrotation)	Dx: Karyotype (alt: FISH) Tx: None. Most die within 1 year (those that survive have severe intellectual defects).
Trisomy 21 (Downs)	- 95% meiotic nondisjunction, 4% Robertsonian translocation <u>Dysmophic features</u>: - **Upslanting palpebral fissures**, small ears, flattened midface - **Epicanthal folds**, redundant nuchal skin - Brushfield spots, protruding tongue, single palmar crease[A], gap between first two toes - CNS: **Intellectual disability**, hypotonia, early-onset dementia - CV: Complete AV septal defect, ASD, VSD - GI: Duodenal atresia, imperforate anus, esophageal atresia - Endo: Hypothyroidism, short stature, obesity, T1DM - Heme: ↑ risk ALL/AML - Atlantoaxial instability	Dx: Karyotype (alt: FISH) Tx: - Monitor for complications (screen patient with CBC, TSH, TTE, hearing/vision tests, cervical MRI) - Life expectancy reduced

Turner (XO)	- Partial or full loss of X chromosome (from paternal nondisjunction, mosaicism, or partial X)
	
	- Short stature, shield chest, widely spaced nipples, webbed neck, cubitus valgus, cystic hygroma/lymphedema
	- Primary hypogonadism (amenorrhea, lack of puberty)
	- <u>Cardiovascular</u>
	  - **Bicuspid aortic valve, aortic coarctation**
	  - High risk for aortic dissection, especially during pregnancy
	- Endocrine (obesity, osteoporosis, insulin resistance, hypothyroidism)
	- Risk for gonadoblastoma (if Y chromosome present)
	- Generally infertile, can become pregnant with IVF/donor eggs
		Dx: Karyotype
		
		Tx:
		- GH replacement during childhood
		- Estradiol therapy (~11-12 y/o to initiate puberty)
		- OCPs in adults
		
		- Screen for common complications (TTE and monitoring for cardiovascular disease)

Klinefelter (47 XXY)	- Due to nondisjunction of sex chromosomes - **Micropenis and small, firm testes** - Subnormal sperm count/infertility - ↓ testosterone, ↑ FSH/LH - Gynecomastia, female hair distribution - Eunuchoid body shape, abnormally tall with long arms/legs - Psychosocially abnormal	Dx: Karyotype
XXX	- Generally normal, with increased likelihood of being tall, and average IQ less than normal	Dx: Karyotype
XYY	- Tall stature, mild intellectual disability, developmental delays	Dx: Karyotype

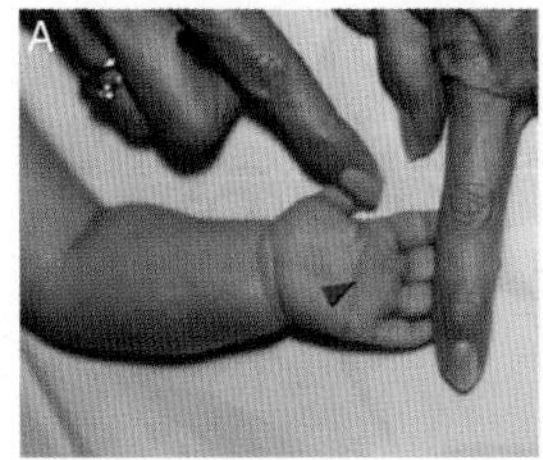

Genetics

	General/Clinical	Management
Fragile X	- FMR1 (CGG repeats→↑ FMR methylation→↓ gene expression) - **Long face, prominent forehead, large ears, macroorchidism** - Moderate intellectual disability - Behavioral abnormalities (ADHD, stereotyped movements) - Girls can be asymptomatic or have mild intellectual disability	Dx: Clinical + genetic testing Tx: Multidisciplinary management of behavioral and cognitive problems
Rett's	- XD disease females in the MECP gene - Normal initial development, followed by **progressive loss of speech and motor skills** starting around 1-2 y/o - Stereotypical hand movements, seizures, autism	Dx: Clinical + genetic testing Tx: Multidisciplinary supportive care
Lesch-Nyhan	- XR HGPRT enzyme deficiency (defective purine metabolism) - Onset at 6 months of hypotonia, developmental delay - Later: Intellectual disability, choreoathetosis, spasticity, **compulsive self injury**, other behavioral abnormalities - Uric acid deposition (gouty arthritis, tophi, nephrolithiasis) - Uric acid "sand-like" crystals in diapers	Dx: Clinical + genetic testing Tx: Allopurinol
Ehlers-Danlos	- AR or AD defects in **collagen synthesis** - Depending on subtype, combination of skin hyperextensibility, joint hypermobility, joint dislocations, scoliosis, poor wound healing, easy bruising, vascular dissection/dilatation - Type I/II (classic, MSK/skin symptoms) - Type III (mostly MSK) - Type IV (high risk for vascular problems, MSK normal)	Dx: Clinical + genetic testing Tx: Supportive care/monitor for complications
Marfan	- AD defect in fibrillin-1 - Cardiovascular: **Aortic dissection/aneurysm**, MVP - **Ectopic lens** - MSK: Joint hypermobility, arachnodactyly, long arms/legs, pectus deformity, kyphosis/scoliosis - Pulm: Lung bullae/spontaneous pneumothorax	Dx: Clinical + genetic testing Tx: - Aortic dilatation: Monitor with TTE, add beta-blocker/ARB, surgery if severely enlarged
Menkes	- XR defect in ATP7A, leading to severe copper deficiency - Brittle kinky hair, growth retardation, hypotonia, epilepsy, progressive neurodegeneration	Tx: Administer Cu
Osteogenesis Imperfecta	- AD defect in COL1A gene - **Bone abnormalities**: Can range from mild (premature osteoporosis/bone loss) to severe (atraumatic fractures) - Other features: Blue sclera[A], short stature, scoliosis, hearing loss, opalescent teeth, easy bruising - Multiple subtypes: Type I (mild), type II (severe/fetal demise), types III-VI (moderate symptoms)	Dx: Clinical + genetic testing Tx: - Multidisciplinary care - Monitor for complications - Bisphosphonates

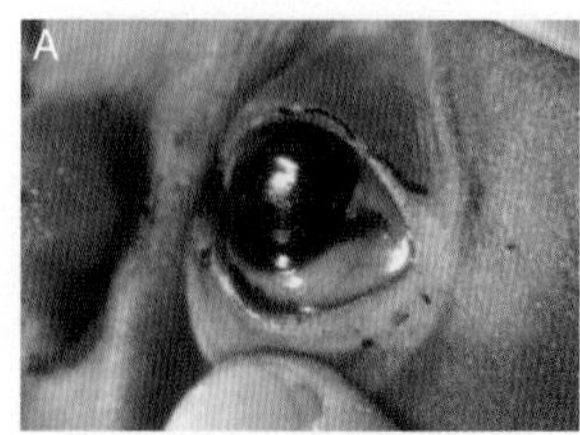

Genetics

	General/Clinical	Management
Xeroderma Pigmentosum	- AR abnormality in repair of pyrimidine dimers from UV light - **Risk for skin cancer** (childhood SCC, BCC, and melanoma) - Keratitis, hypo/hyperpigmentation, opacification of the cornea	Dx: Clinical + genetic testing Tx: Avoid sunlight exposure
Primary Ciliary Dyskinesia (Kartagener)	- AR defect in dynein arms → abnormal ciliary movement - **Chronic rhinosinusitis, bronchiectasis, cough** - Recurrent otitis media - Infertility: Immotile sperm, dysfunctional fallopian tubes - Situs inversus - Screening test: Low nasal NO	Dx: Electron microscopy (showing ciliary dysfunction) Tx: Chest physiotherapy, surgical intervention for advanced disease
McCune Albright	- Sporadic, postzygotic mutation in GNAS gene - **Fibrous dysplasia of bone** - **Multiple café-au lait spots** - **Precocious puberty** - Endocrine: Hyperthyroidism, GH secretion, hypercortisolism	Dx: Clinical + genetic testing Tx: Aromatase inhibitors (letrozole) to prevent precocious puberty
Noonan Syndrome	- Heterogenous AD disorder due to defects in Ras-MAPk - **Short stature** and **congenital heart defects** (pulmonic stenosis) - Facial dysmorphia	Dx: Clinical + genetic testing Tx: Fairly good prognosis for most
Prader-Willi	- Deletion of paternal 15q11-13 or maternal uniparental disomy - **Hypotonia** (earliest sign during infancy) - Obesity, hyperphagia, binge eating - Intellectual disability, hypogonadism, short stature	Dx: Clinical + genetic testing Tx: GH therapy, attempt to prevent weight gain
Angelman	- Deletion of maternal 15q11-13 or paternal uniparental disomy - **Severe intellectual disability**, ataxia, seizures - Frequent smiling/laughing behavior, with hand flapping	Dx: Clinical + genetic testing Tx: Interdisciplinary care, management of complications (e.g., seizures)
Cri-du-chat	- 5p microdeletion - **High-pitched mewing**, hypotonia, microcephaly, intellectual disability, facial dysmorphia	Dx: Clinical + genetic testing
Williams	- 7q microdeletion (includes elastin gene) - **Elfin facies** (wide mouth, small jaw, long philtrum) - Intellectual disability, but good verbal skills/**friendliness** - **Supravalvular aortic stenosis**, renal artery stenosis - Hypercalcemia	Dx: Clinical + genetic testing
DiGeorge Syndrome	- 22q11 microdeletion, causing 3rd/4th branchial arch defects - Thymus/parathyroid hypoplasia (↑ infection risk, hypoCa) - Conotruncal cardiac defects - Facial dysmorphia (cleft lip/palate)	Dx: Clinical (↓ T-cells, cardiac disease) + genetic testing Tx: - Thymic transplantation or HCT - Treat hypocalcemia, cardiac disease

Genetics

	General/Clinical	Management
Glycogen Storage Disease (all AR)		
Type I von Gierke	- Glucose-6-phosphatase deficiency - **Hypoglycemia** (months after birth), lactic acidosis, seizures - Hyperuricemia and hypertriglyceridemia - Thin upper extremities, doll-like face, **hepatosplenomegaly**	Dx: Genetic testing Tx: Maintain glucose levels (cornstarch, commercial glucose polymers)
Type II Pompe	- Lysosomal acid alpha-1,4-glucosidase deficiency - Hypertrophic **cardiomyopathy, hypotonia**, weakness - Death during infancy (in "classic" form)	Dx: Genetic testing Tx: Enzyme replacement therapy
Type III Cori	- 1,6 glucosidase (glycogen debrancher) deficiency - **Hypoglycemia, hepatomegaly**, hypotonia, failure to thrive - Muscle weakness - Normal lactate (vs type I) - Limit dextrans accumulation	Dx: Genetic testing Tx: Maintain glucose levels (cornstarch, commercial glucose polymers)
Type V McArdle	- Glycogen phosphorylase deficiency - Painful **muscle cramps**, myoglobinuria, **exercise intolerance**, presenting in early adolescence - Normal blood glucose and lactate - Second wind phenomenon (due to ↑ muscular blood flow)	Dx: Genetic testing Tx: Pre-exercise carbohydrate loading
Carbohydrate Intolerance Disorders		
Essential Fructosuria	- AR Fructokinase deficiency - Benign condition with fructose found in blood and urine	Dx: (+) urinary reducing sugar test Tx: Benign, none required
Fructose Intolerance	- AR Aldolase B deficiency (Fructose 1-P accumulates in cells, using up intracellular phosphate), resulting in inhibition of glycogenolysis and gluconeogenesis - **Hypoglycemia, emesis following fructose consumption** - Liver failure, failure to thrive - Often appear normal, until new fructose-containing foods introduced to diet	Dx:(+) urinary reducing sugar test, confirm with genetics Tx: Dietary modification (avoid fructose/ sucrose)
Galactokinase Deficiency	- AR galactokinase deficiency - Causes development of **infantile cataracts**	Tx: Treat cataracts, dietary modification
Classic Galactosemia	- AR defect in galactose-1-P uridylyltransferase deficiency - Presents with **infantile cataracts**, hepatomegaly/jaundice, failure to thrive, intellectual disability, ↑ risk for sepsis	Dx: Enzyme activity assay, genetic testing Tx: Dietary modification (avoid galactose)
Urea Cycle Disorders		
Ornithine Transcar-bamylase Deficiency	- XR defect in key urea cycle enzyme - After protein intake, infant develops emesis, lethargy, poor feeding - ↑ Orotic acid, ornithine. ↓ citrulline.	Dx: Clinical + genetic testing

Genetics

	General/Clinical	Management
Amino Acid Disorders		
Phenylketonuria	- AR phenylalanine hydroxylase deficiency (rarely from BH4 deficiency which is an essential cofactor) - **Intellectual disability**, epilepsy, ataxia - Fair complexion, eczema, **"mousy" body odor** - Maternal PKU: If not controlled during pregnancy, infant will suffer from intellectual disability, growth restriction	Dx: ↑ phenylalanine concentration, confirm with genetic testing Tx: Dietary restriction of phenylalanine, enzyme replacement therapy Note: If controlled/recognized early, patients have good prognosis
Maple Syrup Urine	- AR defect in branched-chain ketoacid break down - Within days of birth, develop ketonuria, vomiting, poor feeding, lethargy - Later develop intellectual disability, delayed growth	Dx: ↑ plasma/urine branched AA (leucine, isoleucine, and valine), confirm with genetic testing Tx: Dietary (restrict branched-chain AA), give thiamine
Alkaptonuria	- AR defect in homogentisic acid dioxygenase (part of the degradation pathway of tyrosine) - **Ochronosis**: Black pigment deposition in connective tissues - Urine turns black after long exposure to air	Dx: ↑ HGA in urine/plasma Tx: Dietary (restrict tyrosine)
Homocystinuria	- AR deficiency in cystathionine synthase or methionine synthase - **Marfanoid** body habitus, **ectopic lens** (downward dislocation) - Intellectual disability - **Thrombosis/atherosclerosis**	Dx: Urine/blood homocysteine levels Tx: - Mild: B6 supplementation (+ B9/B12) - Antiplatelets/anticoagulation
Mitochondrial Disorders (maternally inherited mitochondrial DNA conditions)		
MELAS	- Mitochondrial encephalomyopathy with lactic acidosis and stroke-like episodes (results in hemiparesis, hemianopia)	Dx: Mitochondrial DNA testing Tx: Supportive
MERRF	- Myoclonic epilepsy with ragged red fibers - Myoclonus, followed by epilepsy, myopathy, ataxia	
Peroxisomal Disorders		
Zellweger Spectrum	- Includes Zellweger, infantile refsum, and neonatal adrenoleukodystrophy, which are all disorders of abnormal peroxisome biogenesis, with resulting accumulation of very-long chain fatty acids - Causes abnormal CNS development, hypomyelination	- Poor prognosis
Fatty Acid Disorders		
Oxidation Disorders	- Defects in fatty acid oxidation, including AR medium-chain acyl-CoA dehydrogenase deficiency, AR very-long-chain acyl-CoA dehydrogenase deficiency - Presents during infancy or early childhood, with **hypoketotic hypoglycemia** (especially after fasting), ↑ ammonia (decreased urea cycle function)	Dx: Clinical + genetic testing Tx: - Fat-restricted diets - Avoidance of prolonged fasts
Carnitine Deficiency	- Variety of AR mutations in carnitine transport - Toxic accumulation of LCFA in the blood - Causes weakness, severe hypoketotic hypoglycemia, hyperammonemia, cardiomyopathy	Tx: - Fat-restricted diets - Avoidance of prolonged fasts - Carnitine supplementation

Genetics

Lysosomal Storage Disorders

	Enzyme Deficient [substrate accumulates]	Clinical Features	Management/Prognosis
Sphingolipidoses			
Fabry	XR alpha galactosidase A (globotriaosylceramide)	- Slowly progressive painful neuropathy, anhidrosis, angiokeratomas, hypertrophic cardiomyopathy, CKD	- Enzyme replacement therapy - Lives into adulthood
Gaucher	AR glucocerebrosidase (glucocerebroside)	- Hepatosplenomegaly, pancytopenia - Bone: Osteoporosis, avascular necrosis, bone pain	- Enzyme replacement therapy - Can live into adulthood
Niemann-Pick	AR sphingomyelinase (sphingomyelin)	- Progressive neurodegeneration, loss of motor milestones, hypotonia, "cherry-red" macula - Hepatosplenomegaly, areflexia	- Death within few years
Tay-Sachs	AR hexosaminidase A (GM2 ganglioside)	- Progressive neurodegeneration, loss of motor milestones, hypotonia, "cherry-red" macula - Hyperreflexia	- Death within few years
Krabbe	AR galactocerebrosidase (galactocerebroside)	- Presents ~6M old, with progressive neuropathy, developmental delay, hypotonia, optic atrophy	- Death within few years
Metachromatic Leukodystrophy	AR arylsulfatase (cerebroside sulfate)	- Presents ~2 y/o, with progressive neuropathy, gait issues, hypotonia, weakness	- Death within early childhood
Mucopolysaccharidoses			
Hurler	AR iduronidase (heparan sulfate)	- **Coarse facies (" gargoylism")**, short stature, intellectual disability, OSA/airway obstruction - Hepatosplenomegaly - Dysostosis multiplex - Corneal clouding (hurler only) - Behavioral issues, like ADHD (hunter only)	- Enzyme replacement therapy - Live on average to ~10 y/o
Hunter	XR iduronate sulfatase (heparan sulfate)		
Mucolipidosis			
I-Cell Disease	Failure of delivery of key enzymes to lysosomes	- Growth failure, motor delay/hypotonia - Coarse facies - Corneal clouding, dysostosis multiplex - High plasma lysosomal enzymes	- Supportive care

Genetics

Misc. Genetic Disorders

	General/Clinical	Management
Hereditary Hemorrhagic Telangiectasia Osler-Weber-Rendu	- AD condition (endoglin, ALK-1, or SMAD4) - Epistaxis - Mucocutaneous telangiectasia - Mucosal bleeding, leading to anemia - AV malformation (pulmonary can result in paradoxical strokes, polycythemia, shunting) - Venous thrombosis	Dx: Clinical. Confirmatory genetic testing. Tx: - Screen for AVM, consider embolization - Treat anemia
Li-Fraumeni	- Germline p53 predisposition for cancer - Breast cancer, sarcomas, brain tumors, adrenocortical carcinomas	- MRI screening for breast cancer - Colon cancer screening - Consider whole body MRI screens

Genetic Associations	
VACTERL	- Vertebral defects - Anal atresia - Cardiac anomalies - TracheoEsophageal fistula - Renal (+ GU) defects - Limb defects (clubbing[A], radial hypoplasia[B], syndactyly and polydactyly)
CHARGE	- Colobomas: Absence/defect of ocular tissue - Heart (tetralogy of fallot) - Atresia (choanal) - Retarded growth/cognitive development - Genital anomalies - Ear anomalies
Other Genetic Syndromes	
Cornelia de Lange	- Very short stature, small birth weight, and failure to thrive - Single "bushy" eyebrow, micrognathia, microcephaly - Intellectual disability, behavioral abnormalities (autism)
Silver-Russell	- Short stature - Limb asymmetry - Triangular face, small downturned mouth - Excess sweating as infant
Pierre Robin	- Retrognathia - Cleft lip/palate - Backward displacement of tongue (causes airway obstruction)

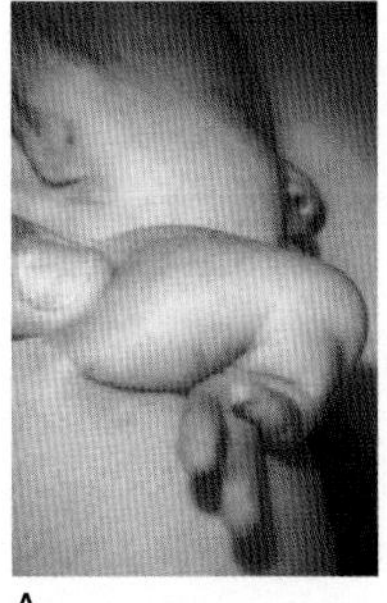
A

Approach to Fevers

Age	DDx/General Considerations	Workup	Management
Fever without source: Acute febrile (rectal temp >100.4°F) illness in which the etiology of fever is not apparent after H&P			
< 7 days old	- [See: Neonatal sepsis]		
Infant (7-28 days)	- High risk for IBI* (risk ↓ with older age) ***Infant bacterial infection** (IBI): Includes meningitis, bone and joint infections, soft tissue, pneumonia, UTI, sepsis/bacteremia, enteritis	- Full workup (CBC w/ diff, blood and urine cultures) - Lumbar puncture with CSF studies	- **Hospitalize all** - Empiric antibiotics (Ampicillin + gentamicin or cefotaxime) - Add Acyclovir (if HSV suspicion)
Infant (28-60 days)	- Viruses (RSV, influenza, parainfluenza, enterovirus) - HSV	- Full workup (CBC w/ diff, blood and urine cultures) +/− Lumbar puncture w/ CSF (only if high risk: see below)	- Hospitalize patients with high risk features - Empiric antibiotics if admitted
Infant (60-90 days)		- Urine culture/urinalysis - Full workup only if significant underlying comorbidities	- (+) UA: Empiric abx for UTI - (−) UA: Close outpatient followup
Children (3-36 months)	- **Self-limited viral infections** - Bacterial infections (UTI, pneumonia)	- Toxic appearing, T ≥ 102°F: - Full workup, hospitalization, empiric antibiotics - Nontoxic, T ≤ 102°F: - No workup, but consider UA in boys < 6-12 months/females < 24 months - Outpatient monitoring with close follow up	

Organisms: Group B *Strep, E. Coli, Listeria, S. pneumoniae, H. influenzae, N. meningitidis, S. aureus, Pseudomonas, Enterococcus*

Risk Stratification: Low risk for IBI if laboratory workup reveals the following
- WBC > 5 K and < 15 K, bands < 1.5 K, normal urinalysis, normal CSF (if LP performed)
- Note: If fever at home, but afebrile now, can safely discharge (if child looks well)

Fever of Unknown Origin

General: Fever (> 101°F) that persists ≥ 8 days, with no clear diagnosis

Etiology:
- Infectious disease (atypical viral presentations, bacterial/fungal infections)
- Connective tissue disease (Juvenile idiopathic arthritis, SLE, Kawasaki)
- Neoplasms (leukemia, lymphoma)

Diagnosis: Workup includes detailed H&P, CBC, ESR/CRP, blood/urine culture, chest x-ray, tuberculosis/HIV screening

Management: Avoid empiric antibiotics (unless septic), but can consider antipyretics (NSAIDs)

Cervical Lymphadenitis

General: Enlarged, inflamed, tender lymph node in the neck

Etiology:
- Bilateral: Viral URI, GAS pharyngitis, HSV, EBV
- Unilateral: *S. aureus* and GAS.

Clinical: > 2 cm, tender lymph node or nodes, possible overlying skin erythema/cellulitis

Diagnosis: Clinical diagnosis. Workup in those with severe symptoms (blood cultures, culture of lesion, throat culture).

Management:
- Bilateral: Most commonly self-limited
- Unilateral: Workup, empiric antibiotic therapy (amoxicillin-clavulanate)

Preoperative Evaluation

General: Evaluate factors that increase risk of surgery
- **Emergency surgery**: In vast majority of cases, benefits of surgery outweigh risks (do not delay for preop evaluation)

System	Evaluation
Cardiovascular	- ECG: Not necessary for low-risk surgery, but obtain in those undergoing medium or high-risk surgery, plus underlying cardiovascular disease/risk factors <u>High-risk groups</u>: - Active acute coronary syndrome, acute heart failure, severe AS (should stabilize prior to surgery) - ACS within last 60 days - Delay after coronary stenting (require at least 6 months of DAPT for drug-eluting stents) <u>Cardiovascular risk stratification</u>: (noncardiac surgery) - RCRI (revised cardiac risk index): Prognosticate perioperative cardiac risk (i.e., give percent risk) - Alternative models include NSQIP MICA, ACS-SRC models - If risk is > 1% for cardiovascular event, may warrant further evaluation (see algorithm below) 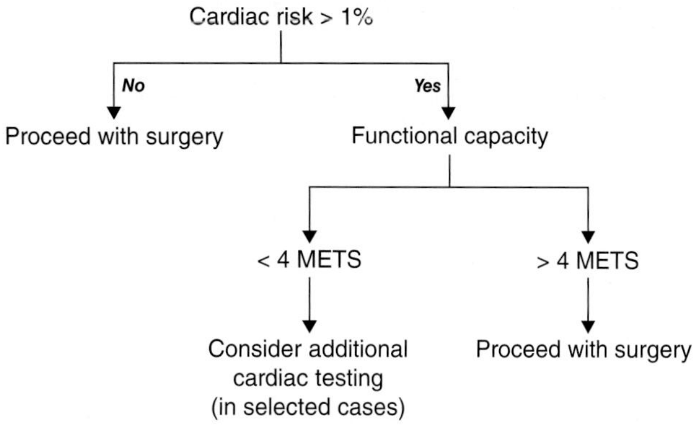 Cardiac risk > 1% *No* → Proceed with surgery *Yes* → Functional capacity → < 4 METS → Consider additional cardiac testing (in selected cases) → > 4 METS → Proceed with surgery - Preoperative stress test indicated if high-risk and **results would change management**
Pulmonary	- Smoking: Ideally quit > 4-8 weeks prior to surgery (reduced postoperative complication rates) - Optimize COPD/asthma/OSA prior to surgery - No indication for CXR or PFTs
Renal	- Creatinine > 2 mg/dL associated with increased surgery risk
Liver	- Surgery generally acceptable for: Child-Pugh class A/B or MELD < 15 - High surgery risk: Child-Pugh class C or MELD > 15
Hematology	<u>Goal blood counts</u>: - Hgb > 7, platelets > 50 K, INR < 1.5 <u>Anticoagulation</u>: - Hold warfarin for 4-5 days prior to surgery (or until INR < 1.5) - Heparin drip (stop hours prior to surgery), LMWH (stop at least 24 hours prior to surgery) - Aspirin, clopidogrel, ticagrelor, prasugrel: Stop 5-7 days prior to surgery
ID	- Cancel elective surgery if current acute infection

<u>Medications</u>
- Drugs to continue:
  - Statins, beta-blockers
  - Insulin (but reduced dose the day of surgery)
- Drugs to hold:
  - ACEi/ARB, diuretics (morning of surgery)
  - NSAIDs (1 week prior to surgery)
  - OCPs (hold in surgery with high risk for thrombotic events)
  - Oral diabetic agents

Postoperative Complications

Postoperative Fever

DDx	General	Diagnosis	Management/PPX
Immediate (< 24 hours)			
Malignant Hyperthermia	- Hypersensitivity to succinylcholine	- Clinical (presents with acute muscle rigidity, rhabdo, hypercapnia, tachycardia, hyperthermia)	- 100% O_2, dantrolene
Blood Product Reaction	- Acute febrile reaction to blood product		- Stop blood product
Other	- Inflammation due to surgery, infections predating the operation		
Early (1-3 days)			
Idiopathic	- Benign, transient fever within first few days after surgery - Often attributed to atelectasis (but no longer believed to cause fever) - Likely related to **inflammation**		- Monitor
Nosocomial Infection	- UTI, pneumonia - Catheter infection (e.g., CLABSI)	- Urinalysis, CXR, check catheters	- Antibiotics
Other	- PE/DVT - Myocardial infarction		
Late (> 3 days)			
Surgical Site Infection	- Most surgical site infections occur during late postop phase - Rarely infection with group A *Strep* and *Clostridium perfringens* can be earlier	- Erythema, warmth, and pain at incision site - Fever, leukocytosis	- Antibiotics - Surgical debridement/cleaning
Surgical Complications	- Abscess, fistula, anastomotic leak		
***C. Difficile* Colitis**	- Severe diarrhea		
Febrile Drug Reaction	- Antibiotics, PPIs, heparin, etc.		- Withdraw drug

Surgical Wound Complications

Surgical Site Infection	- See above
Fascial Dehiscence	- Fascial disruption, most commonly due to **abdominal wall tension** overcoming strength of sutures - Risk: Inadequate closure/technique, or host factors like infection, malnutrition, diabetes - Tx: Abdominal binders, surgical exploration/repair
Evisceration	- Dehiscence with **visceral protrusion through wound** - Tx: Emergent surgery
Hematoma	- Failure of primary hemostasis, resulting in collection of blood near site of incision - Increased risk for surgical site infection - Tx: Drainage of large collections

Fistula

General: Abnormal connection between two organs. Enteric fistulas are communications between bowel lumen and skin or another organ.

Risk:

- Postoperative (**abdominal surgery**, vascular surgery)
- Crohn disease
- **"FETID"** (foreign body, epithelialization, tumor, irradiation/inflamed/IBD/infection, distal obstruction)

Clinical: Variable based on location. Can have skin drainage, diarrhea, fecaluria.

Diagnosis: Either clinical (for obvious cutaneous fistula) OR CT abdomen/pelvis

Management: Initially supportive (give fluid, treat infection, control drainage, etc.)

- Surgical repair: Some enterocutaneous fistulas heal spontaneously, so short trial of supportive care is appropriate prior to surgery

Postoperative Complications

Abdominal Distension/Constipation	
Ileus	- **Paralysis of bowel motility** following surgery. Common in early postoperative period. - Risk: Worse with use of opioids, long/more intensive surgery, GI surgery - Presents with lack of flatus or bowel movements, mild obstructive symptoms (distension), dull pain - KUB XR shows **diffuse bowel dilatation**[A] - Tx: Supportive (fluids, ambulate, etc.)
Obstruction	- Suspicion grows for SBO (vs ileus) with lack of flatus/feces on postop days 4-5 - Caused by **abdominal adhesions** - KUB XR can reveal proximal bowel dilatation, with decompressed bowel distally - Dx: CT abdomen/pelvis - Tx: NG decompression, pain control, consider surgical correction
Ogilvie	- Functional ileus of the colon (acute "pseudo-obstruction" of colon) - Seen in elderly, chronically ill patients - XR/CT shows diffuse large bowel dilatation (vs LBO, which shows a transition at the site of obstruction) - Tx: Supportive care, consider Neostigmine

Other Postop Complications	
Complication	**Etiology/Causes**
Postop Bleeding	- Surgical site bleeding - DIC
Perioperative Myocardial Infarct	- Dx and treat as if normal STEMI/NSTEMI
Decreased Urine Output	- Obstructive (bladder, scan, relieve obstruction) - Renal failure (trial fluids to see if prerenal)
Hypoxemia	- Atelectasis (common after surgery) - Aspiration - PE - Pneumonia - Heart failure

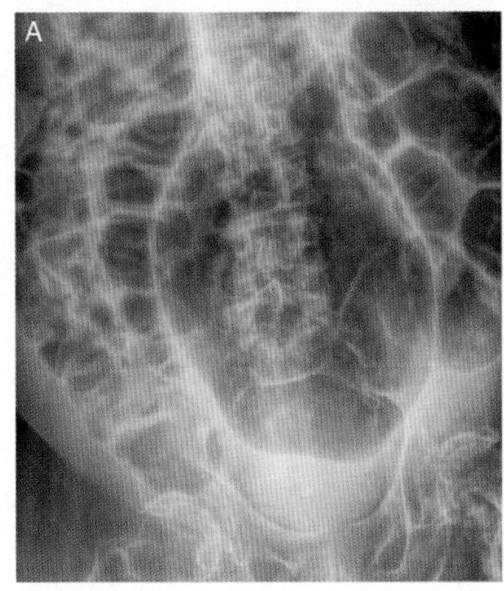

Emergencies/Fractures

Compartment Syndrome

General: Increased pressure within a compartment bound by fascial membranes, resulting in compromised vascular flow and tissue ischemia

Risk: Trauma (e.g., fractures, penetrating, or blunt), ischemia/reperfusion (e.g., vascular injury or arterial insufficiency), prolonged limb compression, IV drugs

Clinical:

- Progressive, tense, swollen extremity compartment
- Pain with passive motion of extremity
- Paresthesias
- Motor symptoms or pulselessness (late findings, poor prognosis)

Diagnosis: Compartment pressure measurement

- < 8 mmHg is normal. Symptoms develop at > 20-30 mmHg.
- Δ Pressure < 30 mmHg (diastolic BP–compartment pressure)

Management: Remove all dressings, keep limb at body level. Emergent fasciotomy.

Fracture Basics

Open Fracture	- Defined as fracture with direct communication externally - Clinically diagnosed (grossly obvious) - Tx: Antibiotics, tetanus PPX, surgery (aggressive irrigation and debridement)
Closed Fracture	- Bone fracture without external communication - Can be traumatic or pathologic (weak bone from osteoporosis, metastasis, etc.) <u>Displacement</u> - Can be nondisplaced OR - Displaced (sideways/translated, angulated, rotated, etc.) <u>Fragments</u> - **Complete**: Bone fully broken into separate pieces - **Incomplete**: Crack in bone, but still partially joined - **Comminuted**: Bone is broken into several pieces <u>Fracture pattern</u> - **Linear**: Parallel to long bone axis - **Transverse**: Perpendicular to long bone axis - **Oblique**: Diagonal to long bone axis - **Spiral**: One part of bone is twisted - **Compression**: Bony collapse (usually vertebrae) - **Impacted**: Fx from bone fragments being driven into each other - **Avulsion**: Fragment of bone ripped from main bone

Fracture Diagnosis/Management

Diagnosis: Plain XR imaging is almost always first step and sufficient for diagnosis

Management:

- Closed, nondisplaced fractures: Treated conservatively with analgesia, ice, and immobilization (splinting, sling)
- Displaced fractures: Require either open or closed reduction prior to immobilization

Fractures

Stress Fractures

General: Small bone fracture from repeated stress from overuse. Common sites include tibial (most common), foot, ankle, femur.

Risk: Sudden increase in intensity of physical activity, low fitness, low bone density, female, irregular menstruation, prior stress fractures

Clinical:

- Insidious onset of pain, associated with recent increase in activity
- Focal tenderness to palpation over bone

Diagnosis:

- XR (insensitive/often negative)
- MRI (highly sensitive, but only used if definitive diagnosis is required)

Management:

- Reduced weight bearing, splinting/boot for protection
- Rest, ice, analgesia
- Gradual return to activity

Rib Fractures

Risk: Blunt chest trauma, severe coughing, pathologic fractures (usually bony mets)

Clinical: Localized pain in the chest wall, which is tender with palpation

Diagnosis: CXR[A] (PA/lateral)

Management:

- Analgesia
    - NSAIDs, opioids. Intercostal nerve blocks
    - Adequate relief required to prevent atelectasis/pneumonia
        - Incentive spirometry
- ≥ 3 rib fractures or rib fractures in high risk patients (i.e., elderly) likely require hospitalization for monitoring/ prevention of complications

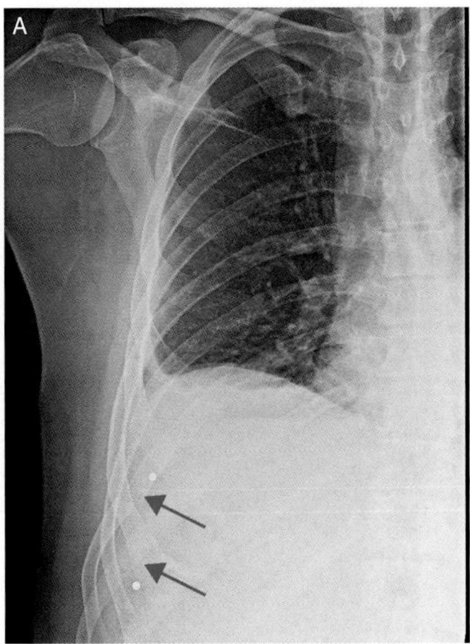

Fractures

Upper Extremity Fractures	
Clavicle	- Most commonly middle third (~70%) with ~25% in the distal third - Usually caused by trauma (fall on shoulder, MVA, etc.) - Tx: Sling, analgesia for minimally displaced fx. Surgical intervention if displaced.
Proximal Humerus[A]	- Often caused by falls - Tx: Conservative (sling). Surgical (if in many pieces).
Mid-Humeral Shaft	- Uncommon. From serious trauma. High risk for neurovascular compromise (especially radial nerve). - Tx: Surgery/splinting (in most cases)
Distal Radius	- **Colles** (with dorsal displacement of distal radius) or **Smith** (with palmar displacement of distal radius) - Risk: Elderly with fall on outstretched hand (Colles is most common) - Tx: Splinting (nondisplaced), closed reduction/splint (displaced)
Monteggia	- Midshaft ulna fracture, with dislocation of radial head
Galeazzi	- Radial midshaft fracture, with instability of radioulnar joint
Scaphoid	- Tenuous, retrograde blood supply. High risk for avascular necrosis, especially with proximal scaphoid. - Fall on outstretched arm with wrist in dorsiflexion - Pain is localized to radial wrist, with focal pain in the anatomic snuff box - Dx: XR. Often negative initially, so if high suspicion, immobilize and repeat imaging in a week. (alt: MRI) - Tx: Surgery (if displaced, or proximal 1/5 of scaphoid). Cast immobilization for others.
Metacarpal Neck	- "Boxer's" fractures (5th metacarpal) - Mechanism: Striking object with clenched fist or hand trauma - Tx: Reduction and splinting in most cases
Lower Extremity Fractures	
Pelvic	- Can occur with minor trauma in elderly or major trauma in healthy adults - Traumatic hip fractures have high risk for injury complications, such as GU, vascular, or spinal
Hip	- Common elderly injury, associated with ↑ morbidity/mortality - Presents after fall, with shortened leg and external hip rotation Classified as: - Intracapsular (femoral neck/head): High risk for complications (e.g., avascular necrosis, due to tenuous blood supply) - Extracapsular (intertrochanteric): Less risk for complication (good blood supply), but high risk for bleeding - Tx: Arthroplasty or open reduction w/ internal fixation. Must prophylaxe for DVT.
Femur	- Related to severe trauma - Risk for fat embolism - Tx: Adults (surgical nailing). Kids (casting).
Patellar	- Blunt knee trauma - Tx: Simple → Immobilization. Displaced or complex → Surgical.
Tibia/ Fibula Shaft	- High speed trauma or sports injury - Often involve both tibia and fibula, requiring ortho consult - Isolated fibula (non-weight-bearing bone) can be treated nonoperatively in most cases
Ankle	- Most commonly unimalleolar, but can be bimalleolar - Similar mechanism to ankle sprains, but severe, focal bone tenderness and inability to bear weight

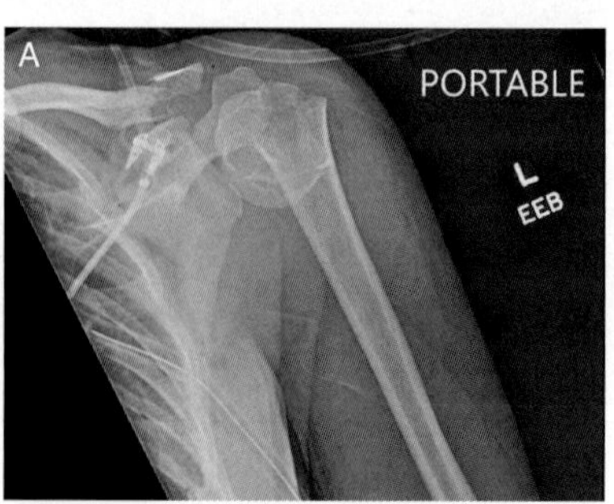

Pediatric Orthopedics

Pediatric Hip Disorders

	General/Clinical	Management
Developmental Dysplasia of Hip	- Abnormal development of acetabulum/femoral head, with resulting instability of the hip joint - Risk factors: Breech, family hx, females <u>Clinical</u> - **Ortolani** (abduction/elevation) - **Barlow** (adduction) - The above maneuvers result in jerks or clunks - Leg length discrepancy, asymmetric inguinal folds	Dx: Clinical, with imaging confirmation (US if < 4 months, XR > 4 months) Tx: - < 6 months: Abduction splint (Pavlik harness) - > 6 months: Often require surgical reduction - Monitor for long-term complications (OA, avascular necrosis)
Slipped Capital Femoral Epiphysis (SCFE)	- Posterior displacement of capital femoral epiphysis from the femoral neck through the growth plate - Commonly affects 10-15-year olds, overweight, males - Presents as groin (or occasionally knee) pain with limp - Limited internal rotation	Dx: XR (ice cream falling off cone) Tx: Surgical femoral head pinning
Legg-Calves-Perthes	- **Avascular necrosis of idiopathic origin** - Peak age ~5-7 - Presents with insidious onset hip pain, worse with activity, and limp (note the subacute, often > 1 month onset, vs other causes)	Dx: XR (often insensitive/normal early). MRI is highly sensitive. Tx: Splinting, with surgery if refractory. Can lead to septic arthritis.
Other Hip Pain	- Septic arthritis, transient synovitis	

Pediatric Orthopedic Disorders

Back	
Scoliosis	- **Excessive lateral curvature of the spine** - Common in young adolescents (usually idiopathic) - Dx: Inspection, Adams forward bend test, measurement of Cobb angle and skeletal maturity - Tx: Monitoring (Cobb < 20°), bracing, or surgery (Cobb > 50°)
Knee	
Osgood-Schlatter	- Overuse injury with strain and **avulsion of the secondary ossification center of the tibial tubercle** - Seen in running/jumping athletes - Presents with pain (generally insidious in onset) over tibial tubercle, exacerbated with contraction of quad muscles - Tx: Conservative (RICE), physical therapy
Foot	
Metatarsus adductus	- Congenital **medial deviation of forefoot** and neutral position of hindfood, so the toes point inward - Often bilateral. Common cause of "pigeon toes" at < 1 y/o. - Tx: Reassurance
Club foot (Talipes equinovarus)	- Pathologic congenital foot deformity, with medial deviation of forefoot, combined with foot supination (plantar surfaces facing inward), ankle plantar flexion, and cavus (high arch) - Tx: Manipulation/casting, followed by achilles tenotomy, bracing to maintain shape. Surgery for refractory cases.
Misc Benign	
Genu varum	- **Bow legged.** Normal before 2-3 y/o. - If older than 3, concern for pathologic variant (rickets, skeletal dysplasias, or Blount disease [disturbance of medial tibial growth plate])
Genu valgum	- **Knock knees.** Normal variant between 4 and 7 y/o.
Flat feet	- Normal in children, as pedal arch is developing in first 8 years - However, if foot does not have full range of motion, then needs referral to orthopedics

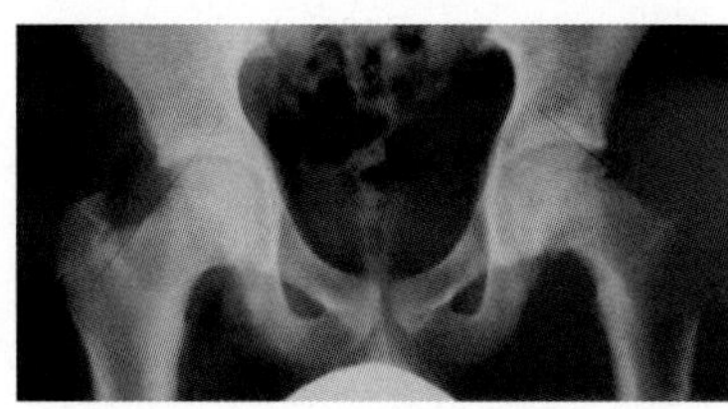

A

Trauma

Initial Evaluation in Trauma	
Airway	- Airway is generally intact if patient is conscious and speaking with normal voice Indications for intubation: (1) GCS < 8 (2) Compromised airway (3) Failure of oxygenation/ventilation (4) Anticipation of rapid deterioration - Cricothyroidotomy reserved for failed intubation and serious need for airway
Breathing	- Check breath sounds and look for symmetric chest wall motion
Circulation	- Evaluation of hemodynamic status (for shock). Check pulses. - Establish IV access (preferably two 16-18 gauge peripheral IVs, but if unable to obtain can place intraosseous or central line) - If signs of shock/hypovolemia, provide boluses of crystalloid fluids - If severe bleeding: - **Massive transfusion protocol** (1:1:1 blood products, including type O blood) - Tourniquet placement for severe extremity bleeding, pelvic binder for hip fracture with possible bleed, and thoracotomy if suspicion for severe aortic injury
Disability	- Focused neurologic examination - GCS evaluation - Pupil assessment, extremity sensation/strength assessment
Exposure	- "**Primary Survey**": Examine for injuries in key areas (back of head, back, buttocks, etc.) - "**Secondary Survey**": Examine the patient entirely for any other wounds or injuries

Shock (in trauma)	
Hypovolemic	- Hemorrhagic is the most common sign of shock - Presents pale and cold with weak pulses and collapsed neck veins
Obstructive	- **Cardiac tamponade**: Requires emergent pericardiocentesis - **Tension pneumothorax**: Requires emergent needle decompression
Cardiogenic	- After trauma, can be caused by myocardial contusion - Cold, clammy, signs of CHF, weak/rapid pulse
Vasomotor (Neurogenic)	- Spinal cord injury can cause ↓ peripheral vascular tone → hypotension. Will appear pink/well perfused.

Five major sources of bleeding:

1. Chest (hemothorax)
2. Abdomen (liver, splenic injury)
3. Pelvis/retroperitoneum (pelvic fracture, kidney injury)
4. Long bones (femur fractures)
5. External (scalp lacerations, other extremity injuries)

Trauma

Head Trauma

[See: Neuro] for full discussion on head trauma

DDx:

- TBI (concussion or more severe injury)
- Bleeds (epidural/subdural hematoma, diffuse axonal injury)
- Skull fractures (linear, basilar)

Diagnosis: CT scan (all with head trauma deserve head CT)

Penetrating Neck Injury

General: Any injury to the neck that penetrates the platysma. Classically anatomically split into three zones, displayed below:

Zone 1	Clavicles up to cricoid	- Great vessels, carotids/jugular, distal trachea, esophagus, lung apex
Zone 2	Cricoid to angle of mandible	- Carotid/jugular/vertebral vessels, vagus/phrenic/recurrent laryngeal nerve, esophagus, larynx, trachea
Zone 3	Angle of mandible to base of skull	- Proximal carotids, jugular vein, vertebral artery, oropharynx, C-spine

Clinical: Variable depending on organ involved

- "Hard signs" of vascular injury: Severe hemorrhage, expanding hematoma, hemodynamic instability
- "Hard signs" of airway/esophageal injury: Hemoptysis, hematemesis, respiratory failure, air bubbling from wound

Diagnosis: Multidetector helical CTA (MDCT-A) is now preferred test (if stable)

- This replaces previous "zone based" method, which (depending on zone involved) employed some combination of arteriography, esophagram, esophagoscopy, bronchoscopy to rule out injury

Management:

- Intubation (for anyone with compromised airway)
- Emergent surgical intervention (hemodynamic instability, expanding hematoma, clear "hard sign" of esophageal, tracheal, or vascular injury)
- If no injury demonstrated on CT, conservative monitoring

Spinal Trauma

General: Acute spinal cord injuries most commonly occur with MVA, but also after falls, sports accidents, and violence. Due to bone fracture, joint dislocation, ligament tear, or disc herniation.

Injury Type	Clinical Features
Complete Cord (ASIA class A)	- Complete loss of motor and sensory below the level of the lesion - Always includes loss of function in sacral segments S4-S5
Incomplete Cord (ASIA classes B-D)	- Incomplete motor and sensory loss - Sacral function present (testing includes preserved anal sensation and contraction)
Spinal Shock	- Like a spinal concussion, with flaccid paralysis, sensory loss, and absent bowel/bladder function below level of injury - Loss of sacral reflexes (bulbocavernosus, anocutaneous) - Recovery is highly variable, from hours to weeks

Diagnosis: CT spine (in suspected areas of injury)

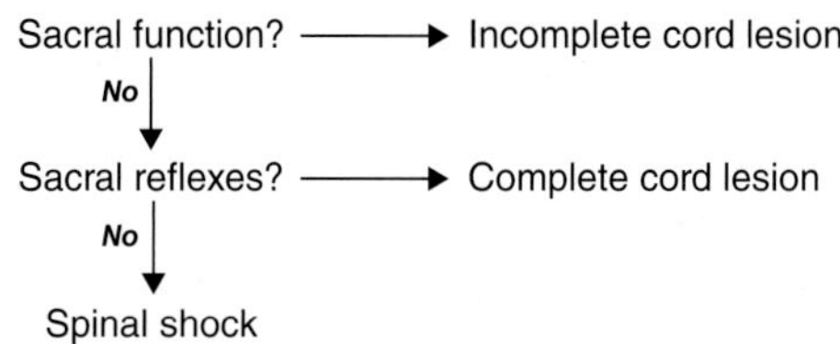

Management:

- Prehospital: Spinal immobilization (cervical collar, backboard)
- ED: Intubation, continued cervical stabilization/immobilization, neuro exam
- Surgery: If unstable fracture, spinal cord compression, or instability

Trauma

Blunt Chest Trauma	
Injury	**Features/Management**
Cardiovascular	
Blunt Cardiac Injury	- Variety of conditions, including ventricular wall rupture, valve damage, myocardial infarction, or "contusion" (presents with myocardial stunning without hemorrhage or structural damage) - **Commotio cordis**: Rare form of injury, sudden cardiac arrest (VFib) from chest trauma - Dx: ECG, TTE, and cardiac enzymes
Traumatic Aortic Rupture	- Often occurs with high-speed deceleration and can create a rapidly expanding hematoma that results in instant death. Most common at isthmus. - A minority of patients can have a contained injury that allows for survival until medical care - Dx: CT - Tx: Urgent surgery
Tamponade	[See: Cards]
Lung	
Pneumothorax [See: Pulm]	- Often due to broken rib - Traumatic pneumothoraces can be under tension, which can cause hemodynamic instability, tracheal deviation away from side of lesion, and contralateral mediastinal shift/ipsilateral diaphragm flattening. Management includes urgent needle decompression (if under tension), followed by chest tube.
Hemothorax	- Bleeding into pleural space from aortic/myocardial rupture, lung parenchyma, or intercostal vessels - Presents similarly to PTX, but dull to percussion on exam - Requires chest tube placement (in low, dependent spot in chest). If > 1.5 L of blood is collected, patient needs emergent surgery.
Rib Fracture	- [See: Ortho] - Risk for pneumothorax, or atelectasis/PNA development
Flail Chest	- Multiple rib fx in different locations that allow a segment of the chest wall to "float" (caves in during inspiration and bulges out during expiration) - Generally three or more ribs fractured in two or more places - Presents with hypoxemia, shallow tachypnea, paradoxical chest movement - Tx: Pain control, supplemental O_2, and positive pressure ventilation (if required)
Pulmonary Contusion	- Occurs within 48 hours of chest trauma (alveolar hemorrhage) - Often associated with flail chest - Presents with hypoxemia, ↓ breath sounds, in setting of trauma - Dx: CXR ("white out" of lungs with patchy infiltrates, which do not follow normal anatomic borders) - Tx: Pain control, supplemental O_2, pulmonary toileting, fluid restriction
Diaphragmatic Rupture	- Presents with respiratory distress - Dx: XR showing bowel in chest - Tx: Surgical repair
Rupture of Trachea or Bronchus	- Usually instantly fatal - Presents with respiratory distress, hemoptysis, dysphonia - Possible subcutaneous emphysema or recurrent pneumothorax (with chest tube air leakage) - Dx: CT chest or bronchoscopy - Tx: Surgical repair

Trauma

Blunt Abdominal Trauma

General: Majority of blunt abdominal trauma associated with MVC, car vs pedestrian, or from falls. Risk for bleeding from laceration or rupture of internal organ.

Liver	- Most common cause of abdominal bleeding post trauma - Tx: Usually no intervention required, unstable patients get surgery, persistent bleeds get IR embolization - Note: Pringle maneuver used during surgery clamps portal triad to control bleeding. If still bleeding, source is hepatic veins.
Spleen	- Most common significant abdominal bleeding post trauma - Often associated with fractured ribs on lower left - Tx: Splenectomy, laceration repair, or IR arterial embolization
Duodenum	- Hematoma formation from compression against posterior ribs - Often occurs in kids due to thin walls/lack of fat - Hematoma causes bowel obstruction, which presents within 1-2 days of injury
Bowel	- Can rupture acutely, or develop ischemia over hours after damage to mesenteric vessels, presenting as bowel ischemia days later
Kidney	- Rare. Includes kidney contusions, lacerations, or renovascular injury. - Can present with gross hematuria

Clinical: Varies from mild symptoms to severe shock/coma. Signs of severe injury:
- Abdominal distension/guarding/rebound tenderness
- Seat belt sign (ecchymosis on abdomen from seat belt)
    - 30% chance of internal injury

Diagnosis/Management:
- See algorithm below
- FAST Scan: Bedside ultrasound, used to identify free fluid[A] (blood). Examines RUQ/LUQ/pelvis/heart.

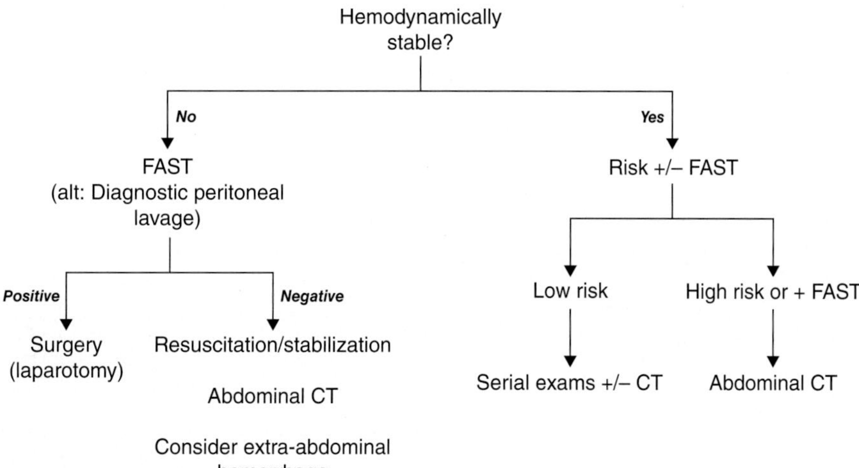

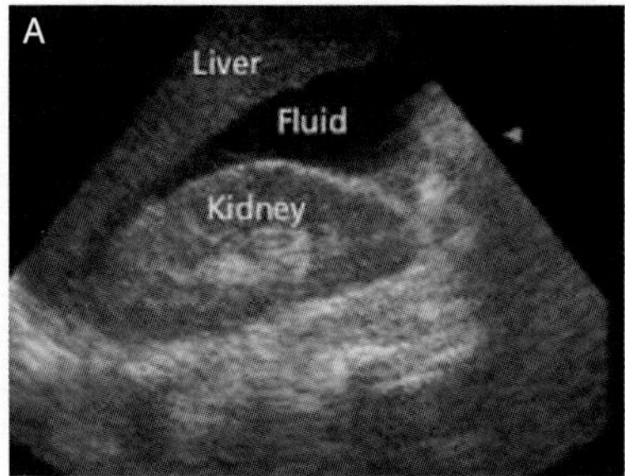

Trauma

Penetrating Abdominal Trauma (Gunshot)

General: Most commonly result in injuries to bowel or liver. The vast majority cause significant intra-abdominal injury that necessitates surgery.

Diagnosis: CT scan w/ contrast (for those without indication for emergent surgery)

Management:

- Emergent laparotomy: Indicated if hypotension, peritonitis, or evisceration
  - If surgery, patient should be given antibiotics
- Surgical management for anyone that is found to have significant injury on CT imaging
- In rare, select circumstances, nonoperative management is chosen for patients without clear injury on CT scan and are hemodynamically stable

Penetrating Abdominal Trauma (Stab Wounds)

General: Compared to gunshot wounds, stab wounds have a wider range of possible pathology, from simple skin/soft tissue injuries that do not penetrate fascia, to injuries to abdominal organs and vasculature

Management:

- Emergent laparotomy: Indicated if hypotension, peritonitis, or evisceration
- Local wound exploration (for fascial penetration)
  - If negative, provide good wound care, and consider discharge
  - If positive, admit for serial abdominal exam and monitoring
    - Consider CT for further workup
    - Surgery if develops peritonitis, hemodynamic instability, anemia, or leukocytosis

Abdominal Compartment Syndrome

General: Defined as elevated intra-abdominal pressure (called intra-abdominal hypertension), that results in organ dysfunction (including impaired cardiac function, renal impairment, ventilation problems, and gut hypoperfusion)

Risk: Trauma, burns, extensive fluid resuscitation (sepsis), abdominal surgery

Clinical: Tensely distended abdomen. Most patients are critically ill and not communicating.

Diagnosis: Measure intra-abdominal pressure (most commonly use bladder pressure)

Management: Surgical decompression (with temporary open abdomen)

Trauma

Pelvic Fracture

General: Pelvic fractures require significant mechanism, such as MVC or car versus pedestrian. Includes pelvic ring, sacral, and acetabular fractures. Often results in significant bleed from damage to iliac vessel branches/venous plexus.

Clinical:
- Instability of pelvis with pelvic compression
- Signs of bleeding, hemodynamic instability

Diagnosis: XR (if unstable) and CT (if stable)
- Note: Must perform rectal exam, vaginal exam, bladder imaging to rule out associated injuries
- FAST exam

Management:
- Pelvic binder, resuscitation/stabilization
- Consideration for operative stabilization, pelvic packing, or embolization of the bleeding vessel (situation specific)

Genitourinary Trauma

Anterior Urethra	- Usually due to direct trauma, including "straddle injuries" - Bleeding into perineum and scrotum may occur - Tx: Conservative (urethral catheter drainage, allowing for spontaneous healing)
Posterior Urethra	- Almost all occur in men. Often occurs with pelvic fractures. - Presents as blood at meatus, difficulty/inability to void, and high-riding prostate on DRE - Dx: Retrograde urethrogram (do not place Foley if complete injury) - Tx: Suprapubic catheter placement for bladder drainage, +/− delayed surgical repair weeks later
Extraperitoneal Bladder	- Presents as suprapubic tenderness, gross hematuria, difficulty voiding - Dx: Retrograde cystography (including post-void) - Tx: Conservative (urethral catheter drainage, allowing for spontaneous healing)
Intraperitoneal Bladder	- Presents as suprapubic tenderness, gross hematuria, difficulty voiding, peritonitis (from urine leakage into peritoneum) - Dx: Retrograde cystography (including post-void) - Tx: Surgical repair
Female Genitalia	- Bruising/lacerations usually occur in setting of sexual abuse
Male Genitalia	- Penile fracture [See: Urology] - Other external injuries include skin/soft tissue injuries, scrotal hematoma - Should use US to rule out testicular rupture or loss of continuity of the tunica albuginea, and retrograde cystogram to rule out urethral injury

Trauma

Extremity/Vascular Injuries

General: Trauma to extremity can include vascular, nervous, bone, and soft tissue damage. If 3/4 of these tissues are involved, the extremity is considered "mangled."

Clinical:

- Fracture: Deformity, point tenderness
- Vascular: Hard signs of injury include active bleed, growing hematoma, absent distal pulses
    - Signs of extremity ischemia ("6 Ps"): Pain, pallor, paresthesias, paralysis, pulselessness, poikilothermia
- Nerve: Weakness or paresthesia (in nerve-specific cutaneous distributions)

Diagnosis:

- XR
- Injured extremity index (IEI) (like ankle-brachial index, but comparing BP between two extremities). < 0.9 abnormal.
    - CT angiography if the IEI is abnormal

Management:

- **Prehospital**: If bleeding, direct pressure, or tourniquet if pressure not sufficient
- **Surgical**: Hard signs of vascular injury → Surgical repair
- **Compartment syndrome**: Common, especially with crush injuries. Requires fasciotomy.
- Traumatic amputation (e.g., of finger)
    - Out of hospital: Patient should clean with saline, wrap in saline-soaked gauze, place in sealed bag on ice
    - Surgical repair at hospital

Select Vascular Injuries

Artery	Mechanism of Injury
Axillary	- Anterior shoulder dislocation
Subclavian	- Clavicular fracture
Brachial	- Supracondylar humeral fracture, elbow dislocation
Iliac branches	- Pelvic fractures
Femoral	- Anterior hip dislocation
Superficial femoral	- Femoral shaft fracture
Popliteal	- Posterior knee dislocation, tibial plateau fracture

Burns

Burns: Overview

General: Injury to skin and possibly underlying tissue from exposure to thermal injury, electricity, chemicals, radiation

Degree	Anatomy	Clinical
1st (Superficial)	- Epidermis only	- Blanching, painful, erythematous skin (looks like sunburn)
2nd (Superficial partial thickness)	- Epidermis and portions of dermis	- Weeping, erythematous skin - Still painful - Blisters present
2nd (Deep partial thickness)	- Epidermis and portions of dermis	- Weeping blisters, variable colors (red and white) - Painless
3rd (Full thickness)	- All epidermis/dermis	- Dry, leathery, waxy white and/or dark charred skin - Painless
4th	- Skin, fat, fascia, muscle, all involved	- Severe, disfiguring injury with deep tissue exposure

Diagnosis: Clinical diagnosis. Important to determine extent of injury through use of scoring system, such as Lund-Browder chart or Rule of Nines (see below).

Burns—Management

Fluids	Parkland formula (estimated fluid requirement): - mL of LR = Kg × % Body surface burned × 4 mL - Fluid given first half over 8 hours and second half over 16 hours - Despite the classic formula above, most burn centers provide fluids to maintain urine output (at least 0.5 mL/kg/hr)
Wound care	- Antimicrobial agents: Silver sulfadiazine, mafenide acetate, Chlorhexidine, others - Covered by gauze or nonadherent film products
Analgesia	- Opioid analgesics
Other	- PPI prophylaxis (curling ulcers) - Ensure proper nutrition (as patients are hypermetabolic). Tube feeds or TPN if necessary.
Surgical	- Escharotomy for circumferential burns (can cause limb ischemia) - Surgical grafting (following conservative therapy, for select severe, but isolated burn wounds)

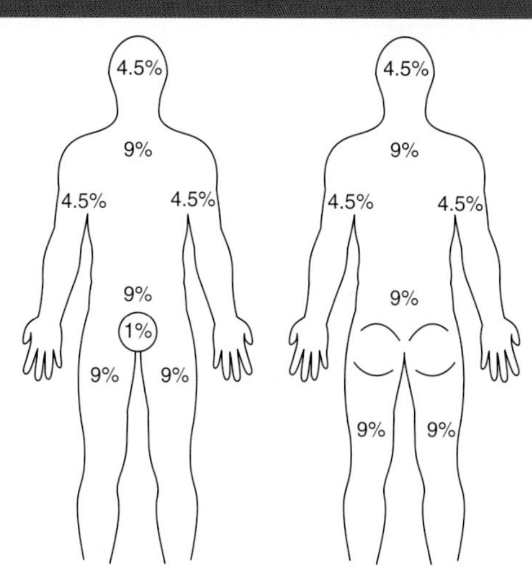

Special situations:

- Inhalation injury
  - Diagnosis: Bronchoscopy
  - Requires intubation if signs of airway edema, blistering, carboxyhemoglobin > 10%, or impending respiratory failure
- Chemical burn: Tap water irrigation
- Electric [See: EM]: Watch for arrhythmia, rhabdo, posterior shoulder dislocation

Note: Burn patients are often in an elevated metabolic state, and are hyperthermic, tachycardic, tachypnic.

Burns: Infection

General: Highest risk for mortality with burns. Organisms:

- Early: *Staphylococcus* and *Streptococcus*
- > 5 days: Gram negatives (*Pseudomonas, E. Coli*, etc.) and fungi (*Candida*)

Clinical:

- Presents as rapid change in clinical condition of patient (increasing pain, change in appearance of burn wound, or systemic signs like hemodynamic changes)
- Note: Traditional sepsis criteria cannot be used due to hypermetabolic state

Diagnosis: Tissue biopsy and culture (> 10^5 colonies per gram tissue)

Management: Surgical debridement, broad spectrum antibiotics, wound care

Anesthesia

	Mechanism	Indication	Side Effects/Management Concerns
Inhaled			
Desflurane Isoflurane Sevoflurane	- Unknown	Unconscious deep sedation	- Most commonly used agents currently due to best side-effect profile
Halothane			- Hepatotoxicity (still used in third world countries)
Enflurane			- Seizures, ↓ myocardial contractility
Methoxyflurane			- Nephrotoxicity
Nitrous oxide		Conscious sedation	- Rapid onset/offset. Frequent nausea/emesis after.
Neuromuscular Blockade			
Succinylcholine	- Depolarizing agent (ACh agonist)	- Endotracheal intubation	- Hyperkalemia, myalgias - Risk for malignant hyperthermia
Rocuronium vecuronium	- Nondepolarizing agent (ACh antagonist)	- Endotracheal intubation - Surgery	- Excreted via hepatic and renal clearance (caution in patients with liver or kidney disease) - Reversed with acetylcholinesterase inhibitors (e.g., neostigmine, edrophonium) or Sugammadex (directly inactivates paralytic agent)
Atracurium cisatracurium	- Nondepolarizing agent (ACh antagonist)	- Endotracheal intubation - Surgery	- Eliminated via Hoffman mxn (spontaneous degradation, not dependent on hepatic or renal clearance)
IV Agents			
Propofol	- GABA potentiation	- Induction	- ↓ BP/HR/cardiac output - Bronchodilation, antiemetic, anticonvulsant
Etomidate	- GABA potentiation/agonist	- Induction	- ↔ BP/HR/cardiac output - Nausea/vomiting
Ketamine	- NMDA antagonist	- Induction	- ↑ BP/HR/cardiac output - Bronchodilation. Hallucinations.
Midazolam	- GABA agonist	- Adjuvant agent - Sedative, amnesia	- Short-acting, used for brief procedures - Respiratory depression (dose-dependent)
Opioids (fentanyl)	- Opioid receptor agonist	- Adjuvant agent - Sedative, analgesic	- Suppression of airway reflexes - Respiratory depression, hypotension

General Anesthesia: Basic Principles

General: General anesthesia aims to create a state of amnesia, analgesia, and muscle paralysis during surgery

Induction	- Initial step: Put patient to sleep - Usually IV agent (e.g., propofol or etomidate) with an opioid (e.g., fentanyl) as adjunct - Once asleep, paralytic agent used prior to intubation
Maintenance	- Inhaled or IV agents (or, most commonly, a combination of both) to keep patient asleep - Neuromuscular blocking agent
Emergence	- Discontinuation of anesthetic agents - Reversal of residual neuromuscular blockade effects, extubation

Inhaled anesthetic pharmacology

- **Blood solubility** (blood:gas partition coefficient) → Determines onset/offset time (↓ solubility → faster onset)
- **Lipid solubility** (oil:gas partition coefficient) → Determines potency (↑ solubility → ↑ potency)
    - Inverse of MAC (minimal alveolar concentration), which is the amount of agent needed to prevent response to noxious stimulus in 50% of people
- Inhaled agents result in:
    - ↑ cerebral blood flow, cerebral vasodilatation
    - ↓ SVR and MAP
    - ↓ Tidal volume, ↑ CO_2, ↓ GFR

Rapid sequence intubation: Etomidate + succinylcholine

Anesthesia

Malignant Hyperthermia

General: Hypermetabolic state that is caused when a susceptible person is exposed to succinylcholine or inhaled anesthetic (e.g., halothane, sevoflurane). Most commonly due to **AD RYR-R mutations** (leading to unregulated amounts of calcium channel activation in muscle).

Clinical:

- **Hyperthermia, tachycardia, hypercapnia**
- Muscle rigidity, rhabdomyolysis
- Mixed metabolic and respiratory acidosis

Management:

- Discontinue anesthetics
- 100% O_2, **dantrolene**
- Monitor and treat arrhythmia, hyperkalemia, rhabdo, acidosis

Spinal/Epidural Anesthesia

General: Injection of anesthetic medication into the subarachnoid space (for spinal) or epidural space (for epidural). Used for lower abdominal, lower extremity, and gynecologic surgery.

Technique: Performed via needle or catheter placed in the lumbar spinal cord. Anesthetic usually **bupivacaine** or lidocaine.

Adverse Events:

High spinal	- Excess anesthetic or improper needle position, resulting in ascending motor/sensory blockade with hypotension, bradycardia, and dyspnea (due to diaphragm paralysis)
Postdural puncture headache	- Headache within 3 days post any dura puncturing procedure - Positional headache (worse when upright), possible nausea/vomiting - Tx: NSAIDs +/− epidural blood patch
Transient neurologic Sx	- Syndrome of painful paresthesias in lower extremity < 24 hours after spinal - Considered benign and transient

Regional Anesthesia

<u>Peripheral nerve block</u>:

- Used for upper and lower extremity procedures
- Injection or infusion of local anesthetic agent
- Specific nerve identified by US or nerve stimulator

<u>Intravenous regional anesthesia</u>:

- Alternative to peripheral nerve block for short procedures (e.g., hand surgery like carpal tunnel release)
- Establish IV, exsanguination of extremity, tourniquet placement, and injection of anesthetic through IV catheter

Local Anesthesia

Esters (duration)	Amides (duration)
Procaine (0.5-1 hour)	Lidocaine (0.75-1.5 hour)
Cocaine (0.5-1 hour)	Mepivacaine (1-2 hour)
Tetracaine (1-6 hour)	Bupivacaine (2-8 hour)

General: Local agents act to prevent nerve cell depolarization/signal propagation through inhibition of Na channels

Adverse Events:

- Each drug has a limited amount of drug that can be injected. If over this amount, risk of systemic toxicity:
  - Early symptoms: Metallic taste, anxiety, perioral numbness
  - Severe symptoms: Seizures, arrhythmia, cardiac arrest
- Methemoglobinemia (rare)

Opiates

	Mechanism	Indication	Side Effects/Management Concerns
Opiates			
Oxycodone (PO) Hydromorphone (PO/IV) Methadone (PO) Morphine (PO/IV) Fentanyl (IV/patch)	- Opioid receptor agonists (especially μ-opioid)	- Pain control - Air hunger (especially morphine)	- Addiction [See: Psych], tolerance - Respiratory/CNS depression - Urinary retention - Nausea, vomiting, headache, lightheadedness - Constipation - Miosis * Tolerance does not develop to constipation or miosis
Codeine		- Antitussive - Pain control	
Dextromethorphan		- Antitussive	
Loperamide Diphenoxylate		- Diarrhea	
Naloxone Naltrexone	- Opioid receptor antagonist	- Reversal of opiate toxicity	- Few side effects if no opioids in system - Can cause signs of withdrawal
Tramadol	- Weak opioid agonist - Serotonin and muscarinic antagonist	- Analgesia	- Common: Nausea/vomiting, dry mouth, dizziness (similar to opiates, but severe respiratory depression less common) - Serotonin syndrome
Buprenorphine	- Partial opioid agonist	- Opioid use disorder (paired with naloxone, so inactive if injected)	- Similar to other opiates

Normal Pregnancy

Basic Terminology of Pregnancy

Gravidity: Total number of pregnancies
Parity: Number of completed pregnancies
- T: **Term** Births (number of pregnancies leading to birth > 37 weeks gestation)
- P: **Preterm** Births (births prior to 37 weeks gestation)
- A: **Abortion**
- L: **Living children**

Developmental age: The number of weeks/days since fertilization
Gestational age (GA): The number of weeks/days since the last menstrual period

Trimesters: (ranges are defined slightly differently depending on source)
1st: Weeks 1-12 weeks GA **2nd**: Weeks 13-27 week GA **3rd**: Weeks 28-birth

Diagnosis of Pregnancy

β-hCG	- Urine or serum (more sensitive) - Generally positive by the time of expected period (~ 2 weeks after ovulation and conception) - β-hCG doubles ~ 48-72 hours during early pregnancy and peaks around 100,000 mIU/mL at 10 weeks GA - β-hCG declines to around 10,000-20,000 mIU/mL at term
Ultrasound	- Used to confirm intrauterine pregnancy - **Gestational sac** visible on transvaginal US at ~ 5 weeks GA (β-hCG ~ 1500 mIU/mL) - **Yolk sac** visible at ~ 5-6 weeks GA - **Fetal heart motion** measurable ~ 6 weeks GA (β-hCG ~ 5000 mIU/mL)

Dating of Pregnancy

Naegele Rule: Estimated date of delivery is last menstrual period + 7 days – 3 months

Ultrasound (if last menstrual period is uncertain):

Test	Timing	Accuracy
Crown-Rump length	< 13 weeks	+/– 5 Days (≤ 9 weeks) to +/– 7 days (9-13 weeks) Most accurate at 7-10 weeks
Biparietal diameter Head-circumference Femur length	> 13 weeks	+/– 7 days (during early second trimester) to +/– 3-4 weeks (by end of third trimester)

Notes:
- If assisted reproduction, can simply add 266 days to date of conception
- If discrepancy between LMP and ultrasound:
    - Can redate (use US date) if the patient's LMP falls outside the above confidence interval for the US test
- Fundal height should be ~ 1 cm/week pregnant
- Fetal heart tones appear ~ 10-12 weeks
- Fetal movements ("quickening") occurs ~ 16-20 weeks

Clinical Signs of Pregnancy

Clinical Symptoms	Examination Findings
- Amenorrhea - Nausea +/– vomiting - General fatigue - Breast enlargement - Mild uterine cramping	- Telangiectasias, palmar erythema, linea nigra - Softening of cervix (Goodell sign) - Softening of uterus (Ladin sign) - Blue discoloration of vagina/cervix (Chadwick sign)

Normal Pregnancy

Physiologic Changes of Pregnancy

Cardiovascular	- ↑ HR, cardiac output, stroke volume; ↓ BP, systemic vascular resistance
Pulmonary	- ↑ Tidal volume, minute/alveolar ventilation; ↓ CO_2
Renal	- ↑ GFR
Heme	- ↑ Plasma volume, ↓ hematocrit. Hypercoagulable state.
Endocrine	- ↑ TBG (increases total T3, T4)
Weight Gain (BMI)	BMI < 18.5: 1 lb/wk (28-40 lb total) BMI 18.5-25: 0.75 lb/wk (25-35 lb total) BMI 25-30: 0.5 lb/wk (15-25 lb total) BMI > 30: 0.25 lb/wk (10-20 lb total)

Common (Benign) Problems During Pregnancy

Back Pain	- Most common in third trimester, as enlarged uterus exaggerates lordosis and changes center of gravity - Tx: Supportive (stretch, heat, massage, acetaminophen)
Constipation	- Tx: Increased PO fluids, bulking agents, laxatives
Edema	- Lower extremity edema from IVC compression - Tx: Positional change (avoid IVC compression), elevate lower extremities
GERD	- Increased relaxation of sphincters - Tx: Antacids
Hemorrhoids	- From venous congestion/IVC compression - Tx: Topical anesthetics/steroids
Round Ligament Pain	- Adnexal pain from stretching of uterus/ligament attachments - Tx: Self-limited
Urinary Frequency	- From increased circulating volume/GFR - Tx: Rule-out UTI

Routine Prenatal Care

First Trimester
 	
(start care by 10 weeks GA)
	- Lab tests:
	  - CBC, blood type/Rh screen, urinalysis and culture
	  - Rubella, varicella antibody screen. RPR/VDRL, chlamydia, HIV, HBsAg, PPD.
	  - TSH, hemoglobin A1C (selected in those at risk)
	- If MCV low AND suspicion for possible **hemoglobinopathy**:
	  - Hemoglobin analysis (via HPLC or IEF) of mom. Test dad if mom carries concerning gene.
	- If concern over family history of genetic condition (**cystic fibrosis, Tay-Sachs**):
	  - Genetically test mom. Test dad if mom carries concerning gene.

Second Trimester	- Aneuploidy screening (either late first or early second trimester) - Neural tube defect screen (US + AFP) - Fetal anatomic US (18-22 weeks) - Diabetes screen (24-28 weeks): 50-g, 1-hour glucose challenge test (GCT)
Third Trimester	- RhoGAM for Rh- women (at 28 weeks) - GBS culture (35-37 weeks) - CBC
Note: OB visits q4 week (up to 28 weeks), q2 week (28-36 weeks), q1 week (36 weeks-birth)	

Vaccinations	- For all: Tdap and influenza (usually 2nd/3rd trimester) - Contraindicated: HPV, MMR, varicella
Nutrition	- Require additional ~ 300 kCal/day (normal woman is ~ 2000) - Note: Avoid undercooked meats, unpasteurized dairy, excessive seafood, deli meats/soft cheeses, limit caffeine - Supplements: Iron supplementation, calcium (1000 mg), folate (0.4-0.8 mg/day, with 4 mg if risk for NT defect)
Exercise	- 20-30 minutes of moderate intensity exercise daily. Avoid high impact sports. - Contraindicated if ruptured membranes, cervical insufficiency, placenta previa, severe preeclampsia

Prenatal Testing

Prenatal Aneuploidy Screening

General: Screening for fetuses at risk for Down syndrome (trisomy 21), trisomy 18, trisomy 13

<table>
<tr><th>Test</th><th>Timing</th><th>Features</th></tr>
<tr><td>First-Trimester Combined</td><td>9-13 weeks</td><td>- Uses PAPP-A, β-hCG, US for nuchal translucency (NT)
<table>
<tr><th></th><th>NT</th><th>PAPP-A</th><th>β-hCG</th></tr>
<tr><td>T21</td><td>↑</td><td>↓</td><td>↑</td></tr>
<tr><td>T18</td><td>↑</td><td>↓</td><td>↓</td></tr>
<tr><td>T13</td><td>↑</td><td>↓</td><td>↓</td></tr>
</table></td></tr>
<tr><td>Second-Trimester Quad</td><td>15-22 weeks</td><td>- Uses AFP, β-hCG, estriol, inhibin
<table>
<tr><th></th><th>AFP</th><th>β-hCG</th><th>Estriol</th><th>Inhibin</th></tr>
<tr><td>T21</td><td>↓</td><td>↑</td><td>↓</td><td>↑</td></tr>
<tr><td>T18</td><td>↓</td><td>↓</td><td>↓</td><td>Variable</td></tr>
<tr><td>T13</td><td colspan="4">Variable findings</td></tr>
</table></td></tr>
<tr><td>Cell Free DNA (cfDNA)</td><td>> 10 weeks</td><td>- Used as both primary screening test and secondary screening test (for + initial screen)
- Has high sensitivity (and high NPV), but is not diagnostic
- Requires adequate circulating cfDNA (low cfDNA if < 10 weeks GA, obese mothers)</td></tr>
</table>

AFP Interpretation:

Reduced AFP (< 0.5 MoM)	Increased AFP (> 2.5 MoM)
- Trisomy 21 and 18 - Fetal demise - Incorrect gestational dating	- Open-neural tube defects: Anencephaly, spina bifida - Abdominal wall defects: Gastroschisis, omphalocele - Multiple gestation - Incorrect gestational dating

Invasive Diagnostic Tests

General: Tests used to obtain fetal DNA, make definitive diagnosis of fetal aneuploidy

	CVS (Chorionic villus sampling)	Amniocentesis
Age	10-13 weeks	15-20 weeks
Gen	Transcervical or transabdominal aspiration of chorionic tissue	Transabdominal aspiration of amniotic fluid (using ultrasound guidance)
Cons	- Risk of fetal loss ~ 1:100 - Risk for maternal bleeding, infection - Limb defects associated with early CVS	- Risk of fetal loss ~ 1:300-500 - Rarely causes leakage of amniotic fluid or direct fetal injury - Note: Discolored (brown) samples are a sign of ↑ risk of fetal demise

Prenatal Testing

<table>
<tr><th colspan="2">Antepartum Fetal Surveillance</th></tr>
<tr><th>Test</th><th>Features</th></tr>
<tr><td>Nonstress Test (NST)</td><td>- Continuous FHR (fetal heart rate) monitoring
- Used after 32 weeks gestation

<u>Reactive NST</u> (for ≥ 32 weeks)
- Two accelerations > 15 bpm above baseline HR lasting > 15 seconds over a 20 minute period
- Reassuring of fetal well-being

<u>Nonreactive NST</u>
- Insufficient (< 2) accelerations over a 40-minute period
- Need to perform further tests (i.e., biophysical profile) or perform longer NST
- Causes: Fetal sleeping (most commonly), fetal CNS anomalies, maternal sedatives
*Can perform vibroacoustic stimulation to try to wake up baby</td></tr>
<tr><td>Contraction Stress Test</td><td>- FHR monitoring with contractions from oxytocin or natural labor (test rarely performed now)
- Observe for late or significantly variable decelerations in FHR occurring with contractions</td></tr>
<tr><td>Biophysical Profile</td><td>- Uses five parameters to score 2 (normal) or 0 (abnormal)

(1) Tone (≥ 1 flexion/extension movement of spine or limb)
(2) Breathing (breathing episode for > 30 seconds)
(3) Fetal movement (≥ 3 limb movements)
(4) Amniotic fluid volume (single deepest vertical pocket ≥ 2 cm)
(5) Nonstress test (reactive)

<u>Score</u>:
8-10 → Reassuring for fetal well being
6 → Equivocal (repeat test soon)
0-4 → Worrisome for asphyxia. Delivery (usually) indicated.</td></tr>
<tr><td>Modified Biophysical Profile</td><td>- Nonstress test and amniotic fluid volume assessment only
- Parameters most predictive of outcome</td></tr>
<tr><td>Amniotic Fluid Index</td><td>- Measure depth of fluid in all 4 quadrants, added together
- > 25 cm polyhydramnios, < 5 cm oligohydramnios</td></tr>
<tr><th colspan="2">Other Tests (used to monitor certain high risk conditions)</th></tr>
<tr><td>Umbilical Artery Velocimetry</td><td>- Determines umbilical artery flow velocity and direction (should be constant and forward)
- Used to assess IUGR/placental insufficiency
- End-diastolic flow can be halted or even reversed with IUGR</td></tr>
<tr><td>Transcranial Doppler</td><td>- US monitoring of cerebral artery flow velocity
- Evaluates for fetal anemia (high rates of flow found in anemic fetuses)</td></tr>
</table>

Teratogenesis

Teratogenic Drugs/Exposures (selected)

Drug	Drug Category	Fetal Findings
ACEi	Class D	- Renal abnormalities - Oligohydramnios (↓ fetal GFR)
Aminoglycoside	Class D	- Neurosensory hearing loss
Androgens	NA	- Virilization (females)
Anticonvulsants	Class D or X	- General class effects: Neural tube defects, congenital heart disease, cleft palate, abnormal facies - **Carbamazepine**, **valproate** at highest risk **Phenytoin** - Fetal hydantoin syndrome: IUGR, facial dysmorphia[A], cleft palate, VSD, intellectual disability
Caffeine	NA	- *Possible* ↑ risk for abortion at > 300 mg/day levels
DES Diethylstilbestrol	Class X	- Genital issues (hypoplastic uterus/cervix, vaginal septa) - Clear cell adenocarcinoma of vagina in adolescents
Fluoroquinolone	Class C	- Fetal cartilage damage
Folate Antagonist (MTX, TMP)	Class X	- Risk for **neural tube defects** - MTX also linked to microcephaly, growth restriction, limb and cranial malformations
Lead	NA	- Increased spontaneous abortion rate (at high levels)
Lithium	Class D	- Ebstein's anomaly, other congenital heart defects
Mercury	NA	- Neurodevelopmental toxicity (at high levels)
Methimazole	Class D	- Aplasia cutis
Radiation	NA	- Risk for microcephaly, growth or intellectual disability at high radiation doses
Statins	Class X	- Possible limb abnormalities, CNS/heart defects
Tetracycline	Class D	- Bone/teeth staining
Thalidomide	Class X	- Bilateral limb malformations (phocomelia), microtia, other cardiac/GI malformations
Vitamin A/ Retinoids	Class X	- Spontaneous abortions, microcephaly, cardiac anomalies - Birth control mandatory for females while using
Warfarin	Class D	- Nasal hypoplasia, limb hypoplasia, stippling of bone epiphysis, optic atrophy - Fetal hemorrhage, spontaneous abortion

Drug Categories:
- Category C: Risk cannot be ruled out
- Category D: Positive evidence of risk
- Category X: Contraindicated in pregnancy

Teratogenesis

Fetal Alcohol Spectrum Disorder

General: Fetal alcohol exposure can result in a highly variable degree of impact on the developing fetus, with multiple phenotypes possible

Clinical:

- Facial abnormalities (short palpebral fissures, thin vermillion border, smooth philtrum)
- Growth retardation (↓ height/weight percentiles)
- Neurologic:
    - Structural: Microcephaly, focal neurologic defects, other structural abnormalities
    - Neurobehavioral impairment: Developmental delay, intellectual disability, behavioral abnormalities
- Heart defects: ASD, VSD, Tetralogy of Fallot

Diagnosis:

Fetal Alcohol Syndrome	- Characteristic facial features (above) plus growth and intellectual impairment
Alcohol-Related Neurodevelopmental Disorder	- Neurobehavioral impairment with documented EtOH exposure - Other features may or may not be present
Alcohol-Related Birth Defects	- Specific malformation with documented EtOH exposure

Other Substances

Opioids	- ↑ risk preterm birth, fetal death/miscarriage, neonatal abstinence syndrome - In mothers with opiate use disorder → use methadone or buprenorphine
Marijuana	- Use discouraged during pregnancy - Evidence is controversial and lacking, but concern for neurodevelopmental impact
Amphetamines **Cocaine**	- ↑ risk of fetal demise, IUGR, preterm birth, placental abruption, miscarriage
Smoking (nicotine, carbon monoxide)	- Placental insufficiency (↑ risk for IUGR, low birthweight) - Placental anomalies (abruption, previa) - Preterm labor, PROM - SIDS

Neonatal Abstinence Syndrome

General: Neonatal withdrawal from maternal opiate use during pregnancy

Clinical:

- Presents within a few days of life
- Irritability, high-pitched cry, poor sleep, feeding difficulty, poor tone, tremors, GI disturbances, failure to thrive

Management:

- Supportive: Adequate nutrition, decreasing sensory stimulation, swaddling
- If supportive care fails, small doses of opiates (methadone or morphine) can be used

Teratogenesis (TORCH)

	General	Clinical	Management/PPX
Toxoplasma	- Protozoan *Toxoplasma gondii* - Fecal-oral transmission of sporozoite on contaminated food/water - Commonly lives in cats - Transplacental transmission	Maternal: Asymptomatic or mild febrile illness Neonates: Often subclinical at birth, then develop fever, maculopapular rash, seizures, jaundice - Classic triad: **Hydrocephalus, intracranial calcifications, chorioretinitis**	Dx: Toxo IgM/IgG Tx: Pyrimethamine + sulfadiazine - Spiramycin (alternative for maternal infection) PPX: Avoid undercooked meats, wash fruit/veg, avoid raw shellfish, avoid cat's litter box
Other (syphilis, varicella-zoster, Zika virus, see below)			
Rubella	- Due to rubivirus that causes "German measles" - Transplacental transmission	Maternal: Self-limited febrile illness, maculopapular rash Neonates: - ↑ risk for fetal demise/abortion and IUGR - Sensorineural deafness, cataracts, microcephaly, congenital heart disease (PDA), rash ("blueberry muffin")	Dx: Rubella IgM/IgG Tx: Supportive PPX: MMR vaccine (before preg)
CMV	- Most common TORCH infection - Transplacental transmission	Maternal: Asymptomatic or mild febrile illness Neonates: - **Sensorineural hearing loss** - Other findings: Small for GA, microcephaly, hepatosplenomegaly, petechiae, seizures - Periventricular intracranial calcifications	Dx: CMV IgM/IgG Tx: - Ganciclovir or valganciclovir (for any symptomatic baby) - No proven maternal treatment or prophylaxis
HSV	- Acquired at birth from actively infected maternal genital tract - Rarely transmitted in utero if mom has primary HSV infection	Neonates: (1) Local: **Vesicular skin, oral, and eye lesions** (2) CNS: Irritability, seizures, lethargy (3) Disseminated: Neonatal sepsis	Dx: HSV PCR (swab lesion) Tx: Acyclovir PPX: - Acyclovir (36 weeks GA to birth, if hx of genital HSV infection) - C-Section: If active genital lesion or prodrome (e.g., vulvar pain)
Syphilis	- Spirochete *T. pallidum* - Transplacental transmission - Most commonly occurs in pregnant women with untreated primary and secondary syphilis (not latent)	Neonates: - ↑ risk of fetal demise, IUGR, prematurity - **Early features**: Maculopapular rash, rhinitis ("snuffles"), fever, jaundice, condyloma lata - **Later features** (> 2 y/o): Frontal bossing, saddle nose, Hutchinson teeth (pegged shaped incisors), mulberry molars, gummas, saber shins (anterior bowing), intellectual disability	Dx: FTA-ABS, RPR/VDRL Tx: Penicillin Note: If allergy, check skin allergy test, and if positive → desensitize
Parvovirus	- DNA virus - Transplacental transmission	Maternal: Febrile illness, polyarthralgias Neonates: - ↑ risk first trimester spontaneous abortions - Infection during 2nd-3rd trimester can cause hydrops fetalis	Dx: Parvo IgM Tx: Monitor fetal MCA velocity for signs of severe anemia. If severe, give intrauterine RBC transfusion.
VZV	- Rare, primary varicella infection - Transplacental transmission during late 1st-2nd trimester (Shingles has no impact on baby)	Neonates: - Vesicular rash/scarring - Microcephaly, hydrocephalus, seizures - Ocular (cataracts, chorioretinitis) - Limb hypoplasia - Intellectual disability	Tx: Acyclovir PPX: - VZV vaccine PRIOR to pregnancy - Varizig, indicated for: - Pregnant, seronegative moms exposed to VZV - Baby exposed at birth
Zika	- Mosquito-transmitted Zika virus - Transplacental transmission, most dangerous in the first trimester	Neonates: Microcephaly, CNS abnormalities, vision/hearing loss, hypertonia, and seizures - Closed anterior fontanelle	Tx: Supportive PPX: Avoid endemic areas

Other Perinatal Infections

Management of Maternal HIV During Pregnancy

General: HIV can be transmitted transplacentally, at the time of delivery, and via breast milk

Prenatal	Initiate **all HIV (+) mothers on ART therapy**: - Dual NRTI backbone (tenofovir/emtricitabine) PLUS - Integrase inhibitor (dolutegravir)
Intrapartum	- Continue ART throughout pregnancy/delivery - If viral load > 1000 copies/mL: Schedule C-section at 38 weeks plus IV Zidovudine
Postnatal	- Moms: Continue ART therapy - Infants: - If low maternal viral load: Zidovudine (2-6 weeks depending on breast vs formula feeding) - If high maternal viral load: ART therapy (full 2-3 drug regimen)

Other Infectious Disease During Pregnancy

Hepatitis B	- Transplacental transmission occurs with active hepatitis B infection - HBeAg (+) moms have ~ 90% transmission rate - Newborns of HBsAg (+) mothers should receive HBIG and hepatitis B vaccine within 12 hours of delivery - Mothers with active hepatitis B can receive tenofovir
Hepatitis C	- Transplacental transmission in ~ 5-10% of HCV infected women (exclusively if HCV RNA (+)) - Babies are usually asymptomatic at birth - Check HCV antibody at ~ 18 months to see if baby infected
Chlamydia	- Maternal infection associated with preterm, PPROM, low birth weight - Causes conjunctivitis (< 2 weeks) and pneumonia (~ 4-12 weeks) in newborns - Tx: Azithromycin (for mother). Erythromycin (for neonate).
Gonorrhea	- Maternal infection associated with spontaneous abortions, PPROM, prematurity - Causes ophthalmia neonatorum (conjunctivitis) - Tx: Ceftriaxone + azithromycin

Abortion

Elective Abortion

General: ~ 50% of pregnancies are unintended, and ~ 20% are terminated electively. Legality in US is state dependent. Procedure:

Type	Timing	Features
Medical	< 10 weeks GA	- Mifepristone, followed by Misoprostol in 24-48 hours
Aspiration	< 14 weeks GA	- Mechanical cervical dilatation and aspiration of uterine contents
Surgical	14-24 weeks GA	- Dilation and evacuation (osmotic or pharm dilators, followed by extraction/curettage)
Induction	14-24 weeks GA	- Misoprostol + mifepristone (Note: Usually use feticidal injection to ensure no live birth)

Management: RhoGAM if Rh (-) [only if > 12 weeks of gestation]. Antibiotic prophylaxis (usually given, but controversial).

Spontaneous Abortion (Miscarriage)

General: Loss of viable uterine pregnancy **prior to the 20th week** of pregnancy. Most common in first trimester, and most commonly due to chromosomal abnormalities.

Risk: ↑ Maternal age (> 35 y/o), smoking/EtOH use, history of spontaneous abortion, maternal systemic disease

Etiology:

Fetal	- **Chromosomal abnormalities** (e.g., aneuploidy [Trisomy 16]) - Trauma - Congenital abnormalities (from teratogens, TORCH infections) - Abnormal implantation
Maternal	- Maternal uterine structural abnormalities - Systemic maternal disease (infection, endocrinopathy, hypercoagulable state)

Diagnosis: **Pelvic exam and TVUS**. US can confirm fetal viability if POC still in utero (assess for cardiac activity).

Management: See below for specifics depending on classification of abortion. RhoGAM if Rh (-).

Complications: Endometritis, septic abortion, hemorrhage

	Symptoms	Findings	Management
Complete	- Uterine bleeding + cramping - Complete passage of POC, followed by resolution of symptoms	- Closed cervical Os - POC absent on US	- Supportive
Threatened	- Uterine bleeding +/– abdominal pain - No POC expulsion	- Closed Cervical Os - Intact membranes - Live fetus	- Supportive care (until symptoms resolve or progress to complete abortion) - ↑ risk for IUGR, preterm, PPROM, fetal death (but can still have viable birth)
Inevitable	- Uterine bleeding + cramping	- Open cervical Os - POC present on US (at level or above os) - Fetus may still have heartbeat	- Can be managed one of three ways, based on preference: (1) Surgery (dilation and curettage) (2) Medically (mifepristone/misoprostol) (3) Expectant management (allow natural passage. Can monitor β-hCG to measure completeness. If spontaneous passage does not occur, can then proceed to surgical or medical intervention.)
Incomplete	- Uterine bleeding + cramping - Passage of large clots/tissue	- Open cervical Os - POC present on US (within/being expelled from cervical canal)	
Missed	- Fetal death without passage of POC - Variable presentation (asymptomatic to uterine bleeding) - Failure of pregnancy to progress	- Closed Cervical Os - US shows nonviable conceptus with no fetal cardiac activity	
Septic	- Foul-smelling vaginal discharge - Most often occurs after elective abortion, but can occur with spontaneous abortion (especially if retained POC)	- Sepsis (fever, hypotension) - Enlarged, tender uterus/cervix	- IV Antibiotics (same as PID) - Suction D&C

Abortion

Intrauterine Fetal Demise

General: Absence of fetal cardiac activity > 20 weeks gestation

Risk: ↑ age, obesity, multiple gestation, smoking, underlying medical conditions

Etiology: Most have no identifiable cause
- Congenital abnormalities, fetal growth restriction
- Maternal infection or systemic disease
- Placental injury (e.g., abruption), uterine abnormalities, fetal cord accident (diagnosis of exclusion)

Clinical: **Uterus small for GA, reported lack of movement**

Diagnosis: US (**without fetal heart activity**, confirmed by 2 MDs)

Management:
- GA 20-24 weeks: Dilation and evacuation or induction and delivery
- GA > 24 weeks: Prostaglandins and Oxytocin for induction and delivery
- Note: If not delivered within a few weeks, risk for maternal DIC

Workup: Autopsy, placental analysis, fetal karyotype, maternal labs (for antiphospholipid, fetomaternal hemorrhage)

Recurrent Spontaneous Abortion

General: Defined as three or more consecutive pregnancy losses

Risk:

Uterine	- Polyps/fibroids/adhesions - Cervical insufficiency
Genetic	- Aneuploidy - Parents with balanced or Robertsonian translocations
Endocrine	- Uncontrolled diabetes - Hypothyroidism, hyperprolactinemia
Hematologic	- Inherited or acquired hypercoagulable states - Antiphospholipid syndrome

Diagnosis:
- Uterine hysterosalpingogram (workup for structure)
- Karyotypes of mom/dad, and abortus if available (for genetic testing)
- Anticardiolipin IgM/IgG, lupus anticoagulant titers, TSH

Management: Treat underlying (surgical correction of structural abnormalities, manage endocrinopathy, etc.)

Cervical Insufficiency

General: Inability of the uterine cervix to retain a pregnancy in the second trimester due to painless dilation of the cervix

Etiology:
- Cervical trauma: Repeated D&C, cervical conization/LEEP, prior labor/delivery
- Congenital cervical abnormalities

Clinical: **Recurrent second trimester pregnancy loss**, cervical dilation and effacement on physical exam
- Can be asymptomatic or present with mild cramping/contractions

Diagnosis: Transvaginal US (cervical length < 25 mm before 24 weeks)

Management:
- **Cerclage** (suture stabilization of the cervical os)
- Vaginal progesterone
- Avoid exercise during pregnancy

Ectopic Pregnancy

Ectopic Pregnancy

General: Implantation at a site other than the endometrium. Locations include:
- Tube ampulla (~ 80%), tube isthmus (~ 10%), fimbriae (~ 5%)
- Abdominal, ovarian, cervical, Cesarean scar (all rare)

Risk: History of ectopic pregnancy, tubal surgery/pathology, history of PID, IVF, endometriosis, smoking
- IUD (lower risk for pregnancy, but elevated risk for ectopic if failure)

Clinical: **Abdominal pain and vaginal bleeding**

Diagnosis: **Serial β-hCG and transvaginal US** (see algorithm below)
- Note: β-hCG should rise by at least 35% in 48 hours (normally it increases by > 50%)

Management:

Surgical Salpingectomy OR salpingostomy	Indicated if: - Hemodynamically unstable or tubal rupture - Ectopic on TVUS, and β-hCG > 5,000 OR fetal cardiac activity present on US - Contraindications to MTX (coexisting intrauterine pregnancy, immunodeficiency, hematologic disease) - Patient not reliable/able to comply with medical follow up
Medical Methotrexate (MTX)	- 50 mg/m^2 dose of MTX given day 1 - β-hCG checked on days 4, 7 - If inadequate decline (< 15%), second dose of MTX given - Follow β-hCG until undetectable

Complications: **Tubal rupture**
- Presents as diffuse abdominal pain (peritonitis), cervical motion tenderness
  - +/– Severe vaginal bleeding
  - Possible hypovolemic shock
- Dx: FAST US
- Tx: Stabilize in ED (ABCs, blood transfusions), emergent laparotomy

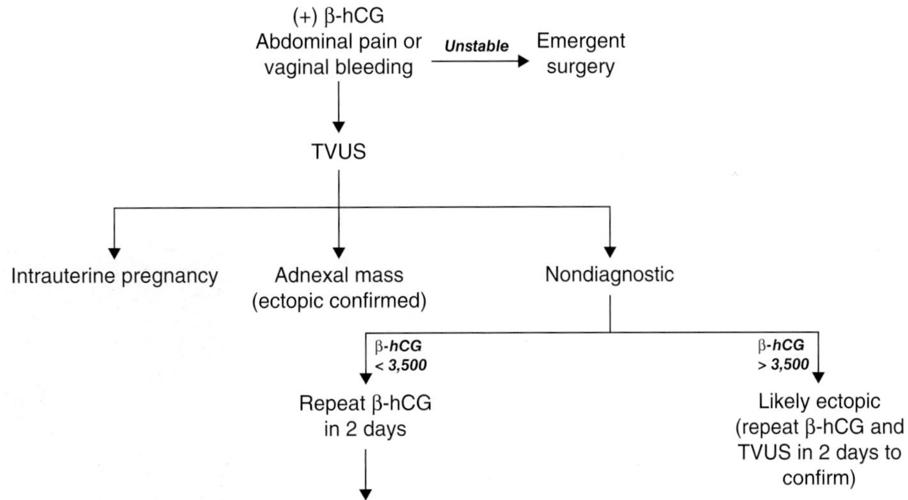

Appropriate β-hCG rise (> 35%): Repeat TVUS (IUP likely)

Inappropriate β-hCG rise (< 35%): Repeat TVUS (ectopic likely)

Decrease in β-hCG: Nonviable pregnancy: Trend β-hCG +/– diagnostic uterine aspiration

Gestational Trophoblastic Disease

Hydatidiform Mole

	Complete Mole (~90% cases)	Partial Mole (~10% cases)
Mxn	- Sperm fertilizes empty ovum	- Normal ovum fertilized by 2 sperm
Karyo	- 46 XX; 46 XY - All paternal chromosomes - p57-negative	- 69 XXY; 69 XXX; (rarely) 69 XYY - Extra paternal chromosome set - p57-positive
Histo	- Diffuse villi swelling/hyperplasia - **No fetal tissue**	- Focal villi swelling/hyperplasia - **Fetal tissue present** (RBC, body parts)
Clin	- Presents with painless uterine bleeding - Uterus enlarged for date - β-hCG high (> 100,000) - Signs of high β-hCG (hyperemesis, preeclampsia, hyperthyroidism, theca lutein cyst)	- Presents as missed abortion - Uterus expected size or small for date - β-hCG mildly elevated
US	- "Snow-storm" pattern, grape-like clusters[A]	- Variable
Prog	- 20% chance of gestational trophoblastic neoplasia - 4% chance of metastatic disease	- < 5% chance of gestational trophoblastic neoplasia - 0% chance of metastatic disease

General: Moles are considered **benign** trophoblastic disease (while invasive moles, placental site trophoblastic tumors, and choriocarcinoma are considered gestational trophoblastic **neoplasia**)

Risk: History of molar pregnancy, age > 35 or < 15

Clinical: See above

Diagnosis: Based on US features, symptoms, and β-hCG. Confirmed with histology.

Management: **Dilation and suction curettage** (alternative: hysterectomy, if done childbearing)
- Follow β-hCG until normalized (+ 6-month period after normalized)
  - Usually 14 weeks for complete mole, 8 weeks partial mole
  - Ensure good contraception during this period of time
  - If β-hCG is elevated → concern for gestational trophoblastic neoplasia

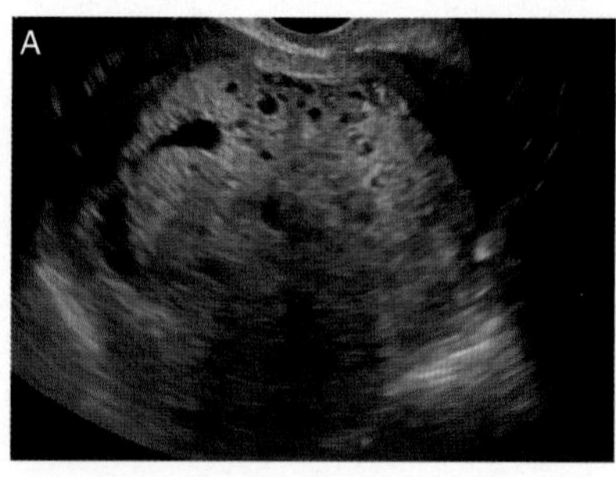

Gestational Trophoblastic Disease

Gestational Trophoblastic Neoplasia (Overview)

General: Refers to a group of malignant trophoblastic neoplasms. Associated with hydatidiform moles or normal pregnancy. Types include:

- Invasive mole
- Placental site trophoblastic tumor
- Choriocarcinoma

Risk: History of molar pregnancy, ↑ maternal age (> 40 y/o), Asian/Native American ancestry

Clinical: Variable depending on subtype of disease

- **Vaginal bleeding**
- Symptoms from ↑ **β-hCG** (hyperthyroidism, theca lutein cysts, pelvic pain)

Diagnosis: Clinical (based on ↑ β-hCG, TVUS, metastatic disease)

- Tissue not required for diagnosis
- Workup (if suspicious) should include CXR (common metastatic site)

Management:

- Low risk: Single-agent chemotherapy (**methotrexate** or actinomycin D)
    - Generally defined as local disease without significant metastasis
- High risk: Multi-agent chemotherapy
    - Generally defined as highly metastatic disease
- Always trend β-hCG and provide effective contraception
- Placental site trophoblastic tumor should be treated with hysterectomy or local resection

Gestational Trophoblastic Neoplasia (Subtypes)

Invasive Mole	- Swollen villi invading into myometrium - Rarely metastasize and can spontaneously regress - Presents as ↑ β-hCG after treatment of molar pregnancy and/or persistent vaginal bleeding - Tx: Chemotherapy (see above) - Note: Hysterectomy is alternative if no desire for fertility
Placental Site Trophoblastic Tumor	- Proliferation of intermediate trophoblasts (no villi) - Usually occurs months or years after a non-molar abortion or pregnancy - Presents as irregular vaginal bleeding and enlarged uterus - Note: β-hCG not significantly elevated (because no syncytiotrophoblast, but hPL is ↑) - Tx: Hysterectomy or resection (poor chemotherapy sensitivity)
Choriocarcinoma	- Can occur with molar pregnancy (50%), abortion, or normal pregnancy - Proliferation of cytotrophoblast and syncytiotrophoblast without chorionic villi - Early metastasis to vagina and lungs (hematogenous spread) - Presents with ↑ β-hCG, vaginal bleeding, possible pulmonary symptoms - Tx: Chemotherapy (see above)

Placental Pathology

Placental Abruption

General: Separation of the placenta prior to delivery of fetus

Risk: History of placental abruption, chronic placental disease (hypertension/eclampsia), abnormal uterus, trauma (blunt trauma, deceleration injury), rapid uterine decompression (e.g., delivery of twin, relief of polyhydramnios)

Clinical: **Severe vaginal bleeding, abdominal pain/contractions**, uterine rigidity/tenderness, fetal distress
- Can be complicated by maternal hemorrhagic shock, DIC, fetal demise

Diagnosis: US (retroplacental hematoma). Note: US findings not consistent, so diagnosis is made clinically.

Management: Stabilization (FHR monitoring, IV access, other supportive care), followed by delivery (depends on stability of mom/baby):
- If both are stable (and > 36 weeks): Vaginal delivery
- If either is unstable: **C-section** (unless vaginal delivery imminent)

Uterine Rupture

General: Complete rupture of uterine wall

Etiology:
- Associated with **prior uterine surgery** (C-section [especially history of rupture, vertical hysterotomy], uterine myomectomy)
- ↑ risk with prolonged labor, excess uterotonic drugs, multiple gestation, ↑ maternal age

Clinical: Presents during labor with sudden worsening of abdominal pain, vaginal bleeding
- Classic signs: **Loss of fetal station, or palpation of fetal parts outside uterus**, symptoms exacerbated by oxytocin
- Can be complicated by urinary tract injury, hemorrhagic shock, fetal distress

Diagnosis: Clinical + US confirmation (disruption of all uterine layers)

Management: Emergent C-section. Hysterectomy. Occasionally uterine repair may be possible.

Other Placental Complications

	General/Risk	Clinical/Diagnosis	Management
Placenta Previa	- **Abnormal placental implantation in lower uterus** Subtypes: - Complete: Covers the cervical os - Partial: Partially covers cervical os - Marginal: Extends to the margin of the os - Low lying: Edge < 2 cm from os - Risk: Prior placenta previa or Cesarean delivery, history of uterine surgery, multiple gestation	- **Painless vaginal bleeding** - Rarely causes uterine contractions - Associated with preterm labor, placenta accreta, vasa previa, PROM - Dx: **Ultrasound** (before digital exam due to risk for hemorrhage) Note: Once placenta is > 2 cm from cervical os, vaginal delivery is considered safe	- If asymptomatic: Follow with US (most previa resolve on own) - Counsel patients to reduce bleeding risk by avoiding sexual activity, strenuous exercise, or prolonged standing - Supportive care/blood transfusions for acute episodes of bleeding - Delivery (at 36-37 weeks) by C-section - C-section also indicated if patient goes into labor, has life-threatening bleed, or severe fetal distress
Vasa Previa	- **Fetal blood vessels covering the cervical os** - Associated with velamentous umbilical cord or succenturiate lobe - Risk: Velamentous cord insertion, low-lying placenta/previa, IVF, multiple gestation	- Painless bleeding after membrane rupture, followed by fetal distress - Apt test to confirm fetal blood (mix NaOH w/ blood → Turns pink if fetal) - Dx: **Transvaginal US** (w/ doppler)	- Antepartum: Fetal surveillance, betamethasone at 28-32 weeks, **schedule C-section at 34-35 weeks** - If labor, bleeding, PROM → Emergent C-section
Placenta Accreta	- Accreta: Anchoring of placental villi to the myometrium - Increta: Chorionic villi invade the myometrium - Percreta: Anchoring of placental villi through the myometrium and into serosa/abdominal organs - Risk: Prior myomectomy, C-section, D&C	- Generally asymptomatic prior to delivery (but may be identified via US) - At delivery: **Lack of placenta delivery** - Retained parts, possible cord avulsion, and severe hemorrhage - Dx: **Ultrasound**	- **Scheduled C-section/hysterectomy at 34-35 weeks** - If diagnosed due to hemorrhage at the time of vaginal delivery → emergent hysterectomy

Multiple Gestation

Overview of Multiple Gestation

General: ~ 30 twin births per 1000 live births in US

Risk: ↑ maternal age, IVF/ assisted reproductive technology

Clinical:
- Moms can experience rapid weight gain, ↑↑ uterus size for age
- ↑ β-hCG, AFP, hPL for expected age

Diagnosis: Most commonly identified on US
- Can see two amniotic sacs or "twin-peaks" sign (fused membranes)

Management:
- **Twin delivery**:
  - Cephalic/cephalic: Vaginal delivery
  - Cephalic/noncephalic: C-section or trial of vaginal delivery
  - Noncephalic/noncephalic: C-section
- **Triplets**: Almost always require C-section

Maternal Complications:
- High risk for gestational hypertension and preeclampsia, placental abnormalities (previa), and C-section

Fetal Complications:
- Prematurity and low birth weight (common, risk ↑ with fetal number)
- Fetal growth restriction (from crowding or uteroplacental insufficiency)
- Increased risk of congenital malformations

- **Twin-twin transfusion**
  - Imbalanced vascular flow to two monochorionic twins
  - "Donor twin": Hypovolemic, growth restriction, oligohydramnios
  - "Recipient twin": Hypervolemia, organomegaly, polyhydramnios
  - Twin anemia polycythemia sequence: Intertwin hemoglobin difference
    - Anemia of one twin and polycythemia of the other twin
  - Management:
    - Mild cases: Expectant management
    - Fetal laser coagulation (corrects flow difference)
    - Amnioreduction (helps prevent preterm contractions)

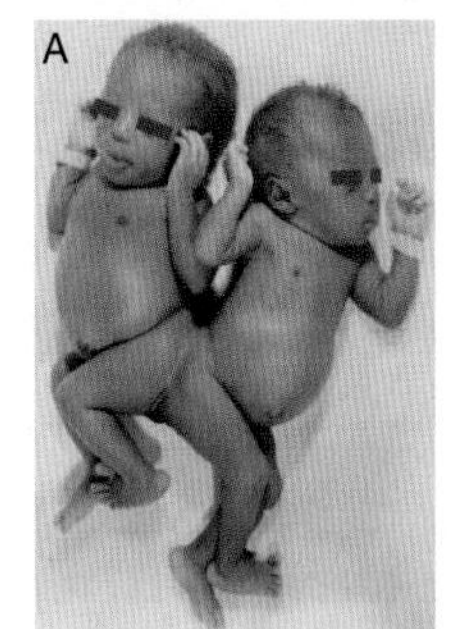

Multiple Gestation (Subtypes)

Class	Features
Dizygotic ("Fraternal twins")	
Dichorionic diamniotic	- Implantation of two separate fertilized ovum - Can be different sexes - Separate placenta/amniotic sacs
Monozygotic ("Identical twins")	
Dichorionic diamniotic	- One fertilized ovum, which splits (~ days 1-3) and implant separately - Separate placenta/amniotic sacs
Monochorionic diamniotic	- One fertilized ovum, which splits after blastocyst forms (~ days 4-8), and implant separately - Share placenta, separate amniotic sac
Monochorionic monoamniotic	- One fertilized ovum, which implants, and then later splits (~ days 8-13) - Same placenta, same amniotic sac - Highest risk for fetal mortality
Conjoined[A]	- Same as monochorionic-monoamniotic, except split occurs at ~ 14 days after embryonic disk has formed

Normal Labor and Delivery

Overview and Definition of Labor

General: Labor is defined as painful **uterine contractions PLUS cervical change**
- Braxton-Hicks contractions: irregular, third trimester contractions with no cervical changes

Stage	Definition	Nulliparous	Multiparous
First (latent)	Onset of labor until 4-6 cm dilation	< 20 hours (average 10-12 hours)	< 14 hours (average 6-8 hours)
First (active)	4-6 cm until complete 10 cm cervical dilation	4-6 hours (> 1-1.2 cm/hr)	2-3 hr (> 1.2-1.5 cm/hr)
Second	Complete cervical dilation to delivery of infant	< 2 hours (3 hours if epidural)	< 1 hour (2 hours if epidural)
Third	From delivery of infant to delivery of placenta	< 30 minutes	< 30 minutes

Evaluation of Labor

Initial Evaluation of Labor:

Fetal Lie/Presentation	- **Lie:** Long axis of fetus compared to long axis of mother (e.g., longitudinal or transverse) - **Presentation:** Part of fetus over pelvic inlet (e.g., cephalic/vertex) - **Leopold maneuvers:** Palpation used to determine fetal lie

Cervical Examination	- **Dilation:** Measured at internal os
	  - Dilation can cause "bloody show" (small cervical bleed)
	- **Effacement:** Thinning of cervix from normal length of 3-5 cm
	- **Station:** Based on position relative to imaginary line between ischial spines
	  - Negative is inside of uterus, positive is outside of uterus
	- **Cervical position** and **consistency**

Speculum Examination	- Evaluate for evidence of **rupture of membranes** (ROM) - Pooling of fluid (asking to bear down), nitrazine paper (amniotic fluid is alkaline), ferning (microscopically) - Other tests: Indigo-carmine dye injection, amnisure immunoassay
Ultrasound	- Can evaluate for effacement or new oligohydramnios (suggests ROM)

Bishop Score: Score predicts likelihood of natural labor, success of labor induction (higher score more favorable)

Cervical Status	0	1	2	3
Dilatation	Closed	1-2 cm	3-4 cm	> 5 cm
Effacement	< 30%	30-50%	50-80%	> 80%
Station	−3	−2	−1 or 0	≥ +1
Consistency	Firm	Intermediate	Soft	
Position	Posterior	Intermediate	Anterior	

Cardinal Movements and Occiput Presentation

Cardinal movements:
- Engagement, descent and internal rotation
- Complete rotation, complete extension
- External rotation
- Anterior shoulder delivery, posterior shoulder delivery

Occiput presentation:
- Vertex presentation with anterior occiput is ideal
- Occiput posterior and transverse can lead to longer delivery time

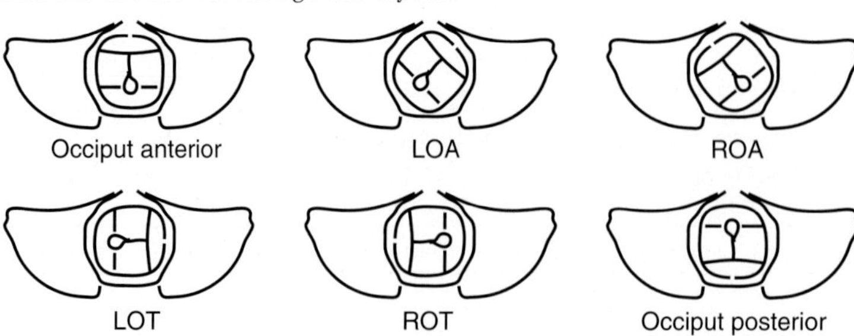

Normal Labor and Delivery

Fetal Heart Rate Monitoring

General: Fetal heart rate can be monitored via **external doppler monitor** or **fetal scalp electrode**. Combined with tocometry, which measures intrauterine pressure to help establish timing, length, and strength of contractions.

Component	Features
Heart Rate	- **Normal**: 110-160/minute **< 110 (bradycardia)**: Congenital heart defects, severe fetal hypoxemia (uterine hyperstimulation, cord prolapse, rapid fetal descent) **> 160 (tachycardia)**: Hypoxia, maternal infection/fever, fetal anemia, drugs
Variability	- **Absent**: Indicates severe fetal distress - **Minimal**: < 6 bpm (indicates fetal hypoxia, drugs, or sleep) - Can attempt fetal scalp stimulation to induce variability - **Normal**: 6-25 bpm - **Marked**: > 25 bpm - **Sinusoidal**[A]: Fetal anemia 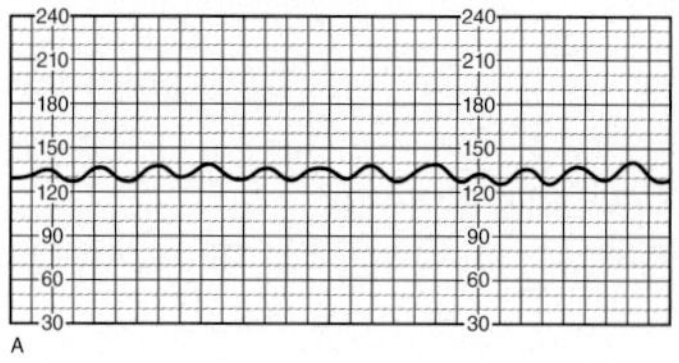
Accelerations	- 15 bpm above baseline for 15 seconds (at least 2 in 20 minutes) Note: At < 32 weeks it is 10 bpm/10 seconds, at least 2 in 20 minutes

Decelerations:

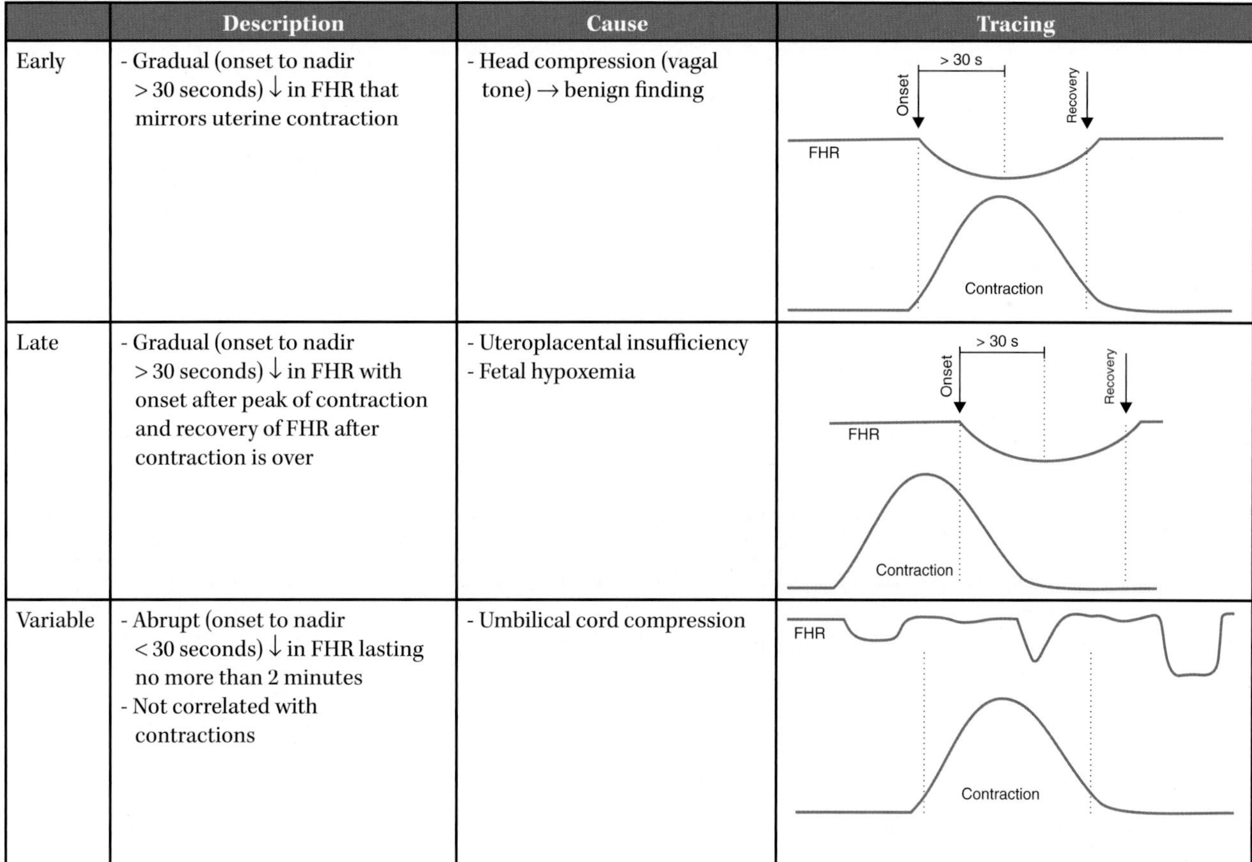

	Description	Cause	Tracing
Early	- Gradual (onset to nadir > 30 seconds) ↓ in FHR that mirrors uterine contraction	- Head compression (vagal tone) → benign finding	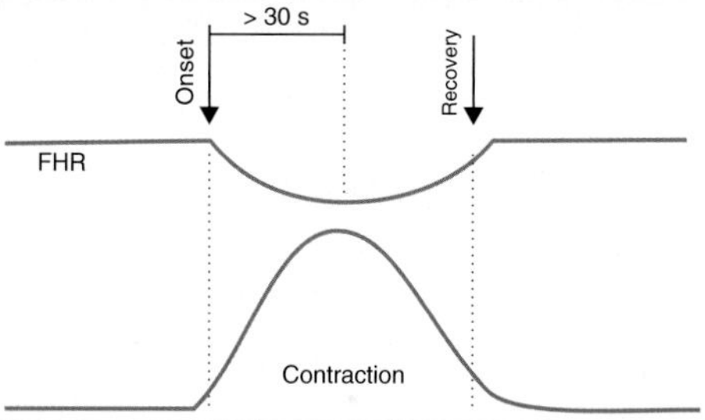
Late	- Gradual (onset to nadir > 30 seconds) ↓ in FHR with onset after peak of contraction and recovery of FHR after contraction is over	- Uteroplacental insufficiency - Fetal hypoxemia	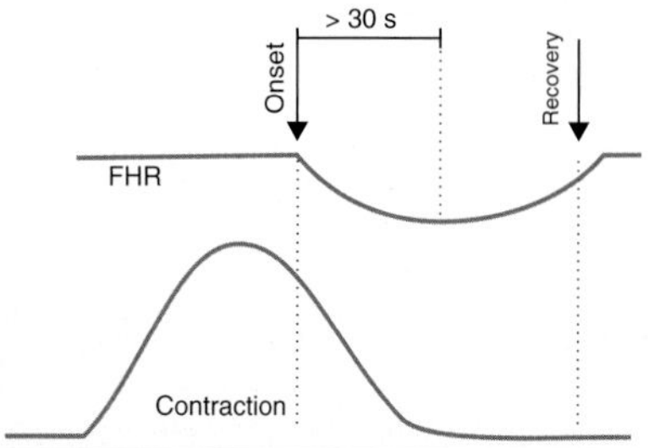
Variable	- Abrupt (onset to nadir < 30 seconds) ↓ in FHR lasting no more than 2 minutes - Not correlated with contractions	- Umbilical cord compression	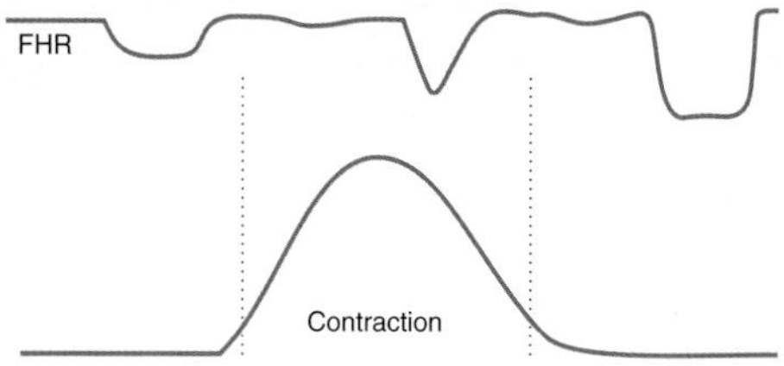

VEAL-CHOP

- **V**ariable → **C**ord compression
- **E**arly → **H**ead compression
- **A**cceleration → **O**kay
- **L**ate → **P**lacental insufficiency

Normal Labor and Delivery

Induction and Augmentation of Labor

Induction: Stimulation of uterine contractions
- Indicated if:
    - Postterm
    - PROM
    - Hypertensive disorders (e.g., preeclampsia)
    - IUGR
    - Oligohydramnios
- Techniques:
    - May begin spontaneously after cervical ripening
    - Oxytocin
    - Amniotomy (artificial rupture of membranes)

Cervical ripening:
- Indicated in those with **poor Bishop score (< 6) prior to induction**
- Methods include:
    - Misoprostol (PGE1)
    - PGE2 gel or vaginal inserts (prepidil/cervidil)
    - Mechanical bulb dilator

Augmentation:
- Indications: Inadequate contractions or prolonged phase of labor
- **Oxytocin**: Stimulates uterus for stronger and more frequent contractions
    - Side effects: Tachysystole, ADH-like effect (hyponatremia), hypotension, maternal fatigue

Analgesia and Pain Management

General: Visceral pain from uterine and cervical distension/cramping (stage 1) and somatic pain from stage 2 of labor as vagina and perineal structures are stretched
- Block must reach T10 for visceral first stage pain, S2-S4 for second stage

Indications: Maternal request (sufficient to provide, assuming no contraindications)

Lamaze	- Coping/relaxation techniques taught in classes during pregnancy
Opiates	- Generally inferior to neuraxial block and avoided - If used, rapid acting agents used (Fentanyl) - Can cause fetal bradycardia and neonatal respiratory depression
Neuraxial	- Options include **epidural, combined spinal-epidural, or spinal** - Generally given continuously via catheter (can be via "single-shot") - Continuous allows easy transition to operative delivery - Drug choice: Local anesthetic (bupivacaine) plus opiate (fentanyl) - [See: Surgery] for discussion of complications
Nerve Block	- Pudendal nerve block: Used as adjunct if patient suffering from somatic vaginal/perineal pain
General Anesthesia	- Reserved for cases of emergent C-section when there is no time for neuraxial block

Operative Labor and Delivery

Cesarean Delivery

Indications:

Maternal	Fetal
Failure to progress, including: - **Cephalopelvic disproportion** - Failed labor induction Structural: - Mechanical obstruction to vaginal birth (e.g., large fibroid) - Placental abruption, previa - Vasa previa or cord prolapse Medical conditions: - HIV infection (untreated) - Active HSV - Cervical cancer	Fetal pregnancy complications: - **Nonreassuring fetal status** - **Fetal malpresentation** - Multiple gestation (triplets or malpresenting first twin) Fetal anomalies: - Macrosomia

Surgical technique:
- Neuraxial anesthesia is preferred (general anesthesia for emergencies)
- Transverse incision (pfannenstiel)
  - Better cosmetics, less postoperative pain
  - Occasionally vertical incisions are used in severe emergencies
- Low transverse hysterotomy
- Delivery of fetus and placenta
- Ensure no retained parts/bleeding (uterine massage/oxytocin)
- Uterine and abdominal wall closure

Postoperative issues:
- Pain, urinary retention, infection, bleeding

Long-term complications:
- Uterine scarring (↑ risk for uterine rupture, placenta previa/accreta, abruption)

Trial of Labor After Cesarean (TOLAC)

General: Primary C-section is often followed by C-section during future pregnancies, some women elect for trial of labor
- TOLAC: Trial of labor after Cesarean
- VBAC: Vaginal birth after Cesarean

- Risk in these patients for uterine rupture at site of C-section scar

Lower risk	- Only 1 prior C-section, via a low transverse hysterotomy - Prior vaginal birth or VBAC
Completely contraindicated	- Prior transfundal uterine incision - Prior uterine rupture

Management:
- Patient-centered decision weighing pros and cons and utilizing prediction calculators
- In general, can encourage TOLAC if lower risk (see above)

Operative Labor and Delivery

Operative Vaginal Delivery

General: Use of forceps or vacuum to assist in the extraction of fetus from vagina

Indications:

- Indicated in select cases when delivery needs to be urgently completed
- Decision must be made on Cesarean delivery vs operative vaginal delivery
- Operative vaginal delivery may be used if:
    - Prolonged second stage of labor (from maternal exhaustion)
    - Fetal compromise (and expeditious vaginal birth is an option)
    - Maternal disorder that contraindicates Valsalva
- Note: In all the above cases, operative delivery must be safe/possible. This means baby has head engaged (with station > 0), full dilation/cervical effacement, membranes ruptured.

Type	Features	Adverse Events
Forceps	- Forceps used to grasp the anterior occiput	- ↑ risk of maternal genital trauma (vs vacuum) - ↑ risk of fetal CN VII injury (vs vacuum)
Vacuum	- Suction cup applied to fetal scalp	- ↑ risk of cephalohematoma, retinal hemorrhage (vs forceps)

*All operative vaginal deliveries have rare risk of fetal CNS hemorrhage

Episiotomy/Lacerations

Episiotomy:

- Surgical enlargement of the vagina via incision into perineum (widens the birth canal to facilitate delivery)
- **Routine episiotomy NOT recommended**
- Occasionally used by some OB physicians when rapid vaginal delivery is needed or for shoulder dystocia
- Approach:
    - Mediolateral (↓ risk of sphincter injury, but harder to repair)
    - Medial (easiest to repair, but painful and ↑ risk of sphincter injury)
- Complications: Sphincter injury, bleeding, infection, rectovaginal fistula

Lacerations:

- Vaginal lacerations are commonplace with vaginal delivery
- Types:
    - Grade 1: Vaginal only
    - Grade 2: Perineal body
    - Grade 3: Into anal sphincter
    - Grade 4: Through anal mucosa
- Complications: Wound abscess, sphincter injury, rectovaginal fistula

Complications of Labor and Delivery

	General/Clinical	Management
Spontaneous Rupture of Membranes (ROM)	- Occurs after the onset of labor - Required for fetal head engagement - Can be confirmed via history of gush of fluid and speculum examination confirming leakage of amniotic fluid	- Normal delivery management Note: Can confirm ROM with nitrazine paper test, fern testing, US (for oligohydramnios), indigo carmine dye injection
Prelabor ROM (PROM)	- **ROM prior to regular contractions** - Occurs at full term (vs PPROM) - ↑ risk of maternal and fetal infections - Confirm with speculum exam +/– testing of fluid	- Induction of labor (Oxytocin)
Preterm Prelabor ROM (PPROM)	- **ROM prior to contractions at < 37 weeks GA** - ↑ risk if prior PPROM, active GU infection - Complications: Intrauterine infection/neonatal sepsis, oligohydramnios, umbilical cord prolapse, fetal malpresentation	- See algorithm below

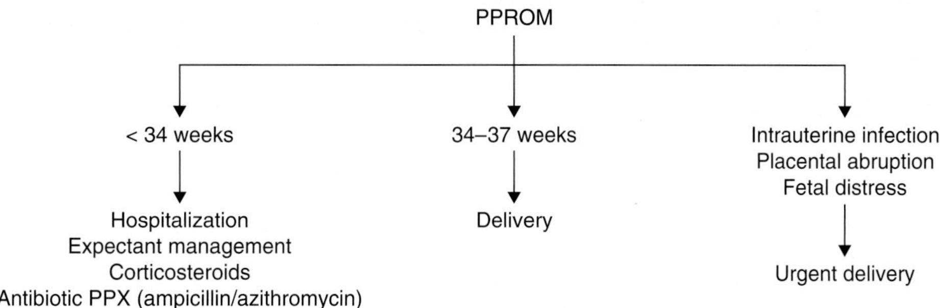

Premature Labor

General: Birth **prior to 37 weeks** gestational age

Risk: Prior premature labor, multiple gestation, smoking, history of cervical surgery, cervical insufficiency

Etiology: Premature labor can be induced by infection, PROM, polyhydramnios, placental abruption

Clinical: Presents similarly to term labor (cramping, contractions, vaginal discharge of clear/blood-tinged fluid)

Diagnosis: **Painful contractions** (> 4 in 20 minutes or > 8 in 60 minutes) AND **cervical change** (dilation > 3 cm or effacement)
- Fetal fibronectin (used between weeks 22 and 34) [High negative predictive value, positive test supports preterm labor]
- TVUS (shortened cervical length supports preterm labor)

Management: All should receive full H&P, speculum exam (r/o ROM), and US

≥ 34 weeks	- **Delivery** - Note: If no progression (and fetal well being is confirmed) then patient can be discharged
32-33 weeks	- Betamethasone - Tocolytic Drugs (48 hours to allow for steroid effects). Drugs include: - β2-mimetics (ritodrine, terbutaline), $MgSO_4$, calcium channel blockers (nifedipine), PG inhibitors (indomethacin) - GBS antibiotic PPX (penicillin G, ampicillin, or clindamycin)
< 32 weeks	- Same as 32-33 weeks, but add $MgSO_4$ (proven neuroprotection)

Fetal complications: Intraventricular hemorrhage, NRDS, PDA, necrotizing enterocolitis, retinopathy, bronchopulmonary dysplasia

Prophylaxis:
- If history of spontaneous preterm birth: Progesterone supplementation
- If short cervix (≤ 25 mm on TVUS at 16-24 weeks):
    - No history of preterm birth: Progesterone
    - Plus history of preterm birth: Progesterone plus cerclage

Complications of Labor and Delivery

Postterm Pregnancy

General: Postterm at ≥ 42 weeks GA

Risk: History of postterm pregnancy, obesity, male fetus, nulliparity

Management: Induce labor if:
- Nonreassuring fetal testing or oligohydramnios
- **≥ 42 weeks**
- Induction encouraged at 41 weeks GA (vs expectant management)

Complications:
- Fetal: Macrosomia, oligohydramnios, meconium aspiration
    - Dysmaturity syndrome (dry peeling nails, flaking skin, lots of hair)
- Maternal: Birth trauma, hemorrhage

GBS Infection

General: Organism that colonizes GU tract in women. Can cause UTI (both cystitis and pyelonephritis), chorioamnionitis, endomyometritis, neonatal sepsis.

Diagnosis: Screened for at **35-37 weeks** in pregnant women (**culture via vaginal/rectal swab**)
- Intrapartum rapid NAAT available if culture not performed in advance of labor

Management:
- Antibiotic PPX: Penicillin G or ampicillin (alt: Cefazolin, clindamycin)
- Started at the onset of labor (but not C-section without labor)
    - Indications include:
        - (+) Routine GBS screening
        - History of infant with neonatal GBS infection
        - GBS bacteriuria during current pregnancy
        - Unknown status, plus:
            - Preterm labor, intrapartum fever, or prolonged ROM (> 18 hours)

Chorioamnionitis

General: Infection of the amniotic fluid, membranes, placenta, and/or decidua. Usually polymicrobial (from vaginal flora in women with ruptured membranes), but can be due to iatrogenically introduced bacteria from procedures.

Clinical: Clinical diagnosis made with **fever >100.4°F** PLUS ≥ 1 of the following:
- Fetal tachycardia (HR > 160 /min)
- Maternal leukocytosis
- Purulent vaginal/cervical discharge
- Uterine tenderness

Diagnosis: Confirmed with positive gram stain/culture of amniotic fluid

Management:
- Antibiotics: **Ampicillin + Gentamicin** (+ Clindamycin or metronidazole if C-section)
- Immediate delivery (labor induction/vaginal delivery is okay unless patient has typical indication for C-section)

Complications of Labor and Delivery

Abnormal Labor Progression

	General	Management
First Stage (Latent)	- Normal: < 20 hours (prima), < 14 hours (multip) - Risk: Unfavorable cervix	- Therapeutic rest (morphine and rest) - Oxytocin and amniotomy - Will eventually pass into active labor or stop having contractions

First Stage (Active)	- Normal: > 6 cm, 1-2 cm/hours progression
	- **Protracted**: Dilating < 1 cm/hours
	- **Arrest**: No cervical change in 4 hours despite adequate contractions
	
	Causes:
	- **Hypocontractile uterine activity** ("lack of power"):
	  - Normal power is > 200 Montevideo units (MVUs)
	    - Defined as peak minus baseline uterine contraction pressure
		- Initial: Oxytocin and amniotomy
		- Arrest: Cesarean delivery

Second Stage	- Normal: < 2-3 hours if nulliparous, <1-2 hours if parous - Longer for those with epidural anesthesia Causes: - **Cephalopelvic disproportion** - Fetal malpresentation - Inadequate contractions, poor maternal effort	- Trial of oxytocin (if infrequent contractions) - Operative delivery OR C-section
Third Stage (Placental Delivery)	- Normal: < 30 minutes - Risk: Prior C-section, D&C, or fibroids	- Oxytocin, uterine massage - Retained placenta: Manual extraction or D&C [See: Postpartum hemorrhage]

Shoulder Dystocia

General: Inability to deliver shoulders after fetal head. Obstetric emergency.

Risk: Maternal obesity, diabetes mellitus, macrosomia, post-term, history of shoulder dystocia
- Note: > 50% of cases are idiopathic and have none of the above risk factors

Clinical: **Recoil of fetal head into the perineum** ("turtle sign")

Management:

B	- Breathe
E	- Elevate legs (McRoberts position: Sharp flexion of the hips)
C	- Call for help
A	- Apply suprapubic pressure (downward to release anterior shoulder)
L	- enLarge vaginal opening with episiotomy
M	- Maneuvers

Complications of Shoulder Dystocia

Erb Palsy	- C5-C6 injury. Presents with "Waiter tip" (arm internally rotated, straight at side; extended elbow, pronated forearm). - Tx: 80% are self-limited and improve over following months. Massage and physical therapy.
Klumpke	- C8-T1 injury. Presents with "claw hand" (extended wrist, extended MCPs, and flexed IPs). - Possible Horner syndrome
Clavicle Fx	- Presents with clavicular bony crepitus, deformity, and/or decreased Moro reflex on the affected side
Humeral Fx	- Presents with upper-arm bony crepitus, deformity, and/or decreased Moro reflex on the affected side
Asphyxia	- Can result in hypoxic-ischemic encephalopathy or death if severe

Complications of Labor and Delivery

Breech Presentation

General: Occurs when buttocks and/or feet are presenting part. 75% spontaneously change to vertex by week 38.

Frank Breech (50-75%)	- Presents rear first, with flexed hips and extended knees
Footling Breech (20%)	- Presents with one or both legs presented first
Complete Breech (5-10%)	- Presents rear first, with flexed hips and flexed knees

Risk: Limited fetal movement (fibroids, oligohydramnios), excess fetal movement (polyhydramnios, fetal growth restriction)

Diagnosis: Leopold maneuvers or ultrasound

Management:

- **External cephalic version**: Performed after week 36
    - Apply directed pressure to abdomen to turn infant to vertex
    - Selection: Normal fetal heart rate, adequate amniotic fluid
    - Risks: Placental abruption, ROM, and cord compression (must be prepared for emergency C-section, give RhoGAM)
    - Contraindications:
        - Absolute: Placenta previa, prior C-section
        - Relative: Active labor with fetal descent, oligohydramnios, nonreassuring fetal monitoring

- **Elective C-section**: Schedule at 39-40 weeks and preferred to vaginal delivery (lower risk of fetal morbidity)

- **Trial of breech vaginal delivery**:
    - Attempt only if low-risk for complications
    - Complications: Cord prolapse or head entrapment

- **Internal podalic version**:
    - Performed to flip around second twin in vaginal delivery of cephalic/non-cephalic twins

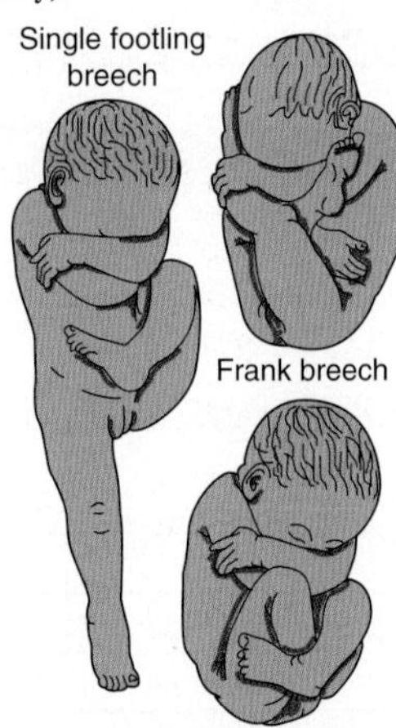

Other Fetal Malpresentation

Face	- Fetal face (from forehead to chin) is leading in birth canal
Brow	- Fetal forehead (from anterior fontanelle to the brow) leading

Transverse	- Fetal longitudinal axis is perpendicular to long axis of uterus
	- Usually converts to cephalic or breech presentation prior to labor
	- If persists, perform external cephalic version at 37 weeks (like breech)
	  - If converts to vertex, deliver vaginally like normal
	  - If does not convert after attempts at external cephalic version → C-section
	- If in active labor and transverse → C-section

Complications of Labor and Delivery

Fetal Distress

Decelerations	Late decelerations: - Late decelerations are always concerning and indicate need for rapid delivery - Causes: Fetal hypoxemia (due to uteroplacental insufficiency) Variable decelerations: - Fetal reflex response to transient umbilical cord compression
Bradycardia	- Heart rate < 110 (averaged over 10 minutes) Causes: - Pre placental (maternal hypoxia, seizure, sedation) - Uteroplacental (abruption, infarction, hemorrhage) - Post placental (cord prolapse, compression, or vasa previa)
Tachycardia	- Heart rate > 160 (averaged over 10 minutes) Causes: - Hypoxia, maternal infection/fever, fetal anemia, drugs

Category I	Category II	Category III
Heart rate 110 to 160/minute Moderate variability No late or variable decelerations	Neither I or III	Recurrent late or variable decelerations Fetal bradycardia Sinusoidal heart rate pattern

Management: For category III tracings
- Turn on left side to decrease IVC compression
- Bolus IV fluids, give oxygen
- Discontinue oxytocin
- If prolonged contraction (hypertonus) or tachysystole (too many contractions): Terbutaline
- Prepare for operative delivery

Cord Emergencies

Nuchal Cord	- Umbilical cord wrapped around fetal neck - Tx: Manually reduce. If unable, but delivery is imminent, clamp in two places and cut.
Cord Prolapse	- Cord protrusion past the presenting part of the fetus and into the cervical canal or vagina - Presents most often with fetal bradycardia/decelerations - Tx: Urgent C-section

Fetal Complications

Fetal (Intrauterine) Growth Restriction (FGR)

General: Defined as weight < 10th percentile or 2500 g
- **Fetal growth restriction**: Failure to reach in-utero growth potential due to genetic/environmental factors
- **Small for gestational age**: Weight < 10th percentile (including both constitutionally small and due to FGR)

	Symmetric FGR	Asymmetric FGR
Clinical	- Reductions in size of all organs - Body, head, and length proportionally affected	- Disproportionate growth restriction - Normal head size, but ↓ length, and ↓↓ **weight**
Timing	- Usually present **before** 20 weeks	- Usually presents **after** 20 weeks
Cause	- Chromosomal defects, genetic disorders - Congenital infections	- Uteroplacental insufficiency - Malnutrition

Management:
- **Prenatal**: Serial ultrasound, monitoring:
  - Fetal growth
  - Biophysical profile (BPP)
  - Umbilical artery doppler (IUGR can result from decreased, absent, or even reversed flow)
- **Delivery**: Try to maximize growth by delaying delivery
  - Deliver at term if no issues with BPP or umbilical doppler
  - Deliver if decreased/reversed flow on umbilical artery doppler and/or BPP becomes abnormal

Complications: Increased risk for prematurity, perinatal asphyxia, hypothermia, hypoglycemia, polycythemia

Large for Gestational Age

General: Weight > 90th percentile or 4000 g

Risk: Maternal diabetes mellitus, excessive weight gain, fetal sex (male), ↑ gestational age

Management: Planned Cesarean delivery, if:
- Estimated fetal weight > 4500 g in women with diabetes
- Estimated fetal weight > 5000 g in women without diabetes

Complications: Hypothermia, hypoglycemia, hypocalcemia, polycythemia
- Birth injuries common (clavicle fracture, brachial plexus injury, facial nerve palsy, shoulder dystocia)

Amniotic Fluid Disorders

	Oligohydramnios	Polyhydramnios
Gen	- AFI < 5	- AFI > 25
Etio	- **Fetal urinary tract abnormalities**: - GU obstruction, renal agenesis - **Rupture of membranes** - Uteroplacental insufficiency	- ↓ **fetal swallowing**: Duodenal atresia, TE fistula - Maternal DM - Multiple gestation, twin-twin transfusion syndrome - **Fetal anemia**, isoimmunization
Dx	- AFI: The sum of the deepest amniotic fluid pocket in all four quadrants - Single deepest pocket: Alternative, arguably better test (< 2 cm oligohydramnios, > 8 cm polyhydramnios)	
Tx	- **Delivery (at 36-37 weeks)** - Amnioinfusion (limited to temporarily increase amniotic fluid volume, for ECV or US imaging)	- Workup for underlying condition - Mild cases resolve without intervention - If severe, amnioreduction +/− Indomethacin (if < 32 weeks)
Comp	- High risk of fetal mortality - Cord compression - Potter sequence - Meconium aspiration	- Prematurity/PROM - Fetal malpresentation - Cord prolapse

Fetal Complications

RhD Alloimmunization

General: **Rh (–) moms** exposed to **fetal Rh (+) blood** in prior pregnancy can lead to maternal anti-Rh IgG that can cross the placenta and result in **fetal hemolytic anemia.** During first pregnancy, IgM builds (which does not pass placenta), but later pregnancies can have IgG that crosses placenta.

Risk: **Prior transplacental fetomaternal bleeding** (more likely if history of pregnancy without prenatal care or in third world country)

Clinical: Generally asymptomatic in mother. Fetal complications:
- Hemolytic anemia
- Kernicterus/jaundice
- Hydrops fetalis: Hyperdynamic state with heart failure, diffuse edema, ascites, pericardial effusion

Diagnosis: **Anti-RhD antibody** in maternal serum (screen at first visit)

Management: **For Rh (–) mothers with detectable anti-Rh(D) antibodies**
- Check father's Rh status:
    - If father is Rh (–), baby must be Rh (–) and not at risk
    - If father is homozygous Rh (+) → baby is Rh (+)
    - If father is heterozygous Rh (+) → test fetus (cell-free DNA)
    - If father not available, confirm fetal Rh typing (cell-free DNA)
- If fetus is Rh (+):
    - Serial maternal IgG Rh titers (≥ 1:16 has high risk for fetal anemia)
    - If high titers, transcranial MCA doppler (high flow → anemia)
    - If ↑ MCA doppler, check fetal CBC via umbilical cord sampling
- If severe fetal anemia:
    - Deliver if ≥ 35 weeks
    - Fetal transfusion < 35 weeks

Prevention: RhoGAM administration. Applies to RhD (–) women plus fetus with possible RhD (+). Indications:
- 28 weeks (beginning of third trimester)
- Within 72 hours of Rh (+) birth (but can be given later if its forgotten)
- Situations with risk of fetomaternal hemorrhage:
    - Abortion
    - Ectopic pregnancy, molar pregnancy
    - CVS/amniocentesis
    - Antepartum vaginal bleeding
    - Placenta previa/abruption
    - External cephalic version
    - Abdominal trauma

Note: If major bleeding suspected, Rosette test can confirm large bleed, with Kleihauer Betke test (measures fetal RBCs in maternal serum) to determine dose of RhoGAM

Other RBC Antigens

General: Maternal alloantibody to non-RhD RBC antigens that can result in hemolytic disease in fetus
- "Kell kills, Duffy dies, Lewis lives"

ABO Incompatibility	- O-type mothers have IgG against AB antigen - Causes mild hyperbilirubinemia within 24 hours of birth
Lewis	- Not associated with fetal hemolysis
Duffy	- Moderate hemolysis
Kell	- Severe hemolysis
Rhc	- Similar to RhD

Maternal Pregnancy Complications

Hyperemesis Gravidarum

General: Disorder of persistent vomiting during early pregnancy

Risk: Nulliparity, multiple gestation, molar pregnancy, history of nausea with estrogen exposure

Clinical:

- **Morning sickness**: Mild nausea and vomiting, common in early pregnancy
- **Hyperemesis gravidarum**: Severe nausea/vomiting, beyond the degree expected from typical morning sickness
  - No clear definition, but the following suggest hyperemesis:
    - Persistence of symptoms into second trimester
    - Ketonuria
    - Starvation and weight loss

Management:

- IV fluids, thiamine (risk for Wernicke encephalopathy), electrolyte repletion
- <u>Antiemetics</u>:
  - **Pyridoxine-doxylamine**
  - Diphenhydramine
  - Promethazine, metoclopramide, ondansetron (if severe)

Fetal and Obstetric Complications from Gestational Diabetes

Fetal Complications:

Exposure	Potential Risks to Fetus
First trimester	- Congenital heart defects (transposition of the great arteries, VSDs, PDA) - Neural tube defects - Small left colon syndrome - Caudal regression syndrome (sacral agenesis, sirenomelia)
Second/third trimester	- Large for gestational age - Macrosomia/organomegaly - Neonatal hypoglycemia - Increased risk for birth trauma (brachial plexus injury, shoulder dystocia, clavicle fracture)

Obstetric Complications:

- Polyhydramnios
- Preeclampsia
- Miscarriage
- Infection
- Postpartum hemorrhage
- ↑ Risk for C-section

Pregestational Diabetes

General: Pregnancy can worsen hyperglycemia in patients with pre existing diabetes mellitus (insulin requirements can ↑)

Management:

Mother	- Strict glucose control with insulin (if necessary) - Basal-bolus insulin dosing preferred (oral agents discontinued) - Ensure weight gain is consistent with expected (careful diet control) - Try to maintain A1C < 6%
Fetus	- Anatomic US at 18-22 weeks (for congenital abnormalities) - Weekly nonstress test, biophysical profile starting at 32 weeks - Delivery ~ 39 weeks (if well-controlled) or earlier if uncontrolled hyperglycemia

Maternal Pregnancy Complications

Gestational Diabetes

General: Glucose intolerance that newly develops during pregnancy, due to increased insulin resistance. Typically diagnosed in late second to third trimester.

Class A1	Gestational diabetes (diet controlled)
Class A2	Gestational diabetes (insulin controlled)
Class B-D	Pregestational diabetes (class depends on onset age and duration)

Risk: ↑ BMI, previous history of gestational DM, prediabetes, Hispanic/Pacific Islander/Native American

Clinical: Typically asymptomatic, but can present due to diabetic complication (large for GA infant, polyhydramnios)

Diagnosis:

- **Screening**: 2-hour 50 g GTT. Performed at 24-28 weeks.
    - Glucose > 140 at 1 hour considered abnormal
- **Diagnostic**: 3-hour 100g GTT (normal cutoffs in table to right)

Fasting	95 mg/dL
1 hour	180 mg/dL
2 hours	155 mg/dL
3 hours	140 mg/dL

Management:

- Nonpharmacologic: Exercise, careful diet, and strict glucose monitoring
    - Diet: ~ 2200 calories, with 40% carbs, 40% fats, 20% protein
    - Glucose targets:
        - Fasting < 95 mg/dL
        - 1 hour postprandial < 140 mg/dL
        - 2 hours postprandial < 120 mg/dL
- If poor control despite above → **Insulin** (alternative: Metformin)
- Delivery:
    - A1 (diet-controlled): No special requirements
    - A2 (insulin-controlled): Deliver at 37-39 weeks
        - Nonstress tests weekly started at 32 weeks
    - Offer C-section if **fetus > 4500 g** (for any class of diabetes)

Note: Mom at increased risk for type II DM after pregnancy, as well as gestational diabetes in future pregnancies. Should have 2-hour 75 g oral glucose tolerance test between 4 and 12 weeks postpartum.

Chronic and Gestational Hypertension

Chronic	- Essential hypertension (> 140/90 mmHg) present **prior to pregnancy or < 20 weeks**
Gestational	- Idiopathic hypertension (> 140/90 mmHg) **after 20 weeks** without proteinuria or organ dysfunction

- Increases risk for: Prematurity, FGR, oligohydramnios, placental abruption, or preeclampsia

Management:

- Monitor blood pressure:
    - Antihypertensive therapy for blood pressure > 140/90 mmHg
    - Drug choices include: **Labetalol, nifedipine, hydralazine (alt: Methyldopa)**
        - Acute blood pressure control with labetalol/hydralazine
        - Avoid ACEi/ARB in pregnancy
    - Careful screening for progression to eclampsia (urine protein, renal function, CBC, LFTs)
- Monitor biophysical profiles starting at 32 weeks
- Delivery:
    - Early term delivery (37-39 weeks) if uncomplicated hypertension
    - Delivery at 34-36 weeks if poorly controlled, severe hypertension

Maternal Pregnancy Complications

Eclampsia and Preeclampsia

General: Clinical syndrome of hypertension, edema, and proteinuria. Believed to be due to abnormal development of the uteroplacental circulation. The resulting ischemic placenta leads to systemic vasoconstriction and ischemia of organs.

Risk:

- History of preeclampsia in prior pregnancy
- Extreme maternal ages (< 20, > 40 y/o), nulliparity
- Multiple gestation
- Black race
- Chronic hypertension, diabetes, kidney disease, obesity, or collagen vascular disease

Clinical:

- Syndrome of hypertension, proteinuria, +/– severe edema
- Occurs after 20 weeks gestation
- Maternal complications: Seizures, DIC, pulmonary edema, intracerebral hemorrhage
- Obstetric complications:
    - Uteroplacental insufficiency
    - Placental abruption
    - Fetal growth restriction
    - Oligohydramnios

Management: Prophylaxis: Low-dose aspirin (used if high-risk)

	Clinical Criteria	Management
Preeclampsia	- **Systolic BP ≥ 140 mmHg or diastolic BP ≥ 90 mmHg** PLUS one of the following: - **Proteinuria** (≥ 2+ on dipstick or > 300 mg/24 hours) OR - New end organ damage (see severe features below)	- Deliver if at term (≥ 37 weeks) - IV magnesium sulfate (seizure ppx at time of delivery)
Preeclampsia with Severe Features	- **Systolic BP ≥ 160 mmHg or diastolic BP ≥ 110 mmHg** OR - New **end organ damage**: - CNS: Severe headache, visual changes (scotomata) - Renal: AKI (Cr > 1.1 or 2× baseline) - GI: ↑ AST/ALT (> 2× normal) - Thrombocytopenia (< 100 K) - Pulmonary edema	- Delivery if ≥ 34 weeks - IV magnesium sulfate - Antihypertensives (for control < 160/110) If < 34 weeks: - Glucocorticoids - Consider delivery
Eclampsia	- **Seizures (generalized tonic-clonic)** PLUS - Underlying preeclampsia - Can be complicated by abruption, DIC, or cardiac arrest	- ABC's, oxygen, place in lateral position - Antihypertensives (for control < 160/110) - IV magnesium sulfate - Lorazepam or phenytoin if refractory seizure - Delivery

Mg Level	Clinical
4-8 mEq/L	Therapeutic range for seizure prophylaxis
7-10 mEq/L	Loss of deep tendon reflexes
10-15 mEq/L	Respiratory paralysis, altered cardiac conduction
> 25 mEq/L	Cardiac arrest

Maternal Pregnancy Complications

Maternal GI Issues

	Clinical	Management
HELLP Syndrome	- Rare complication, associated with preeclampsia - Microangiopathic hemolytic anemia (schistocytes, LDH, ↑ bilirubin) - Elevated liver enzymes (with RUQ abdominal pain) - Thrombocytopenia	- ≥ 34 weeks: Deliver - < 34 weeks: Corticosteroids, deliver if fetal or maternal distress - Antihypertensives, IV $MgSO_4$ (similar to preeclampsia)

Acute Fatty Liver of Pregnancy	- Liver dysfunction and fatty infiltration of hepatocytes
	- Associated with abnormal long-chain fatty acid metabolism
	
	- Presents with **acute liver failure** in third trimester
	  - Jaundice, encephalopathy, coagulopathy
	  - Elevated LFTs (AST/ALT, bilirubin, PT/INR)
		- Delivery (regardless of age)
		- Supportive care
		- May require liver transplantation in severe cases

Intrahepatic Cholestasis of Pregnancy	Presents as diffuse pruritus (palms, soles, worst at night) - ↑ **total serum bile acid levels** - Mildly elevated bilirubin, Alk Phos, AST/ALT	- Delivery near term (~ 36-38 weeks) - Ursodeoxycholic acid
Appendicitis	- Presents with nausea, vomiting, and RLQ abdominal pain - Fever and leukocytosis - Can present with RUQ pain later in pregnancy (due to shifting of GI tract) - Dx: Ultrasound (if inconclusive → MRI)	- Appendectomy

UTI/Pyelonephritis During Pregnancy

General: Women are at an increased risk for UTIs during pregnancy, due to relaxation of smooth muscle in the urinary tract. *E. Coli* most common organism (others include *Staphylococcus saprophyticus*, GBS, *Enterococcus*).

Risk: ↑ risk with multiple gestation, gestational diabetes

Clinical:

- **Asymptomatic bacteriuria**: Generally identified up on routine screening
- **Acute cystitis**: Urgency, increased frequency, dysuria, suprapubic pain
- **Acute pyelonephritis**: Fever, flank pain, CVA tenderness

Diagnosis: > 10^5 colony forming units on culture, plus the above clinical symptoms

Management:

Asymptomatic bacteriuria/UTI	- Antibiotics (nitrofurantoin, amoxicillin, fosfomycin) for 7-day course - Follow up cultures to confirm eradication. If repeat UTI, prophylactic antibiotics likely needed.
Pyelonephritis	- Admission for fluids, parenteral antibiotics (ceftriaxone, cefepime, or ampicillin + gentamicin) - Suppressive antibiotics for the remainder of pregnancy

Thyroid Abnormalities During Pregnancy

Hypothyroidism

- Estrogen causes ↑ in TBG, while hCG causes ↑ in T4 due to TSH receptor stimulation
- If treated for hypothyroidism at baseline → will require increased doses (~ 25%) of levothyroxine

Hyperthyroidism

- Similar symptoms and criteria as hyperthyroidism outside of pregnancy
- Usually due to Graves or β-hCG-induced
- Treatment: Beta-blocker, propylthiouracil (PTU) in first trimester, methimazole in 2nd/3rd trimester

Postpartum

Postpartum Hemorrhage

	Risk	Clinical/Diagnosis	Management
Postpartum Hemorrhage	- Defined as loss of **> 500 mL of blood during vaginal delivery**, or **1000 mL during C-section** - Generally managed with two large bore IVs, fluids, RBC transfusions - If severe, may require intrauterine balloon tamponade, uterine artery embolization, or hysterectomy - Can be complicated by hypovolemic shock and Sheehan syndrome		
Uterine Atony	- Exhausted myometrium - Prolonged labor - Excessive oxytocin - Blockage of contractions - Tocolytics, fibroids, $MgSO_4$ - Macrosomic fetus - Multiparity	- Soft, enlarged, "boggy" uterus - Most common cause of postpartum bleeding	First-line: - Uterine massage - Oxytocin - Methylergonovine (CxI if HTN) - Carboprost (CxI if asthma) Refractory: - Bakri balloon - Uterine artery embolization - Hysterectomy
GU Tract Trauma	- Precipitous labor - Operative vaginal delivery - Macrosomia	- Normal uterus - Visualize bleeding laceration	- Hold pressure over defect - Surgically repair defect
Retained Placenta	- Placenta accreta - Placenta previa - Uterine fibroids - History of C-section, other uterine surgery	- Firm uterus	- Manual removal of retained tissue - Curettage - Hysterectomy (if refractory)

Late (secondary) postpartum hemorrhage:
- Bleeding > 24 hours after delivery
- Causes include: Retained products of conception, endometritis, inadequate involution

Uterine Inversion

General: Uterus turns inside out and "births" itself through the cervix. Occurs with excessive traction (i.e., pulling on placenta), or excessive fundal pressure.

Risk: Macrosomia, rapid L&D, placenta accreta, multiple gestation

Clinical:
- **Absent uterus upon palpation of abdomen**
- Smooth, round mass protruding from vagina
- **Severe hemorrhage**, hemodynamic instability, lower abdominal pain

Management: Manual replacement
- Tocolytics or nitroglycerin (may be required to relax uterus before replacement)
- Uterine atony (occurs after successful replacement): Oxytocin

Sheehan Syndrome

General: Ischemic infarction of the pituitary after hypovolemic shock from postpartum hemorrhage

Clinical: Anterior pituitary insufficiency, including failure to lactate, hypotension, amenorrhea, weight loss, loss of pubic hair

Diagnosis: Hormone testing (TSH, cortisol, estradiol), MRI of pituitary/hypothalamus (to rule out other pathology)

Management: Hormone replacement

Amniotic Fluid Embolism

General: Amniotic fluid enters maternal circulation due to breakdown in the barrier of the uterine vessels, resulting in acute right ventricular failure, respiratory failure, and systemic inflammation

Clinical: Acute onset **cardiogenic shock, hypoxemic respiratory failure, disseminated intravascular coagulation**

Management: Supportive care. Often fatal.

Postpartum

Routine Postpartum Care

Usual findings

- Transient fevers (for 24 hours), chills/shivering
- Breast engorgement
- Uterine involution (returns to nonpregnant state)
- Lochia (vaginal discharge after delivery)
  - Rubra (red for ~ 3-4 days postpartum)
  - Serosa (pink-brown around day ~ 4-14 postpartum)
  - Alba (yellow for weeks postpartum)
- Self-limited hair loss

Pain: NSAIDs, acetaminophen, low dose opioids as necessary

Perineal care: Ice packs, monitor for intact laceration repair

Common Postpartum Complications

Urinary retention

- Presents with inability to void, dribbling, suprapubic pain > 6 hours post delivery
- Bladder scan to confirm
- Tx: Analgesics, ambulation, urinary catheterization as necessary

Pubic symphysis diastasis

- Injury from separation of pubic diaphysis
- Usually due to traumatic delivery of large baby
- Presents with midline abdominal pain with radiation down both legs
  - Pain worse with ambulation
  - Tenderness of symphysis pubis
- Tx: Analgesia, physical therapy, support truss

Postpartum Fever

General: Low-grade fever is normal for first 24 hours post delivery. Postpartum fever is **temperature > 100.4°F 2-10 days post delivery**.

Wound Infection	- Surgical site infection (laceration, episiotomy, C-section) - Presents with swelling and erythema with purulent drainage at wound site - Tx: Requires opening wound, debridement - PPX: Prophylactic antibiotics before Cesarean delivery (cefazolin)
UTI/Cystitis Pyelonephritis	- Common source of persistent fever after delivery - Diagnosis and treatment as in nonpostpartum patients
Mastitis	- Presents with breast erythema, tenderness, fever - [See: Breastfeeding]
Endometritis	- Infection of the uterine lining, usually polymicrobial - Risk: C-section, prolonged labor - Presents with fever, leukocytosis, **abdominal pain, uterine tenderness, purulent discharge** - Rarely can present with toxic shock syndrome - Tx: Broad spectrum antibiotics (gentamicin + clindamycin)
Septic Pelvic Thrombophlebitis	- Rare complication. Endothelial injury results in ovarian deep venous thrombosis and polymicrobial infection. - Presents with **fever +/– abdominal pain, refractory to antibiotics** - Dx: CT or MRI to evaluate for thrombi - Tx: Antibiotics + anticoagulation

Postpartum

Postpartum Depression

Blues	- Presents within 2-3 days of delivery, usually resolving in 2 weeks - Mild depression, irritability, tearfulness - Tx: Reassurance
Depression	- Presents within 4 weeks of delivery - Presents with SIGECAPS symptoms [See: Psych] - Often has ambivalence to the baby - Tx: Antidepressants + psychotherapy
Psychosis	- Most commonly presents within 2 weeks of childbirth - Risk: History of depression with psychotic features, schizophrenia, or bipolar disorder - Presents with delusions, hallucinations, disorganized thoughts - Tx: Antipsychotics, mood stabilizers - Requires hospitalization given risk of infanticide

Breastfeeding

General: After pregnancy, the estrogen and progesterone levels drop, prolactin rises, milk production/lactation is stimulated
- **Colostrum**: Early breast milk. Protein, fat, secretory IgA, and minerals.
- **Mature milk**: Starts ~ 1 week postpartum. Contains protein, fat, lactose, water.

	Benefits	Contraindications
Infant	- Improved immunity (↓ risk of infections, including pneumonia, otitis, gastroenteritis, UTI) - Improvement of GI function/maturity	- Galactosemia
Maternal	- ↓ rates of breast and ovarian cancer - Maternal-infant bonding - Accelerated recovery from childbirth - Quicker return to prepartum weight - Improved child spacing	- Active herpetic breast lesions - HIV (without virologic suppression) - Current chemotherapy or radiation therapy - Use of street drugs or alcohol

Complication	Findings
Engorgement	- Common. Warm, firm, tender, swollen breast. Low-grade fever. - Tx: Continue breastfeeding. Ice packs, analgesia as needed.
Mastitis	- Cellulitis of periglandular tissue caused by nipple trauma - Most commonly MSSA/MRSA - Presents with unilateral breast swelling, tenderness, erythema, purulence, and fever - Tx: Continue breastfeeding. Antibiotics: Dicloxacillin or cephalexin.
Abscess	- Focal area of erythema and fluctuance, often associated with mastitis - Dx: Clinical +/− US - Tx: Antibiotics and needle drainage. I&D if refractory.

Lactation suppression:
- Utilized for those not trying to breastfeed
- Engorgement will have negative feedback and stop prolactin production
- Use supportive bra, minimize nipple stimulation, cold packs, NSAIDs
    - Bromocriptine is not indicated

Menstrual Cycle

Menstrual Phases

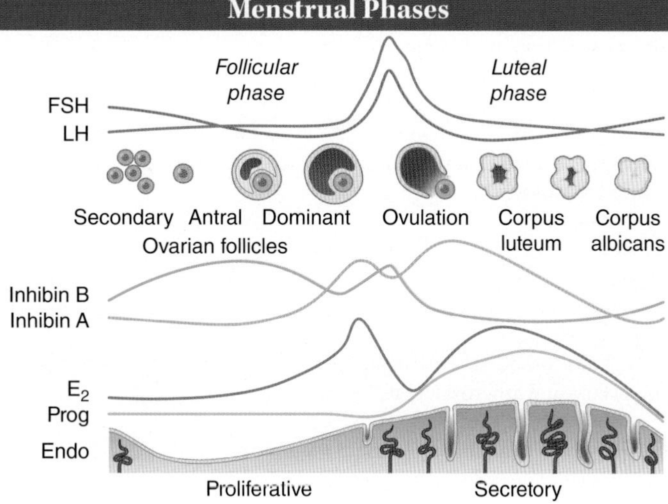

Follicular (Proliferative)	- Starts with menstruation, ends at LH surge/ovulation - Variable in length, but averages 13 days - Development of straight glands and thin secretions - At end of follicular phase, a dominant follicle is selected
Ovulation	- Estradiol reaches a peak, causing positive feedback to the pituitary, resulting in LH surge - Follicle releases ovum, and then transitions to corpus luteum - **Mittelschmerz**: Ovulation pain resulting from ovulation and leakage of blood that irritates peritoneum
Luteal	- Corpus luteum produces progesterone, resulting in endometrial sloughing/ ↓ blood supply - Corpus luteum eventually breaks down without LH or β-hCG, with resulting drop in progesterone - Ends when menses begins

Premenstrual Syndrome (PMS)/Dysphoric Disorder (PMDD)

General: A group of symptoms that can occur within 3-5 days preceding menses
- PMS: Presence of one or more of the below symptoms
- PMDD: Below symptoms, PLUS significant functional impairment

Clinical:
- **Mood swings, irritability, depressed mood, anxiety**
- Anhedonia, problems concentrating, anergia, appetite changes
- Physical symptoms: **Bloating**, breast tenderness

Diagnosis: Prospective symptom diary for at least 2 months, rule out other medical disorders (e.g., hypothyroidism)

Management:
- PMS: Regular exercise, stretching, stress relief techniques
- PMDD: SSRI (alt: OCPs)

Menstrual Cycle

Menopause

General: Physiologic cessation of menstruation in a woman > 45 y/o
- Average age ~ 51

Clinical:
- Irregular menses for years (~ 3-4 years) leading up to final menstrual period
- **Hot flashes (vasomotor symptoms)**
- Vaginal dryness, sexual dysfunction
- Fatigue, sleep disturbance
- Irritability, mood changes

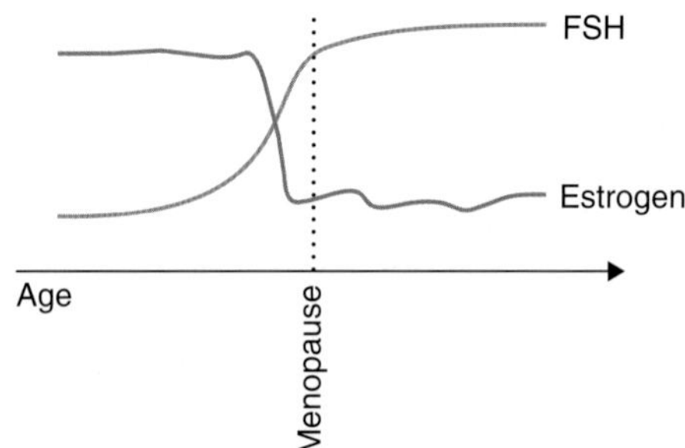

- $\uparrow$ FSH, FSH:LH ratio > 1
- Osteoporosis/progressive bone loss (loss of estrogen)
- $\uparrow$ risk of cardiovascular events and atherosclerosis

Diagnosis: Cessation of menses for 12 months (no further workup required)

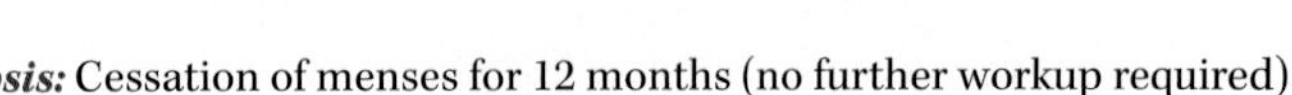

Management:

Vaginal atrophy	- Topical vaginal estrogen
Hot flashes	- Lifestyle modifications for mild symptoms - **Hormone replacement therapy (HRT)** (combo E2/P4) - SSRI, SNRI, gabapentin if HRT contraindicated

Hormone replacement:
- Indicated if moderate-to-severe vasomotor symptoms (< 60 y/o and menopause within last 10 years)
- Transdermal HRT preferred, with combination estrogen/progestin (alternative is OCP)
- Risk: $\uparrow$ risk of cardiovascular events, VTE, breast cancer
- Contraindications:
    - Thromboembolic history (e.g., CVA, DVT/PE)
    - Coronary artery disease
    - Endometrial or breast cancer (ER/PR+)

Primary Ovarian Insufficiency

General: Impaired ovarian function in woman < 40 years old

Etiology:
- Autoimmune oophoritis (positive antiadrenal antibodies)
- Prior chemotherapy or radiation therapy
- Genetic (e.g., fragile X [FMR gene mutation], Turner syndrome)
- Other genetic disorders (often have family history)

Clinical:
- Progressive oligomenorrhea
- Hot flashes, vaginal dryness, fatigue (see menopause symptoms above)

Diagnosis: $\uparrow$ FSH (in menopausal range)

Management:
- Emotional support
- Hormone replacement therapy (combined estrogen/progesterone)

Contraception

Method	Mechanism	Positives/Indications	Side Effects
Surgical			
Vasectomy	- Bilateral vas deferens ligation	- Permanent	- Must use contraception for 3 months - Ensure azoospermia with semen analysis
Tubal ligation	- Occluding or removing the fallopian tubes	- Permanent	- Generally irreversible, but reversal procedures may be able to restore fertility - Increased ectopic pregnancy rate
IUD			
Levonorgestrel Liletta Mirena Kyleena Skyla	- Local hormonal release, increasing cervical mucus viscosity and inducing endometrial atrophy	- Effective for 3-8 years - Immediate fertility when removed - Safe with breastfeeding - Highly efficacious - Induces amenorrhea or irregular periods	- Irregular bleeding/spotting (usually worse in initial 3-6 months, then improves) - Increased ectopic pregnancy rate
Copper (paragard)	- Induces inflammation that creates hostile environment for implantation	- Effective for 10 years - Immediate fertility when removed - Safe with breastfeeding - Highly efficacious	- Cramping, heavier bleeding during periods - Increased ectopic pregnancy rate
<u>IUD contraindications</u>: - Pregnancy, unexplained abnormal uterine bleeding, active gynecologic infection - Relative contraindications include structural uterine abnormality, recent STI, prior ectopic			
Hormonal			
Implant (nexplanon)	- Progestin (etonogestrel) implant in arm - Inhibits ovulation - Increases cervical mucus viscosity	- 3-year lifespan - Immediate fertility when removed - Safe with breastfeeding	- Irregular bleeding
Injections (depo provera)	- Depo progestin (medroxyprogesterone) - Inhibits ovulation - Increases cervical mucus viscosity	- Given every 3 months	- Irregular bleeding - Amenorrhea (develops after ~ 1-2 years) - Possible ↓ bone mineral density (reversible, encourage exercise, Ca/vit D)
Mini-pill	- Progestin only pill - Affects cervical mucus and endometrium - Ovulation not consistently suppressed	- Pill taken daily	- Must be taken at same time every day - Irregular bleeding
Combined oral contraceptive (COC)	- Combined estrogen-progestin - Inhibits gonadotropin surge/ ovulation	- Pill taken daily (+/− hormonal-free period) - ↓ ovarian and endometrial cancer risk - ↓ benign breast conditions - Predictable, lighter menses - Improves acne - Immediate fertility on cessation	- Bloating, nausea, breast tenderness - Breakthrough bleeding - ↑ VTE risk - ↑ stroke, MI risk (especially in those that smoke, older age, or history of migraine with aura) - ↑ blood pressure (mild effect) <u>Estrogen contraindications</u>: - > 35 y/o and daily smoker - Severe, uncontrolled hypertension - History of VTE, stroke, or CAD - Breast cancer - Cirrhosis or hepatocellular adenoma
Ring		- Placed in vagina for 3 weeks, then removed (with 1 week ring-free)	
Patch		- Weekly patch application (wear for 3 weeks, then 1 week off)	

Contraception

Other Contraceptive Methods

Option	Benefits
Male/female condoms	- Provide STI/HIV protection
Fertility awareness	- Timing ovulation via use of a calendar and possibly basal body temperature - Effective way of trying to get pregnant, not preventing it
Spermicide (nonoxynol-9 octoxynol-9)	- Not a primary method of birth control, but can be added to others - Can increase risk of UTI
Lactational amenorrhea	- Must breastfeed every 3 hours and remain amenorrheic - Not 100% reliable, and should use another form of contraception - **Postpartum contraception**: IUDs and progestin-only pills or depots - Estrogen avoided due to VTE risk (within 21 days postpartum)

Emergency Contraception Options

Method	Timing	Efficacy	Mechanism
Copper IUD	Up to 5 days	99%	- Inflammatory reaction that is toxic to sperm and ova, preventing implant
Levonorgestrel 52 mg IUD	Up to 5 days	99%	- Induces endometrial atrophy
Ulipristal ("Ella")	Up to 5 days	98%	- Antiprogestin - Delays ovulation
Levonorgestrel ("Plan B")	Up to 3 days	97%	- Delays ovulation
OCPs (Yuzpe regimen)	Up to 5 days	50-75%	- Delays ovulation - Less effective compared to above methods

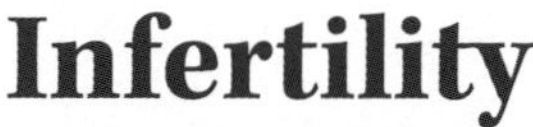

Infertility

Overview of Infertility

General: Inability to conceive within 12 months of active attempts (> 80% of those trying for this period of time will conceive)
- Infertility workup should begin at 12 months, but it is reasonable to start earlier (6 months) in those > 35 y/o

Etiology	Select Examples	Clinical Findings
Male factors - Start with **semen analysis**, which should be repeated if abnormal - If sperm counts are decreased, LH/FSH/testosterone should be checked - If normal semen analysis → female factor infertility or idiopathic male infertility		
Testicular defect	- Testicular insults (toxins, torsion, infection, varicoceles)	- Oligo or azoospermia - Normal endocrine testing
Hypogonadism	Primary hypogonadism (↓ T, ↑ FSH/LH) - Klinefelter, other genetic disorders Secondary hypogonadism (↓T/FSH/LH) - Prolactinoma, hypothyroidism	- Oligo or azoospermia
Sperm abnormalities		- Abnormal sperm morphology or motility
Sperm transport	- Ejaculatory duct obstruction - Congenital absence of vas deferens	- Oligo or azoospermia - Normal endocrine testing - GU ultrasound may reveal structural cause
Female factors - Assessment of ovulatory status (i.e., history of regular menstrual cycles, check midluteal progesterone level) - Hysterosalpingogram (to evaluate tubal patency/uterine cavity abnormalities) - Ovarian reserve analysis: - Day 3 FSH (abnormally elevated with ↓ follicles), estradiol (↑ with low follicle reserve) - Anti-Müllerian hormone level (declines over time with decreasing follicle pool)		
Ovarian factors	- Hypogonadotropism - PCOS - Decreased ovarian reserve	- Abnormal menstrual history, endocrine analysis - Abnormal reserve analysis
Tubal factors	- Pelvic inflammatory disease - Endometriosis - Any other cause of pelvic adhesions	- Hysterosalpingogram abnormalities
Cervical factors	- History of cervical surgery	
Uterine factors	- Fibroids, polyps, or adhesions	- Hysterosalpingogram or TVUS abnormalities

Management of Infertility

Method	Features
Ovulation induction	- Used for ovulatory disorders - Clomiphene is most common drug used (selective SERM at pituitary/hypothalamus, induces ovulation after ~ 1 week) - Alternative agents: Aromatase inhibitors (letrozole), GnRH agonists (leuprolide) - Often associated with hot flashes and ovarian hyperstimulation (syndrome of ovarian enlargement, pain, ascites)
Intrauterine insemination	- Used for cervical dysfunction or severe sexual dysfunction - Concentrated sperm injected into uterus at proper time of cycle OR after stimulation (i.e., with clomiphene)
In-vitro fertilization	- Used in those with severe structural abnormalities (blocked tubes, severe endometriosis), severe male factor infertility, poor response to pharm induction agents, diminished ovarian reserve - Ovaries are stimulated, oocytes aspirated, fertilized in laboratory, then transferred into the uterine cavity

Disorder-specific therapy:

Endometriosis	- Surgical resection and lysis of adhesions - Assisted reproductive technologies
Uterine abnormalities	- Surgical correction (not great data for this either way)
Cervical factor infertility	- Intrauterine insemination

Amenorrhea

Primary Amenorrhea

General: Defined as:

- Absence of menses by 15 years old OR
- Absence of menses and secondary sexual characteristics by age 13

Etiology	Axis	Anatomy	Features	Diagnosis
Central hypogonadism	−	+	<u>Etiology</u>: - Functional (stress/excessive exercise/low BMI) - Hyperprolactinemia - Sellar mass - Kallmann syndrome (low GnRH production, anosmia) - Constitutional pubertal delay	↓ FSH/LH MRI
Ovarian insufficiency	−	+	<u>Etiology</u>: - Turner syndrome - Prior chemotherapy, radiation	↑ FSH/LH karyotype
Outflow tract disorders				
Müllerian agenesis	+	−	- Congenital absence of upper vagina, cervix, and uterus	Ultrasound
Lower GYN	+	+	- Transverse vaginal septum - Imperforate hymen	Clinical exam
Enzyme/hormonal issues				
Complete androgen insensitivity syndrome	+	−	- XR disorder in 46XY patients due to defect in androgen receptor - **Normal external female genitalia**, but no upper vagina, uterus, fallopian tubes - Testes often undescended or in labia majora. Sparse sexual hair, but breast development present. - ↑ Testosterone - Dx: XY karyotype and genetic testing for AR gene - Tx: Gonadectomy (after pubertal development), hormone replacement, vaginal dilation	
5α reductase deficiency	+	−	- AR disorder of lack of male virilization from abnormal conversion of T to DHT - Normal internal male urogenital tract, but **external genitalia is female or indeterminate** - Individual appears male, and will develop further **male sex characteristics during puberty** - Dx: XY karyotype and ↑ T:DHT ratio - Tx: Assign male gender OR gonadectomy/estrogen	

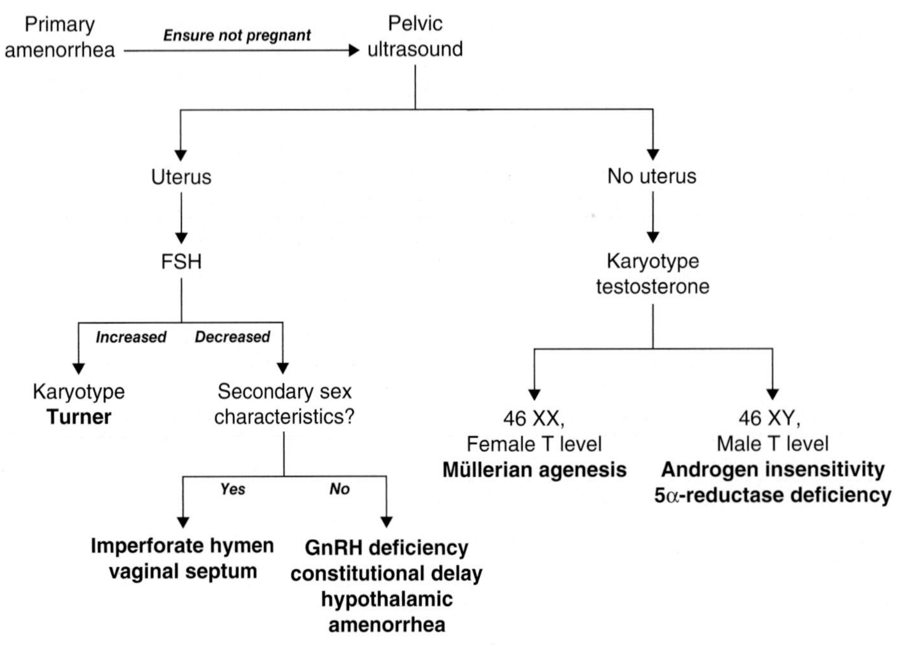

Amenorrhea

Secondary Amenorrhea

General: Absence of menses for 6 consecutive months (if normally irregular) or 3 consecutive months (if previously regular cycles)

Etiology	Features
Pregnancy	- Most common cause
Ovarian	- Primary ovarian insufficiency - PCOS
Hypothalamic	- Functional hypothalamic (eating disorder, excess exercise, weight loss, stress) - Systemic illness
Pituitary	- Hyperprolactinemia (prolactinoma, antipsychotic medication use) - Sheehan syndrome - Other sellar masses
Uterine	- Asherman syndrome (adhesions from prior uterine surgery or infection) - Cervical stenosis
Other	- Menopause - Hypothyroidism - Cushing syndrome

Diagnosis: See workup below
- Always start with urine β-hCG pregnancy test

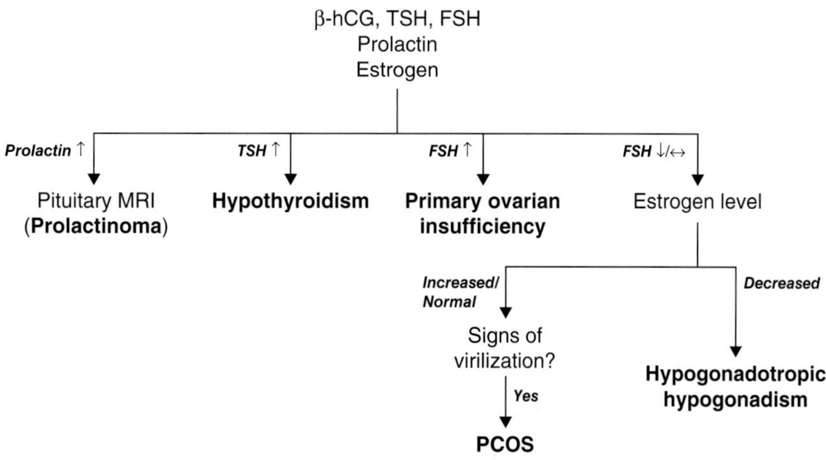

Secondary Amenorrhea—Management

Etiology	Management
Hypothalamic	- Lifestyle changes (increased caloric intake, decreased exercise) - CBT (especially if under stress)
Hyperprolactinemia	- [See: Endocrine] - Bromocriptine or cabergoline
Primary Ovarian Insufficiency	- Estrogen therapy (prevent bone loss)
Asherman	- Hysteroscopic lysis of adhesions
PCOS	- Weight loss, combined oral contraceptives

Hyperandrogenism

Overview of Hirsutism and Virilization

General: Excess androgen production from ovary (testosterone) or adrenal glands (DHEAS)

Clinical:

Hirsutism	- Excess **hair growth (dark, coarse hairs) in androgen-dependent areas** (upper lip, chin, torso, buttocks) - Associated with acne and male-pattern hair loss
Virilization	- Hirsutism as above, PLUS: Clitoral enlargement, increased muscle mass, deepening of voice, male-pattern hair loss

Diagnosis: DHEAS and T levels. Depending on concern for source: Ovarian US or Adrenal CT/MRI.

Differential of Hyperandrogenism

Etiology	T	DHEAS	Features	Management
Ovarian causes				
PCOS	↑	↔	- Hirsutism, insulin resistance, oligomenorrhea	- See below
Sertoli-Leydig tumor	↑↑	↔	- Androgen production from ovarian tumor - Severe virilization, rapid onset	- Surgical excision +/– chemotherapy
Hyperthecosis	↑↑	↔	- Excess active luteinized stromal cells in the ovaries - US demonstrates ↑ size of ovaries (bilateral), ↑ stroma	- Bilateral oophorectomy
Adrenal causes				
Adrenal tumor	↔	↑↑	- Excess androgens from adrenal adenoma or carcinoma - Dx: CT or MRI (unilateral mass)	- Surgical resection
CAH (nonclassical)	↔	↑	- 21-hydroxylase deficiency - Presents similarly to PCOS (hirsutism without virilization) - Dx: ↑ 17-hydroxyprogesterone	- Steroids
Other causes				
Cushing disease				
Idiopathic hirsutism (normal menstrual cycles, labs)				

Polycystic Ovarian Syndrome

General: Syndrome caused by elevated androgens. Occurs in those with genetic susceptibility and insulin resistance, resulting in excessive LH release, abnormal ovarian follicular development, and excessive production of androgens.

Risk: Often comorbid with metabolic syndrome, OSA

Clinical:

- Androgen excess (acne, male pattern hair loss, **hirsutism**)
- Menstrual irregularities (from decreased ovulation or anovulation)
- Obesity, **insulin resistance**
- ↑ risk for endometrial hyperplasia/adenocarcinoma
- Lab findings: ↑ LH/FSH ratio, ↑ testosterone levels, ↑ estrogen levels

Diagnosis: Rotterdam criteria (≥ **2/3** of the following)

- **Oligomenorrhea**
- **Hyperandrogenism** (acne, balding, hirsutism, ↑ serum T)
- **Polycystic ovaries on TVUS**[A]

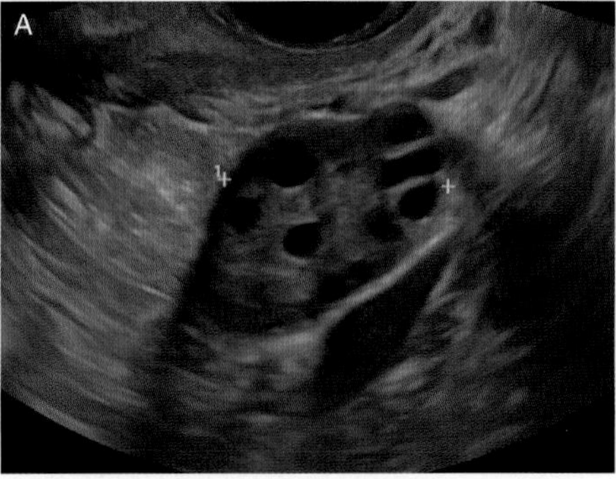

Management:

- Weight loss
- Combined estrogen-progestin contraceptives (for menstrual irregularity, symptoms of excess androgens)
- Infertility: Weight loss, letrozole or clomiphene

Dysmenorrhea

Primary Dysmenorrhea

General: Recurrent, crampy, midline lower abdominal pain that occurs during menses in the absence of other pathology. Caused by uterine ischemia from vasoconstriction associated with prostaglandin release.

Clinical:

- **Low, midline, spasmodic pelvic pain**
- Occurs during first 1-3 days of menstruation
    - Versus endometriosis, which is pain days to weeks before cycle
- Associated with nausea, diarrhea, flushing, headache

Diagnosis: Clinical diagnosis of exclusion

Management:

- NSAIDs (ibuprofen, mefenamic acid)
- Combined oral contraceptives (COC)
- Others: Heat, exercise, massage

Secondary Dysmenorrhea

General: Menstrual pain associated with pathologic process

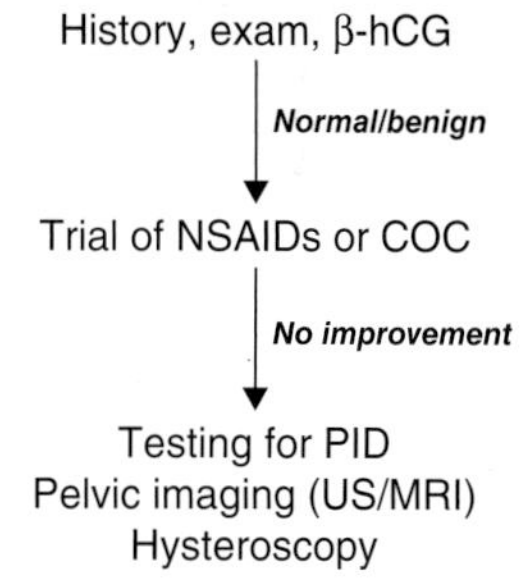

Etiology:

- Adenomyosis
- Endometriosis
- Pelvic inflammatory disease
- **Obstructed menstrual flow:** Cervical stenosis, adhesions, fibroids

Clinical: Historical clues for secondary dysmenorrhea:

- Onset age > 25 years
- Non-midline pain
- No other menstrual symptoms (nausea, fatigue, headache)
- Abnormal uterine bleeding
- Dyspareunia

History, exam, β-hCG
↓ *Normal/benign*
Trial of NSAIDs or COC
↓ *No improvement*
Testing for PID
Pelvic imaging (US/MRI)
Hysteroscopy

Adenomyosis

General: Invasion of endometrial glands/stroma into the uterine musculature

- Myometrium becomes hypertrophic and hyperplastic in response

Risk: Endometriosis, fibroids

Clinical:

- **Dysmenorrhea**
- Menorrhagia
- **Enlarged, boggy uterus**

Diagnosis: TVUS or MRI

- Definitive diagnosis is histologic (but typically imaging is utilized)

Management:

- Progestins (IUDs, pills): Can control menorrhagia short term
- Definitive therapy: **Hysterectomy** or uterine artery embolization

Dysmenorrhea

Endometriosis

General: Functional endometrial glands and stroma outside uterus (e.g., ovary, fallopian tubes, uterosacral ligaments, pelvic peritoneum). Pathophysiology unknown, but current theories include:

- Retrograde menstruation
- Metastasis (lymphatic or vascular spread)
- Metaplastic transformation of tissue

Risk: ↑ risk with nulliparity, early menarche, heavy menstrual bleeding, family history

Clinical:

- Cyclic pelvic and/or rectal pain (classically 1-2 weeks before menses)
- Abnormal uterine bleeding
- **Dyspareunia**
- Dyschezia (painful defecation)
- Ovarian mass (endometrioma, "chocolate brown")
- **Infertility**
- Exam: Posterior vaginal fornix tenderness or nodules, fixation of the uterus from adhesions, or adnexal mass

Diagnosis:

- Laparoscopy (biopsy for histologic confirmation, plus staging of disease)
- Often treated empirically without surgical/histologic diagnosis

Management:

Pain	- First line: NSAIDs plus COC (combined oral contraceptives–hormones used continuously)
	- Second line: GnRH agonist (e.g., Leuprolide) plus add back estrogen/progestin
	- <u>Refractory</u>:
	  - Aromatase inhibitors (anastrozole, letrozole)
	  - Laparoscopic surgical resection

Infertility	- Laparoscopy and lysis of adhesions - Assisted reproduction technologies
Endometrioma	- Laparoscopic cystectomy

Abnormal Uterine Bleeding

Definitions

Normal	- Menses every 28 days (can range from 24- to 38-day cycles) - Up to 8 days of bleeding, up to 80 mL of blood loss
Heavy	- > 80 mL of total blood loss per cycle
Prolonged	- > 8 days of bleeding
Frequent	- Bleeding more often than every 21-24 days
Infrequent	- Bleeding less often than every 35-38 days

Differential Diagnosis of Abnormal Uterine Bleeding

General: Bleeding outside the typical 2-7 days period of a normal 28-day menstrual cycle

Etiology: **"PALMCOEIN"**

- Polyp
- Adenomyosis
- Leiomyoma
- Malignancy
- Coagulopathy
- Ovulatory dysfunction
- Endometrial
- Iatrogenic (IUDs)
- Not yet classified (pregnancy, the most common cause)

Diagnosis:

- Broad workup, including β-hCG, CBC, TSH, prolactin, pap smear
- Pelvic US
- Any postmenopausal women with uterine bleeding deserves endometrial biopsy

AUB due to Ovulatory Dysfunction:

- Menstrual cycle without ovulation (excessive endometrial growth from estrogen)
- Presents with **irregular, infrequent bleeding**
- Causes:
  - Menarche (underdeveloped hypothalamus-pituitary-ovary axis)
  - Menopause (loss of ovulation)
  - PCOS

Management of Abnormal Uterine Bleeding

Acute Bleeding	
Severe bleeding	- Supportive care (2× large bore IV, crystalloids, RBC transfusions) - Uterine tamponade with balloon or gauze - Hemodynamically stable: IV estrogens - Hemodynamically unstable: Uterine curettage
Chronic Abnormal Uterine Bleeding	
Pharm	- Combined oral contraceptives (COC) or progestin IUD/injectable - NSAIDs or tranexamic acid for those with contraindication to COC
Surgical	Definitive: - Endometrial ablation - Uterine artery embolization - Hysterectomy

Vaginitis

	Bacterial Vaginosis	Trichomoniasis	Vulvovaginal Candidiasis
Micro	- Shift in vaginal flora away from lactobacilli, to diverse bacteria including anaerobes - *Gardnerella vaginalis* predominant	- Protozoan *Trichomonas vaginalis*	- Overgrowth of *Candida albicans* (part of normal vaginal flora) - Other *Candida* also possible (e.g., glabrata)
Risk	- Sexual activity - Frequent douching - Smoking	- Unprotected sex (passed person-to-person via sexual contact)	- Diabetes mellitus - Antibiotic use - Immunosuppression
Clin	- Odor, increased discharge	- Increased discharge, odor, pruritus - Dysuria	- Vulvar pruritus - Possible burning, irritation
Exam	- Thin gray-white discharge - "Fishy smell"	- Erythema of the vulva/vaginal mucosa - Punctate hemorrhages of upper vagina/ cervix ("**Strawberry cervix**") - Malodorous yellow-green discharge	- Erythematous, excoriated vagina - Thick, white, discharge with curdy texture without odor
pH	> 4.5	> 4.5	4.0-4.5
Whiff	Positive	Occasionally positive	Negative
Wet Mount	**Clue cells**[A] (epithelial cell with bacteria)	**Motile trichomonads**[B] (bigger than WBC, smaller than epi cells)	**Pseudohyphae**[C]
KOH Prep	Negative	Negative	Positive (pseudohyphae)
Tx	PO metronidazole (5-7 days) Topical metronidazole (5 days) (Vaginal or oral clindamycin can also be used)	PO metronidazole or tinidazole *Partners should also be treated	PO fluconazole (1 time) or topical azoles *Cases of recurrent disease may require longer PO or topical regimens *Glabrata treated with intravaginal boric acid
Other	Amsel criteria (≥ 3/4): Classic vaginal discharge, elevated pH, clue cells, fishy odor		

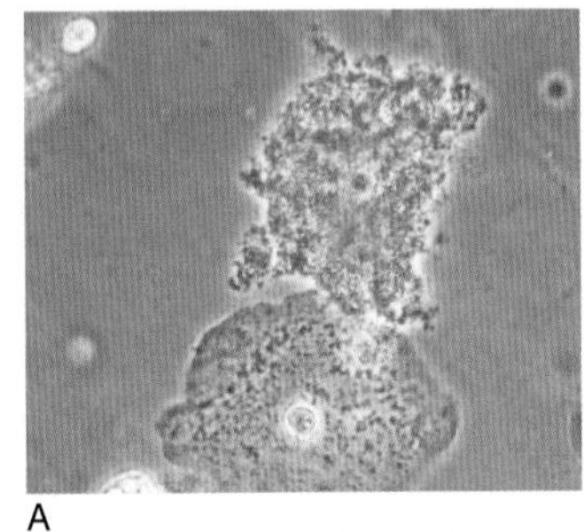
A

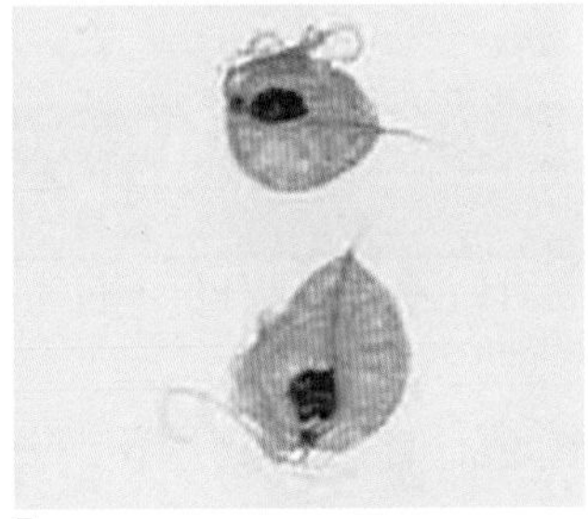
B

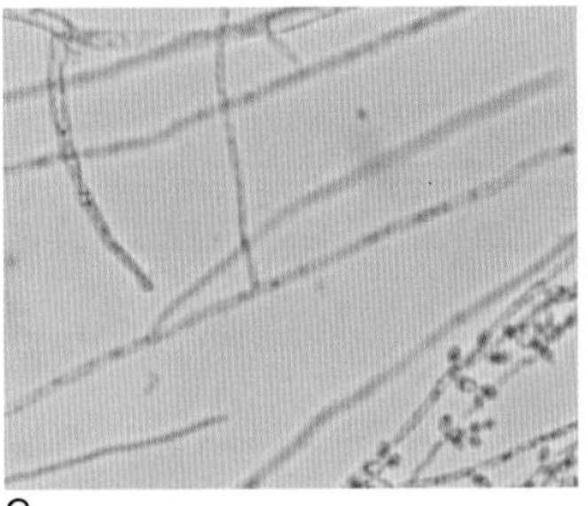
C

Upper Gyn Infection

Pelvic Inflammatory Disease

General: Acute bacterial infection of the **upper genital tract**, including uterus, fallopian tubes (salpingitis), ovaries. Due to ascending infection from lower genital tract.

Etiology:

- Gonorrhea and chlamydia
- Other bacteria: *Mycoplasma genitalium*, group A/B *Strep*, *E. Coli*, *Klebsiella*

Risk: Sexually active, multiple partners, lack of barrier protection, history of PID or STI

- Pregnant women usually not at risk given mucus plug

Clinical:

- Acute onset lower abdominal or pelvic pain
- Uterine, cervical ("Chandelier sign"), and/or adnexal tenderness
- Purulent cervical discharge, possible bleeding/spotting
- Systemic symptoms: Fevers, chills, leukocytosis

Diagnosis: Clinical diagnosis

- Lower abdominal/pelvic pain + uterine, cervical, or adnexal tenderness
- Pelvic imaging (TVUS, CT) supportive, but unnecessary for diagnosis

Management:

Hospitalized	- **"Foxy Doxy": Cefoxitin IV + Doxycycline PO**
	- Clindamycin + gentamicin (alternative regimen)
	- <u>Should hospitalize</u>:
	  - Pregnant women
	  - Poor compliance (e.g., teenagers)
	  - TOA, perihepatitis
	  - Failed outpatient therapy
	  - Unable to tolerate PO
	  - Severe presentations

Outpatient	- Ceftriaxone 1 × IM + doxycycline (14 days)

Complications:

- Infertility, ↑ ectopic pregnancy risk
- Pelvic adhesions

- **<u>Perihepatitis (Fitz-Hugh-Curtis)</u>**
    - Inflammation of the liver capsule/peritoneum
    - RUQ abdominal pain (often pleuritic), possible abnormal LFTs
    - Laparoscopy: Purulent/fibrinous exudates surrounding the liver

- **<u>Tubo-Ovarian Abscess (TOA)</u>**
    - 10% of patients with PID develop TOA, an inflammatory mass of the tubes and/or ovaries
    - Typically polymicrobial
    - Presents like PID, but may be especially sick or not responding to antibiotic therapy
    - Rupture TOA can present with acute abdomen and sepsis
    - Dx: Imaging (TVUS)
    - Tx: Antibiotics for uncomplicated cases, surgical drainage or salpingo-oophorectomy if severe

Congenital Gyn Abnormalities

	General/Clinical	Management
Vaginal Abnormalities		
Imperforate Hymen	- Hymenal epithelium normally degenerates, but can abnormally persist - Obstruction can cause hydrocolpos, mucocolpos, or hematocolpos - Can cause primary amenorrhea	- Surgery
Transverse Vaginal Septum	- Failure of canalization between the lower 2/3 and upper 1/2 of the vagina (Müllerian ducts do not fuse to the urogenital sinus) - Presents with short vagina with blind pouch - Can also present with primary amenorrhea, cyclic pelvic pain	- Surgery
Vaginal Agenesis	- Complete absence of vagina - Associated with Mayer-Rokitansky-Küstner-Hauser (absence of uterus and cervix)	- Vaginal dilators or vaginoplasty
Uterine Abnormalities		
Congenital Uterine Anomalies	- Congenital uterine abnormalities due to abnormal Müllerian duct fusion during embryonic development - Generally idiopathic, but associated with DES exposure - Increased risk for associated renal abnormalities or inguinal hernia - Rarely symptomatic - Dx: TVUS, MRI, or hysterosalpingogram	- Generally no intervention required - Surgical correction if recurrent pregnancy loss

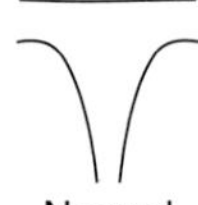
Normal

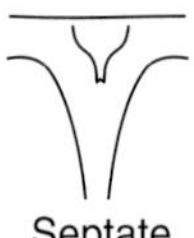
Septate

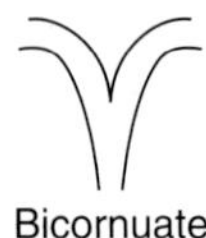
Bicornuate

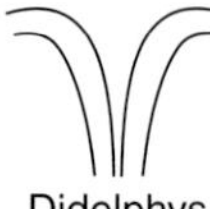
Didelphys

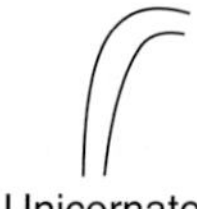
Unicornate

Vaginal/Cervical Lesions

	General/Clinical	Management
Skin Lesions		
Lichen Sclerosus[A]	- Thin, white, wrinkled skin localized on the labia ("paper thin") - Shrinkage and agglutination of labia minora - Severe pruritus, dyspareunia - Increased risk of SCC	Dx: Biopsy Tx: High-potency topical steroids
Lichen Simplex Chronicus	- Localized thickening of the vulvar skin from scratching and pruritus	Tx: Topical steroids (to break itch-scratch cycle)
Vulvar Lichen Planus	- Presents with vulvar pain, pruritus, discharge - Brightly erythematous erosions with "lacy" white striae - Lesions also can be intravaginal or involve other mucosal areas	Dx: Biopsy Tx: High-potency topical steroids
Vulvar Psoriasis	- Classic scaling red plaques, typically also located elsewhere on body - Typically asymptomatic or mild pruritus	Dx: Clinical or biopsy Tx: Topical steroids, UV light
Cysts		
Bartholin Cyst[B]	- Obstruction of Bartholin duct and dilation of the gland - Can occur idiopathically or from trauma - Presents with cyst lateral to the vaginal orifice	If asymptomatic: Observation If infected or symptomatic: - I&D PLUS word catheter placement - Marsupialization (second line) - Antibiotics if recurrent, high risk, or appearing septic
Skene Gland Cyst	- Paraurethral gland cysts, located in the anterior vagina near the opening of the urethra	
Gartner Cyst	- Remnants of mesonephric ducts, located on the lateral vaginal wall - Generally asymptomatic	
Cervical Lesions		
Cervical Cysts	- Nabothian cysts most common, caused when glandular columnar cells become covered by squamous epithelial, but still produce mucus - Generally asymptomatic	- Self-limited
Cervical Polyps	- Polyps often originate from the endocervical canal, appear as broad based or pedunculated lesions - Often asymptomatic, but can cause intermenstrual or postcoital bleed	- Polypectomy if symptomatic
Cervical Stenosis	- Narrowed endocervical canal - Can cause buildup of menstrual flow - Risk: Cervical surgery, cancer - Presents with severe dysmenorrhea, relieved with increased flow - Diagnosis: Clinical exam (try to pass dilator)	- Cervical dilation (laminaria, stent, or surgical dilation)

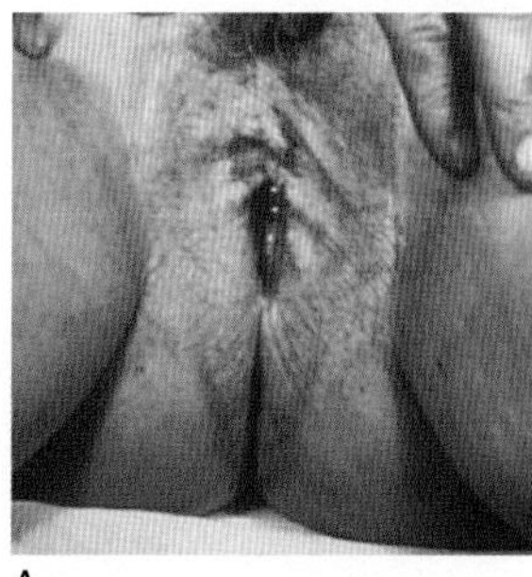
A

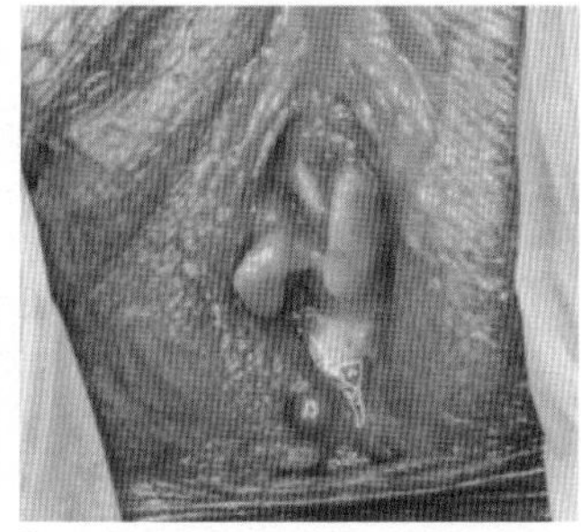
B

Pelvic Organ Prolapse

General: Herniation of the pelvic organs past the vaginal walls. Commonly seen after menopause due to decreased estrogen, vaginal atrophy, and effects of gravity.

Subtype	Definition
Cystocele	- Bladder bulge into the anterior vagina
Rectocele	- Rectum bulge into the posterior vagina
Enterocele	- Protrusion of the small intestines and peritoneum into vagina
Urethrocele	- Prolapse of urethra into the vagina - Often occurs concurrently with cystocele
Uterine prolapse	- Prolapse of the uterus into the vagina

Risk: ↑ age, high parity or history of traumatic delivery, history of pelvic surgery, obesity, chronic constipation

Clinical:

- Pelvic pressure, heaviness or sensation of bulging
- **Protrusion of tissue from the vagina**
- Can be associated with urinary, bowel, or sexual issues (e.g., dyspareunia)
    - Urinary incontinence, a sense of incomplete bladder emptying
    - Defecatory issues (may need to "splint," [apply pressure] to the posterior vagina to allow for defecation)

Diagnosis: Clinical exam. POP-Q score can be utilized to characterize and risk stratify.

Management:

Conservative	- Pelvic floor exercises
	- Vaginal pessaries:
	    - Silicone devices that support the pelvic organs
	    - Regularly remove and clean to avoid infection

Surgical	- Indicated for symptomatic prolapse or failure of conservative treatment Types include: - Hysterectomy with colpopexy (vaginal vault suspension) - Colporrhaphy (fix the hernia) - Colpocleisis: Close the vaginal opening (done in those at high risk of surgery and don't need vagina)

Vesicovaginal Fistula

General: Fistula between vagina and bladder. Associated with recent pelvic surgery, radiation, malignancy, history of traumatic labor.

Clinical: Painless continuous leakage of urine into vagina

Diagnosis: Dye tests, cystoscopy

Management: Surgical correction

Cervical Neoplasia

Cervical Cancer

General: Cancer of the cervix, either squamous cell (~ 70%) or adenocarcinoma (~ 25%). Highly associated with **HPV** (16, 18, 31, 45). Usually originates at the transformation zone (junction between squamous epithelium of ectocervix and glandular epithelium of the endocervix).

Risk: Early onset of sexual activity, multiple or high-risk sex partners, history of other STIs, immunocompromised (e.g., HIV), smoking

Clinical: Often asymptomatic, but **metrorrhagia, postcoital spotting, cervical ulceration** all possible

Diagnosis: Biopsy for definitive diagnosis
- Often first noted on pap smear screening, which should be followed by **colposcopy and directed biopsy**
    - Colpo performed by staining cervix with acetic acid
        - Findings include acetowhite epithelium, mosaicism, punctuations, atypical vessels

Dysplasia Classification:

Dysplasia	Location	Bethesda	CIN
Mild	Bottom 1/3 of cervical epithelium	LSIL	1
Moderate	Bottom and middle 1/3 of cervical epithelium	HSIL	2
Severe or carcinoma in situ	> 2/3 of cervical epithelium	HSIL	3

Cancer Staging:

Stage	Description
I	- Confined to cervix: - IA: Microscopically diagnosed - IB: Macroscopically apparent
II	- Spread beyond cervix (limited to upper vagina or parametrium)
III	- Spread to lower vagina or pelvic side wall
IV	- Invades bladder, rectum, or distant metastasis

Management of Cervical Malignancy

Lesion	Intervention
CIN 1	- **Observation** (monitor Pap +/– HPV q12 months, repeat colposcopy if abnormal) - If CIN 1 persists for 2 years: Consider conization/LEEP
CIN 2	- **Conization/LEEP or observation** (with q6 month serial colposcopy/HPV) - Observation preferred for select CIN 2 patients (e.g., age < 25)
CIN 3	- **Conization/LEEP**
Cancer	- Early disease (stage IA-IB): Surgical conization or hysterectomy - Advanced disease (stage IB2 or higher): Chemotherapy + radiation therapy

If Pregnant:
- LSIL or HSIL pap smears should be investigated with colposcopy
- CIN I: Defer further management to 6 weeks postpartum
- CIN II-III: Monitor serial colposcopy during pregnancy
- Invasive cervical cancer: Can do abortion with treatment, localized excision procedure, or defer treatment until after delivery

Types of procedures:
- Cold knife conization
- LEEP (loop electrical excision procedure)
- Side effects:
    - Cervical stenosis
    - Cervical insufficiency (↑ preterm risk or second trimester loss)

Prophylaxis: HPV 9-valent vaccine (okay to use ages 9-45 y/o)

Cervical Neoplasia

Cervical Cancer Screening

Normal Risk Individuals	
21-29 y/o	- Pap test q3 years
30-65 y/o	- Pap test q3 years OR Pap + HPV cotest q5 years
> 65 y/o	- Discontinue screening if 3 normal paps or 2 normal co-tests within last 10 years
Special Situations	
Smokers	- Reasonable to extend screening to 75-80 y/o
Immunocompromised	- Start screening at 21 y/o - Screen q1 year, extend beyond 65 y/o
Hysterectomy	- If total hysterectomy (cervix removed), no screening needed UNLESS history of CIN grade II or higher lesion (in which case vaginal cytology is reasonable)
Post-ablative for CIN	- After surgery for CIN, requires followup testing (HPV) at 6 months

Interpretation of Screening

ASCCP guidelines from 2019 now use a web/phone application to risk stratify cervical cancer screening results and to determine next best steps (e.g., colposcopy versus repeat testing). General recommendations for average-risk patients below:

AGC (atypical glandular cells)	- Colposcopy, endocervical sampling - Endometrial biopsy if > 35 y/o OR < 35 y/o but at risk for endometrial dysplasia (obesity, PCOS)
ASC-US (≥ 25 y/o)	- Check HPV if available (otherwise, repeat pap in 1 year) - ASC-US + HPV (+): Colposcopy - ASC-US + HPV (−): Cotest in 3 years
LSIL (≥ 25 y/o)	- LSIL + HPV (−): Repeat co-test in 1 year - LSIL + HPV (+ or unknown): Colposcopy
ASC-US or LSIL (21-24 y/o)	- Repeat pap in 12 months - If cytology remains abnormal → colposcopy
HSIL or ASC- H	- Colposcopy - If negative, follow with q6M colposcopy for 2 years
NILM but HPV(+)	- Either repeat cotest in 1 year OR DNA type HPV - If HPV 16 or 18 positive → colposcopy

Endometrial Neoplasia

Endometrial Polyps

General: Hyperplastic overgrowth of endometrial glands/stroma. Generally benign, but are possibly malignant (especially in those that are postmenopausal).

Risk: High estrogen levels (obesity, tamoxifen, hormone replacement therapy)

Clinical: Often asymptomatic, but can cause abnormal uterine bleeding

Diagnosis: TVUS or hysteroscopy is suggestive, but definitive diagnosis on histology

Management:

Premenopausal	- Polypectomy if symptomatic or if at high risk for endometrial hyperplasia/cancer
Postmenopausal	- Polypectomy for all

Uterine Leiomyoma (Fibroids)

General: Benign smooth muscle tumors arising from the myometrium. Sensitive to estrogen and progesterone. Malignant transformation to leiomyosarcoma is very rare.

Subtypes:

Intramural	- Located within uterine wall
Submucosal	- Located beneath endometrium, extending into and distorting uterine cavity - Highest risk for bleeding
Subserosal	- Extend from myometrium to the serosal surface of the uterus
Cervical	- Located within cervix

Risk:

- Black women
- Increased estrogen exposure (low parity, early menarche)
- Alcohol use

Clinical:

- **Abnormal uterine bleeding**
- **Bulk symptoms**: Bloating, constipation, ↑ urinary frequency or retention
- **Pelvic pain**: Dysmenorrhea, dyspareunia
- Exam demonstrates firm, nontender, irregularly shaped uterus

Diagnosis: TVUS (first line)

- Saline sonography or hysteroscopy (can characterize uterine cavity)

Management:

Expectant	- Reasonable to monitor patient if asymptomatic or postmenopausal - Growing fibroid in postmenopausal patient concerning for malignancy
Pharmacologic	- COC, progestin IUDs, GnRH agonists can be trialed for symptomatic patients
Surgical	- Indicated if symptomatic (abnormal uterine bleeding, infertility) - Myomectomy (if patient wishes to maintain fertility) - Hysterectomy or uterine arterial embolization (if done childbearing)

Endometrial Neoplasia

Endometrial Hyperplasia

General: Hyperplastic proliferation of endometrial glands, associated with continuous estrogen exposure.

Subtype	Findings	Cancer Risk
Hyperplasia without atypia	- Mildly crowded glands - Elevated gland-to-stroma ratio	< 10%
Hyperplasia with atypia	- Crowded, disorganized glands - Elevated gland-to-stroma ratio - Nuclear atypia (enlargement, prominent nucleoli)	> 10-20%

Risk: Obesity, PCOS, anovulation, isolated estrogen therapy, tamoxifen, estrogen-producing tumor

Clinical: **Abnormal uterine bleeding, most commonly peri/postmenopausal**
- US may show thickened endometrial stripe (> 4 mm)

Diagnosis: Endometrial biopsy. Indicated if:
- ≥ 45 with abnormal uterine bleeding or postmenopausal bleeding
- < 45 with abnormal uterine bleeding + unopposed estrogen, Lynch syndrome, or failed medical management
- > 35 with atypical glandular cells on pap test

Management:
- Hyperplasia (without atypia): Progestin IUD
- Hyperplasia (with atypia):
    - Hysterectomy
    - Progestin IUD if wish to preserve fertility

Endometrial Carcinoma

General: Most common gynecologic malignancy in US. Subtypes:

Type I	Endometrioid	- Derives from endometrial hyperplasia with atypia - Favorable prognosis (compared to type II)
Type II	Serous clear cell	- Unrelated to estrogen exposure, associated with p53 mutation - See in elderly - Poor prognosis

Risk: Same as hyperplasia (see above), plus:
- Hypertension, diabetes
- Lynch syndrome (should receive regular screening)

Clinical: Asymptomatic or **abnormal uterine bleeding**

Diagnosis: Endometrial biopsy

Management: **Total abdominal hysterectomy**
- Surgery is used to stage patients, establish type of disease (for all patients)
- Adjuvant therapy dictated by stage/risk
    - Radiation therapy for locally invasive tumor (myometrium, cervix)
    - High-risk disease receives chemotherapy +/– radiation

Ovarian Neoplasia

Differential Diagnosis of Adnexal Mass

Etiology	Features	Management
Benign Cysts		
Follicular	- Most common, occurs when follicle fails to rupture after follicular maturation - May cause pain plus irregular bleeding - Thin-walled, fluid-filled, no vascularity	- Self-limited
Corpus luteal	- Corpus luteum failure to involute, continues enlargement after ovulation - Normal in early pregnancy	- Self-limited
Theca-lutein	- Luteinized follicle cysts from overstimulation due to β-hCG - Bilateral cysts occur with gestational trophoblastic disease, multiple gestation	- Self-limited
Benign Mass		
Teratoma (dermoid cyst)	- Ultrasound: Unilocular cystic mass, hyperechoic contents	- Cystectomy
Cystadenoma	- Serous or mucinous cystadenomas are most common benign ovarian tumors - Thin walls with multiple locules possible, > 5 cm in size	- Cystectomy (symptomatic) - Observation
Pathologic Masses		
Endometrioma	- Endometriosis of the ovary. Presents with mass, pelvic pain, dysmenorrhea. - "Chocolate Cyst," appears complex on US (homogeneous internal echoes)	- Cystectomy
Tubo-Ovarian abscess	- Inflammatory mass associated with PID	- Antibiotics, surgery [See: PID]
Malignant Masses		
Epithelial carcinoma	- See next page	
Pregnancy-Associated		
Luteal cyst or luteoma	- Cystic or solid corpus luteum	Self-limited
Ectopic	- Pain, vaginal bleeding, + β-hCG	[See: Ectopic pregnancy]

Workup of Adnexal Mass

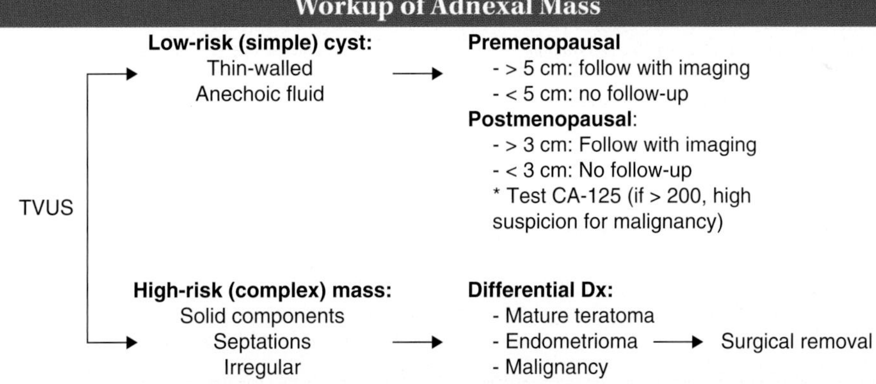

Adnexal Mass Complications

Etiology	Features	Management
Hemorrhagic Cyst	- Most commonly physiologic cyst that **develops internal bleeding** - Often presents with mild to severe abdominal pain - US demonstrates cystic mass with internal echoes	- Usually self-limited (supportive care) - Hospitalization, blood products may be required in more severe cases - Surgery if bleeding continues
Ruptured Cyst	- **Rupture of a cyst, with fluid/blood leakage into peritoneum** - Presents with severe, unilateral lower abdominal pain - US shows ovarian cyst + serous fluid in pelvis	
Ovarian Torsion	- Complete or partial **rotation of ovary around suspensory ligaments**, resulting in ischemia - Risks: Cystic mass (especially > 5 cm) or ovulation induction - Presents as acute onset pelvic pain, adnexal mass, nausea/vomiting - US shows mass, doppler shows limited blood flow	- Ovarian detorsion - Cystectomy - Oophorectomy if fully necrotic

Ovarian Neoplasia

Epithelial Ovarian Neoplasia

General: Most common ovarian cancer, derived from ovarian epithelial lining. Subtypes include serous (most common), mucinous, clear cell, endometrioid.

Risk:

- ↑ age, low parity, early menarche, late menopause, infertility
- Positive family history (first-degree relative), BRCA, Lynch II
- Decreased risk: Oral contraceptive use, multiparity, breast feeding, chronic anovulation

Clinical:

- **Pelvic/abdominal pain, bloating, early satiety**
- Can present with symptoms from advanced disease (bowel obstruction, ascites, pleural effusion)
- US: **Complex, cystic mass** with solid components, thick septations

Diagnosis: Histology after surgical removal

Management: **Total hysterectomy** and salpingo-oophorectomy + lymph node dissection

- Adjuvant chemotherapy in most
- CA-125 surveillance (monitors response to treatment)

Other Ovarian Tumors

	General	Clinical	Management
Germ Cell	- Primarily arise in young women (10-30 y/o) - Associated with β-hCG, AFP, LDH production	- Present with abdominal mass or pain - Bleeding, precocious puberty (β-hCG)	- Oophorectomy/cystectomy
Dysgerminoma	- Tumor of undifferentiated germ cells - LDH, placental AlkPhos production		- Oophorectomy/cystectomy
Mature Teratoma "Dermoid cyst"	- Benign, mature tissues of ectodermal, mesodermal, endodermal origin - Contain hair, squamous cells, sebaceous (oily) material, teeth - < 1% risk of malignant transformation	- Generally asymptomatic - Can lead to ovarian torsion - TVUS: Characteristic appearance	
Immature Teratoma	- Malignant - Immature, trilineage malignancy		
Yolk Sac Tumor	- AFP elevation		
Choriocarcinoma	- Nongestational choriocarcinoma very rare - β-hCG producing	- Precocious puberty (kids) - Postmenopausal bleeding (adults)	
Embryonal	- Undifferentiated, often part of mixed tumor		
Stromal			
Granulosa	- Produce estrogen or inhibin A or B	- Precocious puberty - Endometrial hyperplasia - Postmenopausal bleeding	- Unilateral oophorectomy (if wish to preserve fertility) - TAH-BSO (adults who complete child-bearing)
Sertoli-Leydig	- Produces androgens	- Virilization	
Fibroma	- Benign tumor of fibroblasts	- **Meigs syndrome**: Fibroma + ascites + pleural effusion	- Unilateral oophorectomy
Fallopian Tube	- Adenocarcinoma derived from tubes	- **Latzko triad**: Profuse watery discharge, pelvic pain, mass	- Similar to epithelial ovarian cancer (see above)

Vulvar/Vaginal Neoplasia

Vulvar Neoplasia

General: Most commonly squamous cell carcinoma of the vulva

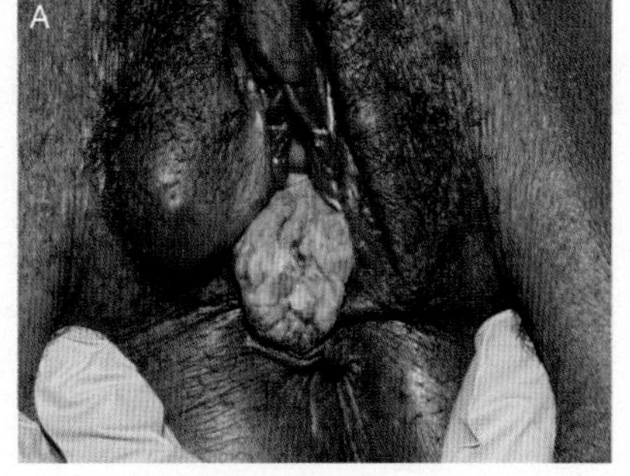

Risk:

- **HPV**, history of cervical cancer
- Vulvar lichen sclerosus
- Immunodeficiency
- Smoking

Clinical:

- **Mass[A] that can cause pruritus, pain, bleeding**
- Varied appearance: Plaque, ulcers, nodular mass

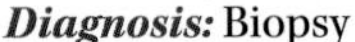

Diagnosis: Biopsy

Management:

- Surgical excision (partial vulvectomy)
- Chemotherapy or radiation for advanced disease

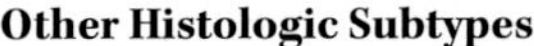

Other Histologic Subtypes:

Melanoma	- Presents as a black itchy mass, with biopsy revealing proliferation of melanocytes - Treated similarly to vulvar SCC with vulvectomy and LN dissection
Extramammary paget	- Rare, intraepithelial adenocarcinoma of the vulva - Presents with pruritus, erythematous "eczematous" appearing lesion - 20% have coexisting adenocarcinoma elsewhere (e.g., breast) - Diagnosis and management with biopsy and excision as above

Vaginal Neoplasia

General: Most commonly squamous cell carcinoma of the vagina, with similar risk factors as cervical cancer. Rarely adenocarcinoma or clear cell carcinoma.

Risk:

- HPV, immunosuppression, chronic inflammation
- DES (diethylstilbestrol) → Adenocarcinoma or clear cell carcinoma

Clinical: Vaginal bleeding, discharge, or postcoital bleeding

Diagnosis: Biopsy

Management:

VAIN (squamous atypia without invasion)	- Excision, laser ablation, or topical therapy
Stage I (limited to vaginal wall)	- Local excision
Stage II-IV	- Chemotherapy and/or radiation therapy

Breast

Evaluation of Nipple Discharge

General: Nipple discharge can range from normal lactation, galactorrhea, or pathologic discharge

Etiology	Presentation	Differential Diagnosis
Lactation	- **Milk production** - Occasionally bloody during pregnancy (benign)	- Pregnancy - Post partum (up to 6 months after cessation of breastfeeding)
Galactorrhea	- **Bilateral milky discharge** - Typically white, clear, or straw colored - Caused by hyperprolactinemia	- Chronic breast stimulation (e.g., from clothing) - Medications (e.g., antipsychotics) - Prolactinoma - Hypothyroidism
Pathologic	- Usually **unilateral production** of fluid from single duct - Can be **serous or blood-tinged**	- Intraductal papilloma - Malignancy - Duct ectasia - Mastitis or abscess

Diagnosis:

- If mass on breast exam: Workup for malignancy (see next page)
- If pathologic features: Ultrasound +/– mammography (if > 30 y/o)
- If galactorrhea: Screening mammogram (if > 40 y/o), medical evaluation (pregnancy test, prolactin, TSH)

Management:

- Physiologic: Treat underlying, remove offending medications
- Pathologic: Surgical excision

Duct Ectasia	- Inflammation and fibrosis of the ductal system - Presents with green, sticky nipple discharge

Breast

Evaluation of New Breast Mass

General: New breast masses can represent benign or malignant processes. Often found on patient self-breast exam.

Diagnosis:

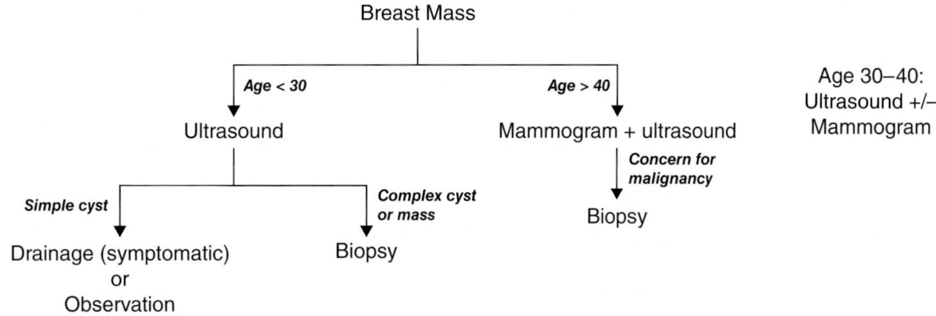

Management:

- **Core needle biopsy (CNB):** Preferred method for tissue diagnosis
- **Fine needle aspiration (FNA):** Reasonable alternative if US highly suggestive of simple cyst
- Surgical excision: Used when CNB is nondiagnostic

	General	Clinical	Management
Nonproliferative Breast Lesions			
Cyst	- **Simple cyst:** Simple fluid filled lesion - **Complex cyst:** Usually benign, but should confirm with FNA, follow with imaging	- Solitary mass - Possibly painful Ultrasound: - Simple: Ovoid, homogenous, anechoic - Complex: Thick-walled, septated, solid components	- Observation (asymptomatic, simple cysts) - FNA (symptomatic or complex) - Surgically remove if recurrent
Fibrocystic Changes	- Nonspecific, nonproliferative breast lesions (cysts, hyperplasia, etc.)	- **Bilateral breast swelling, pain,** tenderness, lumpiness - **Cyclic,** worst before menses occurs, improving after menses	- Reassurance - For pain: Supportive bra, NSAIDs
Galactocele	- Cystic collections of fluid, usually caused by an obstructed milk duct - Common with breastfeeding	- Soft cystic mass on exam - US shows complex cystic mass - Dx: FNA (milky drainage)	- Reassurance
Proliferative Lesions Without Atypia			
Fibroadenoma	- Most common benign breast tumor - Mass of fibrous and glandular tissue - Occurs in premenopausal women	- **Well-defined, mobile, rubbery mass** - Hormone sensitive - US: Well-defined, solid mass - Dx: Core needle biopsy (or repeat imaging in 3-6 months)	- Reassurance or surgical excision
Intraductal Papilloma	- Benign proliferation of ductal epithelium	- Bloody nipple discharge - Dx: Mammography, followed by core needle biopsy	- Surgical excision
Miscellaneous Breast Lesions			
Fat Necrosis	- Benign lesion that occurs after chest trauma, surgery, or radiation	- Presents with irregular breast mass - Appears similar to malignancy on US - Dx: Biopsy (fat, foamy macrophages)	- Reassurance
Phyllodes Tumor	- Rare, breast tumor of fibroblast and stromal proliferation - Occurs in older women (age > 60)	- Large, irregular, painless mass - Rapid growth - Dx: Mammogram, core biopsy	- Surgical excision

Breast

Breast Cancer

General: Most common cancer in women. Most commonly adenocarcinoma derived from epithelial tissues.

Proliferative Lesions with Atypia (Premalignant -- 4-8 × ↑ risk for invasive carcinoma)	
Atypical Ductal Hyperplasia	- Proliferation of atypical ductal cells (similar to DCIS but less extensive) - Tx: Excisional breast biopsy
LCIS	- Often found incidentally on breast biopsy (that was performed for other reason). Can be multicentric and bilateral. - Premalignant expansion of epithelial cells contained within breast lobules
Malignant	
DCIS	- Growth of atypical ductal cells, filling ductal lumen, restricted above the ductal basement membrane - Forms microcalcifications (detected on mammography)
Invasive Ductal	- Most common type of breast cancer - Cords and nests of cells with possible gland formation
Invasive Lobular	- Single-file cellular infiltrate the mammary stroma and adipose tissue (associated with loss of E-cadherin) - Elevated risk for bilateral disease
Inflammatory	- Extremely aggressive subtype with dermal lymphatic invasion - Presents with edema, erythema, peau d'orange[A] (dimpling, pitting). Metastatic disease at presentation.
Paget	- Epidermal spread of malignant ductal cells, resulting in eczematous changes to the nipple - Skin biopsy shows Paget cells (intraepithelial adenocarcinoma cells) - Often concomitant with invasive carcinoma

Risk:

↑ Risk	- Age > 70 (very high relative risk) - First-degree relative with breast cancer, BRCA 1/2 - Excess estrogen exposure (early menarche, age > 30 at first birth, late menopause, history of COC or HRT use) - > 2 EtOH drinks/day
↓ Risk	- Breastfeeding, increased parity, normal BMI, regular exercise

Clinical:

- Early Findings:
  - **Single, nontender, firm mass with ill-defined margins**
  - Mammographic abnormalities on routine screening
- Late Findings: Regional lymphadenopathy, metastatic disease
  - Peau D'Orange skin, dimpling (tethering of Cooper ligament)

Diagnosis: Core needle biopsy (preferred to FNA given higher diagnostic yield, ability to test receptor status [ER/PR/HER2])

Management of Breast Cancer

LCIS	- Observation (if classic LCIS) - Surgically remove (if nonclassic LCIS, i.e. high-risk histologic features)
DCIS	- Mastectomy OR breast-conserving therapy (BCT) (lumpectomy + radiation) - Adjuvant hormonal therapy if ER positive (tamoxifen or anastrozole)
Early stage (stages I, IIA, IIB)	Defined as disease limited to breast with only limited spread to axillary nodes Primary surgery - Mastectomy OR breast conserving therapy - Sentinel lymph node biopsy (for all), with dissection if positive Note: Large or multifocal disease should undergo mastectomy Adjuvant therapy - Endocrine therapy if ER/PR + (tamoxifen) or HER2 + (trastuzumab) - Chemotherapy (if high risk: large tumors, lymph node spread, high 21-gene recurrence score)
Locally advanced (stage III, subset of IIB)	Defined as: extension to chest wall/skin, > 5 cm in size, or extensive regional lymphadenopathy - Neoadjuvant chemotherapy - Surgery (mastectomy or breast-conserving therapy)
Metastatic (stage IV)	- Endocrine therapy and/or systemic chemotherapy

Breast

Screening for Breast Cancer

Age	Screening Recommendation (Average Risk)
< 40	- Not indicated for average risk women
40-50	- **Screening per patient preference**/shared decision-making (guidelines vary by expert group)
50-75	- **Screening recommended for all** (q1-2 years, frequency varies between expert groups)
>75	- Not indicated, unless **life expectancy >10 years**

High-Risk:
- Defined as:
    - BRCA +
    - Personal history of ovarian/breast cancer
    - History of chest radiation therapy
    - Strong family history (as determined by risk calculator with **> 20% risk**)
- Should start screening early, utilizing both mammography and breast MRI (at least annually)

Modality:
- Mammography (primary modality used for all, including dense breasts)
- Ultrasound (used to follow up certain lesions on mammography)
- MRI (used as adjunct is certain high-risk patients)
- Screening clinical or self breast exam: Not indicated for average risk women

Mammography:

BI-RADS Category	Management	Cancer Risk
0: Incomplete	- Additional imaging	N/A
1: Negative	- Continue routine screening	0%
2: Benign	- Continue routine screening	0%
3: Probably benign	- 6-month follow up	< 2%
4: Suspicious	- Core needle biopsy	2-95%
5: Highly suggestive	- Core needle biopsy	> 95%
6: Known malignancy		N/A

Benign findings: Skin or vascular calcifications. Eggshell or rim calcifications.
Pathologic findings: Spiculated mass. Clustered, granular microcalcifications. Fine pleomorphic, linear, or linear-branching calcifications.

BRCA

General: BRCA1 and 2 genes code for tumor suppressor proteins involved in DNA damage detection and repair (double strand breaks). Autosomal dominant inheritance (incomplete penetrance). Mutations place patients at risk for malignancy, especially breast and ovarian.

BRCA 1	- Breast cancer (50-70% risk) - Ovarian cancer (~ 40% risk)
BRCA 2	- Breast cancer (50-70% risk) - Ovarian cancer (~ 15% risk) - Male breast cancer, prostate cancer

Management:

Screening for BRCA mutation	Indicated if: - Personal history of breast cancer at age < 45 - Family history of BRCA gene variant - Strong family history of breast, ovarian cancer
Screening in BRCA patient	- Breast cancer: Annual MRI and mammogram, starting at age 25-30 - Ovarian Cancer: q6 month TVUS + CA125, starting at age 30 Note: Above screening is assuming the patient has not undergone risk-reducing surgery like mastectomy or BSO
Prophylaxis in BRCA +	- Surgical: - Bilateral mastectomy (any age per patient preference) - Bilateral salpingo-oophorectomy (age 35-45 after childbearing) - Pharm: If no mastectomy, can consider tamoxifen

OB-GYN Pharm

	Mechanism	Indication	Side Effects/Management
Reproductive Hormones			
Estrogen Ethinyl estradiol	- Estrogen receptor agonists	- Hormone replacement therapy - Contraception	- Increased risk of venous thromboembolism - Increased risk of endometrial cancer
Progestins Levonorgestrel Medroxyproges-terone Etonogestrel Norethindrone	- Progesterone receptor agonists	- Hormone replacement therapy - Contraception	
GnRH Agonists Leuprolide	- GNRH agonist - If used continuously, acts as an antagonist	- Fibroids, endometriosis - Precocious puberty - Infertility (pulsatile) - Prostate cancer	- Menopausal symptoms when used continuously
SERMs			
Clomiphene	- Antagonist at estrogen receptors in hypothalamus	- Infertility	- Hot flashes - Vision changes (blurring, double vision, scotomata) → warrants discontinuation of therapy
Tamoxifen Raloxifene	- Antagonist of estrogen at breast, but agonist at bone	- ER/PR + breast cancer - Osteoporosis	- Hot flashes - Increased risk of venous thromboembolism - Partial agonist to endometrium (risk for endometrial polyps, cancer)
Other Hormone Antagonists			
Mifepristone Ulipristal	- Progesterone receptor antagonist	- Emergency contraception or abortifacients	- Abdominal pain, uterine cramping, and vaginal bleeding
Anastrozole Letrozole	- Aromatase inhibitors	- ER/PR + breast cancer (if post-menopausal) - Infertility	- Osteoporosis, ↑ fracture risk

Figure Credits

7a Atrial Myxoma. Reproduced with permission from Crawford MH, ed. *Current Diagnosis & Treatment: Cardiology*. 6th ed. New York: McGraw Hill; 2023, Figure 32-1A.

31a Clubbing. From Usatine RP, Smith MA, Mayeaux EJ Jr, Chumley HS. *The Color Atlas and Synopsis of Family Medicine*. 3rd ed. New York, McGraw Hill; 2019, Figure 53-1. Reproduced with permission from Richard P. Usatine, MD.

55a Pharyngitis. From Usatine RP, Smith MA, Mayeaux EJ Jr, Chumley HS. *The Color Atlas and Synopsis of Family Medicine*. 3rd ed. New York, McGraw Hill; 2019, Figure 37-1. Reproduced with permission from Richard P. Usatine, MD.

60a Torus palatinus. From Usatine RP, Smith MA, Mayeaux EJ Jr, Chumley HS. *The Color Atlas and Synopsis of Family Medicine*. 3rd ed. New York, McGraw Hill; 2019, Figure 35-1. Reproduced with permission from Richard P. Usatine, MD.

62a From Knoop KJ, Stack LB, Storrow AB, Thurman R. *The Atlas of Emergency Medicine*. 5th ed. New York, McGraw Hill; 2021. Reproduced with permission from photo contributor: Kevin J. Knoop, MD, MS.

63a Oral candidiasis. From Usatine RP, Smith MA, Mayeaux EJ Jr, Chumley HS. *The Color Atlas and Synopsis of Family Medicine*. 3rd ed. New York, McGraw Hill; 2019, Figure 142-2. Reproduced with permission from Richard P. Usatine, MD.

84a Calcium oxalate stone. From Loscalzo J, Fauci AS, Kasper DL,et al, eds. *Harrison's Principles of Internal Medicine*. 21st ed. New York: McGraw Hill; 2022, Figure 318-1. Reproduced with permission from Dr. Mark Perazella, Yale School of Medicine.

91a Vesicoureteral Reflux. Reproduced with permission from Elsayes KM, Oldham SAA. *Introduction to Diagnostic Radiology*. New York: McGraw Hill; 2014, Chapter 9, Figure C.11.1.

103a Exophthalmos. From Usatine RP, Smith MA, Mayeaux EJ Jr, Chumley HS. *The Color Atlas and Synopsis of Family Medicine*. 3rd ed. New York, McGraw Hill; 2019, Figure 236-7. Reproduced with permission from Richard P. Usatine, MD.

121a Branchial cleft cyst. From Centers for Disease Control and Prevention/ Dr. Carl M. Johnson, Gorgas Memorial Laboratory, Panama City, Panama.

127a Barrett esophagus. Reproduced with permission from Loscalzo J, Fauci AS, Kasper DL, et al, eds. *Harrison's Principles of Internal Medicine*. 21st ed. New York: McGraw Hill; 2022, Figure 323-9C.

134a Bariatric surgery. Reproduced with permission from Loscalzo J, Fauci AS, Kasper DL, et al, eds. *Harrison's Principles of Internal Medicine*. 21st ed. New York: McGraw Hill; 2022, Figure 402-3.

157 Reproduced with permission from G. Bradley Schaefer, James N. Thompson, Jr. Medical Genetics: An Integrated Approach; McGraw Hill; 2017. Figure 8-13.

165a Hirschsprung transition zone. Reproduced with permission from Elsayes KM, Oldham SAA. *Introduction to Diagnostic Radiology*. New York: McGraw Hill; 2014, Chapter 9, Figure C7.1A.

168a Tracheoesophageal fistula. Reproduced with permission from Lalwani AK, ed. *Current Diagnosis & Treatment Otolaryngology— Head and Neck Surgery*. 4th ed. New York: McGraw Hill; 2020, Figure 37-1.

170a Omphalocele. Reproduced with permission from Brunicardi FC, Andersen DK, Billiar TR, et al, eds. *Schwartz's Principles of Surgery*. 11th ed. New York: McGraw Hill; 2019, Figure 39-30.

190b Hairy cell leukemia. Reproduced with permission from Lichtman MA, Shafer MS, Felgar RE, Wang N. *Lichtman's Atlas of Hematology*. New York: McGraw Hill; 2017, Figure VII.G.072.

191a Auer rod. Used with permission from PJF Military Collection/Alamy Stock Photo.

193a Burkitt lymphoma "starry sky." Reproduced with permission from Loscalzo J, Fauci AS, Kasper DL, et al, eds. *Harrison's Principles of Internal Medicine*. 21st ed. New York: McGraw Hill; 2022, Figure A6-21.

206a Used with permission from Michael Lorinsky.

212a Gottron papule. From Usatine RP, Smith MA, Mayeaux EJ Jr, Chumley HS. *The Color Atlas and Synopsis of Family Medicine*. 3rd ed. New York, McGraw Hill; 2019, Figure 189-4. Reproduced with permission from Richard P. Usatine, MD.

217a Gonococcus. From the Centers for Disease Control and Prevention. Available at https://phil.cdc.gov/details.aspx- ?pid=4085. Content provider: CDC/ Joe Millar.

219a Osteosarcoma x-ray. Reprocued with permission from Tehranzadeh J, ed. *Basic Musculoskeletal Imaging*. 2nd ed. New York; McGraw Hill; 2021, Figure 7-1.

232a Café-au-lait spot. From Usatine RP, Smith MA, Mayeaux EJ Jr, Chumley HS. *The Color Atlas and Synopsis of Family Medicine*. 3rd ed. New York, McGraw Hill; 2019, Figure 245-3. Reproduced with permission from Richard P. Usatine, MD.

232b Tinea versicolor. From the Centers for Disease Control and Prevention. Available at https://phil.cdc.gov/Details. aspx?pid=22848. Content provider: CDC/ Dr. Lucille K. Georg.

234a Seborrheic keratosis. From the Centers for Disease Control and Prevention. Available at https://phil.cdc.gov/Details.aspx?pid=5512. Content provider: CDC/Dr. Steve Kraus.

236a Psoriasis. From the Centers for Disease Control and Prevention. Available at https://phil.cdc.gov/Details.aspx?pid=4050. Content provider: CDC/ Dr. N.J. Fiumara.

238a Erythema multiforme. From the Centers for Disease Control and Prevention. Available at https:// phil.cdc.gov/Details.aspx?pid=17523. Content provider: CDC/ Richard S. Hibbets.

243a Lice. From the Centers for Disease Control and Prevention. Available at https://phil.cdc.gov/Details.aspx?pid=19066. Content provider: CDC/ Dr. Dennis Juranek.

243b Bedbugs. From the Centers for Disease Control and Pre- vention. Available at https://phil.cdc.gov/Details.aspx?pid=12703. Content provider: CDC/ CDC-DPDx; Blaine Mathison.

245a Hidradenitis Suppurativa. From Usatine RP, Smith MA, Mayeaux EJ Jr, Chumley HS. *The Color Atlas and Synopsis of Family Medicine*. 3rd ed. New York, McGraw Hill; 2019, Figure 121-1. Reproduced with permission from Richard P. Usatine, MD.

247a Alopecia. From Usatine RP, Smith MA, Mayeaux EJ Jr, Chumley HS. *The Color Atlas and Synopsis of Family Medicine*. 3rd ed. New York, McGraw Hill; 2019, Figure 195-1. Reproduced with permission from Richard P. Usatine, MD.

248a Kaposi sarcoma. From the Centers for Disease Control and Prevention. Available at https://phil.cdc.gov/ Details.aspx?pid=14430. Content provider: CDC.

248b Pyogenic granuloma. From the Centers for Disease Control and Prevention. Available at https://phil.cdc.gov/ Details.aspx?pid=18897. Content provider: CDC/ Donated by Brian Hill, New Zealand.

248c Infantile hemangioma. From the Centers for Disease Control and Prevention. Available at https://phil.cdc.gov/Details.aspx?pid= 14669. Content provider: CDC/ Richard S. Hibbets.

249a Basal cell carcinoma. From the Centers for Disease Control and Pre- vention. Available at https://phil.cdc.gov/Details. aspx?pid=18404. Content provider: National Cancer Institute (NCI); www.cancer.gov.

249b Squamous cell skin cancer. From the Centers for Disease Control and Pre- vention. Available at https://phil.cdc.gov/Details. aspx?pid=18381. Content provider: National Cancer Institute (NCI); www.cancer.gov.

250a Melanoma. From the Centers for Disease Control and Prevention. Available at https://phil.cdc.gov/Details.aspx?pid=18410. Content provider: National Cancer Institute (NCI).

252a Actinomyces. From the Centers for Disease Control and Prevention. Available at https://phil. cdc.gov/Details.aspx?pid=22293. Content provider: Dr. Lucille K. Georg.

255a Rocky mountain fever rash. From the Centers for Disease Control and Prevention. Available at https://phil.cdc. gov/Details.aspx?pid=1962. Content provider: CDC.

256a Leprosy. From the Centers for Disease Control and Prevention. Available at https:// phil.cdc.gov/Details.aspx?pid=19218. Content provider: Dr. Andre J. Lebrun. Photo credit: J. Justin Older, MD.

259a Malaria gametocyte. From the Centers for Disease Control and Prevention. Available at https://phil.cdc.gov/Details.aspx?pid=22817. Content provider: Dr. Mae Melvin.

259b Malaria ring forms. From the Centers for Dis- ease Control and Prevention. Available at https://phil.cdc.gov/ Details.aspx?pid=22811. Content provider: Dr. Mae Melvin.

259c Babesia. From the Centers for Disease Control and Prevention. Available at https://phil. cdc.gov/Details.aspx?pid=20342. Content provider: Dr. R.G. Scholtens.

261a Schistosoma. From the Centers for Disease Control and Prevention. Available at https://phil. cdc.gov/Details.aspx?pid=11193. Content provider: Dr. Shirley Maddison.

262a Molluscum contagiosum. From the Centers for Disease Control and Prevention. Available at https:// phil.cdc.gov/Details.aspx?pid=16695. Content provider: Jim Pledger.

263a Chickenpox. From the Centers for Disease Control and Prevention. Available at https://phil.cdc.gov/Details.aspx?pid=21500. Content provider: K.L. Herrmann.

263b CMV. From the Centers for Disease Control and Prevention. Available at https://phil.cdc.gov/Details.aspx?pid=22070. Content provider: Roger A. Feldman, MD.

266a HIV. From the Centers for Disease Control and Prevention. Available at https://phil.cdc.gov/Details.aspx?pid= 18163. Content provider: National Institute of Allergy and Infectious Diseases (NIAID).

275a Genital herpes. From Usatine RP, Smith MA, Mayeaux EJ Jr, Chumley HS. *The Color Atlas and Synopsis of Family Medicine*. 3rd ed. New York, McGraw Hill; 2019, Figure 135-3. Reproduced with permission from Richard P. Usatine, MD.

288a Brain herniation. Reproduced with permission from Loscalzo J, Fauci AS, Kasper DL, et al, eds. *Harrison's Principles of Internal Medicine*. 21st ed. New York: McGraw Hill; 2022, Figure 28-1.

317a Cholesteatoma. Reproduced with permission from Lalwani AK, ed. *Current Diagnosis & Treatment Otolaryngology—Head and Neck Surgery*. 4th ed. New York: McGraw Hill; 2020, Figure 52-2.

318a Viral conjunctivitis. From Usatine RP, Smith MA, Mayeaux EJ Jr, Chumley HS. *The Color Atlas and Synopsis of Family Medicine*. 3rd ed. New York, McGraw Hill; 2019, Figure 18-1. Reproduced with permission from Richard P. Usatine, MD.

318b Trachoma. From Usatine RP, Smith MA, Mayeaux EJ Jr, Chumley HS. *The Color Atlas and Synopsis of Family Medicine*. 3rd ed. New York, McGraw Hill; 2019, Figure 18-10. Reproduced with permission from Richard P. Usatine, MD.

320a Glaucoma. Reproduced with permission from Loscalzo J, Fauci AS, Kasper DL, et al, eds. *Harrison's Principles of Internal Medicine*. 21st ed. New York: McGraw Hill; 2022, Figure 32-15.

321a CRAO. Reproduced with permission from Loscalzo J, Fauci AS, Kasper DL, et al, eds. *Harrison's Principles of Internal Medicine*. 21st ed. New York: McGraw Hill; 2022, Figure 32-6.

321b Retinal detachment. Reproduced with permission from "Loscalzo J, Fauci A, Kasper D, Hauser S, Longo D, Jameson J. *Harrison's Principles of Internal Medicine*. 21st ed. New York, McGraw-Hill; 2022. Figure 32-14".

321c Diabetic retinopathy. From the Centers for Disease Control and Prevention. Available at https://phil.cdc.gov/Details.aspx?pid=20467. Content provider: Lucille H. Young.

321d Hypertensive retinopathy. From the Centers for Disease Control and Prevention. Available at https://phil.cdc.gov/Details.aspx?pid=20474. Content provider: Lucille H. Young.

324b Dandy-walker MRI. Reproduced with permission from Ropper AH, Samuels MA, Klein JP, Prasad S. eds. *Adams and Victor's Principles of Neurology*. 11th ed. New York: McGraw Hill; 2019, Figure 37-2B.

330a CDC adult vaccination. From the Centers for Disease Control and Prevention. Available at https://www.cdc.gov/vaccines/schedules/hcp/imz/adult.html.

333a Pellagra. From the Centers for Disease Control and Prevention. Public Health Image Library. Available at https://phil.cdc.gov/Details.aspx?pid=3757.

334a Kwashiorkor. From the Centers for Disease Control and Prevention. Public Health Image Library. Available at https://phil.cdc.gov/Details.aspx-?pid=6901. Content provider: CDC/Dr. Lyle Conrad.

369a Umbilical granuloma. From Knoop KJ, Stack LB, Storrow AB, Thurman RJ, eds. *The Atlas of Emergency Medicine*. 5th ed. New York, McGraw-Hill; 2021, Figure 14-10. Reproduced with permission from photo contributor: Anne W. Lucky, MD.

372a Fetal head trauma. Reproduced with permission from Cunningham FG, Leveno KJ, Dashe JS, et al, eds. *Williams Obstetrics*. 26th ed. New York: McGraw Hill; 2022, Figure 33-2.

373a Mongolian spot. From Usatine RP, Smith MA, Mayeaux EJ Jr, Chumley HS. *The Color Atlas and Synopsis of Family Medicine*. 3rd ed. New York, McGraw Hill; 2019, Figure 114-4. Reproduced with permission from Richard P. Usatine, MD.

373b From Usatine RP, Smith MA, Mayeaux EJ Jr, Chumley HS. *The Color Atlas and Synopsis of Family Medicine*. 3rd ed. New York, McGraw Hill; 2019, Figure 115-6. Reproduced with permission from Richard P. Usatine, MD.

373c Gonococcal conjunctivitis. From the Centers for Disease Control and Prevention. Public Health Image Library. Available at https:// phil.cdc.gov/Details.aspx?pid=15899. Content provider: CDC/ J. Pledger.

376a CDC pediatric vaccination table. From the Centers for Disease Control and Prevention. Immunization Schedules. Available at https://www.cdc.gov/vaccines/schedules/hcp/imz/ child-adolescent.html.

385a Single palmar crease. From the Centers for Disease Control and Prevention. Public Health Image Library. Available at https://phil.cdc.gov/Details.aspx?pid=19281. Content provider: CDC.

386a Blue sclera from osteogenesis imperfecta. From the Centers for Disease Control and Prevention. Public Health Image Library. Available at https://phil.cdc.gov/Details.aspx?pid=17951. Content provider: CDC/ Dr. James W. Hansen.

391a Radial hypoplasia. From the Centers for Disease Control and Prevention. Public Health Image Library. Available at https://phil.cdc.gov/ Details.aspx?pid=2635. Content provider: CDC/ Dr. James W. Hansen.

399a Slipped Capital Femoral Epiphysis. Reproduced with permission from McMahon PJ, Skinner HB. *Current Diagnosis & Treatment in Orthopedics*. 6th ed. New York: McGraw Hill; 2021, Figure 12-14A.

425a Conjoined twins. From the Centers for Disease Control and Prevention. Public Health Image Library. Content provider: CDC/ Robert S. Craig. Available at https://phil.cdc.gov/Details.aspx?pid=20314.

434a Breech position. Reproduced with permission from Pernoll ML. *Benson and Pernoll's Handbook of Obstetrics and Gynecology*. 10th ed. New York, NY: McGraw-Hill; 2001.

445a Menstrual cycle. Reproduced with permission from Loscalzo J, Fauci AS, Kasper DL, et al, eds. *Harrison's Principles of Internal Medicine*. 21st ed. New York: McGraw Hill; 2022, Figure 392-8.

456a Clue cells: From the Centers for Disease Control and Prevention. Public Health Image Library. Content provider: CDC/ M. Rein. Available at https://phil.cdc.gov/Details.aspx?pid=14574.

456b Trichomonas. From the Centers for Disease Control and Prevention. DPDx - Laboratory Identification of Parasites of Public Health Concern. Trichomonas: Image Gallery. Available at https://www.cdc.gov/dpdx/trichomoniasis/index.html.

456c Candida: From the Centers for Disease Control and Prevention. Public Health Image Library. Content provider: CDC/ Dr. Hardin. Available at https://phil.cdc.gov/Details.aspx?pid=22947.

459a Lichen sclerosus. From the Centers for Disease Control and Prevention. Public Health Image Library. Content provider: CDC/ Susan Lindsley. Available at https://phil.cdc.gov/Details.aspx?pid=15553.

459b Bartholin cyst. From the Centers for Disease Control and Prevention. Public Health Image Library. Content provider: CDC/ Dr. N.J. Fiumara. Available at https://phil.cdc.gov/Details.aspx?pid=19146.

467a Vulvar cancer. Reproduced with permission from Hoffman BL, Schorge JO, Halvorson LM, et al, eds. *Williams Gynecology*. 4th ed. New York: McGraw Hill; 2020, Figure 31-4.

Index

D

E

F

G

N

O

P

Q

R

S

T

U

V

W

X

Y

Z